Handbook of Experimental Pharmacology

Volume 159

Springer

Berlin
Heidelberg
New York
Hong Kong
London
Milan
Paris
Tokyo

Transgenic Models in Pharmacology

Contributors

M. Bader, A.S. Basile, S. Berger, G. Bernhardt, M. Biel,
B.C. Blaxall, H.H. Bock, O. Brandau, N. Brose, H. Bujard,
F.P. Bymaster, J.-P. Cazenave, Y. Cui, C. Deng, A. Duttaroy,
G. Elizondo, S. Engelhardt, R. Fässler, R. Feil, C.C. Felder,
R. Förster, C. Gachet, J. Gomeza, F.J. Gonzalez, E.F. Greiner,
B. Hechler, L. Hein, H. Herbrand, J. Herz, F. Hofmann,
I.T. Huhtaniemi, B. Isermann, B.L. Kieffer, T. Kleppisch,
W.J. Koch, F. Lanza, C. Léon, S. Mäkelä, P. May, D.L. McKinzie,
G.S. McKnight, T. Miyakawa, S. Narumiya, C.M. Niswender,
S. Offermanns, O. Pabst, J.E. Pintar, M. Poutanen, J. Rettig,
U. Rudolph, S. Rulli, G. Schütz, M. Sendtner, P. Sipilä,
J. Toppari, H. Weiler, J. Wess, T. Wintermantel, M. Yamada,
F.P. Zhang, W. Zhang

Editors
Stefan Offermanns and Lutz Hein

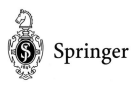 Springer

Professor
Dr. Stefan Offermanns
Pharmakologisches Institut
Universität Heidelberg
Im Neuenheimer Feld 366
69120 Heidelberg, Germany
e-mail: stefan.offermanns@urz.uni-heidelberg.de

Professor
Dr. Lutz Hein
Institut für Pharmakologie und
Toxikologie der Universität
Versbacher Straße 9
97078 Würzburg, Germany
e-mail: hein@toxi.uni-wuerzburg.de

With 43 Figures and 42 Tables

ISSN 0171-2004

ISBN 3-540-00109-3 Springer-Verlag Berlin Heidelberg New York

Library of Congress Cataloging-in-Publication Data
Transgenic models in pharmacology / contributors, M. Bader ... [et al.] ; editors, Stefan Offermanns
and Lutz Hein.   p. ; cm. – (Handbook of experimental pharmacology ; v. 159) Includes bibliographical
references and index
ISBN 3-540-00109-3 (alk. paper)
1. Pharmacology, Experimental. 2. Transgenic animals. 3. Transgenic mice. 4. Mice as laboratory
animals. I. Bader, M. II. Offermanns, Stefan. III. Hein Lutz. IV. Series.
[DNLM: 1. Pharmacology. 2. Animals, Genetically Modified. 3. Models, Animal. QV 34 T772 2004]
QP905.H3 vol. 159   [RM301.25]   [615'.1s–dc2]   [615'.19'0724]   2003054276

Springer-Verlag Berlin Heidelberg New York
a member of BertelsmannSpringer Science+Business Media GmbH

© Springer-Verlag Berlin Heidelberg 2004
Printed in Germany

The use of general descriptive names, registered names, etc. in this publication does not imply, even
in the absence of a specific statement, that such names are exempt from the relevant protective laws
and regulations and free for general use.

Product liability: The publishers cannot guarantee the accuracy of any information about dosage and
application contained in this book. In every individual case the user must check such information by
consulting the relevant literature.

Cover design: design & production GmbH, Heidelberg
Typesetting: Stürtz AG, 97080 Würzburg

Printed on acid-free paper   27/3150 hs – 5 4 3 2 1 0

Preface

Pharmacology has always used methods from neighboring disciplines such as physiology, anatomy, or pathology. At one time, experimental pharmacology was mainly based on animal experiments and clinical observation. Later, important methodological and conceptual influences came especially from biochemistry. Drug actions could *increasingly* be explained on a molecular level as an effect on a receptor, transporter, channel, or an enzyme. However, with the description of more and more protein subtypes and molecular processes, the mechanism of action of individual drugs became *increasingly* complicated. During this development, which has often been called "reductionistic," molecular aspects of drug action and studies in single cells were emphasized. Recently, molecular biology and the different genome projects have provided a plethora of gene products, which represent potential drug targets or which may be involved in the actions of drugs. While the reductionistic approach has broadened our knowledge of the mechanisms of drug action enormously during the last few decades, it conceptually conflicts with an integrative, holistic view embraced by traditional pharmacology and required for a full understanding of drug actions in the context of the whole organism. One of the current challenges for pharmacologists and other scientists working in the biomedical field is therefore the correlation of in silico and in vitro data with in vivo findings. In vitro pharmacology may help to identify novel target proteins, signaling pathways and molecular mechanisms, and this knowledge provides the basis for development and screening of new drugs. However, in most areas of pharmacology, in vivo models are necessary so as to bridge the gap between the effects of drugs in in vitro assay systems and the application of these drugs to humans. Under optimal conditions, transgenic models should help to predict drug actions (and unwanted side effects) in human patients. Transgenic expression and gene targeting methods have progressed at a rapid pace and have opened the way into an exciting new research field that allows us to manipulate individual genes and gene products in the context of a living organism. Consequently, transgenic and gene-targeted animals have revolutionized many areas of biomedical research, including experimental pharmacology, by merging the reductionistic and the holistic approach, which each alone have their limitations.

The aim of this volume—*Transgenic Models in Pharmacology*—of the *Handbook of Experimental Pharmacology* is to provide scientists in biomedicine with up-to-date informa- tion on animal models generated by transgenic or gene-targeting techniques. Naturally, the focus is on the mouse system. Each chapter has been written by leading experts in the field and gives an overview on existing animal models. This is facilitated by tables that list the most important genetically engineered animal models and their phenotypes. We hope that this volume will illustrate the impact of transgenic animal models on the field of experimental pharmacology and toxicology, which includes their role in the understanding of basic cellular mechanisms, the evaluation of potential drug targets, and the testing for drug effects. We are extremely grateful to our colleagues who have written excellent chapters on genetically modified animal models in their fields, giving an impressive overview on the scientific quality as well as on thematic scope of the ongoing research using this methodology. We would also like to thank Susanne Dathe and Doris Walker of Springer-Verlag, who coordinated the production of this volume.

Transgenic Models in Pharmacology is dedicated to the memory of Emeritus Professor Hans Herken (1912–2003). Hans Herken was one of the leading pharmacologists in postwar Germany. After his retirement, he followed the field of experimental pharmacology enthusiastically, and was an important mentor and advisor for many young colleagues until his recent death. Among his numerous activities, he served as an editor of this series for more than three decades. Many volumes, including this one, have been suggested and inspired by Hans Herken.

L. Hein, Würzburg, Germany
S. Offermanns, Heidelberg, Germany

List of Contributors

(their addresses can be found at the beginning of their respective chapters)

List of Contents

Part 1
Transgenic Techniques

Novel Mouse Models in Biomedical Research: The Power of Dissecting Pathways by Quantitative Control of Gene Activities

S. Berger · H. Bujard

Zentrum fuer Molekulare Biologie (ZMBH), Universitaet Heidelberg,
Im Neuenheimer Feld 282, 69120 Heidelberg, Germany
e-mail: h.bujard@zmbh.uni-heidelberg.de

Abstract The last decade has seen significant progress in the development and refinement of genetic approaches applicable to the mouse, making this animal the prime organism for the study of mammalian genetics. Particularly, the potential to control individual gene activities in a temporally defined and tissue-specific manner has allowed us to dissect gene functions and pathways in vivo with unprecedented precision, yielding exciting new insights into such complex biological processes as development, behavior, and disease. For biomedical research, the new approaches of mouse molecular genetics open up new perspectives for modeling human diseases. Particularly methods that allow quantitative and reversible control over disease genes will enable the experimenter to not only study the onset of a disease and its progression but also to examine its potential reversibility and to investigate mechanisms of disease regression. In this chapter, we summarize the principle of Tet regulation as a paradigm for a reversible gene control system and we briefly discuss Tet regulation-based mouse models of human diseases in the area of cancer as well as of neurodegenerative and cardiac diseases.

Keywords Conditional mouse mutants · Tetracycline controlled gene expression · Models of human disease

1
Introduction

During the past decade, experimental approaches have emerged which allow the conditional alteration of individual gene activities in higher eukaryotes in a temporally defined and cell type restricted manner. Applying these approaches to the mouse—thanks to transgenesis and embryonic stem (ES) cell technology, the prime model of mammalian molecular genetics—is increasingly providing new insights into fundamental biological processes. For biomedical research, these technologies are of particular interest as they offer new opportunities for modeling human diseases in transgenic rodents. Such models will more faithfully mimic pathologies and, thus, will enhance our understanding of diseases at the molecular and physiological level, thereby facilitating the development of new strategies for interventions and for prevention.

The crucial precondition for the sensible application of gene activation/inactivation approaches is specificity: interference should exclusively affect the gene under study. This demanding prerequisite is met, to different extent, by systems based either on elements heterologous to, e.g., the mammalian cell, or on modified endogenous components. The most commonly applied strategies presently, which apparently fulfill the required criteria best, exploit prokaryotic elements, evolutionarily most distant to higher eukaryotes.

Thus, the CRE/LoxP recombination system of *Escherichia coli* phage P1 has been successfully applied, and the conditional knock-out approach in transgenic mice has yielded a wealth of information. A second widely applied strategy, which aims at controlling transcription of target genes in eukaryotes, is based on regulatory elements of the *E. coli* tetracycline resistance operon.

When the two basic strategies—site-specific recombination and control with gene expression—are compared, genetic analysis via temporally and spatially restricted recombination has proven to be enormously successful. Nevertheless, the potential of reversibly and quantitatively interfering with a gene's activity, e.g., at the level of transcription, adds another quality to the study of gene function in vivo: the well-defined and reversible perturbation of a system allows not only comparisons between the normal and the perturbed state, but also monitoring of the system's reaction when interference is terminated. Therefore, for modeling human diseases in transgenic animals, the fully reversible control of target genes appears to be particularly informative as will be shown below.

For these reasons we restrict our review to what one may call "truly conditional," i.e., reversible approaches. Moreover, being fully aware of the various methods developed, we will focus on the Tet regulatory system as a paradigm for which, due to its widespread application, an extended experience has accumulated. For information on various other approaches, we refer the reader to some informative recent reviews (Sauer 1998; Lewandoski 2001; Gossen and Bujard 2002; Kuehn and Schwenk 2002).

The Tet regulatory systems meet two essential criteria for genetic conditionality: (1) They allow the experimenter to reversibly alter the expression of a gene and, thus, to study the impact of timely limited perturbations of gene activities; (2) they enable the experimenter to not only switch a gene on and off, but also to adjust its activity to intermediate levels, which often mimics pathological states more closely than total gene inactivation. Thus, the activity of a disease gene can be altered at a given time within an animal's lifespan to different degrees and, if required, for a defined time period only. These features permit us to address a number of important questions regarding such issues as:

– Early events during the onset of a disease
– Disease progression
– Potential reversibility of pathologies upon inactivation of the disease-initiating gene
– Disease regression

Disease models with such properties will be most suitable for the identification and validation of genes and their products as targets for pharmacological interventions. They will also be valuable as in vivo systems for preclinical drug efficacy studies.

In the following, we will describe the principle of Tet regulation and some recent technological advances before we highlight some conditional mouse models in the area of oncology as well as neurodegenerative and cardiac diseases. Obviously, we cannot give a comprehensive survey and apologize to colleagues whose excellent work could not be included in the context of this chapter.

2
The Tet Regulatory System—Principles, Components, and Approaches

The Tet regulatory systems act at the level of transcription whereby a gene of interest is controlled via an artificial control circuit superimposed on the enormously complex regulatory network of an eukaryotic cell. This circuit can be controlled from outside, preferably by the tetracycline derivative doxycycline (Dox). When properly set up, the circuit by itself will not at all or only marginally affect the metabolism of the host cell, thereby relying on the Tet systems' exquisite specificity. The favorable properties of the Tet systems are based on three crucial parameters (for reviews see Gossen and Bujard 2001; Baron and Bujard 2000):

– The evolutionary distance between the regulatory core elements of the system which are of prokaryotic origin and which appear not to engage in interactions with essential components of the eukaryotic cell

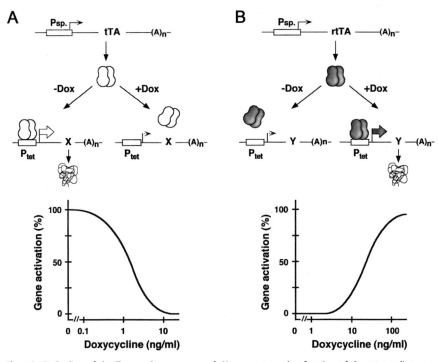

Fig. 1A, B Outline of the Tet regulatory system. **A** *Upper part*, mode of action of the tetracycline con-trolled transactivator (tTA). In absence of the effector substance Dox, tTA binds to *tet* operator se-quences within P_{tet} and activates transcription of gene X. In the presence of Dox, tTA is prevented from binding and activating P_{tet}. *Lower part* illustrates the response of tTA-dependent gene expression at different concentrations of Dox. Gene activity is maximal in the absence of the antibiotic and is gradu-ally downregulated at the single-cell level by increasing concentrations. **B** *Upper part*, mode of action of the reverse tetracycline controlled transactivator (*rtTA*). The original rtTA differs from tTA in 4 amino acids within the TetR moiety, resulting in the reverse phenotype which requires Dox for binding to *tet* operator sequences and, thus, to P_{tet}. *Lower part*, response of rtTA-mediated gene expression using the improved rtTA2^S-M2 to different concentrations of Dox. By increasing effector concentrations beyond 10 ng/ml, transcription is gradually enhanced until it reaches the maximum at 80–100 ng/ml. In both systems, tissue or cell-type specificity is brought about by the promoter P_{sp} driving tTA/rtTA expression

Fig. 2A–C Schematic outline of the tetracycline-controlled transcription factors, their responsive pro-moters, and induction profiles of rtTAs. **A** Fusions between the repressor protein (TetR) of the *E. coli Tn10* tetracycline resistance operon and domains capable of either activating or silencing transcription. tTA is a fusion between the 207 amino acid TetR and the 128 amino acid long C-terminal portion of VP16 of *Herpes simplex* virus. In all tTA2 and rtTA2 versions, the VP16 moiety is replaced by three 13 amino acid-long minimal activation domains (*F*). rtTA2^S-S2 and rtTA2^S-M2 are improved versions of

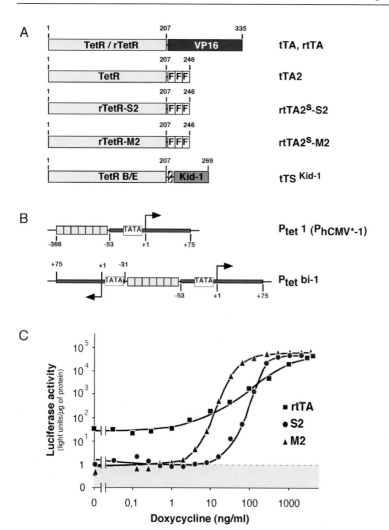

rtTA, based on novel TetR mutants. tTA2 and the new rtTA versions are encoded in synthetic polynucleotides optimized for expression in mammalian cells. tTS^{kid}-1 is a fusion between TetR$^{B/E}$ and a 61 amino acid-long repression domain (KRAB) from the human kidney protein Kid-1. A nuclear localization sequence is placed between TetR and the silencing domain. The TetR$^{B/E}$ version prevents heterodimerization between tTS and rtTA monomers when coexpressed in one cell. **B** tTA/rtTA-responsive promoters. P_{tet} is a fusion between seven *tetO* operators (*gray boxes*) and a minimal promoter derived from the human cytomegalovirus promoter IE (P_{hCMV}). The bidirectional promoter P_{tet}bi-1 consists of a core of heptamerized *tet* operators which is flanked by two divergently oriented P_{hCMV}-derived minimal promoters. Bidirectional promoters allow the coregulation of two genes. Positions spanning promoter regions and operator sequences are indicated with respect to the transcriptional start site (+1). **C** Induction of luciferase activity by rtTA, rtTA2^S-S2, and rtTA2^S-M2 at different Dox concentrations. HeLa cell lines were used, which stably synthesize the respective transactivators under P_{hCMV} control and which also contain the stably integrated luciferase gene under P_{tet} control. Both new rtTAs (S2, M2) do not show intrinsic background activities under these conditions. rtTA2^S-M2 exhibits, in addition, an around tenfold higher sensitivity towards Dox

- The unusual specificity of interaction between the Tet repressor (TetR) and the *tet* operator (*tet*O) as well as between TetR and its inducer, Dox
- The well-studied chemical and physiological properties of the inducing agents, i.e., various tetracyclines of which some, particularly Dox, have been widely used in human and animal medicine

As outlined in Figs. 1 and 2, there are two complementary Tet control systems which consist of three elements each: (1) the tetracycline-controlled transactivators (tTAs) or reverse tetracycline-controlled transactivators (rtTAs) which are fusions between TetR and transcriptional activation domains; (2) a minimal, i.e., enhancerless RNA polymerase II promoter, fused downstream to an array of seven *tet*O sequences designated P_{tet}; and (3) the inducing compound Dox or other tetracycline derivatives. In the tTA system, Dox prevents binding of tTA to P_{tet} and, thus, abolishes transcription (Gossen and Bujard 1992). By contrast, rtTA requires Dox for binding to and activation of P_{tet} (Gossen et al. 1995).

In transgenic animals, the rtTA approach is to be preferred whenever a gene should be activated rapidly, since saturating a system with a small effector substance is an intrinsically more rapid process than its depletion (as required for the tTA system). For the same reason, the tTA principle is advantageous whenever a fast shut off of a gene's expression is required.

2.1
Operating the Tet Control Circuit with Dox

Dox penetrates cell membranes by diffusion. Therefore, P_{tet}-controlled genes can be activated at the single-cell level in a ridgeless manner by properly adjusting Dox concentrations. In cultured cells, Dox concentrations far below toxicity levels (5–10 μg/ml for HeLa cells) are required. Thus, tTA is gradually inactivated between 0.05 and 5 ng/ml, whereas 20–100 ng/ml are sufficient for activating the novel rtTA2^S-M2 (Fig. 2 and below). To establish proper Dox concentration in the mouse, the antibiotic is most conveniently supplied via drinking water where 50–200 μg/ml are sufficient for switching off the tTA system in any organ (Kistner et al. 1996). Higher concentrations are required even for the rtTA2^S-M2 system (Fig. 2), but 2 mg/ml (in the water supply), an amount unproblematic also over long periods of time, are usually sufficient. Rapid induction may be achieved by i.p. injection (Fig. 3) whereby up to 2 mg of Dox in 0.2 ml of isotonic saline every 24 h is a well-tolerated dosage in short term experiments (1 to 2 weeks; Hasan et al. 2001). Due to the excellent cell and tissue penetration properties of Dox, appropriate concentrations for tTA inactivation and activation of rtTA2^S-M2 are readily achieved in different compartments of the animal including the placenta and the milk of lactating mothers. Thus, Tet regulation can be imposed onto the developing embryo as well as on offspring before and during weaning. Partial induction of Tet-controlled genes may be achieved by adjusting the amount of Dox delivered, though it has to be reconciled that tissue distribution and biological half-life of Dox differ from organ to organ (Kistner

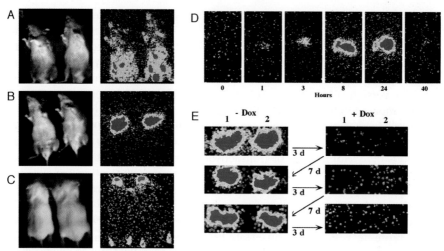

Fig. 3A–E In vivo imaging of Tet-regulated luciferase expression in live animals. **A–C** Animals of 3 mouse lines expressing the tTA gene under the control of P_{hCMV}, P_{LAP} and P_{CamKII}, respectively, were crossed to individuals of the LC-1 strain (Schoenig et al. 2002) where the luciferase and the *cre* gene are coregulated by P_{tet}bi-1 (Fig. 2). To demonstrate organ-/tissue-specific expression directed by the different promoters driving the transactivators, luciferase expression of double transgenic animals was analyzed non-invasively via luciferase bioluminescence. **A** P_{hCMV}, several organs/tissues. **B** P_{LAP} hepatocytes. **C** P_{CamKII}, brain. **D** Kinetics of induction for hepatocyte-specific luciferase synthesis. Luciferase of rTA^{LAP}/LC-1 double transgenic animals was non-invasively monitored after i.p. injection of 2 mg of Dox at the times indicated. First signs of luciferase activity can be detected after 1 h. **E** Switching luciferase expression in the liver. As shown in multiple cycles of gene activation, exposure of TA^{LAP}-2/LC-1 mice to Dox abolishes luciferase activity within 3 days. Reactivation can be monitored after 2 days (in the experiment shown 7 days) after Dox withdrawal. The identical cycle of activation/inactivation is observed when the same animals are re-examined after 3 months

et al. 1996). Accordingly, proper calibration of experimental conditions is required. The various organs differ also in the kinetics of induction (Kistner et al. 1996), kidney and brain being the slowest, but as is shown in Fig. 3, luciferase activity in the liver is detectable already 1 h after Dox injection (Hasan et al. 2001).

The brain poses a particular problem, as Dox penetrates the blood–brain barrier less efficiently. For operating the tTA system, the amount of Dox that reaches the brain under the above feeding conditions is, however, sufficient (see work described below) while, for the rtTA system, the novel M2 transactivator version which is tenfold more sensitive towards Dox (Fig. 2) is expected to ameliorate problems encountered with the originally described rtTA.

2.2
Modifications of the Tet System

Several significant modifications and improvements of the original tTA system have been developed over the years, particularly the generation of the rtTA, which is based on a TetR mutant that exhibits fundamentally different DNA binding characteristics: it requires Dox or anhydrotetracycline for its association with *tet*O. The originally described rtTA has been replaced by greatly improved versions (Urlinger et al. 2000) which are more sensitive towards Dox and which exhibit negligible residual affinities towards *tet*O. Particularly, the transactivator version rtTA2^S-M2 senses Dox at around tenfold lower concentrations when compared to the original rtTA (Fig. 2).

Several further modifications are worth mentioning. For a number of reasons, the VP16 domain of the original tTA/rtTA was replaced by minimal activation domains yielding a set of transactivators with graded activation potential (Baron et al. 1997). Moreover, all tTA/rtTAs of the new generation are encoded in synthetic sequences optimized in various ways for expression in human cells (Urlinger et al. 2000).

A development that had considerable impact was the generation of bidirectional promoters, P_{tet}bi (Baron et al. 1995). Here, the heptamerized *tet*O sequences are flanked on both sides by minimal promoters (Fig. 2) which allow for the simultaneous regulation of two genes, whereby the respective transcription units face in opposite directions. These constructs are particularly useful when one gene is used for a reporter function. Thus, the initial characterization of functional transgenic animals is facilitated, particularly when expression of the actual gene of interest is difficult to detect. By using the luciferase gene as reporter, the range of regulation and the tightness of control can be readily assessed, whereas, e.g., the *lacZ* or GFP gene allows monitoring of expression in situ. As will be shown below, the luciferase gene appears particularly useful since it permits the monitoring of gene activities in live animals in a non-invasive way (Hasan et al. 2001).

A problem sometimes encountered is the so-called "leakiness," which refers to a basal level of expression of the P_{tet}-controlled transcription unit in the uninduced state. Although this issue caught considerable attention, it has only rarely been addressed in a correct way. A thorough discussion of this topic can be found elsewhere (Freundlieb et al. 1999) but in essence, one has to discriminate between (1) P_{tet}-dependent and (2) integration site-dependent background activity.

Ad (1): P_{tet}-1 is not necessarily silent in all cellular environments. It may have an intrinsically elevated activity in cells which contain particular transcription factors capable of binding to the promoter itself or to neighboring sequences of the vector. This leakiness is, however, typical for episomal states of the DNA carrying the transcription unit and for transient expression situations in cell culture. As pointed out previously (Gossen and Bujard 1992), an adaptation of P_{tet} to particular cellular environments may sometimes be advantageous.

Ad (2):   The basal activity of a chromosomally integrated minimal promoter depends strongly on its integration site. When inserted into an appropriate locus, P_{tet}-1 will be transcriptionally silent even though it may be activated by tTA or rtTA to high levels resulting in regulation factors of up to 10^6 (Kistner et al. 1996; Schoenig et al. 2002). By contrast, when the P_{tet}-controlled transcription unit is located close to a nearby enhancer, it may be activated even in the absence of its cognate activator tTA or rtTA. This problem can be circumvented by increasing the number of clones (i.e., the number of independent integration events) to be screened, or, more actively, by reducing the activity of P_{tet}-1 in the uninduced state by shielding it via Tc-controlled transcriptional silencer (tTS) proteins (Freundlieb et al. 1999). Ideally, tTS (Fig. 2) and rtTA bind in a mutually exclusive manner to the *tet*O sequences within P_{tet}, depending on the presence and absence of Dox. This approach was shown to substantially reduce the basal activity of P_{tet} in a number of cell lines (Freundlieb et al. 1999) and in transgenic mice (Zhu et al. 2001a).

As the latter approach allows active suppression of potential unregulated background activity of P_{tet} even when caused by elements which are proximal to the integration site of the minimal promoter, it seems to be more versatile than the adaptation of P_{tet} as proposed above. However, it requires the inclusion of one more component.

An issue that has raised concern is the potential toxicity of tTA and rtTA. Like any other transcription factor, tTA and rtTA, when overexpressed induce undesired pleiotropic effects by "squelching" (Gill and Ptashne 1988) which may even lead to cell death. Thus, tTA or rtTA must not exceed a certain intracellular concentrations. When generating tTA/rtTA in cell or mouse lines, there will automatically be a selection for well-tolerated, integration site-dependent expression levels. Thus, simple screening for proper clones or founder animals will be sufficient as demonstrated by dozens of well functioning tTA/rtTA cell lines and mouse strains. The situation changes, however, when a tTA or rtTA encoding gene is to be integrated into a specific chromosomal locus, e.g., by homologous recombination following the so-called knock-in strategy. Here, the result of integration is not subject to subsequent physiological pre-selection of a proper integration site. Instead, the expression level of the *tTA/rtTA* gene is locus-specific and might be too high to be tolerated or too low to be effective. In such cases, tTAs and rtTAs with a graded activation potential may be chosen which compensate for different expression levels (Baron et al. 1997).

Finally, a remark regarding strategies for setting up Tet regulation is helpful at this point. It is frequently attempted to establish the Tet regulation in cultured cells or in mice in a one-step procedure, i.e., by coinjection (or cotransfection in case of a cellular system) of the two essential DNA constructs. Even though such an experimental shortcut may appear attractive, one should be aware that the two DNAs preferably cointegrate at the same chromosomal locus—frequently in multiple copies—which generally leads to considerable crosstalk between enhancers driving the expression of the transactivator gene and the minimal promoter within P_{tet}, resulting in elevated background activities. This approach is, therefore, only sensible if efficient screening or selection systems are available. In addition, it has to be kept in mind that it is of great value to separately generate and characterize mouse strains which tissue-specifically produce tTA or rtTA as well as mouse lines containing various genes of interest under P_{tet} control as the combination of these various lines offer a higher degree of freedom in the design of experiments.

2.3
Non-invasive Monitoring of Tet-Controlled Transcription Units

The possibility of detecting luciferase activity via bioluminescence in life animals (Contag 1997) can be exploited to monitor the activity of a target gene noninvasively. By coregulating a gene of interest with the luciferase gene via a bidirectional promoter like P_{tet}bi (Fig. 2), luciferase bioluminescence can be exploited as an indicator for the activity of the target gene (Hasan et al. 2001; Fig. 3). This approach is particularly useful in long-term experiments in which the expression of a target gene may be subjected to regulatory regimens with repeated on-and-off cycles or in which partial induction of a gene is intended. Furthermore, since the intensities of target gene expression can vary considerably even among litter mates (Kistner et al. 1996), quantifying luciferase bioluminescence and correlating this activity with the expression of the target gene in individuals enrolled in an experiment will permit a more precise interpretation of the action of the gene under study.

For further methodological and technical information, we like to refer the reader to some recent reviews dealing with various aspects of Tet regulation (Baron and Bujard 2000; Gossen and Bujard 2001; Gossen and Bujard 2002; Schoenig and Bujard 2002).

3
Mouse Models for Human Diseases

Pathologies generally arise through mutations that result in either misexpression of genes or the synthesis of mutated gene products, whereby misexpression refers to deviations from physiological expression levels as well as from temporal programs and spatial (cell-type) restrictions, while mutated gene products may be effective by loss of function or by gaining dominant qualities.

Experimental approaches, which permit the quantitative control of individual gene activities in a temporal and cell type-specific manner, are, therefore, suited to model pathological condition that may rather faithfully mimic respective diseases in transgenic animals. Like most conditional systems acting at the level of gene expression, the Tet regulatory principle is binary in nature. Accordingly, most researchers have followed the strategy of separately generating transgenic tTA or rtTA mouse lines that produce the respective transactivator under the control of a promoter which should relay tissue or cell-type specificity to the system. As the function of promoters is frequently affected by the site of integration, they may loose their specificity, to a different extent, the most common result being position-effect variegation. Sometimes, loss of specificity is accompanied with a highly defined artificial activity pattern, which may be exploited for studying respective subpopulations of cells.

The second mouse line required should contain the target gene under P_{tet} control. The function of P_{tet} is again dependent on the integration site as discussed above. Thus, for tight control and wide range of regulation of a target gene, one has to screen for an appropriate founder line. The identification of such lines is greatly facilitated by the bidirectional promoter P_{tet}bi where, e.g., the luciferase gene is coregulated with the gene of interest and used for monitoring the regulation potential of a newly generated mouse line (Hasan et al. 2001; Schoenig et al. 2002). In any case, numerous mouse lines were described where tight regulation was achieved, of which, in this regard, the most spectacular one was generated by Glenn Fishman and colleagues (Lee et al. 1998) who placed the gene encoding the diphtheria toxin A chain under Tet control in order to induce ablation of specific cell populations.

More than 50 tTA/rtTA and about 80 "receiving" mouse lines containing target genes under P_{tet} control have been published so far (Tables 1, 2, and 3), and numerous further lines are in the state of being characterized in various laboratories. The synergism that could be created when these rapidly increasing pools of mouse lines would be freely exchangeable within the academic community is certainly worth a call to our colleagues and to organizations maintaining repositories for cooperation.

The generation of useful transgenic animals will greatly profit from experimental approaches that would allow us to generate mouse lines with defined properties in a more efficient and predictable manner. In case of transactivator lines, the integration of tTA/rtTA genes behind specific promoters via homologous recombination may sometimes be of advantage as it has led to animals that express the transactivator faithfully (Bond et al. 2000; Perea 2001). But even with this apparently safe approach, it cannot be excluded that the insertion of the transactivator genes in close vicinity of the promoter may disturb the functional program of some regulatory regions. For "receiving" mouse lines, it appears feasible to identify "silent but activatable loci" where a P_{tet}-controlled transcription unit may, upon integration, function in a predictable manner (K. Schoenig, PhD dissertation 2003). Such loci could be targeted via homologous recombination or by using the BAC technology converted into a vector for transgenesis. Eventually, we might learn more about transcriptional insulators in mammalian systems, which could then be used with similar success, as in drosophila (Burgess-Beusse et al. 2002). Thus, it appears likely that the integrated use of various novel approaches will in the near future significantly increase the efficiency of generating defined mouse lines with largely predictable regulatory properties.

Table 1 Mouse lines expressing tTA or rtTA genes

Promoter	Tissue specificity	tTA	rtTA	Reference(s)
Albumin	Liver	+		Manickan et al. 2001; Raben et al. 2001
α CaMKII[a]	Brain	+		Mayford et al. 1996
α CaMKII	Brain		+	Mansuy et al. 1998
CD2	T cell lineage		+	Legname et al. 2000
CD34	Early bone marrow Progenitor and stem cells	+		Radomska et al. 2002
Clara cell 10-kDa protein (CC10)	Lung airway (parenchyma)		+	Mehrad et al. 2002
Clara cell secretory protein (CCSP)	Respiratory epithelial cells		+	Tichelaar et al. 2000
hCMV	Various tissues	+	+	Kistner et al. 1996; Wiekowski et al. 2001
Endothelin receptor B (EDNRB)	Melanocytes, neural crest	+	+	Shin et al. 1999
Fatty acid binding protein (Fbp)	Small intestine, cecum, colon, bladder		+	Saam et al. 1999
Growth hormone (GH)	Pituitary gland		+	Roh et al. 2001
Intronic IgH enhancer, minimal promoter	Thymus, bone marrow	+		Hess et al. 2001
Immunoglobulin heavy chain enhancer and SRα promoter	Hematopoietic system	+		Felsher et al. 1999
Insulin	Pancreatic β-cells	+		Efrat et al. 1995
Insulin	Pancreatic β-cells		+	Thomas et al. 2001; Milo-Landesmann et al. 2001
Interphotoreceptor retinoid-binding protein (IRBP)	Photoreceptor cells	+		Chang et al. 2000
Keratin 5 (K5)	Epidermis, hair follicle	+	+	Diamond et al. 2000
Keratin 6 (K6)	keratinocytes	+		Guo et al. 1999
Keratin 14 (K14)	Epidermis, squamous epithelia		+	Xie et al. 1999
Keratin 14 (K14)	Mammary gland	+		Dunbar et al. 2001
Keratin 18 (K18)	Trachea, upper bronchi, submucosal glands		+	Ye et al. 2001
Lck	T cell lineage	+		Leenders et al. 2000; Labrecque et al. 2001
Liver-enriched activator protein (LAP)[a]	Liver	+		Kistner et al. 1996
Liver-enriched activator protein (LAP)	Liver		+	Schoenig et al. 2002
Major histocompatibility complex (MHC) class II Eα	Thymic, epithelial, Dendritic, B cells, macrophages,	+		Witherden et al. 2000
α-Myosin heavy chain (MHCα)[a]	Heart muscle	+		Passman et al. 1994
α-Myosin heavy chain (MHCα)	Heart muscle		+	Valencik et al. 2001

Table 1 (continued)

Promoter	Tissue specificity	tTA	rtTA	Reference(s)
Major urinary protein (MUP)	Liver	+		Manickan et al. 2001
MMTV long terminal repeat[a]	Mammary gland, salivary gland, seminal vesicle	+		Henninghausen et al. 1995
MMTV long terminal repeat	Mammary gland, salivary gland, seminal vesicle		+	D'Cruz et al. 2001; Hsu et al. 2001; Gunther et al. 2002
Muscle creatine kinase (MCK)	Muscle	+		Ghersa et al. 1998; Ahmad et al. 2000
Nestin	Various tissues		+	Mitsuhashi et al. 2001
Neuron-specific enolase (NSE)[a]	Brain	+		Chen et al. 1998
P0	Schwann cells		+	Pot et al. 2002
P2	Olfactory sensory neurons		+	Gogos et al. 2000
pdx-1	Pancreas	+		Holland et al. 2002
Peripheral myelin protein 22 (PMP22)	Schwann cells	+		Perea et al. 2001
PrP	Brain	+		Tremblay et al. 1998
Prolactin	Pituitary gland	+		Roh et al. 2001
Retinoblastoma gene (Rb)	Brain, lung, spleen		+	Nikitin et al. 2001
Rhodopsin	Photoreceptor cells		+	Chang et al. 2000
SM22α	Smooth muscle cells	+		Ju et al. 2001
Surfactant protein-C (SP/C)	Respiratory epithelial cells		+	Tichelaar et al. 2000
Tek	Endothelial cells	+		Sarao et al. 1998
Tie	Endothelial cells	+		Sarao et al. 1998
Tie2	Vascular endothelium		+	Teng et al. 2002
Tyrosinase	Melanocytes		+	Chin et al. 1999

[a] Mouse line available at The Jackson Laboratory, Bar Harbor, ME 04609, USA.

Table 2 tTA/rtTA responsive mouse lines

Genes under Tet control	tTA/rtTA-responsive promoter		Reference(s)
	P_{tet}-1	P_{tetbi}	
Reporter genes			
Luciferase (L7)[a]	+		Kistner et al. 1996
LacZ, nls/luciferase (nZL-2)[a]		+	Kistner et al. 1996b
LacZ	+		Mayford et al. 1996
LacZ nls	+		Sarao et al. 1998
GFP and lacZ		+	Krestel et al. 2001
Luciferase/Cre recombinase (LC-1)		+	Schoenig et al. 2002
Cre recombinase	+		Saam et al. 1999; Lindeberg et al. 2002; Radomska et al. 2002; Perl et al. 2002
Cre-IRES-tau/lacZ	+		Gogos et al. 2000
Genes of interest			
Adenylylcyclase type VI	+		Gao et al. 2002
AML1-ETO fusion	+		Rhoades et al. 2000
Axin	+		Hsu et al. 2001
BCR-ABL1 fusion	+		Huettner et al. 2000
BOB.1-OBF.1/luc		+	Hess et al. 2001
α-CaMKII-Asp[286]	+		Mayford et al. 1996
Calcineurin autoinhibitory domain	+		Malleret et al. 2001
Calcineurin (mutant)	+		Mansuy et al. 1998
cAMP response protein (CREB)	+		Chen et al. 1998; Sakai et al. 2002
cAMP response protein (CREB)-VP16 fusion	+		Barco et al. 2002
cAMP response protein (CREB) (mutant)	+		Pittenger et al. 2002
β-Catenin/eGFP		+	Cheon et al. 2002
Chemokine KC/lacZ		+	Wiekowski et al. 2001
Colony stimulation factor-1 (CSF-1)	+		van Nguyen et al. 2002
CYP1B1	+		Hwang et al. 2001
Diphtheria toxin A chain (DTA)	+		Lee et al. 1998
Diphteria toxin A chain (mutant)	+		Gogos et al. 2000

Table 2 (continued)

Genes under Tet control	tTA/rtTA-responsive promoter		Reference(s)
	P_{tet}-1	P_{tet}bi	
Dystrophin	+		Ahmad et al. 2000
Endothelin receptor B (EDNRB)	+		Shin et al. 1999
Epidermal growth factor receptor (EGFR) (truncated)	+		Roh et al. 2001
ErbB2 receptor tyrosine kinase	+		Xie et al. 1999
Estrogen receptor α	+		Hruska et al. 2002
FGF-receptor 2 (soluble dn mutant)	+		Hokuto et al. 2002
Fibroblast growth factor-7 (FGF 7)	+		Tichelaar et al. 2000
Fibroblast growth factor-10 (FGF 10)	+		Clark et al. 2001
Fibroblast growth factor-18 (FGF 18)	+		Whitsett et al. 2002
Forkhead transcription factor (FKHR) (truncated)	+		Leenders et al. 2000
ΔFosB[a]	+		Chen et al. 1998
Acid α-glucosidase (GAA)	+		Raben et al. 2001
GATA 6	+		Liu et al. 2002
GluR-A (eGFP-tagged)/lacZ		+	Mack et al. 2001
Glycogen synthase kinase-3β/lacZ		+	Lucas et al. 2001
Hormone-sensitive lipase (HSL)	+		Suzuki et al. 2001
Hox A10	+		Bjornsson et al. 2001
Huntingtin fragment and lacZ		+	Yamamoto et al. 2000
Id1	+		Passman et al. 1994
Idx-1 Hammerhead ribozyme	+		Thomas et al. 2001
α-Integrin/luciferase		+	Valencik et al. 2001
Lymphocyte specific protein tyrosine kinase p56[lck]	+		Legname et al. 2000
MHC class I H-2K[b]	+		Nagaraju et al. 2000
MHC class II Eα	+		Witherden et al. 2000
Met receptor	+		Wang et al. 2001
Mineralocorticoid receptor antisense RNA	+		Beggah et al. 2002
c-myc	+		Felsher et al. 1999; D'Cruz et al. 2001
Nogo A/lacZ	+	+	Pot et al. 2002
Inducible NO-synthetase (iNOS)/eGFP	+	+	Mungrue et al. 2002

Table 2 (continued)

Genes under Tet control	tTA/rtTA-responsive promoter		Reference(s)
	P_{tet}-1	P_{tet}bi	
NR1/*lacZ*		+	Jerecic et al. 1999
NR1 (N598R)/*lacZ*		+	Jerecic et al. 2001
κ Opioid receptor (RASSL) /*lacZ*[a]	+		Redfern et al. 1999
Ornithine decarboxylase (ODC)	+		Guo et al. 1999
p27[KIP1]/eGFP		+	Mitsuhashi et al. 2001
Parathyroid hormone related protein PThrP	+		Dunbar et al. 2001
Pdx1	+		Holland et al. 2002
Peripheral myelin protein 22 (PMP22)	+		Perea et al. 2001
Prion (PrP[C])	+		Tremblay et al. 1998
Protein kinase C-β	+		Bowman et al. 1997
Protein kinase C-ε	+		Choi et al. 2002
Protein phosphatase 1	+		Genoux et al. 2002
H-Ras[V12G]	+		Chin et al. 1999
K-Ras[G12D]	+		Fisher et al. 2001
Retinoblastoma	+		Nikitin et al. 2001
Serotonin 1A receptor	+		Ghavami et al. 1999; Gross et al. 2002
Serotonin 1B receptor	+		Ghavami et al. 1999
Surfactant protein D (SP-D)	+		Zhang et al. 2002
SV40 large T antigen	+		Efrat et al. 1995; Manickan et al. 2001
T cell receptor α OT1	+		Labrecque et al. 2001
TAC-β-integrin fusion/luciferase		+	Valencik et al. 2001
TGF-β	+		Liu et al. 2001
TrK B	+		Ghersa et al. 1998
Urokinase-like plasminogen activator (uPA)		+	Sisson et al. 2002
Utropin	+		Squire et al. 2002
Vascular chymase (RVCH)	+		Ju et al. 2001
Vascular endothelial growth factor (VEGF)	+		Ohno-Matsui et al. 2002; Dor et al. 2001

Nls, nuclear localization signal.

[a] Mouse line available at The Jackson Laboratory, Bar Harbor, ME 04609, USA.

Table 3 Mouse lines with cointegrated tTA/rtTA and P$_{tet}$-controlled genes

Promoter	Tissue	tTA/ rtTA	Gene under P$_{tet}$ control	Reference
Clara cell 10 kd protein	Lung parenchyma	rtTA	Interferon-γ	Wang et al. 2001
Clara cell 10 kd protein	Lung parenchyma	rtTA	Interleukin-9	Temann et al. 2002
Clara cell 10 kd protein	Lung parenchyma	rtTA	Interleukin-11	Ray et al. 1997
Clara cell 10 kd protein	Lung parenchyma	rtTA	Interleukin-13	Zheng et al. 2000
Clara cell 10 kd protein	Lung parenchyma	rtTA	RANTES	Pan et al. 2000
Collagen type II	Chondrocytes	tTA	MMP-13	Neuhold et al. 2001
Insulin gene II	Pancreas	rtTA	TNF-α	Green et al. 2000
Insulin gene II	Pancreas	rtTA	pdx-1 Antisense RNA	Lottmann et al. 2001
LcK	T cells	rtTA	GATA3 (KRR)	Zhang et al. 1999
β-Lactoglobulin	Mammary gland	rtTA	α-Lactoglobulin	Soulier et al. 1999
Retinoblastoma (RB)	Thalamus, muscle, cerebrellum, eye	rtTA	Cre recombinase	Utomo et al. 1999
SK-channel 3 (SK3)	Brain	tTA	SK-channel 3 SK3	Bond et al. 2000
Whey acidic protein (WAP)	Mammary gland	rtTA	Cre recombinase	Utomo et al. 1999

3.1
Modeling Cancer in Mice

A new generation of mouse tumor models became reality with the advent of approaches that allowed for the control of the activity of oncogenes and tumor suppressor genes in a temporally defined and tissue-specific manner. Tumor initiation, progression, and maintenance could now be experimentally dissected with unprecedented precision. The most striking and exciting discovery made with these conditional tumor models is the complete regression of many, even highly invasive, tumors after turning down the activity of the initiating oncogene. Nearly all oncogenes examined to date, including *Myc, H-ras, K-ras, ErbB2, Bcr-Abl1, Fgf7*, and *SV40 Tag*, appear to be not only required for tumor initiation but also for tumor maintenance. Thus, as first shown for *Myc* (Felsher and Bishop 1999), inactivation of a single initiating oncogene can lead to complete regression of 90% of tumors in the hematopoietic system. Similarly, malignant melanomas which developed in an *Ink4a-* and *Arf*-tumor suppressor-deficient background underwent complete regression when the initiating oncogene H-*ras* was inactivated by Dox withdrawal (Chin et al. 1999). These and other groups' findings convey an important and unexpected message: Mutations accumulating in developing tumors do not necessarily introduce functional redundancies that stabilize tumor development. These findings imply that targeting the activity of a single oncogene could result in an effective therapy of a tumor. This reasoning is most impressively supported by a recent report (Jain et al. 2002) describing a conditional mouse model for *Myc*-induced tumors. The authors show that brief inactivation of *Myc* leads to sustained regression of osteogenic sarcoma and differentiation of osteogenic sarcoma cells into mature osteocytes. Subsequent reactivation of *Myc* did not restore the malignant state of the cells, as would be predicted, but instead induced apoptosis.

Together, the results emerging from several laboratories studying the conditional activation/inactivation of various oncogenes shed new light on mechanisms governing induction and commitment of tumorigenesis. They suggest that many tumors are rather rigidly dependent on expression patterns that are established under the governance of the initiating oncogene whose continued function is required. This "oncogene addiction" apparently makes tumors vulnerable to interference with single oncogenes as shown by Felsher and coworkers, where a brief interruption of *Myc* expression caused the breakdown of the malignant state. On the other hand, when *Myc* is induced in mammary gland, only 30% of the tumors arising regress upon inactivation of the oncogene, whereas around 60% have acquired a *Myc*-independent but preferred secondary pathway via mutations in *K-ras* gene (D'Cruz et al. 2001). This finding would suggest that targeting of *Myc* and *K-ras* will result in the regression of many known tumors.

It is likely that numerous human cancers will be modeled in conditional mouse lines in the near future, yielding new insights into functions of genes which contribute to tumor development, thereby revealing new pharmacological targets.

3.2
Conditional Mouse Models for Neurodegenerative Diseases

The first impressive example for applying Tet control to brain functions stems from the laboratory of Eric Kandel. Placing the tTA gene under control of the αCamKII promoter yielded mouse lines which expressed the tTA gene in defined areas of the forebrain, particularly in the hippocampus, cortex, amygdala, and striatum. Crossing such mice with animals that contained a Ca^{2+}-independent version of the *αCamKII* gene under P_{tet} control resulted in double transgenic individuals suitable for the study of synaptic plasticity. In a first set of experiments, Mayford et al. (1996) demonstrated that expression of the dominant active gene product caused a loss of long-term potentiation in the hippocampus and a deficit in spatial learning, whereas repression of the transgene reversed both the physiological and memory deficit.

The same tTA mouse line was used by René Hen and colleagues to model the human Huntington's disease (HD) in the mouse. HD is an inherited progressive neurological disorder caused by an expansion of repeated CAG codons in the huntingtin gene. In the genetic model described by Yamamoto et al. (2000), a chimeric mouse/human huntingtin gene containing 94 CAG repeats was placed under P_{tet} control. When respective mice were crossed with animals expressing tTA via the αCamKII promoter, it was found that in double transgenic animals the expression of the huntingtin gene in the adult brain led to neuroanatomical abnormalities typical for HD. These neuropathological changes resulted in severe progressive motor dysfunction. Strikingly, however, in symptomatic adult animals, the shut off of huntingtin gene expression via Dox could reverse the HD phenotype. Specifically, the nuclear and cytoplasmic aggregates disappeared and the behavioral phenotype approached again the one of control animals. In a further publication (Martin-Aparicio et al. 2001), it was shown that aggregate formation is dependent on the balance between huntingtin synthesis and its degradation via proteasomes. Interestingly, neither mutant huntingtin nor its aggregates are lethal to the cell, demonstrating that HD is due to neuronal dysfunction and not to cell death. These results have yielded significant insights as they show that (1) for progressive HD the continued expression of the huntingtin gene is required, (2) the plasticity of the brain is likely to be sufficient for recovery even from severe symptoms if one could influence the balance between huntingtin production and degradation and, thus, (3) pharmacological interventions may be successful even after symptoms have become visible.

Obviously, corresponding questions can be addressed to prion diseases which result from transformation of cellular prion protein (PrP^c) into a pathogenic scrapie isoform (PrP^{sc}). Indeed, Stanley Prusiner and his group described a mouse model in which PrP^c production was controlled via tTA in a PrP^c-deficient background. They found that high levels of PrP^c are lethal during embryogenesis and postnatal development, whereas in the adult animal neither induction nor repression of PrP^c was detrimental. By contrast, the development of the prion disease upon infection of the animals with low amounts of PrP^{sc} was strongly dependent on the expression level of the transgene encoding PrP^c. These results indicate that while PrP^c may not play an essential role in the brain of adult animals, its continued presence is a prerequisite for acquiring the disorder. It will be interesting to learn whether neurodegenerative symptoms can be halted or even reversed also in this disease by turning down the activity of the PrP^c gene. Mouse models as described by Tremblay et al. (1998) should, in principle, be suitable to examine such questions.

3.3
Modeling Cardiac Diseases

Several routes have been followed in the quest of modeling cardiac pathologies. A number of laboratories have made use of Fishman's mouse line expressing the tTA gene under the control of the αMHC promoter, highly specifically in heart muscle (Passman et al. 1994). Cardiomyopathies were, for example, induced by limited cell ablation via tTA-controlled diphtheria toxin induction (Lee et al. 1998), by conditional expression of specifically designed G_i-coupled receptors (Redfern et al. 1999), or by controlling the expression of the mineralocorticoid receptor (MR). Here, we would like to briefly discuss the recent work of Frédéric Jaisser and colleagues (Beggah et al. 2002), a particularly interesting example representative of the approach. MR, a ligand-dependent transcription factor of the steroid receptor family, is a target for hypertension therapy. It is produced in the kidney, where it is involved in sodium reabsorption and potassium excretion. It is also present in the heart, where its physiological role is not clear. To study MR function exclusively in the heart, the production of antisense mRNA directed towards the murine transcript of the *MR* gene was placed under heart muscle-specific tTA control. The resulting mouse model allowed for reversibly inhibited expression of *MR* in cardiomyocytes. Inhibition resulted in dramatic cardiac hypertrophy, ventricular dysfunction, fibrosis, and heart failure. However, when expression of MR-specific antisense RNA was turned off by Dox administration, heart failure and cardiac remodeling were reversed and heart/body weight ratios returned to control values within one month. Most impressively, interstitial cardiac fibrosis regressed as well, indicating that the pathological extracellular matrix depositions were reversible, in contrast to previous observations (Redfern et al. 2000).

The different conditional mouse models for cardiac diseases will continue to yield novel and complementing insights into complex pathological pathways. Some of these models may develop into useful tools for drug efficacy studies in not too distant future.

4
Concluding Remarks

The disease models briefly discussed herein just give a glimpse into a rapidly growing area of biomedical research, where advances in the genetic manipulation of the mouse are being exploited and begin to yield novel insights into pathways and dynamics of pathological conditions. This is also underlined by work compiled in Table 1–3, in which numerous other pathologies were modeled in the mouse including the induction of autoimmune myositis (Nagaraju et al. 2000), the study of autoimmunity in diabetes type I (Green and Flavell 2000; Christen et al. 2001), lung development (Tichelaar et al. 2000), airway remodeling in asthma (Zhu et al. 2001b), osteoarthritis (Neuhold et al. 2001), and Alzheimer's disease (Lucas et al. 2001) to mention a few. In all these models, the temporal program of pathological processes and its potential reversibility was examined, and in an unexpected high number of cases, pathological states could, despite severe symptoms, be abrogated by repressing the disease-causing gene. Thus, already some of the first truly conditional disease models, which demonstrated the reversibility of even advanced pathological conditions, have changed our views on respective diseases, sparking at the same time new ideas for pharmacological interventions.

Obviously, the mouse is by far the genetically most accessible mammalian system with significant physiological similarities to humans and has become the experimental animal of choice for studying gene functions in vivo and for uncovering molecular mechanisms underlying pathological conditions. Indeed, we can expect a wealth of new information on in vivo gene functions in the near future. On the other hand, one has to keep in mind the physiological differences between humans and mice, which limit the value of mouse models. Future efforts have, therefore, to be directed towards "humanizing" the mouse, and making other suitable mammalian systems such as the rat more readily accessible for defined genetic alterations.

Progress is also required in methods and technologies, which allow us to control from outside individual genes in vivo with high precision. Despite the great potential of various experimental approaches available today, many problems remain. Thus, as long as we know little about the influence of chromatin structure on gene expression and its sensitivity towards perturbations caused, e.g., by recombination events, reliable experimental designs where cell type specificity is maintained and position effect variegation is prevented will remain difficult. Precise and minimal disturbance, gene targeting, as well as the application of the BAC technology may ameliorate some of these shortcomings in future. On the other hand, approaches that leave the gene of interest totally untouched in its genomic context would be highly valuable and may be available soon. For example, controlling custom-made zinc finger-based transcription factors recognizing specific sequences within the promoter of a target gene or regulated synthesis of RNAs interfering with the expression of mRNA or polypeptides that attack specific gene products may develop into systems of choice. Finally, many biological processes are governed by kinetics too fast to be resolved by methods currently available. Progress in the development of noninvasive monitoring systems will overcome some of the present limitations. Obviously, in our strive towards a better understanding of in vivo gene function, there is a broad spectrum of problems waiting for good ideas.

Acknowledgements. Ms. Sibylle Reinig is recognized for help in the preparation of this manuscript. Work in the authors' laboratory has been supported by the Volkswagen-Stiftung (Program: "Conditional mutagenesis") and the European Community ("Development of novel gene expression and genome modification strategies").

References

Ahmad A, Brinson M, Hodges B L, Chamberlain J S, Amalfitano A (2000) Mdx mice inducibly expressing dystrophin provide insights into the potential of gene therapy for duchenne muscular dystrophy. Hum Mol Genet 9:2507—2515

Barco A, Alarcon J M, Kandel E R (2002) Expression of constitutively active CREB protein facilitates the late phase of long-term potentiation by enhancing synaptic capture. Cell 108:689–703

Baron U, Bujard H (2000) The Tet repressor-based system for regulated gene expression in eukaryotic cells: principles and advances. Methods Enzymol 327:659–686

Baron U, Gossen M, Bujard H (1997) Tetracycline controlled transcription in eukaryotes: novel transactivators with graded transactivation potential. Nucl Acids Res 25:2723–2729

Baron U, Freundlieb S, Gossen M, Bujard H (1995) Coregulation of two gene activities by tetracycline via a bidirectional promoter. Nucl Acids Res 23:3605–3606

Beggah A T, Escoubet B, Puttini S, Cailmail S, Delage V, Ouvrard-Pascaud A, Bocchi B, Peuchmaur M, Delcayre C, Farman N, Jaisser F (2002) Reversible cardiac fibrosis and heart failure induced by conditional expression of an antisense mRNA of the mineralocorticoid receptor in cardiomyocytes. Proc Natl Acad Sci USA 99:7160—7165

Bjornsson J M, Andersson E, Lundstrom P, Larsson N, Xu X, Repetowska E, Humphries R K, Karlsson S (2001) Proliferation of primitive myeloid progenitors can be reversibly induced by HOXA10. Blood 98:3301–3308

Bond C T, Sprengel R, Bissonnette J M, Kaufmann W A, Pribnow D, Neelands T, Storck T, Baetscher M, Jerecic J, Maylie J, Knaus H G, Seeburg P H, Adelman J P (2000) Respiration and parturition affected by conditional overexpression of the Ca2+-activated K+ channel subunit, SK3. Science 289:1942—1946

Bowman J C, Steinberg S F, Jiang T, Geenen D L, Fishman G I, Buttrick P M (1997) Expression of protein kinase C beta in the heart causes hypertrophy in adult mice and sudden death in neonates. J Clin Invest 100:2189—2195

Burgess-Beusse B, Farrell C, Gaszner M, Litt M, Mutskov V, Recillas-Targa F, Simpson M, West A, Felsenfeld G (2002) The insulation of genes from external enhancers and silencing chromatin. Proc Nat Acad Sci USA 99:16433–16437

Chang M A, Horner J W, Conklin B R, DePinho R A, Bok D, Zack D J (2000) Tetracycline-inducible system for photoreceptor-specific gene expression. Invest Ophthalmol Vis Sci 41:4281–4287

Chen J, Kelz M B, Zeng G, Sakai N, Steffen C, Shockett P E, Picciotto M R, Duman R S, Nestler E J (1998) Transgenic animals with inducible, targeted gene expression in brain. Mol Pharmacol 54:495–503

Cheon S S, Cheah A Y, Turley S, Nadesan P, Poon R, Clevers H, Alman B A (2002) beta-Catenin stabilization dysregulates mesenchymal cell proliferation, motility, and invasiveness and causes aggressive fibromatosis and hyperplastic cutaneous wounds. Proc Natl Acad Sci USA 99:6973–6978

Chin L, Tam A, Pomerantz J, Wong M, Holash J, Bardeesy N, Shen Q, O'Hagan R, Pantginis J, Zhou H, Horner J W 2nd, Cordon-Cardo C, Yancopoulos G D, DePinho R A (1999) Essential role for oncogenic Ras in tumour maintenance. Nature 400:468–472

Choi D S, Wang D, Dadgar J, Chang W S, Messing R O (2002) Conditional rescue of protein kinase C epsilon regulates ethanol preference and hypnotic sensitivity in adult mice. J Neurosci 22:9905–9911

Clark J C, Tichelaar J W, Wert S E, Itoh N, Perl A K, Stahlman M T, Whitsett J A (2001) FGF-10 disrupts lung morphogenesis and causes pulmonary adenomas in vivo. Am J Physiol Lung Cell Mol Physiol 280:L705–715

Christen U, Wolfe T, Mohrle U, Hughes A C, Rodrigo E, Green E A, Flavell R A, Herrath M G (2001) A dual role for TNF-alpha in type 1 diabetes: islet-specific expression abrogates the ongoing autoimmune process when induced late but not early during pathogenesis. J Immunol 166:7023–7032

Contag C H, Spilman S D, Contag P R, Oshiro M, Eames B, Dennery P, Stevenson D K, Benaron D A (1997) Visualizing gene expression in living mammals using a bioluminescent reporter. Photochem Photobiol 66:523–531

D'Cruz C M, Gunther E J, Boxer R B, Hartman J L, Sintasath L, Moody S E, Cox J D, Ha S I, Belka G K, Golant A, Cardiff R D, Chodosh L A (2001) c-MYC induces mammary tumorigenesis by means of a preferred pathway involving spontaneous *Kras2* mutations. Nat Med 7:235–239

Diamond I, Owolabi T, Marco M, Lam C, Glick A (2000) Conditional gene expression in the epidermis of transgenic mice using the tetracycline-regulated transactivators tTA and rTA linked to the keratin 5 promoter. J Invest Dermatol 115:788–794

Dor Y, Camenisch T D, Itin A, Fishman G I, McDonald J A, Carmeliet P, Keshet E (2001) A novel role for VEGF in endocardial cushion formation and its potential contribution to congenital heart defects. Development 128:1531–1538

Dunbar M E, Dann P, Brown C W, Van Houton J, Dreyer B, Philbrick W P, Wysolmerski J J (2001) Temporally regulated overexpression of parathyroid hormone-related protein in the mammary gland reveals distinct fetal and pubertal phenotypes. J Endocrinol171:403–416

Efrat S, Fusco-DeMane D, Lemberg H, al Emran O, Wang X (1995) Conditional transformation of a pancreatic beta-cell line derived from transgenic mice expressing a tetracycline-regulated oncogene. Proc Natl Acad Sci USA 92:3576—3580

Felsher D W, J M Bishop (1999) Reversible tumorigenesis by MYC in hematopoietic lineages. Mol Cell 4:199—207

Fisher G H, Wellen S L, Klimstra D, Lenczowski J M, Tichelaar J W, Lizak M J, Whitsett J A, Koretsky A, Varmus H E (2001) Induction and apoptotic regression of lung adenocarcinomas by regulation of a K-Ras transgene in the presence and absence of tumor suppressor genes. Genes Dev 15:3249-3262

Freundlieb S, Schirra-Mueller C, Bujard H (1999) A tetracycline controlled activation/ repression system for mammalian cells. J Gene Med 1:4—12

Gao M H, Bayat H, Roth D M, Yao Zhou J, Drumm J, Burhan J, Kirk Hammond H (2002) Controlled expression of cardiac-directed adenylylcyclase type VI provides increased contractile function. Cardiovasc Res 56:197-204

Genoux D, Haditsch U, Knobloch M, Michalon A, Storm D, Mansuy I M (2002) Protein phosphatase 1 is a molecular constraint on learning and memory. Nature 418:970–975

Ghavami A, Stark K L, Jareb M, Ramboz S, Segu, L, Hen R (1999) Differential addressing of 5-HT1A and 5-HT1B receptors in epithelial cells and neurons. J Cell Sci 112(Pt 6):967–976

Ghersa P, Gobert R P, Sattonnet-Roche P, Richards C A, Merlo Pich E, Hooft van Huijsduijnen R (1998) Highly controlled gene expression using combinations of a tissue-specific promoter, recombinant adenovirus and a tetracycline-regulatable transcription factor. Gene Ther 5:1213–1220

Gill G, Ptashne M (1988) Negative effect of the transcriptional activator GAL4. Nature. 334:721–4.

Gogos J A, Osborne J, Nemes A, Mendelsohn M, Axel R (2000) Genetic ablation and restoration of the olfactory topographic map. Cell 103:609–620

Gossen M, Bujard H (2002) Studying gene function in eukaryotes by conditional gene inactivation. Ann Rev Genet 36:153–173

Gossen M, Bujard H (2001) Tetracyclines in the control of gene expression in eukaryotes. In: M Nelson, W Hillen, R A Greenwald (eds) Tetracyclines as molecular probes for micro and mammalian biology. Birkhäuser Verlag, Basel pp. 139–157

Gossen M, Bujard H (1992) Tight control of gene expression in mammalian cells by tetracycline responsive promoters. Proc Natl Acad Sci USA 89:5547-5551

Gossen M, Freundlieb S, Bender G, Müller G, Hillen W, Bujard H (1995) Transcriptional activation by tetracycline in mammalian cells. Science 268:1766—1769

Green E A, Flavell R A (2000) The temporal importance of TNFalpha expression in the development of diabetes. Immunity 12:459–469

Gross C, Zhuang X, Stark K, Ramboz S, Oosting R, Kirby L, Santarelli L, Beck S, Hen R (2002) Serotonin1A receptor acts during development to establish normal anxiety-like behaviour in the adult. Nature 416:396–400

Gunther E J, Belka G K, Wertheim G B, Wang J, Hartman J L, Boxer R B, Chodosh L A (2002) A novel doxycycline-inducible system for the transgenic analysis of mammary gland biology. Faseb J 16:283–292

Guo Y, Harris R B, Rosson D, Boorman D, O'Brien T G (2000) Functional analysis of human ornithine decarboxylase alleles. Cancer Res 60:6314–6317

Hasan M T, Schoenig K, Graewe W, Bujard H (2001) Long-term, non-invasive imaging of regulated gene expression in living mice. Genesis 29:116—122

Hennighausen L, Wall R J, Tillmann U, Li M, Furth P A (1995) Conditional gene expression in secretory tissues and skin of transgenic mice using the MMTV-LTR and the tetracycline responsive system. J Cell Biochem 59:463–472

Hess J, Nielsen P J, Fischer K D, Bujard H, Wirth T (2001) The B lymphocyte-specific coactivator BOB.1/OBF.1 is required at multiple stages of B-cell development. Mol Cell Biol 21:1531–1539

Hokuto I, Perl A K, Whitsett J A (2002) Prenatal, but not postnatal inhibition of FGF-receptor signaling causes emphysema. J Biol Chem: in press

Holland A M, Hale M A, Kagami H, Hammer R E, MacDonald R J (2002) Experimental control of pancreatic development and maintenance. Proc Natl Acad Sci USA 99:12236–12241

Hruska K S, Tilli M T, Ren S, Cotarla I, Kwong T, Li M, Fondell J D, Hewitt J A, Koos R D, Furth PA, Flaws J A (2002) Conditional over-expression of estrogen receptor alpha in a transgenic mouse model. Transgenic Res 11:361—372

Hsu W, Shakya R, Costantini F (2001) Impaired mammary gland and lymphoid development caused by inducible expression of Axin in transgenic mice. J Cell Biol 155:1055–1064

Huettner C S, Zhang P, Van Etten R A, Tenen D G (2000) Reversibility of acute B-cell leukaemia induced by BCR-ABL1. Nat Genet 24:57–60

Hwang D Y, Chae K R, Shin D H, Hwang J H, Lim C H, Kim Y J, Kim B J, Goo J S, Shin Y Y, Jang I S, Cho J S, Kim Y K (2001) Xenobiotic response in humanized double transgenic mice expressing tetracycline-controlled transactivator and human CYP1B1. Arch Biochem Biophys 395:32–40

Jain M, Arvanitis C, Chu K, Dewey W, Leonhardt E, Trinh M, Sundberg C D, Bishop J M, Felsher D W (2002) Sustained loss of a neoplastic phenotype by brief inactivation of MYC. Science 297:102–104

Jerecic J, Schulze C H, Jonas P, Sprengel R, Seeburg P H, Bischofberger J (2001) Impaired NMDA receptor function in mouse olfactory bulb neurons by tetracycline-sensitive NR1 (N598R) expression. Brain Res Mol Brain Res 94:96–104

Jerecic J, Single F, Kruth U, Krestel H, Kolhekar R, Storck T, Kask K, Higuchi M, Sprengel R, Seeburg P H (1999) Studies on conditional gene expression in the brain. Ann NY Acad Sci 868:27–37

Ju H, Gros R, You X, Tsang S, Husain M, Rabinovitch M (2001) Conditional and targeted overexpression of vascular chymase causes hypertension in transgenic mice. Proc Natl Acad Sci USA 98:7469–7474

Kistner A, Gossen M, Zimmermann F, Jerecic J, Ullmer C, Lübbert H, Bujard H (1996) Doxycycline-mediated, quantitative and tissue-specific control of gene expression in transgenic mice. Proc Natl Acad Sci USA 93:10933–10938

Krestel H E, Mayford M, Seeburg P H, Sprengel R (2001) A GFP-equipped bidirectional expression module well suited for monitoring tetracycline-regulated gene expression in mouse. Nucl Acids Res 29:E39

Kuehn R, Schwenk F (2002) Conditional knockout mice. In: J van Deursen, M Hofker (eds) The Transgenic Mouse: Methods and Protocols. Humana Press Inc., Totowa, NJ, USA, pp 159—186

Labrecque N, Whitfield L S, Obst R, Waltzinger C, Benoist C, Mathis D (2001) How much TCR does a T cell need? Immunity 15:71–82

Lee P, Morley G, Huang Q, Fischer A, Seiler S, Horner J W, Factor S, Vaidya D, Jalife J, Fishman G I (1998) Conditional lineage ablation to model human diseases. Proc Natl Acad Sci USA 95:11371–11376

Leenders H, Whiffield S, Benoist C, Mathis D (2000) Role of the forkhead transcription family member, FKHR, in thymocyte differentiation. Eur J Immunol 30:2980–2990

Legname G, Seddon B, Lovatt M, Tomlinson P, Sarner N, Tolaini M, Williams K, Norton T, Kioussis D, Zamoyska R (2000) Inducible expression of a p56Lck transgene reveals a central role for Lck in the differentiation of CD4 SP thymocytes. Immunity 12:537–546

Lewandoski M. (2001) Conditional control of gene expression in the mouse. Nature Rev Genet 2:743—755

Lindeberg J, Mattsson R, Ebendal T (2002) Timing the doxycycline yields different patterns of genomic recombination in brain neurons with a new inducible Cre transgene. J Neurosci Res 68:248–253

Liu C, Morrisey E E, Whitsett J A (2002) GATA-6 is required for maturation of the lung in late gestation. Am J Physiol Lung Cell Mol Physiol 283:L468–475

Liu X, Alexander V, Vijayachandra K, Bhogte E, Diamond I, Glick A (2001) Conditional epidermal expression of TGFbeta 1 blocks neonatal lethality but causes a reversible hyperplasia and alopecia. Proc Natl Acad Sci USA 98:9139–9144

Lottmann H, Vanselow J, Hessabi B, Walther R (2001) The Tet-On system in transgenic mice: inhibition of the mouse pdx-1 gene activity by antisense RNA expression in pancreatic beta-cells. J Mol Med 79:321–328

Mack V, Burnashev N, Kaiser K M, Rozov A, Jensen V, Hvalby O, Seeburg P H, Sakmann B, Sprengel R (2001) Conditional restoration of hippocampal synaptic potentiation in Glur-A-deficient mice. Science 292:2501–2504

Malleret G, Haditsch U, Genoux D, Jones M W, Bliss T V, Vanhoose A M, Weitlauf C, Kandel E R, Winder D G, Mansuy I M (2001) Inducible and reversible enhancement of learning, memory, and long-term potentiation by genetic inhibition of calcineurin. Cell 104:675–686

Manickan E, Satoi J, Wang T C, Liang T J (2001) Conditional liver-specific expression of simian virus 40 T antigen leads to regulatable development of hepatic neoplasm in transgenic mice. J Biol Chem 276:13989–13994

Mansuy I M, Mayford M, Jacob B, Kandel E R, Bach M E (1998) Restricted and regulated overexpression reveals calcineurin as a key component in the transition from short-term to long-term memory. Cell 92:39–49

Mansuy I M, Winder D G, Moallem T M, Osman M, Mayford M, Hawkins R D, Kandel E R (1998) Inducible and reversible gene expression with the rtTA system for the study of memory. Neuron 21:257–265

Martin-Aparicio E, Yamamoto A, Hernandez F, Hen R, Avila J and Lucas JJ (2001) Proteasomal-dependent aggregate reversal and absence of cell death in an conditional mouse model of Huntington's disease. J Neorosci 21:8772–8781

Mayford M, Bach M E, Huang Y Y, Wang L, Hawkins R D, Kandel E R (1996) Control of memory formation through regulated expression of a CaMKII transgene. Science 274:1678–1683

Mehrad B, Wiekowski M, Morrison B E, Chen S C, Coronel E C, Manfra D J, Lira S A (2002) Transient lung-specific expression of the chemokine KC improves outcome in invasive aspergillosis. Am J Respir Crit Care Med 166:1263–1268

Milo-Landesman D, Surana M, Berkovich I, Compagni A., Christofori G, Fleischer N, Efrat S (2001) Correction of hyperglycemia in diabetic mice transplanted with reversibly immortalized pancreatic beta cells controlled by the tet-on regulatory system. Cell Transplant 10:645–650

Mitsuhashi T, Aoki Y, Eksioglu Y Z, Takahashi T, Bhide P G, Reeves S A, Caviness V S Jr (2001) Overexpression of p27Kip1 lengthens the G1 phase in a mouse model that targets inducible gene expression to central nervous system progenitor cells. Proc Natl Acad Sci USA 98:6435–6440

Mungrue I N, Gros R, You X, Pirani A, Azad A, Csont T, Schulz R, Butany J, Stewart D J, Husain M (2002) Cardiomyocyte overexpression of iNOS in mice results in peroxynitrite generation, heart block, and sudden death. J Clin Invest 109:735–743

Nagaraju K, Raben N, Loeffler L, Parker T, Rochon P J, Lee E, Danning C, Wada R., Thompson C, Bahtiyar G, Craft J, Hooft Van Huijsduijnen R, Plotz P (2000) Conditional up-regulation of MHC class I in skeletal muscle leads to self-sustaining auto-immune myositis and myositis-specific autoantibodies. Proc Natl Acad Sci USA 97:9209–9214

Neuhold L A, Killar L, Zhao W, Sung M L, Warner L, Kulik J, Turner J, Wu W, Billinghurst C, Meijers T, Poole A R, Babij P, DeGennaro L J (2001) Postnatal expression in hyaline cartilage of constitutively active human collagenase-3 (MMP-13) induces osteoarthritis in mice. J Clin Invest 107:35—44

Nikitin A, Shan B, Flesken-Nikitin A, Chang K H. Lee W H (2001) The retinoblastoma gene regulates somatic growth during mouse development. Cancer Res 61:3110–3118

Ohno-Matsui K, Hirose A, Yamamoto S, Saikia J, Okamoto N, Gehlbach P, Duh E J, Hackett S, Chang M, Bok D, Zack D J, Campochiaro P A (2002) Inducible expression of vascular endothelial growth factor in adult mice causes severe proliferative retinopathy and retinal detachment. Am J Pathol 160:711–719

Pan Z Z, Parkyn L, Ray A, Ray P (2000) Inducible lung-specific expression of RANTES: preferential recruitment of neutrophils. Am J Physiol Lung Cell Mol Physiol 279:L658–666

Passman R S, Fishman G I (1994) Regulated expression of foreign genes in vivo after germline transfer. J Clin Invest 94:2421–2425

Perea J, Robertson A, Tolmachova T, Muddle J, King R H, Ponsford S, Thomas P K, Huxley C (2001) Induced myelination and demyelination in a conditional mouse model of Charcot-Marie-Tooth disease type 1A. Hum Mol Genet 10:1007–1018

Perl A K, Wert S E, Nagy A, Lobe C G, Whitsett J A (2002) Early restriction of peripheral and proximal cell lineages during formation of the lung. Proc Natl Acad Sci USA 99:10482–10487

Pittenger C, Huang Y Y, Paletzki R F, Bourtchouladze R, Scanlin H, Vronskaya S, Kandel E R (2002) Reversible inhibition of CREB/ATF transcription factors in region CA1 of the dorsal hippocampus disrupts hippocampus-dependent spatial memory. Neuron 34:447–462

Pot C, Simonen M, Weinmann O, Schnell L, Christ F, Stoeckle S, Berger P, Rulicke T, Suter U, Schwab M E (2002) Nogo-A expressed in Schwann cells impairs axonal regeneration after peripheral nerve injury. J Cell Biol 159:29–35

Raben N, Lu N, Nagaraju K, Rivera Y, Lee A, Yan B, Byrne B, Meikle P J., Umapathysivam K, Hopwood J J, Plotz P H (2001) Conditional tissue-specific expression of the acid alpha-glucosidase (GAA) gene in the GAA knockout mice: implications for therapy. Hum Mol Genet 10:2039–2047

Radomska H S, Gonzalez D A, Okuno Y, Iwasaki H, Nagy A, Akashi K, Tenen D G, Huettner C S (2002) Transgenic targeting with regulatory elements of the human CD34 gene. Blood 100:4410–4419

Redfern C H, Coward P, Degtyarev M Y, Lee E K, Kwa A T, Hennighausen L, Bujard H, Fishman G I, Conklin B R (1999) Conditional expression and signaling of a specifically designed G(i)-coupled receptor in transgenic mice. Nat Biotechnol 17:165—169

Redfern C H, Degtyarev M Y, Kwa A T, Salomonis N, Cotte N, Nanevicz T, Fidelman N, Desai K, Vranizan K, Lee E K, Coward P, Shah N, Warrington J A, Fishman G I, Bernstein D, Baker A J, Conklin B R (2000) Conditional expression of a Gi-coupled receptor causes ventricular conduction delay and a lethal cardiomyopathy. Proc Natl Acad Sci USA 97:4826–4831

Rhoades K L, Hetherington C J, Harakawa N, Yergeau D A, Zhou L, Liu L Q, Little M T, Tenen D G, Zhang D E (2000) Analysis of the role of AML1-ETO in leukemogenesis, using an inducible transgenic mouse model. Blood 96:2108–2115

Roh M, Paterson A J, Asa S L, Chin E, Kudlow J E (2001) Stage-sensitive blockade of pituitary somatomammotrope development by targeted expression of a dominant negative epidermal growth factor receptor in transgenic mice. Mol Endocrinol 15:600–613

Saam J R, Gordon J I (1999) Inducible gene knockouts in the small intestinal and colonic epithelium. J Biol Chem 274:38071–38082

Sakai N, Thome J, Newton S S, Chen J, Kelz M B, Steffen C, Nestler E J, Duman R S (2002) Inducible and brain region-specific CREB transgenic mice. Mol Pharmacol 61:1453–1464

Sarao R, Dumont D J (1998) Conditional transgene expression in endothelial cells. Transgenic Res 7:421–427

Sauer B (1998) Inducible gene targeting in mice using the Cre/loxP system. Methods Enzymol 14:381—392

Schoenig K (2003) PhD dissertation, University of Heidelberg, Germany

Schoenig K, Bujard H (2002) Generating conditional mouse mutants via tetracycline controlled gene expression. In: J van Deursen, M Hofker (eds) The Transgenic Mouse: Methods and Protocols. Humana Press Inc., Totowa, NJ, USA, pp 69–104

Schoenig K, Schwenk F, Rajewsky K, Bujard H (2002) Stringent doxycycline dependent control of CRE recombinase in vivo. Nucl Acids Res 30:e134

Shin M K, Levorse J M, Ingram R S, Tilghman S M (1999) The temporal requirement for endothelin receptor-B signalling during neural crest development. Nature 402:496–501

Sisson T H, Hanson K E, Subbotina N, Patwardhan A, Hattori N, Simon R H (2002) Inducible lung-specific urokinase expression reduces fibrosis and mortality after lung injury in mice. Am J Physiol Lung Cell Mol Physiol 283:L1023—1032

Soulier S, Stinnakre M G, Lepourry L, Mercier J C, Vilotte J L (1999) Use of doxycycline-controlled gene expression to reversibly alter milk-protein composition in transgenic mice. Eur J Biochem 260:533–539

Squire S, Raymackers J M, Vandebrouck C, Potter A, Tinsley J, Fisher R, Gillis J M, Davies K E (2002) Prevention of pathology in mdx mice by expression of utrophin: analysis using an inducible transgenic expression system. Hum Mol Genet 11:3333–3344

Suzuki J, Shen W J, Nelson B D, Patel S, Veerkamp J H, Selwood S P, Murphy G M Jr, Reaven E, Kraemer F B (2001) Absence of cardiac lipid accumulation in transgenic mice with heart-specific HSL overexpression. Am J Physiol Endocrinol Metab 281:E857–866

Temann U A, Ray P, Flavell R A (2002) Pulmonary overexpression of IL-9 induces Th2 cytokine expression, leading to immune pathology. J Clin Invest 109:29–39

Teng P I, Dichiara M R, Komuves L G, Abe K, Quertermous T, Topper JN (2002) Inducible and selective transgene expression in murine vascular endothelium. Physiol Genomics 11:99–107

Thomas M K, Devon O N, Lee J H, Peter A, Schlosser D A, Tenser M S, Habener J F (2001) Development of diabetes mellitus in aging transgenic mice following suppression of pancreatic homeoprotein IDX-1. J Clin Invest 108:319–329

Tichelaar J W, Lu W, Whitsett J A (2000) Conditional expression of fibroblast growth factor-7 in the developing and mature lung. J Biol Chem 275:11858–11864

Tremblay P, Meiner Z, Galou M, Heinrich C, Petromilli C, Lisse T, Cayetano J, Torchia M, Mobley W, Bujard H, DeArmond S J, Prusiner S B (1998) Doxycycline control of prion protein transgene expression modulates prion disease in mice. Proc Natl Acad Sci USA 95:12580–12585

Urlinger S, Baron U, Thellmann M, Hasan M T, Bujard H, Hillen W (2000) Exploring the sequence space for tetracycline dependent transcriptional activators: novel mutations yield expanded range and sensitivity. Proc Natl Acad Sci US:7963—7968

Utomo A R, Nikitin A Y, Lee W H (1999) Temporal, spatial, and cell type-specific control of Cre-mediated DNA recombination in transgenic mice. Nat Biotechnol 17, 1091—1096

Valencik M L, McDonald J A (2001) Codon optimization markedly improves doxycycline regulated gene expression in the mouse heart. Transgenic Res 10:269–275

Van Nguyen A, Pollard J W (2002) Colony stimulating factor-1 is required to recruit macrophages into the mammary gland to facilitate mammary ductal outgrowth. Dev Biol 247:11–25

Wang Z, Zheng T, Zhu Z, Homer R J, Riese R J, Chapman H A Jr, Shapiro S D, Elias J A (2000) Interferon gamma induction of pulmonary emphysema in the adult murine lung. J Exp Med 192:1587—1600

Wang R, Ferrell L D, Faouzi S, Maher J J, Bishop J M (2001) Activation of the Met receptor by cell attachment induces and sustains hepatocellular carcinomas in transgenic mice. J Cell Biol 153:1023–1034

Whitsett J A, Clark J C, Picard L, Tichelaar J W, Wert S E, Itoh N, Perl A K, Stahlman M T (2002) Fibroblast growth factor 18 influences proximal programming during lung morphogenesis. J Biol Chem 277:22743–22749

Wiekowski M T, Chen S C, Zalamea P, Wilburn B P, Kinsley D J, Sharif W W, Jensen K K, Hedrick J A, Manfra D, Lira S A (2001) Disruption of neutrophil migration in a conditional transgenic model: evidence for CXCR2 desensitization in vivo. J Immunol 167:7102–7110

Witherden D, van Oers N, Waltzinger C, Weiss A, Benoist C, Mathis D (2000) Tetracycline-controllable selection of CD4(+) T cells: half-life and survival signals in the absence of major histocompatibility complex class II molecules. J Exp Med 191:355–364

Xie W, Chow L T, Paterson A J, Chin E, Kudlow J E (1999) Conditional expression of the ErbB2 oncogene elicits reversible hyperplasia in stratified epithelia and up-regulation of TGFalpha expression in transgenic mice. Oncogene 18, 3593–3607

Yamamoto A, Lucas J J, Hen R (2000) Reversal of neuropathology and motor dysfunction in a conditional model of Huntington's disease. Cell 101:57–66

Ye L, Chan S, Chow Y H, Tsui L C, Hu J (2001) Regulated expression of the human CFTR gene in epithelial cells. Mol Ther 3:723–733

Zhang D H, Yang L, Cohn L, Parkyn L, Homer R, Ray P, Ray A (1999) Inhibition of allergic inflammation in a murine model of asthma by expression of a dominant-negative mutant of GATA-3. Immunity 11:473–482

Zhang L, Ikegami M, Dey C R, Korfhagen T R, Whitsett J A (2002) Reversibility of pulmonary abnormalities by conditional replacement of surfactant protein D (SP-D) in vivo. J Biol Chem 277:38709–38713

Zheng T, Zhu Z, Wang Z, Homer R J, Ma B., Riese R J Jr, Chapman H A Jr, Shapiro S D, Elias J A (2000) Inducible targeting of IL-13 to the adult lung causes matrix metalloproteinase- and cathepsin-dependent emphysema. J Clin Invest 106:1081–1093

Zhu Z, Ma B, Homer R J, Zheng T, Elias J A (2001a) Use of the tetracycline controlled silencer (tTS) to eliminate transgene leak in inducible overexpression transgenic mice. J Biol Chem 276:25222–25229

Zhu Z, Lee C G, Zheng T, Chupp G, Wang J, Homer R J, Noble P W, Hamid Q, Elias J A (2001b) Airway inflammation and remodeling in asthma. Lessons from interleukin 11 and interleukin 13 transgenic mice. Am J Respir Crit Care Med 164:67–70

Part 2
Molecular Systems

Adrenergic System

S. Engelhardt · L. Hein

Institut für Pharmakologie und Toxikologie, Universität Würzburg,
Versbacher Strasse 9, 97078 Würzburg, Germany,
e-mail: hein@toxi.uni-wuerzburg.de

Abstract The adrenergic system is an essential regulator of cardiovascular, endocrine, neuronal, vegetative, and metabolic function. The biological effects of the endogenous catecholamines epinephrine and norepinephrine are mediated by nine distinct G protein-coupled receptor subtypes. These adrenergic receptors can be divided into three different groups, the α_1-receptors (α_{1A}, α_{1B}, α_{1D}), α_2-receptors (α_{2A}, α_{2B}, α_{2C}) and β-receptors (β_1, β_2, β_3). In the absence of sufficiently subtype-selective ligands, transgenic mouse models with targeted deletions in the individual receptor genes as well as mouse lines with tissue-specific overexpression of adrenergic receptors have been generated recently. Most adrenergic receptor subtypes have distinct physiological functions. Within the α_2-

receptor group, α_{2A}- and α_{2C}-receptors operate together to control catechol-amine release from adrenergic neurons, whereas α_{2B}-receptors are essential for angiogenesis in the developing placenta. Transgenic models of β_1- and β_2-adrenergic receptors in the heart have revealed differences in signal transduction between these receptors. Whereas both receptors may increase cardiac contractility, chronic signaling via β_1-receptors in cardiac myocytes causes hypertrophy, fibrosis, and heart failure. The α_1-adrenergic receptor subtypes α_{1A}, α_{1B}, α_{1D} are primarily involved in the regulation of vascular tone and may have partially overlapping functions in vivo. Transgenic mouse models have revealed a number of novel and distinct physiological functions for adrenergic receptors, neurotransmitter transporters, and enzymes, and they may lead to novel therapeutic applications for subtype-selective drugs.

Keywords Adrenergic receptors · Transgenic mice · Gene targeting

Abbreviations

αMHC	α-Myosin heavy chain
AADC	Aromatic L-amino acid decarboxylase
AR	Adrenergic receptor
CAM	Constitutively active receptor mutant
COMT	Catechol-O-methyltransferase
DβH	Dopamine β-hydroxylase
EMT	Extraneuronal monoamine transporter
KO	Knockout
MAO	Monoamine oxidase
NET	Norepinephrine transporter
NHE	Na^+-H^+-exchanger
PNMT	Phenylethanolamine N-methyltransferase
TH	Tyrosine hydroxylase
VMAT	Vesicular monoamine transporter
WT	Wild-type

1
Introduction

The adrenergic system is an essential regulator to increase cardiovascular and metabolic capacity during situations of stress, exercise, and disease. Nerve cells in the central and peripheral nervous system synthesize and secrete the neurotransmitters norepinephrine and epinephrine. In the peripheral nervous system, norepinephrine and epinephrine are released from two different sites (Fig. 1): norepinephrine is the principal neurotransmitter of sympathetic neurons which innervate many organs and tissues. In contrast, epinephrine—and to a smaller degree also norepinephrine—are produced and secreted from the adrenal gland

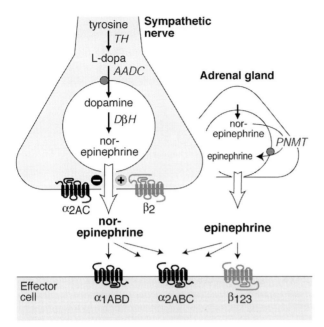

Fig. 1 Functional organization of the adrenergic system in sympathetic nerves and in the adrenal gland. In sympathetic nerves, norepinephrine is synthesized from the precursor tyrosine and stored in synaptic vesicles. In the chromaffin cells of the adrenal gland, most of the norepinephrine is further converted into epinephrine by PNMT. Both catecholamines mediate their biological actions via nine different G protein-coupled receptor subtypes, which are differentially distributed between pre- and post-synaptic sites

into the circulation. Thus, the actions of norepinephrine are mostly restricted to the sites of release from sympathetic nerves, whereas epinephrine acts as a hormone to stimulate many different cells via the blood stream.

The biological actions of epinephrine and norepinephrine are mediated via nine different G protein-coupled receptors, which are located in the plasma membrane of neuronal and non-neuronal target cells (Fig. 1). These receptors are divided into two different groups, α-adrenergic receptors and β-adrenergic receptors. The distinction between α- and β-adrenergic receptors was first proposed based on experiments with various catecholamine derivatives to produce excitatory (α) or inhibitory (β) responses in isolated smooth muscle systems (Ahlquist 1948). Altogether, nine adrenergic receptors have been identified by molecular cloning (Bylund et al. 1994): three α_1-adrenergic receptors (α_{1A}, α_{1B}, α_{1D}), three α_2-subtypes (α_{2A}, α_{2B}, α_{2C}), and three β-adrenergic receptors (β_1, β_2, β_3) (Fig. 1). Due to the lack of sufficiently subtype-selective ligands, the unique physiological properties of the α-receptor subtypes, for the most part, have not been fully elucidated. However, recent studies in mice carrying deletions in the genes encoding for individual adrenergic receptor subtypes have greatly advanced the knowledge about the specific functions of these receptors (for re-

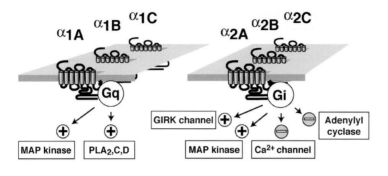

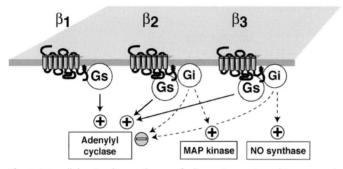

Fig. 2 Intracellular signaling pathways of adrenergic receptor subtypes. α_1-adrenergic receptors couple to several intracellular second messengers via G_q proteins, whereas α_2-receptors engage G proteins of the G_i family to transmit signals. β-Adrenergic receptors may couple to G_s and G_i proteins, dependent on the receptor subtype

views, see Rohrer and Kobilka 1998; Hein et al. 1999b; Rohrer 2000; Kalsner 2001; Philipp et al. 2002b).

In addition to the adrenergic receptors, many of the enzymes which are involved in the synthesis and degradation of catecholamines as well as catecholamine transporters are important drug targets which have been studied in transgenic mouse models (for review see Carson and Robertson 2002).

2
α_1-Adrenergic Receptors

α_1-Adrenergic receptors mediate contraction and hypertrophic growth of smooth muscle cells. Due to discrepancies between the pharmacological subtype classification, mRNA and protein expression data, and experiments with cloned α_1-receptor subtypes, some confusion exists in the literature with respect to the nomenclature of α_1-receptor subtypes. In the present terminology, α_{1A} (cloned α_{1c}), α_{1B} (cloned α_{1b}) and α_{1D}-receptors (cloned α_{1d}) can be distinguished (Bylund et al. 1998). The α_1-receptor subtypes can all activate G_q proteins, resulting in intracellular stimulation of phospholipases C, A_2, and D, mobilization of Ca^{2+}

Table 1 Overview of transgenic models with altered α_1-adrenergic receptor (α_1-AR) expression

Protein	Gene	Genetic model	Phenotype	Reference(s)
α_{1A}-AR	Adra1a	Targeted deletion	Decreased resting blood pressure	Rokosh and Simpson 2002
α_{1B}-AR	Adra1b	Targeted deletion	Blunted blood pressure response and cardiovascular hypertrophy to norepinephrine	Cavalli et al. 1997; Spreng et al. 2001; Vecchione et al. 2002
		αMHC-promotor-α_{1B}AR	No cardiac hypertrophy at young age, dilated cardiomyopathy in older mice	Akhter et al. 1997a; Grupp et al. 1998; Lemire et al. 2001
		αMHC-promotor-CAMα_{1B}AR	Cardiac hypertrophy, heart failure after aortic constriction	Milano et al. 1994b; Wang et al. 2000
		thyroglobulin-promotor-CAMα_{1B}AR	Malignant transformation of thyroid follicular cells	Ledent, 1997
		α_{1B}-promotor-α_{1B}AR	Cardiac hypertrophy, autonomic failure, apoptotic neurodegeneration	Zuscik et al. 2000, 2001
α_{1D}-AR	Adra1d	Targeted deletion	Decreased resting blood pressure, normal cardiac function	Tanoue et al. 2002

from intracellular stores, and activation of mitogen-activated protein kinase and PI3 kinase pathways (Fig. 2). Recently, phenotypes of mice carrying deletions in all three genes encoding for α_1-receptor subtypes have been described (Cavalli et al. 1997; Rokosh and Simpson 2002; Tanoue et al. 2002; summarized in Table 1).

2.1
Blood Pressure Regulation

Based on experiments with pharmacological ligands, all three subtypes of α_1-adrenergic receptors seem to be involved in the regulation of vascular tone. Knockout of the α_{1A}- and α_{1D}-receptor subtypes caused reduced blood pressure at rest and following injection of vasoconstrictory catecholamines (Rokosh and Simpson 2002; Tanoue et al. 2002) whereas in mice lacking α_{1B}-receptors, resting blood pressure was normal but vasoconstriction to α-agonists was blunted (Cavalli et al. 1997). Interestingly, α_{1A}-receptors were not expressed in large conduit arteries (thoracic aorta and carotid arteries) but in smaller arteries of the gut, kidney, and skin, indicating that α_{1A}-receptor-selective antagonists might be useful to treat hypertension. The α_{1B}-receptor may be responsible for vasoconstriction and cardiovascular remodeling evoked by chronic adrenergic activation (Vecchione et al. 2002). These results suggest that α_1-receptor subtypes have overlapping functions in the vascular system.

2.2
Cardiac Hypertrophy Induced by α_1-Adrenergic Receptors

In addition to their role in the regulation of vascular tone, α_1-adrenergic receptors exert important trophic and contractile effects on cardiac myocytes. Several transgenic models with cardiac-specific or general overexpression of either wild-type or constitutively active α_{1B}-receptors have been generated (Table 1). Whereas some transgenic lines with overexpression of wild-type α_{1B}-receptors did not show any cardiac hypertrophy (Akhter et al. 1997a; Grupp et al. 1998; Lemire et al. 1998), others demonstrated massive dilated cardiomyopathy at older age (Lemire et al. 2001). When α_{1B}-receptors were overexpressed under control of their own promotor, transgenic mice with constitutively active α_{1B}-receptors developed greater cardiac hypertrophy than wild-type receptors (Zuscik et al. 2001). These results demonstrate that α_{1B}-receptors can induce cardiac hypertrophy and are thus potential drug targets in human post-myocardial infarction and heart failure hypertrophy and remodeling.

2.3
Neuronal Function of α_1-Adrenergic Receptors

While norepinephrine exerts a wide spectrum of effects in the central nervous system, the contribution of the α_1-receptor system to these neuronal functions is largely unknown. Mice lacking α_{1B}-receptors showed an enhanced reactivity to new situations (Drouin et al. 2002). In contrast, in the water maze, α_{1B}-receptor-deficient mice were unable to learn the task. They were perfectly able, however, to escape in a visible platform procedure. These results confirm previous findings showing that the noradrenergic pathway is important for the modulation of behaviors such as reaction to novelty and exploration, and suggest that this behavior is mediated, at least partly, through α_{1B}-adrenergic receptors (Spreng et al. 2001). Locomotor hyperactivities induced by D-amphetamine, cocaine, or morphine were dramatically decreased in mice lacking the α_{1B}-subtype when compared with wild-type littermates (Drouin et al. 2002). Moreover, behavioral sensitizations induced by D-amphetamine, cocaine, or morphine were also decreased in α_{1B}-deficient mice. These data indicate a critical role of α_{1B}-adrenergic receptors and noradrenergic transmission in the vulnerability to addiction. In contrast, transgenic overexpression of wild-type or constitutively active α_{1B}-receptors under control of their own promotor resulted in an unexpected phenotype which was characterized by severe neurological degeneration with Parkinson-like locomotor deficits and grand mal seizures (Zuscik et al. 2000).

3
α_2-Adrenergic Receptors

Similar to the other subfamilies of adrenergic receptors, three genes encoding for α_2-adrenergic receptor subtypes, α_{2A}, α_{2B} and α_{2C}, have been identified (Fig. 1). Initially, an additional α_{2D}-receptor was proposed based on affinity profiles for an array of pharmacological ligands. However, after cloning of the α_2-receptor genes from several species, the α_{2D}-receptor was shown to be a species variant of the human α_{2A}-receptor in rat, mouse, and guinea pig (Bylund et al. 1994). Part of the pharmacological difference between α_{2A}- and α_{2D}-receptors could be attributed to a Ser to Ala variation in the fifth transmembrane domain of the α_{2A}-receptor rendering this receptor less sensitive to the antagonists rauwolscine and yohimbine (Link et al. 1992). All three α_2-receptor subtypes modulate several intracellular signaling cascades including inhibition of adenylyl cyclase, stimulation of phospholipase D, stimulation of mitogen-activated protein kinases, stimulation of K^+ currents, and inhibition of Ca^{2+} currents (Fig. 2).

Several mouse lines have been generated by gene-targeting in embryonic stem cells which do not express functional α_2-adrenergic receptors (Link et al. 1995, 1996; Altman et al. 1999). All of these mice developed apparently normally, although mice lacking α_{2B}-adrenergic receptors were not born at the expected Mendelian ratios, indicating that this receptor may play a role during embryonic development (Link et al. 1996; Cussac et al. 2001; for an overview, see Table 2). Combined deletion of all three α_2-receptor subtypes in mice caused embryonic lethality due to severe defects of placental angiogenesis (Philipp et al. 2002a). During early placenta development, α_{2B}-receptors in trophoblast giant cells are required for activation of the mitogen-activated protein (MAP) kinase pathway,

Table 2 Transgenic mouse models with altered α_2-adrenergic receptor (α_2-AR) expression

Protein	Gene	Genetic model	Phenotype	Reference(s)
α_{2A}-AR	Adra2a	Targeted deletion	Tachycardia, hypertension, increased sympathetic norepinephrine release	Altman et al. 1999; Hein et al. 1999a
		Insulin promotor-α_{2A}-AR	Enhanced α_2-mediated inhibition of insulin secretion	Link et al. 1996; Devedjian et al. 2000
		Adipocyte promotor-α_{2A}-AR x β_3-KO	High-fat diet-induced obesity	Valet et al. 2000
α_{2B}-AR	Adra2b	Targeted deletion	Abolished hypertensive response to α_2-agonists	Link et al. 1996
α_{2C}-AR	Adra2c	Targeted deletion	Enhanced aggression	Link et al. 1995; Scheinin et al. 2001
		α_{2C}-promotor-α_{2C}AR	Altered behavior	Scheinin et al. 2001
α_{2ABC}-AR	Adra2a,b,c	Targeted deletion	Embryonic lethal due to defective placental angiogenesis	Philipp et al. 2002a

which is a key signaling cascade in the formation of a vascular labyrinth of fetal and maternal vessels in the placenta.

In addition, a point mutation has been introduced into the α_{2A}-receptor gene (α_{2A}-D79 N) in order to evaluate the physiological role of separate intracellular signaling pathways of this receptor in vivo (MacMillan et al. 1996). In vitro, the α_{2A}-D79 N receptor was defective in coupling to K^+ channel activation (Surprenant et al. 1992). In vivo this point mutation prevented K^+ current activation and Ca^{2+} channel inhibition by α_2-agonists (Lakhlani et al. 1997). Surprisingly, introduction of this point mutation into the mouse genome led to a reduction of α_{2A}-D79 N receptor expression by 80% in vivo (MacMillan et al. 1996). Because of the decreased receptor density, α_{2A}-D79 N mice behaved as "functional knockouts" in most experiments (MacMillan et al. 1998). However, the presynaptic α_2-receptor function was largely preserved in these mice, indicating that the remaining α_{2A}-D79 N receptors were still fully functional at this site (Altman et al. 1999).

3.1
Presynaptic Feedback Inhibition of Neurotransmitter Release

Feedback inhibition is an essential mechanism to control transmitter release from neurons. In adrenergic neurons, α_2-adrenergic receptors sense the transmitter concentration in the synaptic cleft and inhibit further secretion of norepinephrine, i.e., they function as "autoreceptors" (Starke et al. 1975). Experiments in tissues from gene-targeted mice suggest that two α_2-receptor subtypes, α_{2A} and α_{2C}, operate together as presynaptic inhibitory regulators in sympathetic nerves (Hein et al. 1999a). These two receptor subtypes inhibited neurotransmitter release in several central and peripheral nervous system locations (Trendelenburg et al. 1999; Trendelenburg et al. 2001; Bücheler et al. 2002).

Presynaptic α_2-autoreceptor subtypes can be distinguished functionally: α_{2A}-receptors inhibited transmitter release significantly faster and at higher action potential frequencies than the α_{2C}-receptors (Hein et al. 1999a; Scheibner et al. 2001b; Bücheler et al. 2002). When α_{2A}- and α_{2C}-receptors were stably expressed together with N-type Ca2+ channels or G protein-gated inwardly-rectifying potassium channel (GIRK) channels, deactivation kinetics after removal of norepinephrine was greatly different between these two subtypes (Bünemann et al. 2001). The α_{2C}-receptor was active for a significantly longer time after agonist removal than the α_{2A}-subtype. This difference in α_2-receptor deactivation kinetics could be explained by the higher affinity of norepinephrine for the α_{2C}- than for the α_{2A}-receptor subtype. This property makes the α_{2C}-receptor particularly suited to control neurotransmitter release at low action potential frequencies (Hein et al. 1999a). In contrast, the α_{2A}-receptor seems to operate primarily at high stimulation frequencies in sympathetic nerves and may thus be responsible for control of norepinephrine release during maximal sympathetic activation.

In addition to their function as autoreceptors, α_2-adrenergic receptors can also regulate the exocytosis of a number of other neurotransmitters in the central and peripheral nervous system, and thus operate as "heteroreceptors." In the brain, α_{2A}- and α_{2C}-receptors can inhibit dopamine release in basal ganglia (Bücheler et al. 2002) as well as serotonin secretion in mouse hippocampus and brain cortex (Scheibner et al. 2001a). In contrast, the inhibitory effect of α_2-agonists on gastrointestinal motility was mediated solely by the α_{2A}-subtype (Scheibner et al. 2002).

3.2
Cardiovascular Control by α_2-Adrenergic Receptors

α_2-Receptors are essential regulators of the cardiovascular system. Activation of α_2-receptors by intravenous application of α_2-agonists causes a biphasic blood pressure response: after a transient hypertensive phase arterial pressure falls below the baseline. After oral application of α_2-agonists, the hypotensive action dominates and is being used to treat elevated blood pressure in hypertensive patients. In mice, the two phases of the pressure reponse are mediated by two different α_2-receptor subtypes: α_{2B}-receptors are responsible for the initial hypertensive phase, whereas the long-lasting hypotension is mediated by α_{2A}-receptors (Link et al. 1996; MacMillan et al. 1996; Altman et al. 1999). Thus, the α_{2A}-receptor is a therapeutic target for subtype-selective antihypertensive agents.

Some evidence indicates that α_{2A}-receptors may also participate in the vasoconstriction mediated by α_2-agonists in mice (MacMillan et al. 1996). Bolus injection of norepinephrine caused transient hypertension in wild-type mice and in α_{2B}- and α_{2C}-deficient mice but not in mice lacking the α_{2A}-receptor (Duka et al. 2000).

In addition to its role as a vasoconstrictor, α_{2B}-receptors in the central nervous system are required for the development of salt-sensitive hypertension (Makaritsis et al. 1999a,b; Makaritsis et al. 2000; Gavras et al. 2001; Kintsurashvili et al. 2001). Nephrectomy followed by salt loading has been established as a model of hypertension in mice (Gavras et al. 2001). In this system, the development of hypertension depends on increased vasopressin release and sympathetic activation (Gavras and Gavras 1989). Bilateral nephrectomy and saline infusion raised blood pressure in wild-type, α_{2A}-, and α_{2C}-receptor-deficient mice. However, in α_{2B}-deficient animals a small fall in arterial pressure was observed (Makaritsis et al. 1999a).

Under certain conditions, even the α_{2C}-receptor subtype may contribute to vascular regulation: when kept below 37°C for a while, cutaneous arteries of the mouse tail showed an α_{2C}-receptor-dependent vasoconstriction which could not be observed when the vessel segments were incubated at body temperature (Chotani et al. 2000). This finding may be of great therapeutic interest for the treatment of Raynaud's disease. Patients with Raynaud's phenomenon suffer from severe vasoconstrictory periods of their fingers and toes which are usually triggered by exposure to cold. Treatment of these patients with α_2-adrenergic antagonists diminished the vasoconstriction (Freedman et al. 1995). Thus, inhibition of α_{2C}-receptors may prove an effective treatment for Raynaud's phenomenon.

3.3
Analgesia, Sedation, and Other CNS Effects

In the mouse, all three α_2-receptor subtypes are involved in the regulation of pain perception. The α_{2A}-receptor mediates the antinociception induced by systemically applied α_2-agonists, including clonidine and dexmedetomidine (Hunter et al. 1997; Stone et al. 1997; Fairbanks and Wilcox 1999). Interestingly, α_{2A}-receptor-deficient mice showed a reduced antinociceptive effect to isoflurane (Kingery et al. 2002). In contrast, the imidazoline/α_2-receptor ligand moxonidine caused spinal antinociception which was at least partially dependent on α_{2C}-receptors (Fairbanks et al. 2002).

Surprisingly, spinal α_{2B}-receptors are required for the antinociceptive effect of nitrous oxide which is used as a potent inhalative analgesic during anesthesia (Guo et al. 1999; Sawamura et al. 2000). Activation of endorphin release in the periaqueductal gray by nitrous oxide stimulates a descending noradrenergic pathway which releases norepinephrine onto α_{2B}-receptors in the dorsal horn of the spinal cord (Zhang et al. 1999). In mice lacking α_{2B}-receptors, the analgesic effect of nitrous oxide was completely abolished (Sawamura et al. 2000).

In human patients, α_2-agonists are used in the postoperative phase or in intensive care as sedative, hypnotic, and analgesic agents (Scholz and Tonner 2000; Maze et al. 2001). The sedative effects of α_2-agonists in mice are solely mediated by the α_{2A}-receptor subtype (Lakhlani et al. 1997). Mice lacking α_{2B}- or α_{2C}-receptors did not differ in their sedative response from wild-type control mice (Hunter et al. 1997; Sallinen et al. 1997). Similarly, the anesthetic-sparing effect of α_2-agonists was completely abolished in α_{2A}-D79 N mice (Lakhlani et al. 1997). The hypnotic effect of α_2-agonists is most likely mediated in the locus coeruleus. Neurons of the locus coeruleus express α_{2A}-adrenergic receptors at very high density (Wang et al. 1996). Furthermore, α_{2A}-antisense oligonucleotide injection into the locus coeruleus in rats attenuated the sedative effects of exogenous α_2-agonists (Mizobe et al. 1996).

α_2-Adrenergic receptors affect a number of behavioral functions in the central nervous system (Sallinen et al. 1998; Sallinen et al. 1999; Bjorklund et al. 2000; Schramm et al. 2001). In particular, the α_{2C}-receptor subtype has been demonstrated to inhibit the processing of sensory information in the central nervous system of the mouse (for a recent review see Scheinin et al. 2001). Activation of α_{2C}-receptors disrupts execution of spatial and non-spatial search patterns, whereas stimulation of α_{2A}- and/or α_{2B}-receptors may actually improve spatial working memory in mice (Bjorklund et al. 2001). It may be concluded that novel agonists devoid of α_{2C}-receptor affinity can modulate cognition more favorably than non-subtype selective drugs.

In contrast, drugs acting via the α_{2C}-receptor may gain therapeutic value in disorders associated with enhanced startle responses and sensorimotor gating deficits, such as schizophrenia, attention deficit disorder, post-traumatic stress disorder, and drug withdrawal (Sallinen et al. 1998). In addition to the α_{2C}-subtype, the α_{2A}-receptor has an important role in modulating behavioral functions. Experiments using gene-targeted mice indicate that the α_{2A}-receptor may play a protective role in some forms of depression and anxiety and this receptor may mediate part of the antidepressant effects of imipramine (Schramm et al. 2001). Thus, α_{2A}- and α_{2C}-receptors complement each other to integrate central nervous system function and behavior.

In addition, α_2-receptors are involved in the regulation of seizure threshold. Activation of central α_{2A}-receptors causes a powerful anti-epileptogenic effect in mice (Janumpalli et al. 1998).

4
β-Adrenergic Receptors

Activation of cardiac β-adrenergic receptors by the endogenous catecholamines epinephrine and norepinephrine represents the strongest stimulus to increase myocardial performance (Brodde 1993). The β_2-adrenergic receptor was the first G protein-coupled receptor to be cloned (Dixon et al. 1986) and served as the prototype to study the function and regulation of seven transmembrane domain-containing receptors. In the field of cardiac β-adrenergic signaling a multitude of transgenic mouse models has been generated that has contributed to our understanding of β-adrenergic signaling (Table 3).

Table 3 Overview of transgenic models with altered β-adrenergic receptor (β-AR) expression

Receptor	Gene	Genetic model	Phenotype	Reference(s)
β_1-AR	*Adrb1*	Atrial specific overexpression	Decreased heart rate variability	Bertin et al. 1993; Mansier et al. 1996
		Ventricular specific overexpression	Leftward-shift of frequency-response to isoproterenol	Zolk et al. 1998
			Progressive myocyte hypertrophy, fibrosis, heart failure	Engelhardt et al. 1999; Bisognano et al. 2000
			Early impairment of cardiomyocyte Ca^{2+} handling	Engelhardt et al. 2001a
			Enhanced beating frequency of isolated atria indicating constitutive activity of the β_1-AR	Engelhardt et al. 2001b
			Reduced hypertrophy and fibrosis after inhibition of Na^+/H^+-exchange	Engelhardt et al. 2002
		Targeted gene deletion	Cardiac response to isoproterenol abolished, alterations in dynamic heart rate control	Rohrer et al. 1996; Rohrer et al. 1998
			Biphasic response of right atrial beating frequency to isoproterenol stimulation	Devic et al. 2001
			Reduced vascular relaxation	Chruscinski et al. 2001
			Absence of isoproterenol-induced modulation of long-term potentiation	Winder et al. 1999
β_2-AR	*Adrb2*	Ventricular-specific overexpression	Very high overexpression: hypertrophy, fibrosis; moderate overexpression: enhanced contractility	Milano et al. 1994a; Liggett et al. 2000
			Enhanced beating frequency and force of isolated atria indicating constitutive activity of the β_2-AR	Bond et al. 1995
		Targeted gene deletion	Blunted hypotensive response to isoproterenol, lower body fat content	Chruscinski et al. 1999
			Impairment of chronotropic range, contractility and metabolic rate in $\beta_1\beta_2$-KO	Rohrer et al. 1999

Table 3 (continued)

Receptor	Gene	Genetic model	Phenotype	Reference(s)
β_3-AR	*Adrb3*	Targeted gene deletion	Moderate increase in body fat content	Susulic et al. 1995; Revelli et al. 1997
			Increase of β-adrenergic cardiac inotropy	Varghese et al. 2000
		Lung-specific overexpression (vascular smooth muscle cells)	Blunted response to bronchoconstrictive stimuli	McGraw et al. 1999
		Lung-specific overexpression (endothelial cells)	Enhanced bronchodilation after β-adrenergic stimulation	McGraw et al. 2000
		Lung-specific overexpression (alveolar type II cells)	Enhanced clearance of alveolar fluid	McGraw et al. 2001
		Ventricular-specific overexpression	Enhanced myocardial contractility	Kohout et al. 2001
β_{1-3}-AR	*Adrb1,2,3*	Targeted gene deletion	Impairment of diet-induced thermogenesis	Bachman et al. 2002

4.1
β-Adrenergic Receptors in the Cardiovascular System

Traditionally it has been assumed, that the β_1-subtype mediates the myocardial effects of β-adrenergic stimulation and that β_2-adrenergic receptors would exert their actions primarily in the smooth muscle cells of the lung, uterus, and blood vessels. This view has been challenged as it is clear now that cardiomyocytes co-express all three β-adrenergic receptor subtypes.

4.1.1
Transgenic Models for the β_1-Adrenergic Receptor

The β_1-adrenergic receptor (β_1AR) is the predominant subtype on cardiac myocytes. It accounts for about 60%–80% of the β-adrenergic receptor population on cardiac myocytes and also dominates functionally in the non-failing myocardium. Atrial overexpression of the β_1-AR under control of the ANF promotor led to enhancement of basal beating frequency (Bertin et al. 1993) and a decrease in heart rate variability (Mansier et al. 1996). Studies on isolated atria from these mice showed a shift of the dose–response curve for isoproterenol-induced force of contraction to the left with unchanged maximal effects, indicating that the overexpressed receptors acted mainly as functional spare receptors (Zolk et al. 1998).

Two groups have independently generated transgenic mice with cardiac-restricted overexpression of the human β_1-adrenergic receptor under control of the αMHC-promotor (Engelhardt et al. 1999; Bisognano et al. 2000). Moderate overexpression of the human β_1-adrenergic receptor (up to 46-fold compared to wild-type animals) led to a phenotype resembling human heart failure with cardiomyocyte hypertrophy and apoptosis, interstitial fibrosis, contractile dysfunction, and finally clinically overt heart failure between 10 and 12 months of age (Fig. 3a; Engelhardt et al. 1999). Very early in the course of the disease, alterations in cardiomyocyte calcium handling occurred which correlated with reduced expression of junctin, which is an important regulator of calcium transport in the sarcoplasmic reticulum (Engelhardt et al. 2001a).

β_1-AR transgenic mice showed upregulation of the cardiac Na^+/H^+-exchanger 1 (NHE1) on mRNA and protein level before fibrosis and contractile dysfunction become apparent in these mice (Engelhardt et al. 2002). Pharmacologic NHE1-inhibition by cariporide prevented the development of β_1-adrenergic receptor-induced hypertrophy, fibrosis, and heart failure. Thus, the cardiac Na^+/H^+-exchanger 1 is essential for the detrimental effects of chronic β_1-receptor stimulation in the heart and may, in addition, become an important target for the treatment of human heart failure.

Apart from defining the role of β-adrenergic receptor subtypes in myocardial hypertrophy, β_1-AR transgenic mice confirmed the occurrence of spontaneous activity of the human β_1-AR (Engelhardt et al. 2001b). This spontaneous activation in the absence of endogenous agonists could be clinically relevant, as

a

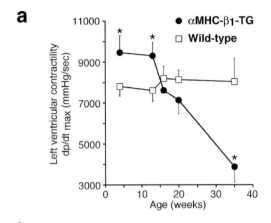

b

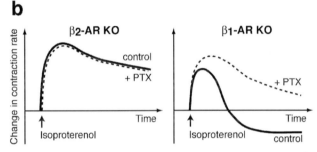

Fig. 3a, b Cardiac effects of β_1- and β_2-adrenergic receptors. **a** Left ventricular contractility is enhanced in young mice with cardiac overexpression of the human β_1-adrenergic receptor as compared with wild-type mice. Long-term enhancement of cardiac β_1-adrenergic signaling leads to progressive deterioration of cardiac function with overt heart failure at 35 weeks of age. (Data taken with permission from Engelhardt et al. 1999.) **b** Different effects of β_1- and β_2-adrenergic receptors on contraction rate of isolated cardiomyocytes from neonatal mice lacking either β_2-AR (*left*) or β_1-AR (*right*). Activation of β_1-AR by isoproterenol in β_2-AR KO myocytes led to an increase in contraction rate which was not altered after pretreatment with pertussis toxin (*PTX*). In contrast, stimulation of β_2-AR in β_1-receptor-deficient myocytes showed a transient positive chronotropic response which was followed by a longer-lasting negative chronotropic effect. The negative chronotropic effect of β_2-AR stimulation was mediated by G_i proteins, as this effect was completely abolished after PTX pretreatment. (Data adapted from Devic et al. 2001)

among the pure β-receptor blocking agents used for the treatment of heart failure those with measurable inverse agonistic activity in the β_1-AR transgenic model were associated with a significant decrease in mortality in clinical trials. On the contrary, xamoterol and bucindolol, agents which lack this property or even display partial agonistic activity (Bristow 2000; Andreka et al. 2002), did not lead to a reduction in mortality from heart failure. Thus, while the spontaneous activity of the human β_1-adrenergic receptor is comparably small compared to the β_2-subtype (Bond et al. 1995), such small differences in activation of β_1-adrenergic receptors may become important for cardiac function in the long run.

Disruption of the genes of all three β-adrenergic receptors has been described (Susulic et al. 1995; Rohrer et al. 1996; Revelli et al. 1997; Chruscinski et al. 1999). β_1-adrenergic receptor knockout mice displayed embryonic lethality which was dependent on the genetic background (Rohrer et al. 1996). In β_1-AR KO mice which survived until adulthood, the inotropic response to β-adrenergic stimulation with isoproterenol was completely lost in β_1-AR-knockout mice, indicating that the β_2-subtype may not contribute significantly to β-adrenergically mediated increases of contractility in the murine heart. While one has to keep in mind that the three β-adrenergic receptor subtypes might display compensatory expression changes when one or more of them is genetically deleted (Susulic et al. 1995; Hutchinson et al. 2001), this model led to new insights about β-adrenergic signaling in cardiac myocytes.

4.1.2
Transgenic Models for the β_2-Adrenergic Receptor

Transgenic overexpression of the human β_2-adrenergic receptor (20–30 pmol of receptor/mg membrane protein) in the ventricles of transgenic mice led to marked enhancement of basal cardiac contractility, which could not be further augmented by β-agonist treatment (Milano et al. 1994a). Given that the β_2-subtype constitutes about 25%–30% of the total β-adrenergic receptor number which is normally 50–70 fmol/mg of membrane protein, this corresponds to over 1,000-fold overexpression compared to endogenous receptor levels. In contrast to overexpression of the β_1-receptor, this dramatic level of receptor density remarkably did not result in overt cardiac pathology. Even at more than 1 year of age these animals were reported to show only minimal morphological alterations of the myocardium (Koch et al. 2000). Thus, β_2-adrenergic receptor gene therapy was proposed to enhance myocardial function of failing hearts (Lefkowitz et al. 2000). At least on a short-term basis, this concept was proven to effectively enhance myocardial contractility in a rabbit model of heart failure (Akhter et al. 1997b) and in human cardiac myocytes isolated from failing hearts.

Overexpression of the human β_2-adrenergic receptor in surgical or genetic heart failure models led to ambiguous results, however. While high-density β_2-AR overexpression worsened cardiac function after aortic banding (Du et al. 2000a), it preserved cardiac contractility after myocardial infarction without adverse consequences (Du et al. 2000b). In mice with cardiac overexpression of $G\alpha_q$ (Dorn et al. 1999) and in mice carrying a mutation in the gene for cardiac troponin T (Freeman et al. 2001), high-level overexpression of the β_2-AR led to further impairment of cardiac structure and function. However, if lower levels of β_2-AR-overexpression were used (30- to 60-fold), beneficial effects of β_2-AR overexpression could be demonstrated in the same model (Dorn et al. 1999; Liggett et al. 2000). These observations were confirmed by a study of Liggett et al. which showed that moderate (i.e., 60-fold) overexpression was well tolerated, while very high densities of transgenic β_2-AR receptors (350-fold) induced cardiac pathology (Liggett et al. 2000).

Several reports using transgenic or knockout mice indicate, that β_1- and β_2-receptors differ in their intracellular signaling pathways (Fig. 2). In addition to its activation of the G_s pathway, coupling of the β_2-AR to G_i proteins could be demonstrated in mice with cardiac overexpression of the β_2-receptor (Xiao et al. 1999, Gong et al. 2000; Heubach et al. 2003). Dual coupling of cardiac β_2-adrenergic receptors to G_s (within 10 min) and G_i proteins (from 10 min onwards) also occurred in isolated neonatal cardiomyocytes from mice lacking β_1- or β_2-receptors (Fig. 2b, Devic et al. 2001). However, contrary to what has been described initially in HEK293 cells (Daaka et al. 1997), this switch from G_s to G_i-coupling did not appear to be protein kinase A (PKA)-mediated (Devic et al. 2001). In isolated cardiomyocytes from gene-targeted mice, β_1-AR stimulation induced apoptosis but β_2-AR stimulation had a protective effect on β_1-AR induced apoptosis (Zhu et al. 2001). At present, it is unclear whether β_2-AR-mediated stimulation of p38 MAP kinase (Communal et al. 2000) or G_i-mediated activation of Akt-kinase (Chesley et al. 2000) is responsible for the anti-apoptotic effect of β_2-receptor activation.

β_2-AR knockout mice display no overt pathology (Chruscinski et al. 1999). While their heartfunction is normal both under basal and under stimulated conditions, these mice show a blunted hypotensive response to isoproterenol. A detailed analysis of the β-adrenergic subtypes responsible for the regulation of vascular tone in mice was then carried out on isolated vessels from mice with deletion of the β_1AR and the β_2AR (Chruscinski et al. 2001). In most isolated arterial and venous blood vessel segments, the β_1-receptor induced vasodilation prevailed over β_2-mediated vasorelaxation.

$\beta_1\beta_2$-double knockout animals had normal basal cardiac function and even showed preserved maximum exercise capacity (Rohrer et al. 1999). Mice lacking β_1- and β_2-receptor subtypes have also helped to clarify a longstanding question as to whether a fourth β-receptor subtype exists (Kaumann and Molenaar 1997). The putative β_4-adrenergic receptor has been postulated, based on functional assays on isolated organs and ligand binding assays, where in the presence of high concentrations of the β-receptor antagonist CGP12177 cardiostimulatory effects became apparent. In isolated atria from β_1- and β_2-knockout mice, it has been demonstrated that the pharmacology of the putative β_4-adrenergic receptor subtype is entirely dependent on the presence of the β_1-adrenergic receptor, i.e., must be an atypical state of the β_1-AR (Konkar et al. 2000; Kaumann et al. 2001).

4.1.3
Transgenic Models for the β_3-Adrenergic Receptor

Although the β_3-AR was the last of the three receptor subtypes to be cloned, the β_3-subtype was the first to be inactivated genetically in the mouse (Susulic et al. 1995). As expected from the expression pattern of the β_3-AR, the phenotypic analysis concentrated on the regulation of lipolysis in these mice (see below). More recently, the function of the β_3-AR in the myocardium has been studied by the use of β_3-AR knockout mice. In experiments on isolated organs, the β_3-adrenergic receptor has been demonstrated to couple to inhibitory G proteins in the heart (Gauthier et al. 1996) and to elicit a negative inotropic response via the release of NO (Gauthier et al. 1998). Interestingly, the negative inotropic effect of nitric oxide release after β-adrenergic stimulation was dependent on the presence of the β_3-adrenergic receptor (Varghese et al. 2000). In neonatal cardiomyocytes from β_1-AR/β_2-AR knockout animals, dual coupling of the β_3-AR to both G_s and G_i, with the G_i component dominating, was described (Fig. 3b, Devic et al. 2001). Recently, Kohout et al. have generated transgenic mice with cardiac-restricted overexpression of the human β_3-adrenergic receptor (Kohout et al. 2001). In marked contrast to the above-mentioned findings, the β_3-AR mediated positive inotropic responses in this mouse model. This effect was G_s-mediated without measurable G_i coupling being present (Kohout et al. 2001).

4.2
β-Adrenergic Receptors in the Pulmonary System

β-adrenergic receptors play an important role in regulating the function of the respiratory tract. Their activation has been shown to promote bronchodilation (reviewed by Barnes 1995) mainly through the β_2-subtype located on bronchial smooth muscle cells and airway epithelial cells. Liggett and co-workers have investigated the role of the β_2-adrenergic receptor in various cell-types of the lung by overexpression of this receptor with tissue-specific promotors. By targeted overexpression of the β_2-AR to smooth muscle cells, they identified the β_2-AR as the limiting factor in the signal transduction cascade mediating epinephrine-induced bronchial relaxation (McGraw et al. 1999). Mice with 75-fold overexpression of the receptor showed markedly enhanced relaxation to β-agonist treatment and a blunted response to bronchoconstrictor treatment (McGraw et al. 1999). Subsequently, the same group studied the role, which is much less defined, of β_2-adrenergic receptor signal transduction on alveolar epithelial cells. By the use of the Clara cell secretory cell promotor they achieved a twofold increase in β_2-adrenergic receptor density in airway epithelial cells (McGraw et al. 2000). Again, these mice were more resistant to bronchoconstrictive stimuli than their wild-type littermates. These results support a role for the epithelial cells in the regulation of airway responsiveness in vivo. Recently, McGraw et al. overexpressed the β_2-adrenergic receptor also in alveolar type II cells by the use of the rat surfactant protein C promotor (McGraw et al. 2001). In the absence of exogenous β-agonists, the authors detected a marked increased alveolar fluid clearance from the alveolar lumen.

4.3
Role of β-Adrenergic Receptors in Metabolic Pathways

All three β-adrenergic receptors have been implicated in the regulation of metabolism. The β-adrenergic receptors regulate insulin secretion (β_2-AR), glycogenolysis (β_2-AR), and lipolysis (β_1-AR and β_3-AR). Some of these aspects have been addressed with the use of transgenic animals. β_2-AR knockout mice have a lower body fat content (Chruscinski et al. 1999) and show a lower respiratory exchange ratio. The authors propose that this might be indicative of a defect in glycogen mobilization which results in a shift from glycogen to fat metaboliza-tion (Chruscinski et al. 1999). Two independent groups have generated mice with targeted deletion of the β_3-adrenergic receptor (Susulic et al. 1995; Revelli et al. 1997). Both groups detected a moderate increase in body fat content, sup-porting a role for the β_3-adrenergic receptor in lipolysis. On the contrary, β_{1-3}-subtype triple knockout mice exhibited a more pronounced phenotype with re-spect to metabolism (Bachman et al. 2002). These mice display impaired diet-induced thermogenesis in response to a high-fat diet and subsequently develop marked obesity.

4.4
Function of β-Adrenergic Receptors in the CNS

The adrenergic system plays a central role in regulating numerous functions of the central nervous system including regulation of sympathetic tone, learning and memory, mood, and food intake. A single study so far used transgenic mod-els with altered β-adrenergic receptor expression to study β-adrenergic recep-tors' role in long-term potentiation. By the use of mice with deletion of the β_1- and/or the β_2-adrenergic receptor, the β_1-subtype was found to be involved in the modulation of long-term potentiation (Winder et al. 1999).

5
Enzymes and Transporters of the Adrenergic System

The endogenous catecholamines, dopamine, norepinephrine, and epinephrine, are synthesized from the precursor amino acid tyrosine(Fig. 4). In the first bio-synthetic step, tyrosine hydroxylase (TH) generates L-dopa, which is further converted to dopamine by the aromatic L-amino acid decarboxylase (AADC). Dopamine is then transported from the cytosol into synaptic vesicles by a vesic-ular monoamine transporter (VMAT). In these vesicles, dopamine β-hydroxyl-ase (DβH) generates norepinephrine, which is further converted to epinephrine in the adrenal gland by phenylethanolamine N-methyltransferase (PNMT). A detailed review about genetic mouse models (Table 4) and human mutations in genes involved in synthesis and degradation of catecholamines has been pub-lished recently (Carson and Robertson 2002).

Catecholamines are essential for embryonic development as targeted deletion of the genes for tyrosine hydroxylase and dopamine β-hydroxylase in mice led to embryonic lethality during mid-gestation (Thomas et al. 1995; Zhou et al. 1995). TH-deficient embryos died between embryonic days 11.5 and 15.5 with bradycardia, disorganized cardiomyocytes, and blood congestion in liver and large blood vessels. In mice that survived with a targeted disruption of the DβH

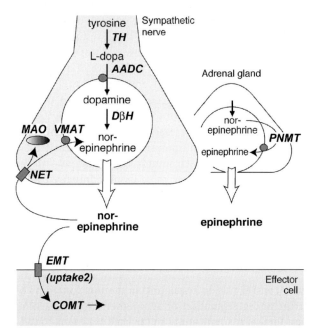

Fig. 4 Enzymes and transporters for catecholamine biosynthesis, uptake, and metabolism. As catecholamines do not cross the lipid phase of the plasma membrane, specific transporter proteins are required for concentration of catecholamines in synaptic/storage vesicles (*VMAT*) and for reuptake into presynaptic neurons (*NET*) or neighboring cells (*EMT*). Two enzymes, monoamine oxidase (*MAO*) and catechol-*O*-methyltransferase (*COMT*) are required for metabolic degradation of catecholamines

gene, maternal behavior was greatly impaired (Thomas and Palmiter 1997b). Deletion of the TH gene led to deficiency in dopamine, norepinephrine, and epinephrine. When the synthesis of norepinephrine in sympathetic neurons was selectively restored by transgenic overexpression of TH under control of the DβH promotor, the embryonic lethality of TH-knockout mice could be rescued (Kim et al. 2000). However, these mice were still lacking TH in their dopaminergic neurons and thus were "dopamine"-knockouts and were hypoactive and hypophagic and died by 3 weeks of age.

The vesicular monoamine transporter operates to accumulate cytosolic monoamines into synaptic vesicles, using the proton gradient maintained across the synaptic vesicular membrane. Until now, two separate vesicular monoamine transporters have been cloned, VMAT1 and VMAT2. The brain vesicular monoamine transporter (VMAT2) pumps monoamine neurotransmitters and Parkinsonism-inducing dopamine neurotoxins such as 1-methyl-4-phenyl-phenypyridinium (MPP$^+$) from the neuronal cytoplasm into synaptic vesicles. Mice lacking functional VMAT2 died by the second week after birth (Takahashi et al. 1997). Heterozygous VMAT2-KO mice displayed prolonged QT intervals during telemetric ECG recording and were thus more prone to die from spontaneous arrhythmia (Itokawa et al. 1999).

Table 4 Transgenic mouse models with altered expression of catecholamine synthesizing or metabolizing enzymes and transporters

Protein	Gene	Genetic model	Phenotype	References(s)
Tyrosine hydroxylase, TH	*Th*	Targeted deletion	Embryonic lethal (E11.5–15.5)	Zhou et al. 1995
Dopamine β-hydroxylase, DβH	*Dbh*	Targeted deletion	Embryonic lethal, impaired maternal behavior	Thomas et al. 1995; Thomas and Palmiter, 1997a
Vesicular monoamine transporter, MAT-2	*Slc18a2*	Targeted deletion	Perinatal lethality, increased QT interval	Takahashi et al. 1997; Itokawa et al. 1999
Norepinephrine transporter, NET	*Slc6a2*	Targeted deletion	Reduced body weight and emperature, hypersensitivity towards amphetamine	Xu et al. 2000
Extraneuronal monoamine transporter, EMT	*Orct3*	Targeted deletion	Normal development, impaired extraneuronal uptake of catecholamines	Zwart et al. 2001
Monoamine oxidase A, MAO-A	*Maoa*	Targeted deletion	Aggressive behavior	Cases et al. 1995
Monoamine oxidase B, MAO-B	*Maob*	Targeted deletion	Resistance to neurotoxic effects of MPTP	Grimsby et al. 1997
Catecholamine-O-methyltransferase, COMT	*Comt*	Targeted deletion	Increased anxiety	Gogos et al. 1998

The action of norepinephrine in the synaptic cleft is mostly terminated by re-uptake into neurons by the norepinephrine transporter (NET) or by extraneu-ronal uptake via the extraneuronal monoamine transporter (EMT, "uptake2"). NET is the target of many pharmacological drugs, including tricyclic antide-pressants (e.g., desipramine), selective norepinephrine reuptake inhibitors (e.g., reboxetine), and the psychostimulant amphetamine. NET-deficient animals be-haved like antidepressant-treated wild-type mice. Mutants were hyper-respon-sive to locomotor stimulation by cocaine or amphetamine (Xu et al. 2000).

Norepinephrine that is not recycled into its neuron via NET may be taken up by another transport mechanism into surrounding cells, the EMT, which was also termed "uptake-2" or organic cation transporter 3 (OCT-3). Homozygous mutant mice lacking EMT were viable and fertile with no obvious physiological defect and also showed no significant imbalance of norepinephrine or dopa-mine. However, EMT-deficient mice showed an impaired uptake-2 activity as measured by accumulation of intravenously administered MPP^+ (Zwart et al. 2001).

Several mouse lines lacking enzymes required for catecholamine degradation have been generated (for review see Carson and Robertson 2002). MAO-A-defi-cient mice had increased brain levels of 5-HT, norepinephrine, and dopamine and were more aggressive than control mice (Cases et al. 1995). In contrast, MAO-B deficiency did not lead to altered 5-HT, NE, or dopamine levels (Grims-by et al. 1997), but mutant mice were resistant to the neurodegenerative effects of 1-methyl-4-phenyl-1,2,3,6-tetrahydropyridine (MPTP), a toxin that induces a condition reminiscent of Parkinson's disease.

Catechol O-methyltransferase (COMT) is one of the major mammalian en-zymes involved in the metabolic degradation of catecholamines and is consid-ered a candidate for several psychiatric disorders and symptoms, including the psychopathology associated with the 22q11 microdeletion syndrome. Mutant mice lacking COMT demonstrated sexually dimorphic and region-specific changes of dopamine levels, notably in the frontal cortex. In addition, homozy-gous COMT-deficient female (but not male) mice displayed impairment in emo-tional reactivity in the dark/light exploratory model of anxiety (Gogos et al. 1998).

6
Pharmacological Relevance of Transgenic Models of the Adrenergic System

Transgenic and knockout mice with altered expression of adrenergic receptors, enzymes, and transporters are essential tools (1) to identify the specific func-tion of closely related proteins of the adrenergic system and (2) to explore novel drug targets in those mouse models which resemble human diseases. Gene tar-geting has led to the identification of specific, non-redundant functions of indi-vidual receptor subtypes for the α_2- and β-receptor subfamilies. Despite the fact that there is some functional overlap between α_2-receptor subtypes (Philipp et al. 2002b), the most important physiological roles of these receptors have been identified: whereas α_{2A}- and α_{2C}-receptors operate together to control catecholamine release from adrenergic neurons, α_{2B}-receptors are essential for angiogenesis in the developing placenta labyrinth (Hein et al. 1999; Philipp et al. 2002a). Novel drugs with subtype selectivity for individual α_2-receptor subtypes may improve drug therapy for analgesia, hypertension, Raynaud's syndrome, postoperative sedation, psychiatric disorders, as well as chronic heart failure and other diseases with enhanced sympathetic activity. Similarly, transgenic models have added significant knowledge to our understanding of the function of cardiac β-receptor subtypes. Most importantly, differences in signal transduction between cardiac β_1- and β_2-receptors may unravel novel drug targets for the treatment of human heart failure. The fact that some transgenic mouse models are also useful as disease models to test novel treatment strategies is highlighted by the observation that increased activity of the cardiac Na^+-H^+-exchanger 1 can be inhibited by cariporide to prevent hypertrophy, fibrosis and heart failure in transgenic mice with cardiac overexpression of the β_1-adrenergic receptor (Engelhardt et a. 2002). Additional mouse models are currently being generated to extend these observations to the family of three α_1-adrenergic receptors. Furthermore, genetic mouse models may, in the future, be useful to identify the relevance of genetic variants of adrenergic receptors, enzymes, and transporters for the development or susceptibility for human diseases.

Acknowledgements. The authors own work was supported by the Deutsche Forschungsgemeinschaft (SFBs 355 and 487).

References

Ahlquist RP (1948) A study of the adrenotropic receptors. Am J Physiol 153: 586–600

Akhter SA, Milano CA, Shotwell KF, Cho MC, Rockman HA, Lefkowitz RJ, Koch WJ (1997a) Transgenic mice with cardiac overexpression of α_{1B}-adrenergic receptors. In vivo α_1-adrenergic receptor-mediated regulation of β-adrenergic signaling. J Biol Chem 272: 21253–21259

Akhter SA, Skaer CA, Kypson AP, McDonald PH, Peppel KC, Glower DD, Lefkowitz RJ, Koch WJ (1997b) Restoration of β-adrenergic signaling in failing cardiac ventricular myocytes via adenoviral-mediated gene transfer. Proc Natl Acad Sci USA 94: 12100–12105

Altman JD, Trendelenburg AU, MacMillan L, Bernstein D, Limbird L, Starke K, Kobilka BK, Hein L (1999) Abnormal regulation of the sympathetic nervous system in α_{2A}-adrenergic receptor knockout mice. Mol Pharmacol 56: 154–161

Andreka P, Aiyar N, Olson LC, Wei JQ, Turner MS, Webster KA, Ohlstein EH, Bishopric NH (2002) Bucindolol displays intrinsic sympathomimetic activity in human myocardium. Circulation 105: 2429–2434

Bachman ES, Dhillon H, Zhang CY, Cinti S, Bianco AC, Kobilka BK, Lowell BB. (2002) βAR signaling required for diet-induced thermogenesis and obesity resistance. Science 297:843–845

Barnes PJ (1995)β-adrenergic receptors and their regulation. Am J Respir Crit Care Med 152: 838–860

Bertin B, Mansier P, Makeh I, Briand P, Rostene W, Swynghedauw B, Strosberg AD (1993) Specific atrial overexpression of G protein coupled human β_1 adrenoceptors in transgenic mice. Cardiovasc Res 27: 1606–1612.

Bisognano JD, *et al.* (2000) Myocardial-directed overexpression of the human β_1-adrenergic receptor in transgenic mice. J Mol Cell Cardiol 32: 817–830

Bjorklund M, Sirvio J, Riekkinen M, Sallinen J, Scheinin M, Riekkinen P, Jr. (2000) Overexpression of α_{2C}-adrenoceptors impairs water maze navigation. Neuroscience 95: 481–487

Bjorklund M, Siverina I, Heikkinen T, Tanila H, Sallinen J, Scheinin M, Riekkinen P, Jr. (2001) Spatial working memory improvement by an α_2-adrenoceptor agonist dexmedetomidine is not mediated through α_{2C}-adrenoceptor. Prog Neuropsychopharmacol Biol Psychiatry 25: 1539–1554

Bond RA, Leff P, Johnson TD, Milano CA, Rockman HA, McMinn TR, Apparsundaram S, Hyek MF, Kenakin TP, Allen LF, et al. (1995) Physiological effects of inverse agonists in transgenic mice with myocardial overexpression of the β_2-adrenoceptor. Nature. 374: 272–276.

Bristow MR (2000) What type of β-blocker should be used to treat chronic heart failure? Circulation 102: 484–486

Brodde OE (1993) β-adrenoceptors in cardiac disease. Pharmacol Ther 60: 405–430

Bücheler M, Hadamek K, Hein L (2002) Two α_2-adrenergic receptor subtypes, α_{2A} and α_{2C}, inhibit transmitter release in the brain of gene-targeted mice. Neuroscience 109: 819–826

Bünemann M, Bücheler MM, Philipp M, Lohse MJ, Hein L (2001) Activation and Deactivation kinetics of α_{2A}- and α_{2C}-adrenergic receptor-activated G protein-activated inwardly rectifying K$^+$ channel currents. J Biol Chem 276: 47512–47517

Bylund DB, Bond RA, Clarke DE, Eikenburg DC, Hieble JP, Langer SZ, Lefkowitz RJ, Minneman KP, Molinoff PB, Ruffolo RR, Strosberg AD, Trendelenburg UG (1998) Adrenoceptors, in: The IUPHAR compendium of receptor characterization and classification, IUPHAR Media: London, 58–74

Bylund DB, Eikenberg DC, Hieble JP, Langer SZ, Lefkowitz RJ, Minneman KP, Molinoff PB, Ruffolo RR, Trendelenburg U (1994) International Union of Pharmacology nomenclature of adrenoceptors. Pharmacol Rev 46: 121–136

Carson RP, Robertson D (2002) Genetic manipulation of noradrenergic neurons. J Pharmacol Exp Ther 301: 410–417

Cases O, Seif I, Grimsby J, Gaspar P, Chen K, Pournin S, Muller U, Aguet M, Babinet C, Shih JC, et al. (1995) Aggressive behavior and altered amounts of brain serotonin and norepinephrine in mice lacking MAOA. Science 268: 1763–1766

Cavalli A, Lattion AL, Hummler E, Nenniger M, Pedrazzini T, Aubert JF, Michel MC, Yang M, Lembo G, Vecchione C, Mostardini M, Schmidt A, Beermann F, Cotecchia S (1997) Decreased blood pressure response in mice deficient of the α_{1B}-adrenergic receptor. Proc Natl Acad Sci USA 94: 11589–11594

Chesley A, Lundberg MS, Asai T, Xiao RP, Ohtani S, Lakatta EG, Crow MT (2000) The β_2-adrenergic receptor delivers an antiapoptotic signal to cardiac myocytes through G(i)-dependent coupling to phosphatidylinositol 3'-kinase. Circ Res 87: 1172–1179.

Chotani MA, Flavahan S, Mitra S, Daunt D, Flavahan NA (2000) Silent α_{2C}-adrenergic receptors enable cold-induced vasoconstriction in cutaneous arteries. Am J Physiol Heart Circ Physiol 278: H1075–1083

Chruscinski A, Brede ME, Meinel L, Lohse MJ, Kobilka BK, Hein L (2001) Differential distribution of β-adrenergic receptor subtypes in blood vessels of knockout mice lacking β_1- or β_2-adrenergic receptors. Mol Pharmacol 60: 955–962

Chruscinski AJ, Rohrer DK, Schauble E, Desai KH, Bernstein D, Kobilka BK (1999) Targeted disruption of the β_2-adrenergic receptor gene. J Biol Chem 274: 16694–16700.

Communal C, Colucci WS, Singh K (2000) p38 mitogen-activated protein kinase pathway protects adult rat ventricular myocytes against β-adrenergic receptor-stimulated apoptosis. Evidence for Gi-dependent activation. J Biol Chem 275: 19395–19400.

Cussac D, Schaak S, Denis C, Flordellis C, Calise D, Paris H (2001) High level of α_2-adrenoceptor in rat foetal liver and placenta is due to α_{2B}-subtype expression in haematopoietic cells of the erythrocyte lineage. Br J Pharmacol 133: 1387–1395

Daaka Y, Luttrell LM, Lefkowitz RJ (1997) Switching of the coupling of the β_2-adrenergic receptor to different G proteins by protein kinase A. Nature 390: 88–91.

Devedjian JC, Pujol A, Cayla C, George M, Casellas A, Paris H, Bosch F (2000) Transgenic mice overexpressing α_{2A}-adrenoceptors in pancreatic β-cells show altered regulation of glucose homeostasis. Diabetologia. 43: 899–906

Devic E, Xiang Y, Gould D, Kobilka B (2001) β-adrenergic receptor subtype-specific signaling in cardiac myocytes from β_1 and β_2 adrenoceptor knockout mice. Mol Pharmacol 60: 577–583.

Dixon RA, Kobilka BK, Strader DJ, Benovic JL, Dohlman HG, Frielle T, Bolanowski MA, Bennett CD, Rands E, Diehl RE, et al. (1986) Cloning of the gene and cDNA for mammalian β-adrenergic receptor and homology with rhodopsin. Nature 321: 75–79.

Dorn GW, 2nd, Tepe NM, Lorenz JN, Koch WJ, Liggett SB (1999) Low- and high-level transgenic expression of β_2-adrenergic receptors differentially affect cardiac hypertrophy and function in Gαq- overexpressing mice. Proc Natl Acad Sci USA 96: 6400–6405.

Drouin C, Darracq L, Trovero F, Blanc G, Glowinski J, Cotecchia S, Tassin JP (2002) α_{1B}-adrenergic receptors control locomotor and rewarding effects of psychostimulants and opiates. J Neurosci 22: 2873–2884

Du XJ, Autelitano DJ, Dilley RJ, Wang B, Dart AM, Woodcock EA (2000a) β_2-adrenergic receptor overexpression exacerbates development of heart failure after aortic stenosis. Circulation 101: 71–77.

Du XJ, Gao XM, Jennings GL, Dart AM, Woodcock EA (2000b) Preserved ventricular contractility in infarcted mouse heart overexpressing β_2-adrenergic receptors. Am J Physiol Heart Circ Physiol 279: H2456–2463.

Duka I, Gavras I, Johns C, Handy DE, Gavras H (2000) Role of the postsynaptic α_2-adrenergic receptor subtypes in catecholamine-induced vasoconstriction. Gen Pharmacol 34: 101–106

Engelhardt S, Boknik P, Keller U, Neumann J, Lohse MJ, Hein L (2001a) Early impairment of calcium handling and altered expression of junction in hearts of mice overexpressing the β_1-adrenergic receptor. Faseb J 15: 2718–2720

Engelhardt S, Grimmer Y, Fan GH, Lohse MJ (2001b) Constitutive activity of the human β_1-adrenergic receptor in β_1-receptor transgenic mice. Mol Pharmacol 60: 712–717

Engelhardt S, Hein L, Keller U, Klambt K, Lohse MJ (2002) Inhibition of Na$^+$-H$^+$ exchange prevents hypertrophy, fibrosis, and heart failure in β_1-adrenergic receptor transgenic mice. Circ Res 90: 814–819.

Engelhardt S, Hein L, Wiesmann F, Lohse MJ (1999) Progressive hypertrophy and heart failure in β1-adrenergic receptor transgenic mice. Proc Natl Acad Sci USA 96: 7059–7064

Fairbanks CA, Stone LS, Kitto KF, Nguyen HO, Posthumus IJ, Wilcox GL (2002) α_{2C}-adrenergic receptors mediate spinal analgesia and adrenergic-opioid synergy. J Pharmacol Exp Ther 300: 282–290

Fairbanks CA, Wilcox GL (1999) Moxonidine, a selective α_2-adrenergic and imidazoline receptor agonist, produces spinal antinociception in mice. J Pharmacol Exp Ther 290: 403–412

Freedman RR, Baer RP, Mayes MD (1995) Blockade of vasospastic attacks by α_2-adrenergic but not α_1-adrenergic antagonists in idiopathic Raynaud's disease. Circulation 92: 1448–1451

Freeman K, Lerman I, Kranias EG, Bohlmeyer T, Bristow MR, Lefkowitz RJ, Iaccarino G, Koch WJ, Leinwand LA (2001) Alterations in cardiac adrenergic signaling and calcium cycling differentially affect the progression of cardiomyopathy. J Clin Invest 107: 967–974

Gauthier C, Leblais V, Kobzik L, Trochu JN, Khandoudi N, Bril A, Balligand JL, Le Marec H (1998) The negative inotropic effect of β_3-adrenoceptor stimulation is mediated by activation of a nitric oxide synthase pathway in human ventricle. J Clin Invest 102: 1377–1384

Gauthier C, Tavernier G, Charpentier F, Langin D, Le Marec H (1996) Functional β_3-adrenoceptor in the human heart. J Clin Invest 98: 556–562

Gavras H, Gavras I (1989) Salt-induced hypertension: the interactive role of vasopressin and of the sympathetic nervous system. J Hypertens 7: 601–606

Gavras I, Manolis AJ, Gavras H (2001) The α_2-adrenergic receptors in hypertension and heart failure: experimental and clinical studies. J Hypertension 19: 2115–2124

Gogos JA, Morgan M, Luine V, Santha M, Ogawa S, Pfaff D, Karayiorgou M (1998) Catechol-O-methyltransferase-deficient mice exhibit sexually dimorphic changes in catecholamine levels and behavior. Proc Natl Acad Sci USA 95: 9991–9996

Gong H, Adamson DL, Ranu HK, Koch WJ, Heubach JF, Ravens U, Zolk O, Harding SE (2000) The effect of Gi-protein inactivation on basal, and β_1- and β_2AR-stimulated contraction oy myocytes from transgenic mice overexpressing the β_2-adrenoceptor. Br J Pharmacol 131:594–600

Grimsby J, Toth M, Chen K, Kumazawa T, Klaidman L, Adams JD, Karoum F, Gal J, Shih JC (1997) Increased stress response and β-phenylethylamine in MAOB-deficient mice. Nat Genet 17: 206–210

Grupp IL, Lorenz JN, Walsh RA, Boivin GP, Rindt H (1998) Overexpression of α_{1B}-adrenergic receptor induces left ventricular dysfunction in the absence of hypertrophy. Am J Physiol 275: H1338–1350

Guo TZ, Davies MF, Kingery WS, Patterson AJ, Limbird LE, Maze M (1999) Nitrous oxide produces antinociceptive response via α_{2B} and/or α_{2C} adrenoceptor subtypes in mice. Anesthesiology 90: 470–476

Hein L, Altman JD, Kobilka BK (1999a) Two functionally distinct α_2-adrenergic receptors regulate sympathetic neurotransmission. Nature 402: 181–184

Hein L, Limbird LE, Eglen RM, Kobilka BK (1999b) Gene substitution/knockout to delineate the role of α_2-adrenoceptor subtypes in mediating central effects of catecholamines and imidazolines. Ann N Y Acad Sci 881: 265–271

Heubach JF, Blaschke M, Harding SE, Ravens U, Kaumann AJ (2003) Cardiostimulant and cardiodepressant effects through overexpressed human β_2-adrenoceptors in murine heart: regonal differences and functional role of β_2-adrenoceptors. Nauyn Schmiedebergs Arch Pharmacol 367:380–390

Hunter JC, Fontana DJ, Hedley LR, Jasper JR, Lewis R, Link RE, Secchi R, Sutton J, Eglen RM (1997) Assessment of the role of α_2-adrenoceptor subtypes in the antinociceptive, sedative and hypothermic action of dexmedetomidine in transgenic mice. Br J Pharmacol 122: 1339–1344

Hutchinson DS, Evans BA, Summers RJ (2001) β_1-adrenoceptors compensate for β_3-adrenoceptors in ileum from β_3-adrenoceptor knock-out mice. Br J Pharmacol 132: 433–442.

Itokawa K, Sora I, Schindler CW, Itokawa M, Takahashi N, Uhl GR (1999) Heterozygous VMAT2 knockout mice display prolonged QT intervals: possible contributions to sudden death. Brain Res Mol Brain Res 71: 354–357

Janumpalli S, Butler LS, MacMillan LB, Limbird LE, McNamara JO (1998) A point mutation (D79 N) of the α_{2A} adrenergic receptor abolishes the antiepileptogenic action of endogenous norepinephrine. J Neurosci 18: 2004–2008

Kalsner S (2001) Autoreceptors do not regulate routinely neurotransmitter release: focus on adrenergic systems. J Neurochem 78: 676–684

Kaumann AJ, Engelhardt S, Hein L, Molenaar P, Lohse M (2001) Abolition of (-)-CGP 12177-evoked cardiostimulation in double β_1/β_2-adrenoceptor knockout mice. Obligatory role of β_1-adrenoceptors for putative β_4-adrenoceptor pharmacology. Naunyn Schmiedeberg's Arch Pharmacol 363: 87–93

Kaumann AJ, Molenaar P (1997) Modulation of human cardiac function through 4 β-adrenoceptor populations. Naunyn Schmiedeberg's Arch Pharmacol 355: 667–681.

Kim DS, Szczypka MS, Palmiter RD (2000) Dopamine-deficient mice are hypersensitive to dopamine receptor agonists. J Neurosci 20: 4405–4413

Kingery WS, Agashe GS, Guo TZ, Sawamura S, Frances Davies M, David Clark J, Kobilka BK, Maze M (2002) Isoflurane and Nociception: Spinal α_{2A} adrenoceptors mediate antinociception while supraspinal α_1 adrenoceptors mediate pronociception. Anesthesiology 96: 367–374

Kintsurashvili E, Gavras I, Johns C, Gavras H (2001) Effects of antisense oligodeoxynucleotide targeting of the α_{2B}-adrenergic receptor messenger RNA in the central nervous system. Hypertension 38: 1075–1080

Koch WJ, Lefkowitz RJ, Rockman HA (2000) Functional consequences of altering myocardial adrenergic receptor signaling. Annu Rev Physiol 62: 237–260

Kohout TA, Takaoka H, McDonald PH, Perry SJ, Mao L, Lefkowitz RJ, Rockman HA (2001) Augmentation of cardiac contractility mediated by the human β_3- adrenergic receptor overexpressed in the hearts of transgenic mice. Circulation 104: 2485–2491.

Konkar AA, Zhai Y, Granneman JG (2000) β_1-adrenergic receptors mediate β_3-adrenergic-independent effects of CGP 12177 in brown adipose tissue. Mol Pharmacol 57: 252–258.

Lakhlani PP, MacMillan LB, Guo TZ, McCool BA, Lovinger DM, Maze M, Limbird LE (1997) Substitution of a mutant ?$_{2A}$-adrenergic receptor via "hit and run" gene targeting reveals the role of this subtype in sedative, analgesic, and anesthetic-sparing responses in vivo. Proc Natl Acad Sci USA 94: 9950–9955

Ledent C, Denef JF, Cotecchia S, Lefkowitz R, Dumont J, Vassart G, Parmentier M (1997) Costimulation of adenylyl cyclase and phospholipase C by a mutant α_{1B}-adrenergic receptor transgene promotes malignant transformation of thyroid follicular cells. Endocrinology 138:369–378.

Lefkowitz RJ, Rockman HA, Koch WJ (2000) Catecholamines, cardiac beta-adrenergic receptors, and heart failure. Circulation 101: 1634–1637

Lemire I, Allen BG, Rindt H, Hebert TE (1998) Cardiac-specific overexpression of α_{1B}AR regulates βAR activity via molecular crosstalk. J Mol Cell Cardiol 30: 1827–1839

Lemire I, Ducharme A, Tardif JC, Poulin F, Jones LR, Allen BG, Hebert TE, Rindt H (2001) Cardiac-directed overexpression of wild-type α_{1B}-adrenergic receptor induces dilated cardiomyopathy. Am J Physiol Heart Circ Physiol 281: H931–938

Liggett SB, Tepe NM, Lorenz JN, Canning AM, Jantz TD, Mitarai S, Yatani A, Dorn GW 2nd (2000) Early and delayed consequences of β_2-adrenergic receptor overexpression in mouse hearts: critical role for expression level. Circulation 101: 1707–1714

Link RE, Daunt D, Barsh G, Chruscinski A, Kobilka BK (1992) Cloning of two mouse genes encoding α_2-adrenergic receptor subtypes and identification of a single amino acid in the mouse α_2-C10 homolog responsible for an interspecies variation in antagonist binding. Mol Pharmacol 42: 16–27

Link RE, Desai K, Hein L, Stevens ME, Chruscinski A, Bernstein D, Barsh GS, Kobilka BK (1996) Cardiovascular regulation in mice lacking α_2-adrenergic receptor subtypes b and c. Science 273: 803–805

Link RE, Stevens MS, Kulatunga M, Scheinin M, Barsh GS, Kobilka BK (1995) Targeted inactivation of the gene encoding the mouse α_{2C}-adrenoceptor homolog. Mol Pharmacol 48: 48–55

MacMillan LB, Hein L, Smith MS, Piascik MT, Limbird LE (1996) Central hypotensive effects of the α_{2A}-adrenergic receptor subtype. Science 273: 801–803

MacMillan LB, Lakhlani PP, Hein L, Piascik M, Guo TZ, Lovinger D, Maze M, Limbird LE (1998) In vivo mutation of the α_{2A}-adrenergic receptor by homologous recombination reveals the role of this receptor subtype in multiple physiological processes. Adv Pharmacol 42: 493–496

Makaritsis KP, Handy DE, Johns C, Kobilka B, Gavras I, Gavras H (1999a) Role of the α_{2B}-adrenergic receptor in the development of salt-induced hypertension. Hypertension 33: 14–17

Makaritsis KP, Johns C, Gavras I, Altman JD, Handy DE, Bresnahan MR, Gavras H (1999b) Sympathoinhibitory function of the α_{2A}-adrenergic receptor subtype. Hypertension 34: 403–407

Makaritsis KP, Johns C, Gavras I, Gavras H (2000) Role of α_2-adrenergic receptor subtypes in the acute hypertensive response to hypertonic saline infusion in anephric mice. Hypertension 35: 609–613

Mansier P, et al. (1996) Decreased heart rate variability in transgenic mice overexpressing atrial β_1-adrenoceptors. Am J Physiol 271: H1465–1472

Maze M, Scarfini C, Cavaliere F (2001) New agents for sedation in the intensive care unit. Crit Care Clin 17: 881–897

McGraw DW, Forbes SL, Kramer LA, Witte DP, Fortner CN, Paul RJ, Liggett SB (1999) Transgenic overexpression of β_2-adrenergic receptors in airway smooth muscle alters myocyte function and ablates bronchial hyperreactivity. J Biol Chem 274: 32241–32247

McGraw DW, Forbes SL, Mak JC, Witte DP, Carrigan PE, Leikauf GD, Liggett SB (2000) Transgenic overexpression of β_2-adrenergic receptors in airway epithelial cells decreases bronchoconstriction. Am J Physiol Lung Cell Mol Physiol 279: L379–389

McGraw DW, Fukuda N, James PF, Forbes SL, Woo AL, Lingrel JB, Witte DP, Matthay MA, Liggett SB (2001) Targeted transgenic expression of β_2-adrenergic receptors to type II cells increases alveolar fluid clearance. Am J Physiol Lung Cell Mol Physiol 281: L895–903

Milano CA, Allen LF, Rockman HA, Dolber PC, McMinn TR, Chien KR, Johnson TD, Bond RA, Lefkowitz RJ (1994a) Enhanced myocardial function in transgenic mice overexpressing the β_2-adrenergic receptor. Science. 264: 582–586

Milano CA, Dolber PC, Rockman HA, Bond RA, Venable ME, Allen LF, Lefkowitz RJ (1994b) Myocardial expression of a constitutively active α_{1B}-adrenergic receptor in transgenic mice induces cardiac hypertrophy. Proc Natl Acad Sci USA 91: 10109–10113

Mizobe T, Maghsoudi K, Sitwala K, Tianzhi G, Ou J, Maze M (1996) Antisense technology reveals the α_{2A} adrenoceptor subtype to be the subtype mediating the hypnotic response to the highly selective agonist, dexmedetomidine, in the locus coeruleus of the rat. J Clin Invest 98: 1076–1080

Philipp M, Brede M, Hadamek K, Gessler M, Lohse MJ, Hein L (2002a) Placental α_2-adrenoceptors control vascular development at the interface between mother and embryo. Nat Genet 31:311–315

Philipp M, Brede M, Hein L (2002b) Physiological significance of α_2-adrenergic receptor subtype diversity: one receptor is not enough. Am J Physiol 283:R287–R295

Revelli JP, Preitner F, Samec S, Muniesa P, Kuehne F, Boss O, Vassalli JD, Dulloo A, Seydoux J, Giacobino JP, Huarte J, Ody C (1997) Targeted gene disruption reveals a leptin-independent role for the mouse β_3-adrenoceptor in the regulation of body composition. J Clin Invest 100: 1098–1106

Rohrer DK (2000) Targeted disruption of adrenergic receptor genes. Methods Mol Biol 126: 259–277

Rohrer DK, Chruscinski A, Schauble EH, Bernstein D, Kobilka BK (1999) Cardiovascular and metabolic alterations in mice lacking both β_1- and β_2-adrenergic receptors. J Biol Chem 274: 16701–16708

Rohrer DK, Desai KH, Jasper JR, Stevens ME, Regula DP, Jr., Barsh GS, Bernstein D, Kobilka BK (1996) Targeted disruption of the mouse β_1-adrenergic receptor gene: developmental and cardiovascular effects. Proc Natl Acad Sci USA 93: 7375–7380

Rohrer DK, Kobilka BK (1998) Insights from in vivo modification of adrenergic receptor gene expression. Annu Rev Pharmacol Toxicol 38: 351–373

Rohrer DK, Schauble EH, Desai KH, Kobilka BK, Bernstein D (1998) Alterations in dynamic heart rate control in the β_1-adrenergic receptor knockout mouse. Am J Physiol 274: H1184–1193

Rokosh DG, Simpson PC (2002) Knockout of the $\alpha_{1A/C}$-adrenergic receptor subtype: The $\alpha_{1A/C}$ is expressed in resistance arteries and is required to maintain arterial blood pressure. Proc Natl Acad Sci USA 99:9474–9479

Sallinen J, Haapalinna A, MacDonald E, Viitamaa T, Lahdesmaki J, Rybnikova E, Pelto-Huikko M, Kobilka BK, Scheinin M (1999) Genetic alteration of the α_2-adrenoceptor subtype c in mice affects the development of behavioral despair and stress-induced increases in plasma corticosterone levels. Mol Psychiatry 4: 443–452

Sallinen J, Haapalinna A, Viitamaa T, Kobilka BK, Scheinin M (1998) Adrenergic α_{2C}-receptors modulate the acoustic startle reflex, prepulse inhibition, and aggression in mice. J Neurosci 18: 3035–3042

Sallinen J, Link RE, Haapalinna A, Viitamaa T, Kulatunga M, Sjoholm B, Macdonald E, Pelto-Huikko M, Leino T, Barsh GS, Kobilka BK, Scheinin M (1997) Genetic alteration of α_{2C}-adrenoceptor expression in mice: influence on locomotor, hypothermic, and neurochemical effects of dexmedetomidine, a subtype-nonselective α_2-adrenoceptor agonist. Mol Pharmacol 51: 36–46

Sawamura S, Kingery WS, Davies MF, Agashe GS, Clark JD, Kobilka BK, Hashimoto T, Maze M (2000) Antinociceptive action of nitrous oxide is mediated by stimulation of noradrenergic neurons in the brainstem and activation of α_{2B} adrenoceptors. J Neurosci 20: 9242–9251

Scheibner J, Trendelenburg AU, Hein L, Starke K (2001a) α_2-adrenoceptors modulating neuronal serotonin release: a study in α_2-adrenoceptor subtype-deficient mice. Br J Pharmacol 132: 925–933

Scheibner J, Trendelenburg AU, Hein L, Starke K (2001b) Stimulation frequency-noradrenaline release relationships examined in α_{2A}-, α_{2B}- and α_{2C}-adrenoceptor-deficient mice. Naunyn Schmiedeberg's Arch Pharmacol 364: 321–328

Scheibner J, Trendelenburg AU, Hein L, Starke K, Blandizzi C (2002) α_2-adrenoceptors in the enteric nervous system: a study in α_{2A}-adrenoceptor-deficient mice. Br J Pharmacol 135: 697–704

Scheinin M, Sallinen J, Haapalinna A (2001) Evaluation of the α_{2C}-adrenoceptor as a neuropsychiatric drug target studies in transgenic mouse models. Life Sci 68: 2277–2285

Scholz J, Tonner PH (2000) α_2-Adrenoceptor agonists in anaesthesia: a new paradigm. Curr Op Anesthesiol 13: 437–442

Schramm NL, McDonald MP, Limbird LE (2001) The α_{2A}-adrenergic receptor plays a protective role in mouse behavioral models of depression and anxiety. J Neurosci 21: 4875–4882

Spreng M, Cotecchia S, Schenk F (2001) A behavioral study of α_{1B} adrenergic receptor knockout mice: increased reaction to novelty and selectively reduced learning capacities. Neurobiol Learn Mem 75: 214–229

Starke K, Endo T, Taube HD (1975) Pre- and postsynaptic components in effect of drugs with alpha adrenoceptor affinity. Nature 254: 440–441

Stone LS, MacMillan LB, Kitto KF, Limbird LE, Wilcox GL (1997) The α_{2A} adrenergic receptor subtype mediates spinal analgesia evoked by α_2 agonists and is necessary for spinal adrenergic-opioid synergy. J Neurosci 17: 7157–7165

Surprenant A, Horstman DA, Akbarali H, Limbird LE (1992) A point mutation of the α_2-adrenoceptor that blocks coupling to potassium but not to calcium currents. Science. 257: 977–980

Susulic VS, Frederich RC, Lawitts J, Tozzo E, Kahn BB, Harper ME, Himms-Hagen J, Flier JS, Lowell BB (1995) Targeted disruption of the β_3-adrenergic receptor gene. J Biol Chem 270: 29483–29492

Takahashi N, Miner LL, Sora I, Ujike H, Revay RS, Kostic V, Jackson-Lewis V, Przedborski S, Uhl GR (1997) VMAT2 knockout mice: heterozygotes display reduced amphetamine-conditioned reward, enhanced amphetamine locomotion, and enhanced MPTP toxicity. Proc Natl Acad Sci USA 94: 9938–9943

Tanoue A, Nasa Y, Koshimizu T, Shinoura H, Oshikawa S, Kawai T, Sunada S, Takeo S, Tsujimoto G (2002) The α_{1D}-adrenergic receptor directly regulates arterial blood pressure via vasoconstriction. J Clin Invest 109:765–775

Thomas SA, Matsumoto AM, Palmiter RD (1995) Noradrenaline is essential for mouse fetal development. Nature 374: 643–646

Thomas SA, Palmiter RD (1997a) Disruption of the dopamine β-hydroxylase gene in mice suggests roles for norepinephrine in motor function, learning, and memory. Behav Neurosci 111: 579–589

Thomas SA, Palmiter RD (1997b) Impaired maternal behavior in mice lacking norepinephrine and epinephrine. Cell 91: 583–592

Trendelenburg AU, Hein L, Gaiser EG, Starke K (1999) Occurrence, pharmacology and function of presynaptic α_2- autoreceptors in $\alpha_{2A/D}$-adrenoceptor-deficient mice. Naunyn Schmiedeberg's Arch Pharmacol 360: 540–551

Trendelenburg AU, Klebroff W, Hein L, Starke K (2001) A study of presynaptic α_2-autoreceptors in $\alpha_{2A/D}$-, α_{2B}- and α_{2C}-adrenoceptor-deficient mice. Naunyn Schmiedeberg's Arch Pharmacol 364: 117–130

Valet P, Grujic D, Wade J, Ito M, Zingaretti MC, Soloveva V, Ross SR, Graves RA, Cinti S, Lafontan M, Lowell BB (2000) Expression of human α_2-adrenergic receptors in adipose tissue of β_3-adrenergic receptor-deficient mice promotes diet-induced obesity. J Biol Chem 275: 34797–34802

Varghese P, Harrison RW, Lofthouse RA, Georgakopoulos D, Berkowitz DE, Hare JM (2000) β_3-adrenoceptor deficiency blocks nitric oxide-dependent inhibition of myocardial contractility. J Clin Invest 106: 697–703.

Vecchione C, Fratta L, Rizzoni D, Notte A, Poulet R, Porteri E, Frati G, Guelfi D, Trimarco V, Mulvany MJ, Agabiti-Rosei E, Trimarco B, Cotecchia S, Lembo G (2002) Cardiovascular influences of α_{1B}-adrenergic receptor defect in mice. Circulation 105: 1700–1707

Wang BH, Du XJ, Autelitano DJ, Milano CA, Woodcock EA (2000) Adverse effects of constitutively active α_{1B}-adrenergic receptors after pressure overload in mouse hearts. Am J Physiol Heart Circ Physiol 279: H1079–1086

Wang R, Macmillan LB, Fremeau RT, Jr., Magnuson MA, Lindner J, Limbird LE (1996) Expression of α_2-adrenergic receptor subtypes in the mouse brain: evaluation of spatial and temporal information imparted by 3 kb of 5' regulatory sequence for the α_{2A} AR-receptor gene in transgenic animals. Neuroscience 74: 199–218

Winder DG, Martin KC, Muzzio IA, Rohrer D, Chruscinski A, Kobilka B, Kandel ER (1999) ERK plays a regulatory role in induction of LTP by theta frequency stimulation and its modulation by β-adrenergic receptors. Neuron. 24: 715–726

Xiao RP, Avdonin P, Zhou YY, Cheng H, Akhter SA, Eschenhagen T, Lefkowitz RJ, Koch WJ, Lakatta EG (1999) Coupling of β_2-adrenoceptor to Gi proteins and its physiological relevance in murine cardiac myocytes. Circ Res 84: 43–52

Xu F, Gainetdinov RR, Wetsel WC, Jones SR, Bohn LM, Miller GW, Wang YM, Caron MG (2000) Mice lacking the norepinephrine transporter are supersensitive to psychostimulants. Nat Neurosci 3: 465–471

Zhang C, Davies MF, Guo TZ, Maze M (1999) The analgesic action of nitrous oxide is dependent on the release of norepinephrine in the dorsal horn of the spinal cord. Anesthesiology 91: 1401–1407

Zhou QY, Quaife CJ, Palmiter RD (1995) Targeted disruption of the tyrosine hydroxylase gene reveals that catecholamines are required for mouse fetal development. Nature 374: 640–643

Zhu WZ, Zheng M, Koch WJ, Lefkowitz RJ, Kobilka BK, Xiao RP (2001) Dual modulation of cell survival and cell death by β_2-adrenergic signaling in adult mouse cardiac myocytes. Proc Natl Acad Sci USA 98: 1607–1612

Zolk O, Kilter H, Flesch M, Mansier P, Swynghedauw B, Schnabel P, Böhm M (1998) Functional coupling of overexpressed β_1-adrenoceptors in the myocardium of transgenic mice. Biochem Biophys Res Commun 248: 801–805

Zuscik MJ, et al. (2001) Hypotension, autonomic failure, and cardiac hypertrophy in transgenic mice overexpressing the α_{1B}-adrenergic receptor. J Biol Chem 276: 13738–13743

Zuscik MJ, Sands S, Ross SA, Waugh DJ, Gaivin RJ, Morilak D, Perez DM (2000) Overexpression of the α_{1B}-adrenergic receptor causes apoptotic neurodegeneration: multiple system atrophy. Nat Med 6: 1388–1394

Zwart R, Verhaagh S, Buitelaar M, Popp-Snijders C, Barlow DP (2001) Impaired activity of the extraneuronal monoamine transporter system known as uptake-2 in Orct3/Slc22a3-deficient mice. Mol Cell Biol 21: 4188–4196

Muscarinic Acetylcholine Receptor Knockout Mice

J. Wess[1] · W. Zhang[2] · A. Duttaroy[2] · T. Miyakawa[3] · J. Gomeza[2] · Y. Cui[2] · A. S. Basile[2]
F. P. Bymaster[4] · D. L. McKinzie[4] · C. C. Felder[4] · C. Deng[5] · M. Yamada[2]

[1] Molecular Signaling Section, Laboratory of Bioorganic Chemistry,
National Institute of Diabetes and Digestive and Kidney Diseases, Bldg. 8A,
Room B1A-05, 8 Center Drive, Bethesda, MD 20892, USA,
e-mail: jwess@helix.nih.gov
[2] Laboratory of Bioorganic Chemistry, National Institute of Diabetes and Digestive
and Kidney Diseases, Bethesda, MD 20892, USA
[3] Center for Learning and Memory, MIT, Cambridge, MA 02139–4307, USA
[4] Lilly Research Laboratories, Eli Lilly and Company, Indianapolis, IN 46285, USA
[5] Laboratory of Biochemistry and Metabolism, National Institute of Diabetes and Digestive
and Kidney Diseases, Bethesda, MD 20892, USA

Abstract Muscarinic acetylcholine receptors (mAChRs) play critical roles in regulating the activity of many important functions of the central and peripheral nervous system. However, identification of the physiological and pathophysiological roles of the individual mAChR subtypes (M$_1$–M$_5$) has proven a difficult task, primarily due to the lack of ligands endowed with a high degree of receptor subtype selectivity and the fact that most tissues and organs express multiple mAChRs. To circumvent these difficulties, we and others have used gene targeting strategies to generate mutant mouse lines containing inactivating mutations of the M$_1$–M$_5$ mAChR genes. The different mAChR mutant mice and the corresponding wild-type control animals were subjected to a battery of physiological, pharmacological, behavioral, biochemical, and neurochemical tests. The M$_1$–M$_5$ mAChR mutant mice (MXR$^{-/-}$ mice) were all viable and reproduced normally. However, each mutant mouse line displayed distinct phenotypical changes. For example, M1R$^{-/-}$ mice showed a pronounced increase in locomotor activity, probably due to the increase in dopamine release in the striatum. In addition, pilocarpine-induced epileptic seizures were absent in M1R$^{-/-}$ mice. Pharmacological analysis of M2R$^{-/-}$ mice indicated that the M$_2$ subtype plays a key role in mediating three of the most striking central muscarinic effects: tremor, hypothermia, and analgesia. As expected, muscarinic agonist-mediated bradycardia was abolished in M2R$^{-/-}$ mice. M3R$^{-/-}$ mice displayed a significant decrease in food intake, reduced body weight and peripheral fat deposits, and very low serum leptin and insulin levels. Additional studies showed that the M$_3$ receptor subtype also plays a key role in mediating smooth muscle contraction and glandular secretion. Behavioral analysis of M4R$^{-/-}$ mice suggested that M$_4$ receptors mediate inhibition of D$_1$ dopamine receptor-mediated locomotor stimulation, probably at the level of striatal projection neurons. Studies with M5R$^{-/-}$ mice indicated that vascular M$_5$ receptors mediate cholinergic relaxation of cerebral arteries and arterioles. Behavioral and neurochemical studies showed that M$_5$ receptor activity modulates both morphine reward and withdrawal processes, probably through activation of M$_5$ receptors located on midbrain dopaminergic neurons. These results offer promising new perspectives for the rational development of novel muscarinic drugs.

Keywords Acetylcholine · Analgesia · Gene targeting · Knockout mice · Morphine · Muscarinic agonists · Muscarinic receptors · Oxotremorine · Parasympathetic nervous system · Pilocarpine

Abbreviations

ACh	Acetylcholine
AGRP	Agouti-related peptide
CNS	Central nervous system
i.c.v.	Intracerebroventricular
i.t.	Intrathecal
LDT	Laterodorsal tegmental nucleus
M1R$^{-/-}$ (M2R$^{-/-}$, etc.)	M$_{1(2, etc.)}$ muscarinic receptor-deficient (mice)
mAChR	Muscarinic acetylcholine receptor
MCH	Melanin-concentrating hormone
POMC	Proopiomelanocortin
s.c.	Subcutaneous
VTA	Ventral tegmental area
WT	Wild-type

1
Introduction

Acetylcholine (ACh) is a major neurotransmitter both in the central and in the peripheral nervous system (Wess et al. 1990). ACh exerts its diverse physiological functions through activation of two distinct classes of plasma membrane receptors, the nicotinic and muscarinic ACh receptors. Whereas the nicotinic ACh receptors function as ligand-gated ion channels, the muscarinic ACh receptors (mAChRs) are prototypical members of the superfamily of G protein-coupled receptors (Wess 1996). Molecular cloning studies have revealed the existence of five molecularly distinct mAChR subtypes (M$_1$–M$_5$) (Caulfield 1993; Wess 1996; Caulfield and Birdsall 1998). Based on their differential G protein coupling properties, the five receptors can be subdivided into two major functional classes. Whereas the M$_2$ and M$_4$ receptors are preferentially coupled to G proteins of the G$_i$ family, the M$_1$, M$_3$, and M$_5$ receptors are selectively linked to G$_{q/11}$ proteins (Caulfield 1993; Wess 1996; Caulfield and Birdsall 1998).

Receptor localization studies have shown that mAChRs are present in virtually all organs, tissues, or cell types (Caulfield 1993; Levey 1993; Vilaro et al. 1993; Wolfe and Yasuda 1995). It is well known that peripheral mAChRs mediate the actions of ACh at parasympathetically innervated effector tissues (organs), including reduction in heart rate and stimulation of glandular secretion and smooth muscle contraction (Wess et al. 1990; Caulfield 1993). Central mAChRs are involved in a very large number of vegetative, sensory, cognitive, behavioral, and motor functions (Wess et al. 1990; Levine et al. 1999, 2001). Moreover, a considerable body of evidence indicates that disturbances in the central mAChR system may play a role in a number of pathophysiological conditions including Alzheimer's and Parkinson's disease, depression, schizophrenia, and epilepsy (Coyle et al. 1983; Wess et al. 1990; Janowsky et al. 1994; Bymaster et al. 1999; Eglen et al. 1999; Levine et al. 1999, 2001; Felder et al. 2000).

A key question is which specific mAChR subtypes (M_1–M_5) are involved in mediating the diverse physiological actions of ACh. Such information is not only of theoretical interest but also of considerable therapeutic relevance for the development of novel muscarinic drugs. In the past, identification of the physiological roles of the individual mAChR subtypes has been a difficult task, primarily due to the lack of ligands that can activate or inhibit individual receptor subtypes with a high degree of selectivity (Wess 1996; Caulfield and Birdsall 1998; Felder et al. 2000). This task is further complicated by the fact that most organs, tissues, or cell types express multiple mAChRs (Caulfield 1993; Levey 1993; Vilaro et al. 1993; Wolfe and Yasuda 1995). To overcome these obstacles, we recently used gene-targeting techniques to generate mouse lines deficient in each of the five mAChR genes (Gomeza et al. 1999a,b; Yamada et al. 2001a,b; Miyakawa et al. 2001; Fisahn et al. 2002). M_1 (Hamilton et al. 1997; Gerber et al. 2001), M_3 (Matsui et al. 2000), and M_5 (Takeuchi et al. 2002) receptor mutant mice have also been generated by other laboratories.

In this chapter, we will summarize the results of recent studies carried out with M_1–M_5 mAChR-mutant mice. While we will focus in some more detail on our own work in this area, all other relevant studies will also be outlined (see Table 1 for a summary of major phenotypes). The clinical implications of the newly generated data will be discussed throughout the text.

2
General Strategy Used to Generate mAChR-Mutant Mice

During the past few years, we used gene ablation techniques to generate mutant mouse strains lacking M_1 (Miyakawa et al. 2001; Fisahn et al. 2002), M_2 (Gomeza et al. 1999a), M_3 (Yamada et al. 2001a), M_4 (Gomeza et al. 1999b), or M_5 mAChRs (Yamada et al. 2001b). All mutant mouse strains were obtained by using a similar strategy which is summarized briefly below.

To generate M_1–M_5 receptor mutant mice, we initially cloned the murine M_1–M_5 mAChR genes from a 129SvJ mouse genomic library (Genome Systems). Subsequently, we constructed targeting vectors containing two copies of the herpes simplex virus thymidine kinase gene and a phosphoglycerate kinase (PGK)-neomycin resistance cassette which replaced functionally essential segments of the receptor coding sequences. The targeting vectors were linearized and introduced into embryonic stem cells by electroporation. The M_1, M_3, M_4, and M_5 receptor constructs were electroporated into TC1 (129SvEv) cells (Deng et al. 1996), and the M_2 receptor construct was introduced into 129'J1' cells (Gomeza et al. 1999a). Clones resistant to G418 and ganciclovir were tested for the occurrence of homologous recombination via Southern hybridization. Properly targeted embryonic stem cell clones were microinjected into C57BL/6 J blastocysts to generate male chimeric offspring, which in turn were mated with female CF-1 (Charles River Laboratories), C57BL/6 J (The Jackson Laboratories), or 129SvEv mice (Taconic Farms) to generate F1 offspring. F1 animals heterozygous for the desired mAChR mutation were then intermated to produce homozygous

Table 1 Major phenotypes displayed by M_1–M_5 mAChR-mutant mice

Inactivated mAChR gene	Major phenotypes	Reference(s)
M_1	Absence of pilocarpine-induced seizures; loss of muscarinic agonist-mediated M current (I_m) inhibition in sympathetic ganglion neurons	Hamilton et al. 1997
	Lack of slow, voltage-independent muscarinic inhibition of N- and P/Q-type Ca^{2+} channels in sympathetic ganglion neurons	Shapiro et al. 1999
	Increased locomotor activity	Miyakawa et al. 2001
	Loss of muscarinic agonist-induced MAPK activation and drastic reduction of muscarinic agonist-mediated PI ydrolysis in primary cortical cultures	Hamilton and Nathanson 2001
	Lack of carbachol-mediated MAPK activation in CA1 hippocampal pyramidal neurons	Berkeley et al. 2001
	Increased locomotor activity and increased extracellular dopamine levels in the striatum	Gerber et al. 2001
	Lack of muscarine-mediated γ oscillations in area CA3 of the hippocampus	Fisahn et al. 2002
	Absence of muscarinic agonist-induced $GTP\gamma S$ binding to G proteins of the G_q family in hippocampus and cerebral cortex	Porter et al. 2002
	Lack of cardiovascular stimulation following systemic administration of McN-A-343	Hardouin et al. 2002
	Lack of pilocarpine-stimulated in vivo PI hydrolysis in hippocampus and cerebral cortex	F.P. Bymaster et al., unpublished results
M_2	Absence of oxotremorine-mediated tremor responses; reduced oxotremorine-mediated hypothermic and analgesic responses	Gomeza et al. 1999a
	Loss of fast, voltage-dependent muscarinic inhibition of N- and P/Q-type Ca^{2+} channels in sympathetic ganglion neurons	Shapiro et al. 1999
	Lack of carbachol-mediated bradycardic effects in isolated spontaneously beating atria; slight impairment of carbachol-mediated contractions of ileal, bladder, and tracheal smooth preparations (in vitro)	Stengel et al. 2000
	Absence of oxotremorine-mediated inhibition of $[^3H]ACh$ release from K^+-depolarized hippocampal and cortical slices	Zhang et al. 2002a
	Failure of the partial muscarinic agonist, BuTAC, to trigger increased serum corticosterone levels	Hemrick-Luecke et al. 2002
	Loss of muscarine-mediated desensitization of peripheral nociceptors	Bernardini et al. 2002
	Reduced carbachol-mediated inhibition of electrically stimulated $[^3H]$norepinephrine release from heart atria, urinary bladder, and vas deferens	Trendelenburg et al. 2002

Table 1 (continued)

Inactivated mAChR gene	Major phenotypes	Reference(s)
M_3	Increase in pupil size, bladder distension, and greatly impaired carbachol-mediated contractions of ileal and bladder smooth muscle preparations (in vitro); lack of salivation following administration of a low dose of pilocarpine (1 mg/kg, s.c.)	Matsui et al. 2000
	Reduced body weight and mass of peripheral fat pads, associated with low serum insulin and leptin levels and reduced food intake; reduced salivation following administration of an intermediate dose of pilocarpine (5 mg/kg, s.c.)	Yamada et al. 2001a
	carbachol-induced contractions in various smooth preparations (in vitro)	Stengel et al. 2002; Stengel and Cohen 2002
M_4	Increased oxotremorine-stimulated [^{3}H]dopamine outflow from K$^+$-depolarized striatal slices	Zhang et al. 2002b
	Increased locomotor activity under basal conditions and after administration of a D_1 dopamine receptor agonist	Gomeza et al. 1999b
	Absence of oxotremorine-mediated inhibition of [^{3}H]ACh release from K$^+$-depolarized striatal slices	Zhang et al. 2002b
	Loss of oxotremorine-stimulated [^{3}H]dopamine outflow from K$^+$-depolarized striatal slices	Zhang et al. 2002b
	Reduced autoinhibition of ACh release in heart atria and urinary bladder	Zhou et al. 2002
	Lack of muscarinic agonist-mediated analgesic responses in the simultaneous absence of M_2 receptors	Duttaroy et al. 2002
M_5	Lack of ACh-mediated dilation of cerebral arteries and arterioles; reduced efficiency of oxotremorine-stimulated [^{3}H]dopamine outflow from K$^+$-depolarized striatal slices	Yamada et al. 2001b
	Lack of sustained increase in dopamine levels in the nucleus accumbens normally observed after electrical stimulation of the laterodorsal tegmental nucleus	Forster et al. 2002
	Decreased sensitivity to the rewarding effects of morphine and reduced severity of naloxone-precipitated morphine withdrawal symptoms	Basile et al. 2002
	Slightly impaired pilocarpine-induced salivation response; increased water intake following an extended period of food and water deprivation	Takeuchi et al. 2002

mAChR mutant mice (F2). Most studies reviewed in the following were carried out with littermates of the F2 or F3 generation.

To examine whether disruption of a specific mAChR gene led to secondary changes in the expression levels of the remaining four mAChRs, we (Gomeza et al. 1999a,b; Miyakawa et al. 2001; Yamada et al. 2001a; Fisahn et al. 2002) and Hamilton et al. (1997) carried out a series of immunoprecipitation studies. For these studies, mAChR-containing membrane preparations were labeled with the non-subtype-selective muscarinic antagonist, [^{3}H]quinuclidinyl benzilate, followed by receptor solubilization and immunoprecipitation by subtype-selective antisera. These studies showed that the inactivation of a specific mAChR gene did not lead to significant changes in the expression levels of the remaining four mAChR subtypes (Hamilton et al. 1997; Gomeza et al. 1999a,b; Miyakawa et al. 2001; Yamada et al. 2001a; Fisahn et al. 2002).

Mutant mice lacking M_1, M_2, M_3, M_4, or M_5 mAChRs were viable and were obtained at the expected Mendelian frequency. None of the mutant mouse strains displayed any gross behavioral or morphological abnormalities. Moreover, the different mAChR mutant mouse strains did not differ from their wild-type (WT) littermates in fertility and longevity.

3
M1R$^{-/-}$ Mice

3.1
M1R$^{-/-}$ Mice Are Hyperactive

In the central nervous system (CNS), M_1 mAChRs are abundantly expressed in all major forebrain areas including cerebral cortex, hippocampus, and striatum (Levey et al. 1991; Levey 1993; Vilaro et al. 1993; Wolfe and Yasuda 1995). An initial behavioral analysis of M_1 muscarinic receptor-deficient (M1R$^{-/-}$) mice showed that the lack of M_1 receptors did not lead to any significant deficits in sensory-motor gating, nociception, motor coordination, and anxiety-related behavior (Miyakawa et al. 2001). However, M1R$^{-/-}$ mice displayed a pronounced increase in locomotor activity that was consistently observed in all tests that included locomotor activity measurements (Miyakawa et al. 2001). M_1 receptors are abundantly expressed in the striatum (Weiner et al. 1990; Levey et al. 1991; Bernard et al. 1992; Hersch et al. 1994), a region known to play a key role in the regulation of locomotor activity (Di Chiara et al. 1994). We therefore speculated that the lack of striatal M_1 receptors might be responsible for the hyperactivity phenotype displayed by the M1R$^{-/-}$ mice. M_1 receptors represent the predominant mAChR subtype expressed by striatal projection neurons giving rise to the so-called striatopallidal pathway (Weiner et al. 1990; Bernard et al. 1992; Hersch et al. 1994), activation of which is thought to reduce locomotor activity (Di Chiara et al. 1994). It is therefore possible that this inhibitory striatal outflow is reduced in M1R$^{-/-}$ mice, resulting in the observed hyperactivity phenotype.

Interestingly, Gerber et al. (2001) recently reported that the hyperactivity phenotype of M1R$^{-/-}$ mice is associated with a significant increase (~2-fold) in extracellular striatal dopamine concentrations, most probably due to an increase in dopamine release. These authors proposed that the lack of stimulatory M_1 receptors present on a subset of inhibitory striatal (striosomal) neurons projecting to the dopamine-containing neurons of the substantia nigra pars compacta may be responsible for the observed increase in striatal dopamine levels displayed by the M1R$^{-/-}$ mice.

Independent of the precise molecular mechanisms by which the lack of M_1 receptors leads to an increase in locomotor activity, these recent findings suggest that blockade of striatal M_1 mAChRs may represent a useful strategy to improve locomotor activity in patients suffering from Parkinson's disease, a disease characterized by drastically reduced striatal dopamine levels. Since at least some forms of schizophrenia are associated with increased dopaminergic transmission in various areas of the brain, Gerber et al. (2001) also proposed that M_1 receptor dysfunction might be involved in the pathophysiology of certain forms of schizophrenia.

3.2
M1R$^{-/-}$ Mice Perform Well in Learning and Memory Tasks

A considerable body of behavioral and pharmacological data suggests that M_1 mAChRs play an important role in learning and memory processes (Hagan et al. 1987; Quirion et al. 1989; Fisher et al. 1996; Iversen 1997). To further test this concept, we subjected M1R$^{-/-}$ mice to several hippocampus-dependent learning and memory tasks. Somewhat surprisingly, we found that the lack of M_1 receptors did not lead to major cognitive deficits (Miyakawa et al. 2001).

M1R$^{-/-}$ mice performed equally well as their WT littermates in the Morris water maze, a test which is frequently used to assess spatial reference memory in rodents (Miyakawa et al. 2001). Moreover, in fear conditioning studies, M1R$^{-/-}$ mice displayed normal freezing levels during context testing carried out 24 h after conditioning. Similarly, the lack of M_1 receptors did not lead to significant cognitive deficits in the eight-arm radial maze test during training with a 30–120 s delay time between individual trials (Miyakawa et al. 2001).

However, we noted that M1R$^{-/-}$ mice exhibited reduced freezing in auditory-cued testing carried out 48 h after fear conditioning and during context testing carried out 4 weeks after conditioning (Miyakawa et al. 2001). Moreover, in the eight-arm radial maze test, M1R$^{-/-}$ mice displayed an increased number of revisiting errors during trials without delay (Miyakawa et al. 2001). This phenotype is therefore somewhat reminiscent of human attention deficit-hyperactivity disorder in which hyperactivity is often accompanied by cognitive deficits (Paule et al. 2000). However, since the M1R$^{-/-}$ mice showed an excellent correlation between increased locomotor activity and impaired performance in the fear conditioning and eight-arm radial maze tests, it is likely that the behavioral deficits displayed by the M1R$^{-/-}$ mice are primarily caused by their hyperactivity phenotype. Nevertheless, the possibility exists that the observed hyperactivity phenotype masks minor cognitive deficits caused by the absence of M_1 mAChRs. Consistent with this notion, Greene et al. (2001) observed that $M1R^{-/-}$ mice exhibit deficits in some measures of spatial learning and memory.

Based on the many behavioral and pharmacological studies implicating M_1 receptor activity in many cognitive functions, our finding that $M1R^{-/-}$ mice did not show major cognitive impairments was somewhat surprising. It is therefore conceivable that compensatory developmental changes have occurred in the $M1R^{-/-}$ mice that restore normal cognitive function even in the absence of M_1 receptors. This hypothesis could be tested in future studies by using novel gene targeting techniques that allow the ablation of specific genes in an inducible fashion.

3.3
Pilocarpine-Induced Epileptic Seizures Are Absent in $M1R^{-/-}$ Mice

Interestingly, Hamilton et al. (1997) showed that high doses of systemically administered pilocarpine, a non-subtype-selective muscarinic agonist, consistently induced epileptic seizures in WT mice but failed to do so in $M1R^{-/-}$ mice. However, the lack of M_1 receptors had no significant effect on the initiation and maintenance of seizures induced by kainic acid. We recently found that the lack of M_2–M_5 receptors does not interfere with pilocarpine-induced seizure responses (F.P. Bymaster et al., unpublished observations). These results raise the possibility that increased M_1 receptor activity may contribute to the pathophysiology of at least certain forms of epileptic seizures (Hamilton et al. 1997).

3.4
$M1R^{-/-}$ Mice Show Distinct Electrophysiological Deficits

Electrophysiological studies demonstrated that muscarinic agonist-mediated M current (I_m) inhibition was abolished in sympathetic ganglion neurons derived from $M1R^{-/-}$ mice (Hamilton et al. 1997). Since muscarinic suppression of I_m increases the firing rate of sympathetic neurons (Cole and Nicoll 1984), the lack of this activity in $M1R^{-/-}$ mice is likely to lead to reduced neuronal excitability in response to preganglionic stimulation. Consistent with this concept, the stimulatory cardiovascular effects following systemic administration of the muscarinic agonist McN-A-343, which preferentially activates M_1 mAChRs on postsynaptic sympathetic neurons in vivo, were absent in $M1R^{-/-}$ mice (Hardouin et al. 2002).

Somewhat surprisingly, patch-clamp studies showed that the lack of M_1 receptors had no significant effect on muscarinic agonist-mediated inhibition of I_m in mouse hippocampal CA1 pyramidal cells (Rouse et al. 2000). Likewise, hippocampal pyramidal cells derived from WT and $M1R^{-/-}$ mice displayed a similar degree of inhibition of two additional potassium conductances, the after-hyperpolarization current, I_{ahp}, and the leak potassium conductance, I_{leak} (Rouse et al. 2000).

Patch-clamp studies using sympathetic ganglion neurons derived from mAChR mutant mice also demonstrated that the slow, voltage-independent muscarinic inhibition of N- and P/Q-type Ca^{2+} channels was absent in $M1R^{-/-}$ mice (Shapiro et al. 1999). On the other hand, the fast, voltage-dependent muscarinic inhibition of N- and P/Q-type Ca^{2+} channels remained intact in $M1R^{-/-}$ mice but was lacking in $M2R^{-/-}$ mice (Shapiro et al. 1999). These results indicate that distinct mAChR subtypes are involved in mediating fast and slow muscarinic inhibition of voltage-gated Ca^{2+} channels in mouse sympathetic neurons.

Interestingly, Fisahn et al. (2002) recently showed that muscarine failed to induce γ-oscillations in the CA3 area of hippocampi from $M1R^{-/-}$ mice. On the other hand, this activity remained unaffected by the lack of M_2–M_5 receptors. Fisahn et al. (2002) also demonstrated that M_1 receptor activation depolarizes hippocampal CA3 pyramidal neurons by increasing the mixed Na^+/K^+ current, I_h, and the Ca^{2+}-dependent nonspecific cation current, I_{cat}, but not by inhibition of I_m. γ-Oscillations involve the synchronized firing of large ensembles of neurons at high frequency (20–80 Hz). Such oscillations occur in different areas of the brain under various behavioral conditions including the performance of certain cognitive tasks (see Fisahn et al. 2002 and references cited therein). Whether or not the absence of hippocampal γ-oscillations in $M1R^{-/-}$ mice is associated with specific behavioral deficits remains to be investigated.

3.5
$M1R^{-/-}$ Mice Display Distinct Biochemical Deficits

Activation of brain mAChRs leads to pronounced increases in the breakdown of phosphoinositide (PI) lipids and the activation of the mitogen-activated protein kinase (MAPK) pathway (Hamilton and Nathanson 2001, and references therein). It is well known that MAPK activation plays an important role in neuronal plasticity, differentiation, and survival. Strikingly, muscarinic agonist-induced MAPK activation was virtually abolished in primary cortical cultures from newborn $M1R^{-/-}$ mice (Hamilton and Nathanson 2001). Consistent with this finding, Berkeley et al. (2001) reported that muscarinic agonist-mediated MAPK activation was absent in CA1 hippocampal pyramidal neurons from $M1R^{-/-}$ mice. On the other hand, this activity remained unaffected by the lack of M_2–M_4 mAChRs (Berkeley et al. 2001).

Hamilton and Nathanson (2001) also demonstrated that muscarinic agonist-stimulated PI hydrolysis was reduced by more than 60% in primary cortical cultures from newborn $M1R^{-/-}$ mice. In a related study, Porter et al. (2002) used an antibody capture/guanosine triphosphate (GTP)γS binding assay for the $G\alpha_q$/$G\alpha_{11}$ G protein subunits (this class of G proteins is linked to activation of the PI pathway) to study mAChR-mediated activation of G_q/G_{11} in the mouse hippocampus and cerebral cortex. They found that muscarinic agonist-induced GT-

PγS binding to G_q/G_{11} was virtually abolished in tissues prepared from M1R$^{-/-}$ mice (Porter et al. 2002). In contrast, no significant loss in signaling was observed in the corresponding tissues from M3R$^{-/-}$ mice (Porter et al. 2002). Consistent with these in vitro studies, muscarinic agonist-induced in vivo PI hydrolysis in cortex and hippocampus was found to be specifically eliminated in M1R$^{-/-}$ mice (F.P. Bymaster et al., unpublished results).

In conclusion, the lack of M_1 receptors is associated with pronounced electrophysiological and biochemical deficits in mouse cerebral cortex and hippocampus. The behavioral correlates, if any, of these deficits remain to be elucidated.

4
M_2 and M_4 mAChR-Deficient Mice

As indicated in the introduction, the M_2 and M_4 mAChRs are both coupled to G proteins of the G_i family. At a cellular level, activation of these two receptors therefore results in similar biochemical and electrophysiological responses (Caulfield 1993; Wess 1996; Caulfield and Birdsall 1998). However, while M_2 receptors are widely expressed both in the CNS and in the body periphery, M_4 receptors are clearly more abundant in the CNS, where they are expressed at particularly high levels in the forebrain (Levey 1993; Wolfe and Yasuda 1995).

4.1
Role of M_2 Receptors in Cardiac and Smooth Muscle Function

In the body periphery, M_2 mAChRs are abundantly expressed in the heart and in smooth muscle organs (Caulfield 1993; Eglen et al. 1996; Brodde and Michel 1999). Stengel et al. (2000, 2002) recently reported that the cholinergic agonist, carbachol, induced concentration-dependent bradycardic effects in isolated spontaneously beating mouse atria prepared from WT, M3R$^{-/-}$, and M4R$^{-/-}$ mice. Strikingly, this activity was completely abolished in atrial preparations from M2R$^{-/-}$ mice (Stengel et al. 2000). This observation is consistent with the outcome of many previous pharmacological studies and the fact that the vast majority of cardiac mAChRs represent M_2 receptors (Caulfield 1993; Brodde and Michel 1999).

In order to examine the potential functional role of smooth muscle M_2 receptors, Stengel et al. (2000) studied carbachol-induced contractile responses in isolated smooth muscle preparations from stomach fundus, urinary bladder and trachea of WT and M2R$^{-/-}$ mice. In these experiments, carbachol proved to be roughly twofold more potent in WT than in M2R$^{-/-}$ preparations, suggesting that the M_2 receptor subtype contributes to the efficiency of mAChR-mediated smooth muscle contraction. In contrast, the lack of M_4 receptors had no significant effect on the magnitude of the contractile responses observed in the different smooth muscle preparations (Stengel et al. 2000). Recent studies (Matsui et al. 2000; Stengel et al. 2002) carried out with isolated tissues from M3R$^{-/-}$ mice indicate that M_3 receptors play a predominant role in muscarinic agonist-mediated smooth muscle contraction, consistent with a vast body of pharmacological evidence (Caulfield 1993; Eglen et al. 1996; see Sect. 5.2).

4.2
M$_2$ Receptors Mediate Tremor and Hypothermic Responses

Systemic administration of oxotremorine or other centrally active muscarinic agonists results in several pharmacological effects including akinesia and tremor (Ringdahl et al. 1988; Sanchez and Meier 1993), two of the key symptoms of Parkinson's disease. Oxotremorine-induced tremor responses can be suppressed by pretreatment of animals with widely used anti-Parkinson drugs such as muscarinic antagonists and L-dopa (Horst et al. 1973; Korczyn and Eshel 1979; Quock and Lucas 1983). For these reasons, oxotremorine-induced tremor has often been used as an animal model to identify new anti-Parkinson drugs. In WT mice, as expected, systemic administration of oxotremorine, a non-subtype-selective muscarinic agonist, resulted in dose-dependent tremor responses (Gomeza et al. 1999a). Strikingly, this response was totally abolished in M2R$^{-/-}$ mice (Gomeza et al. 1999a). On the other hand, the lack of M$_1$ (Hamilton et al. 1997), M$_3$ (F.P. Bymaster et al., unpublished results), M$_4$ (Gomeza et al. 1999b), or M$_5$ (Yamada et al. 2001b) mAChRs had essentially no effect on oxotremorine-induced tremor responses. These findings convincingly demonstrate that muscarinic agonist-induced tremor responses are mediated by the M$_2$ receptor subtype. The molecular mechanisms by which M$_2$ receptor activation triggers Parkinson-like symptoms remain unclear at present.

A considerable body of evidence indicates that mAChRs located in thermoregulatory centers of the hypothalamus contribute to the regulation of body temperature (Myers 1980). Consistent with the concept, systemic administration of oxotremorine leads to dose-dependent decreases in body temperature in WT mice (Gomeza et al. 1999a,b). Studies with mAChR-mutant mice showed that the oxotremorine-induced hypothermia responses were significantly reduced in M2R$^{-/-}$ but not in M4R$^{-/-}$ mice (Gomeza et al. 1999a,b), suggesting that central M$_2$ receptors play a key role in cholinergic regulation of body temperature. Since oxotremorine-induced hypothermia was reduced but not abolished in M2R$^{-/-}$-mutant mice, other mAChR subtypes also appear to be involved in this activity.

4.3
Role of M$_2$ Receptors in Muscarinic Stimulation
of the Hypothalamic–Pituitary–Adrenocortical Axis

Hemrick-Luecke et al. (2002) recently studied mAChR-mediated increases in corticosterone levels in WT and mAChR-mutant mice. Consistent with previous pharmacological studies, systemic administration of the partial muscarinic agonist, BuTAC ([5R-(exo)]-6-[4-butylthio-1,2,5-thiadiazol-3-yl]-1-azabicyclo-[3.2.1]-octane) led to robust increases in serum corticosterone levels in WT mice. This response remained unaffected in M4R$^{-/-}$ mice but was abolished in M2R$^{-/-}$ mice (Hemrick-Luecke et al. 2002). These data suggest that the M_2 receptor subtype plays a key role in mediating muscarinic activation of the hypothalamic–pituitary–adrenocortical axis in mice.

4.4
M4R$^{-/-}$ Mice Show Increases in Basal and D$_1$ Dopamine Agonist-Stimulated Locomotor Activity

The M_4 mAChR, like the M_1 receptor subtype, is expressed at particularly high levels in the striatum (Levey 1993; Hersch et al. 1994; Wolfe and Yasuda 1995). Interestingly, studies with M4R$^{-/-}$ mice showed that the lack of M_4 receptors was associated with a slight but statistically significant increase in basal locomotor activity (Gomeza et al. 1999b). We also demonstrated that the locomotor stimulation following the administration of a centrally active D_1 dopamine receptor agonist was greatly enhanced in M4R$^{-/-}$ mice (Gomeza et al. 1999b). Previous studies have shown that virtually all D_1 dopamine receptor-expressing striatal projection neurons also express M_4 mAChRs (Bernard et al. 1992; Ince et al. 1997) and that activation of this set of neurons facilitates locomotion (Di Chiara et al. 1994). Moreover, Olianas et al. (1996) recently demonstrated that D_1 receptor-mediated increases in cyclic adenosine monophosphate (cAMP) levels in striatal membrane preparations can be inhibited by concomitant stimulation of M_4 mAChRs. Taken together, these findings are consistent with the concept that activation of striatal M_4 receptors inhibits D_1 receptor-stimulated locomotor responses, suggesting that blockade of striatal M_4 receptor might be beneficial in the treatment of Parkinson's disease and related extrapyramidal movement disorders by potentiating the stimulatory locomotor effects of dopamine receptor agonists. On the other hand, M_4 receptor agonists may become useful in the treatment of schizophrenia and related psychoses by suppressing the hyperactivity of limbic dopamine systems which also coexpress D_1 dopamine and M_4 muscarinic receptors (Bymaster et al. 1999; Felder et al. 2000).

4.5
Role of M$_2$ and M$_4$ Receptors in Mediating Analgesic Effects

4.5.1
M$_2$ and M$_4$ Receptors Mediate Analgesic Effects at Spinal and Supraspinal Sites

Many laboratories have shown that systemic administration of centrally active muscarinic agonists induces pronounced analgesic effects and that this activity is dependent on both spinal and supraspinal mechanisms (Yaksh et al. 1985; Green and Kitchen 1986; Hartvig et al. 1989; Iwamoto and Marion 1993; Swedberg et al. 1997). Interestingly, it has been suggested that the potential use of muscarinic agonists as analgesic drugs is less likely to lead to tolerance and addiction associated with the use of classical opioid analgesics (Widman et al.

1985; Swedberg et al. 1997). Identification of the mAChR subtype involved in this activity is therefore of considerable therapeutic interest.

Since activation of G proteins of the G_i family frequently results in reduced neuronal activity, we considered it likely that M_2 and/or M_4 receptors are involved in mediating muscarinic agonist-dependent antinociceptive responses. To test this hypothesis, we studied the pain sensitivity of M2R$^{-/-}$ and M4R$^{-/-}$ mice, using the tail-flick and hot-plate analgesia tests (Gomeza et al. 1999a,b). In the first set of studies, analgesia was induced by systemic (subcutaneous) administration of oxotremorine. As expected, oxotremorine induced dose-dependent analgesic effects in WT mice (Gomeza et al. 1999a,b). Interestingly, these effects were markedly reduced, but not abolished, in M2R$^{-/-}$ mice (Gomeza et al. 1999a), indicating that the M_2 receptor subtype plays a key role in mediating muscarinic agonist-dependent analgesia. On the other hand, M4R$^{-/-}$ mice showed analgesic responses that were similar to those observed with WT mice (Gomeza et al. 1999b). Moreover, a recent study demonstrated that oxotremorine was completely devoid of analgesic activity in mutant mice lacking both M_2 and M_4 receptors (M2R$^{-/-}$/M4R$^{-/-}$ mice; Duttaroy et al. 2002). Similar results were obtained with other centrally active muscarinic agonists (Duttaroy et al. 2002). These findings indicate that muscarinic agonist-induced antinociception is mediated predominantly by M_2 receptors but that M_4 receptors also contribute to this activity. In fact, we recently demonstrated that maximum analgesia can be achieved even in the absence of M_2 receptors by simply increasing the dose of the administered agonist (Duttaroy et al. 2002). It is likely that the antinociceptive activity of M_4 receptors remained undetected in the M_4 receptor single knockout mice (M4R$^{-/-}$ mice) due to the presence of the predominant M_2 receptor pathway (Gomeza et al. 1999b).

To assess the relative contribution of spinal versus supraspinal mechanisms to muscarinic agonist-mediated analgesic effects, Duttaroy et al. (2002) also carried out a series of intrathecal (i.t.) and intracerebroventricular (i.c.v.) injections studies. Independent of the route of application, the analgesic activity of oxotremorine (10 μg/mouse; i.t. or i.c.v.) was greatly reduced in M2R$^{-/-}$ mice (by ~50–90%), little changed in M4R$^{-/-}$ mice, and essentially abolished in M2R$^{-/-}$/M4R$^{-/-}$ mice (shown for the i.t. injection experiments in Fig. 1). This pattern was very similar to that observed after systemic administration of oxotremorine (Gomeza et al. 1999a,b; Duttaroy et al. 2002).

These data indicate that both M_2 and M_4 receptors are involved in mediating the analgesic effects of muscarinic agonists at the spinal and supraspinal level. Clearly, the M_2 receptor-dependent analgesic pathway predominates, most likely to the high expression levels of this receptor subtype in the spinal cord (Duttaroy et al. 2002). However, the results of the i.c.v. injection studies indicate that activation of supraspinal (brain) M_2 and M_4 receptors also leads to robust analgesic effects. Several lines of evidence suggest that both presynaptic and postsynaptic mechanisms contribute to the mAChR-mediated analgesic responses (discussed in Duttaroy et al. 2002). Since M_4 receptors, unlike M_2 receptors, do not appear to play a significant role in cardiac and smooth muscle function, the

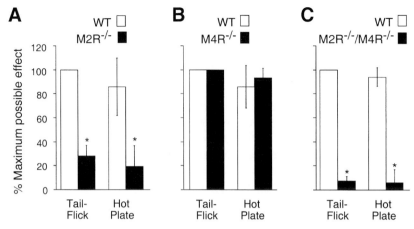

Fig. 1A–C Pain sensitivity of WT and mAChR-mutant mice following intrathecal (i.t.) administration of oxotremorine. **A** M2R$^{-/-}$ and WT control mice. **B** M4R$^{-/-}$ and WT control mice. **C** M$_2$/M$_4$ receptor double-knockout mice (M2R$^{-/-}$/M4R$^{-/-}$ mice) and WT control animals. Adult male mice (n=5–6/group) were injected i.t. with a single dose (10 μg/mouse) of oxotremorine, and analgesic effects were determined using the tail-flick and hot-plate assays as described (Duttaroy et al. 2002). Data are given as mean±SD (*p<0.05, compared to WT). (Data were taken from Duttaroy et al. 2002)

development of selective M$_4$ receptor agonists as novel analgesic agents appears to be an attractive goal.

4.5.2
M$_2$ Receptors Mediate Desensitization of Peripheral Nociceptors

Recent studies have shown that activation of mAChRs present on peripheral nociceptors of the skin can also suppress the transmission of pain impulses (Bernardini et al. 2001a,b). Electrophysiological and neurochemical studies with skin or skin-saphenous nerve preparations showed that muscarine-induced peripheral antinociception was abolished in M2R$^{-/-}$ mice (Bernardini et al. 2002). In contrast, muscarine-mediated peripheral antinociceptive responses were similar in WT and M4R$^{-/-}$ mice (Bernardini et al. 2002). It is possible that this peripheral M$_2$ receptor activity contributes to the analgesic effects observed after systemic administration of muscarinic agonists in the hot-plate and tail-flick experiments (see above). Several studies suggest that ACh is synthesized and released by different cell types of the skin (Grando et al. 1993; Buchli et al. 1999), raising the possibility that non-neuronally released ACh might be involved in modulating peripheral nociception via activation of M$_2$ mAChRs.

4.6
Role of M_2 and M_4 Receptors as Muscarinic Autoreceptors and Heteroreceptors

4.6.1
Central Muscarinic Autoreceptors

ACh, like many other neurotransmitters, can inhibit its own release via stimulation of so-called inhibitory autoreceptors present on cholinergic nerve endings (Kilbinger 1984; Starke et al. 1989). Physiologically, this mechanism probably serves to fine-tune ACh release at cholinergic synapses. Classical pharmacological studies have often led to contradictory results regarding the identity of the inhibitory muscarinic autoreceptors expressed in a given peripheral or central tissue (Kilbinger 1984; Starke et al. 1989), probably primarily due to the limited receptor subtype selectivity of the ligands used in these studies.

Since autoinhibition of neurotransmitter release is most frequently mediated by receptors coupled to G proteins of the G_i family, we initially studied whether autoinhibition of ACh release was altered in tissues from M2R$^{-/-}$ and M4R$^{-/-}$ mice. We first examined the identity of the muscarinic autoreceptors in various central mouse tissues (Zhang et al. 2002a). Specifically, we studied oxotremorine-mediated inhibition of potassium-stimulated [^{3}H]ACh release using superfused hippocampal, cortical, and striatal slices that had been preincubated with [^{3}H]choline to label cellular ACh pools. Proper regulation of ACh release in these brain regions is known to be important for a number of important CNS functions including cognitive processes and the control of locomotor activity and coordination.

In WT preparations, oxotremorine inhibited potassium-stimulated [^{3}H]ACh release in all three tissues in a concentration-dependent fashion (by up to ~80%), probably due to stimulation of presynaptic release-inhibitory muscarinic autoreceptors (Zhang et al. 2002a). In the absence of M_2 receptors (M2R$^{-/-}$ mice), the release-inhibitory activity of oxotremorine was abolished in hippocampal and cortical preparations but remained largely intact in striatal slice preparations. Reciprocally, in the absence of M_4 receptors (M4R$^{-/-}$ mice), the release-inhibitory activity of oxotremorine was not significantly affected in hippocampal and cortical preparations but was no longer detectable in striatal slice preparations (Zhang et al. 2002a).

These findings demonstrate that autoinhibition of ACh release is mediated predominantly by M_2 receptors in the mouse hippocampus and cerebral cortex, but primarily by M_4 receptors in the mouse striatum, indicating that autoinhibition of ACh release can involve different mAChRs in different regions of the brain. These results should provide a rational basis for the development of novel muscarinic drugs designed to enhance or decrease muscarinic cholinergic transmission in a variety of pathophysiological conditions including Alzheimer's and Parkinson's disease.

4.6.2
Peripheral Muscarinic Autoreceptors and Heteroreceptors

Zhou et al. (2002) recently used isolated tissues from mAChR-mutant mice to characterize the release-inhibitory muscarinic autoreceptors in two peripheral tissues, mouse heart atria and urinary bladder. They demonstrated that both M_4 and non-M_4 (probably M_2) mAChRs are involved in mediating autoinhibiton of ACh release in mouse heart atria. On the other hand, autoinhibition of ACh release was found to be mediated predominantly by M_4 receptors in the mouse urinary bladder (Zhou et al. 2002).

It is well known that activation of mAChRs located on peripheral sympathetic nerve terminals (so-called heteroreceptors) leads to the inhibition of norepinephrine (Fuder and Muscholl 1995). In a recent study, Trendelenburg et al. (2002) carried out a series of in vitro [^{3}H]norepinephrine release studies to determine the molecular identity of the muscarinic heteroreceptors mediating inhibition of sympathetic transmitter release in mouse atria, urinary bladder, and vas deferens. Specifically, electrically evoked norepinephrine release was assessed using tissue preparations from WT, M2R$^{-/-}$, and M4R$^{-/-}$ mice, following preincubation of tissues with [^{3}H]norepinephrine. This analysis showed that the release-inhibitory muscarinic heteroreceptors represent mixtures of M_2 and non-M_2 receptors in all three tissues studied (Trendelenburg et al. 2002). Whereas the identity of the non-M_2 heteroreceptors in the cardiac and bladder preparations could not be assessed with a sufficient degree of certainty, the non-M_2 heteroreceptors present in the vas deferens are likely to represent primarily M_4 receptors (Trendelenburg et al. 2002). These results should contribute to a better understanding of the molecular mechanisms governing the interplay between the sympathetic and parasympathetic nervous systems under physiological and pathophysiological conditions.

5
M3R$^{-/-}$ Mice

The M_3 mAChR subtype is widely expressed throughout the CNS (Levey et al. 1994). At present, however, little is known about the physiological roles of these central M_3 receptors. In the periphery, M_3 mAChRs play a role in mediating muscarinic stimulation of smooth muscle contraction and glandular secretion (Wess et al. 1990; Caulfield 1993; Matsui et al. 2000; Stengel et al. 2002).

5.1
M3R$^{-/-}$ Mice Show Reduced Body Weight, Peripheral Fat Deposits, and Food Intake

Analysis of M3R$^{-/-}$ mice showed that the lack of M_3 receptors was not associated with any obvious behavioral deficits (Yamada et al. 2001a; T. Miyakawa et al., unpublished results). Immediately after birth, WT and M3R$^{-/-}$ mice showed

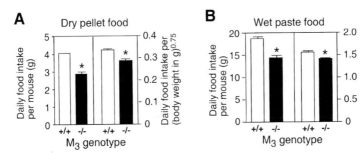

Fig. 2A, B M3R$^{-/-}$ mice consume less food than their WT (+/+) littermates. Daily consumption of (**A**) standard dry food pellets and (**B**) wet mash food by adult male mice. Food intake was measured daily over a 5-day observation period. Data are expressed as food intake per mouse or as food intake per (body weight in g)$^{0.75}$ ("metabolic body weight"; Kleiber 1975). Data are given as mean±SEM (n=10 per group; data were taken from Yamada et al. 2001a). *$p<0.05$ (compared to WT)

similar body weights. However, starting at about 2–3 weeks after birth, M3R$^{-/-}$ mice showed a significant reduction in body weight (Yamada et al. 2001a). This difference in body weight continued to increase during the following weeks and persisted throughout the life of the animals. Generally, adult male or female M3R$^{-/-}$ mice weigh about 25% less than their WT littermates. However, the lack of M$_3$ receptors did not interfere with linear growth (Yamada et al. 2001a).

More detailed studies showed that that the mass of peripheral fat deposits was significantly reduced (by ~50%) in M3R$^{-/-}$ mice (Yamada et al. 2001a). Moreover, serum triglyceride levels were found to be reduced by approximately 25% in M3R$^{-/-}$ mice. The lack of M$_3$ receptors also led to pronounced reductions (~5–10-fold) in serum leptin and insulin levels, consistent with the concept that the levels of these two hormones usually correlate well with the amount of total body fat (Schwartz et al. 2000). However, it is possible that the absence of pancreatic M$_3$ receptors, which are thought to play a role in facilitating insulin release (Boschero et al. 1995), also contributes to the observed reduction in serum insulin levels. Despite reduced insulin levels, M3R$^{-/-}$ mice did not develop hyperglycemia, probably because the insulin sensitivity of peripheral tissues is increased in lean individuals (Schwartz et al. 2000).

Additional studies showed that locomotor activity patterns, metabolic rate, and gastrointestinal motor activity in vivo were similar in WT and M3R$^{-/-}$ mice (Yamada et al. 2001a). On the other hand, systematic food intake studies demonstrated that M3R$^{-/-}$ mice consumed considerably less food than their WT littermates. This difference in food intake was observed not only with standard dry pellet food but also with a wet mash diet (Fig. 2). This latter finding suggests that it is unlikely that impaired salivation associated with dry mouth (see Sect. 5.3) is a major factor responsible for the reduced food intake displayed by the M3R$^{-/-}$ mice.

Radioligand binding studies showed that M$_3$ receptors are expressed at high levels (~1 pmol/mg membrane protein) in the hypothalamus (Yamada et al.

2001a), the key control center for the regulation of appetite. To test the hypothesis that the lack of M_3 receptors was associated with altered expression levels of appetite-regulating hypothalamic neuropeptides, we measured the expression levels of proopiomelanocortin (POMC), agouti-related peptide (AGRP), preproorexin, and melanin-concentrating hormone (MCH) which are considered critical regulators of feeding and energy balance and act downstream of the hypothalamic leptin system (Elmquist et al. 1999; Schwartz et al. 2000). Whereas POMC- and AGRP-containing neurons are present in the arcuate nucleus and are the primary leptin targets, MCH and the orexins are synthesized by second-order neurons in the lateral hypothalamus which receive innervation from the POMC and AGRP neurons (Elmquist et al. 1999; Schwartz et al. 2000).

RT-PCR studies (Yamada et al. 2001a), complemented by Northern blotting experiments, demonstrated that M3R$^{-/-}$ mice showed increased expression levels of the appetite-stimulating peptide, AGRP, and reduced levels of the appetite-suppressing peptide, POMC, both of which are expressed in so-called first-order leptin-sensitive hypothalamic neurons in the arcuate nucleus. This pattern is typically seen in fasted mice or under conditions of leptin deficiency and serves to stimulate food intake by reducing the activity of hypothalamic melanocortin receptors (Elmquist et al. 1999; Schwartz et al. 2000).

Interestingly, M3R$^{-/-}$ mice displayed a significant decrease in the expression of MCH (Yamada et al. 2001a), an appetite-stimulating peptide synthesized virtually exclusively in second-order neurons of the lateral hypothalamus. This was a surprising observation since increased AGRP levels and reduced POMC levels usually trigger an increase in MCH levels resulting in increased food intake (Elmquist et al. 1999; Schwartz et al. 2000). It should be noted in this context that hypothalamic MCH neurons receive abundant cholinergic innervation from lower brain regions and that muscarinic agonists can stimulate hypothalamic MCH expression (Bayer et al. 1999). Consistent with this latter observation, in situ hybridization/immunohistochemistry double labeling studies showed that M_3 receptors are found on most hypothalamic MCH-containing neurons (Yamada et al. 2001a).

I.c.v. infusion experiments indicated that M3R$^{-/-}$ mice failed to increase their food intake following administration of AGRP. In contrast, the appetite-stimulating effects of MCH remained fully intact in M3R$^{-/-}$ mice (Yamada et al. 2001a), suggesting that MCH-dependent downstream signaling pathways remain unaffected in M3R$^{-/-}$ mice.

Taken together, these findings strongly suggest that hypothalamic M_3 receptors are required for maintaining proper MCH expression and proper responsiveness of MCH neurons to input from first-order hypothalamic neurons. It is likely that the loss of this activity is a key factor responsible for the reduced food intake displayed by the M3R$^{-/-}$ mice. In agreement with this proposal, MCH-deficient mice show a phenotype that is very similar to that of the M3R$^{-/-}$ mice (Shimada et al. 1998). Pharmacological manipulation of this newly identified hypothalamic cholinergic pathway may represent a novel strategy for the control of food intake.

5.2
Role of M$_3$ Receptors in Smooth Muscle Function

Consistent with a large body of pharmacological evidence (Wess et al. 1990; Caulfield 1993; Eglen et al. 1996), Matsui et al. (2000) recently showed that M3R$^{-/-}$ mice showed deficits in mAChR-mediated smooth muscle contraction. These authors reported, for example, that M3R$^{-/-}$ mice had enlarged pupils, consistent with the predicted involvement of M$_3$ receptors in parasympathetic stimulation of the tone of the pupillary sphincter muscle. It was noted, however, that M3R$^{-/-}$ mice retained a weak light reflex and that atropine further increased the pupil size of M3R$^{-/-}$ mice (Matsui et al. 2000), indicating that non-M$_3$ mAChRs also make a contribution to the contractility of ocular smooth muscles.

Matsui et al. (2000) also found that male M3R$^{-/-}$ mice exhibited severely distended urinary bladders, which, however, did not seem to affect renal function. Consistent with this observation, carbachol-induced contractile responses of isolated urinary bladder strips were almost completely abolished in tissues derived from male or female M3R$^{-/-}$ mice (Matsui et al. 2000; Stengel et al. 2002). However, for reasons that are unclear at present, the degree of bladder distension was much less severe in female than in male M3R$^{-/-}$ mice (Matsui et al. 2000).

Additional studies examined whether the lack of M$_3$ receptors also affected mAChR-mediated contractions of smooth muscle preparations from mouse ileum, stomach fundus, trachea, and gallbladder (Matsui et al. 2000; Stengel et al. 2002; Stengel and Cohen 2002). These studies showed that the magnitude of carbachol-mediated contractile responses were significantly reduced (by ~40%–80%) in all four preparations studied, suggesting that both M$_3$ and non-M$_3$ receptors play a role in mediating smooth muscle contraction in these tissues. On the other hand, M3R$^{-/-}$ mice did not display any apparent gastrointestinal complications in vivo such as diarrhea, constipation, hemorrhage, and histological abnormalities (Matsui et al. 2000) or decreased gastrointestinal transit time, as studied in a charcoal transit test (Yamada et al. 2001a). These findings indicate that the presence of M$_3$ receptors is not essential for gastrointestinal function in vivo, probably due to the presence of many other receptor systems regulating gastrointestinal function.

5.3
Role of M$_3$ Receptors in Salivary Secretion

Two studies reported that the oral cavity of M3R$^{-/-}$ mice was moist, suggesting that M3R$^{-/-}$ mice were not severely impaired in basal salivary flow (Matsui et al. 2000; Yamada et al. 2001a). Matsui et al. (2000) first reported that pilocarpine (1 mg/kg, s.c.) failed to stimulate salivary secretion in M3R$^{-/-}$ mice. In contrast, we found, by using three different doses of pilocarpine (1, 5, and 15 mg/kg, s.c.) that pilocarpine-induced salivation was significantly reduced (by ~50%) only at the intermediate dose (5 mg/kg), suggesting that both M_3 and non-M_3 mAChRs (M_1 receptors?) mediate muscarinic stimulation of salivary secretion. One possible explanation for these discrepant results is that Matsui et al. (2000) only examined one single low dose (1 mg/kg, s.c.) of pilocarpine and used a different method to quantitate salivary flow (note that the strategy used to disrupt the M_3 receptor gene was identical in both studies).

6
M5R$^{-/-}$ Mice

The M_5 receptor was the last mAChR subtype to be cloned (Bonner et al. 1988). M_5 receptors are expressed, at rather low levels, in both neuronal and non-neuronal cells (Caulfield and Birdsall 1998; Eglen and Nahorski 2000). Until very recently, the physiological roles of the M_5 receptor remained obscure. However, recent studies with M5R$^{-/-}$ mice have revealed several important physiological functions that are mediated by activation of M_5 receptors (Yamada et al. 2001b; Basile et al. 2002; Forster et al. 2002; Takeuchi et al. 2002).

6.1
M5 Receptors Facilitate Dopamine Release in the Striatum

Receptor localization studies (Vilaro et al. 1990; Weiner et al. 1990) have shown that the M_5 receptor is the major mAChR subtype expressed by the dopamine-containing neurons of the midbrain (substantia nigra pars compacta and ventral tegmental area). The dopamine-containing neurons of the substantia nigra pars compacta provide the major dopaminergic innervation of the striatum. Since muscarinic agonists are known to facilitate striatal dopamine release (Lehmann and Langer 1982; Raiteri et al. 1984), Weiner et al. (1990) suggested that M_5 receptors located on dopaminergic nerve terminals may mediate this activity. To test this hypothesis, we carried out a series of in vitro dopamine release studies using striatal slice preparations prelabeled with [^{3}H]dopamine. In agreement with previous studies (Lehmann and Langer 1982; Raiteri et al. 1984), incubation of WT striatal slices with increasing concentrations of oxotremorine resulted in concentration-dependent increases in potassium-stimulated [^{3}H]dopamine release (Yamada et al. 2001b). In M5R$^{-/-}$ mice, the oxotremorine concentration-response curve was shifted to the right by a factor of about 5–10 (Yamada et al. 2001b), suggesting that both M_5 and non-M_5 mAChRs are involved in facilitating striatal dopamine release. In agreement with this notion, oxotremorine-mediated increases in striatal dopamine release were totally abolished in striatal slices prepared from M4R$^{-/-}$ mice (Zhang et al. 2002b), indicating that the presence of striatal M_4 receptors is essential for this activity. In this latter study (Zhang et al. 2002b), we also demonstrated that activation of striatal M_3 receptors inhibits oxotremorine-mediated dopamine release, indicating that at least three mAChR subtypes are involved in modulating striatal dopamine outflow. The precise neuronal pathways through which the individual mAChRs exert their modulatory effects on striatal dopamine release remain to be elucidated.

6.2
M5 Receptors Mediate ACh-Induced Dilation of Cerebral Arteries and Arterioles

ACh is a powerful dilator of most vascular beds. This activity is known to be mediated by activation of endothelial mAChRs triggering the release of NO, the actual vasorelaxing agent (Furchgott and Zawadzki 1980; Rosenblum 1986; Huang et al. 1995; Faraci and Sigmund 1999). Recently, M_5 receptor mRNA has been identified in various peripheral and cerebral blood vessels (Phillips et al. 1997; Elhusseiny et al. 1999). To test the hypothesis that vascular M_5 receptors are involved in mediating the vasorelaxing effects of ACh, we investigated whether the lack of M_5 receptors led to changes in vascular tone using several in vivo and in vitro vascular preparations. These studies showed that ACh-mediated dilation of extra-cerebral arteries (carotid and coronary arteries) remained fully intact in M5R$^{-/-}$ mice (Yamada et al. 2001b). Strikingly, however, ACh virtually lost the ability to dilate cerebral arteries and arterioles in M5R$^{-/-}$ mice, as studied with the basilar artery and pial arterioles as model systems (Yamada et al. 2001b; Fig. 3). These findings support the concept that cerebral arteries and arterioles are endowed with endothelial M_5 receptors which mediate the vasorelaxing effects of ACh. On the other hand, this activity is mediated by non-M_5 mAChRs (M_3?) in extra-cerebral arteries.

A considerable body of evidence indicates that neuronally released ACh is involved in the regulation of cerebral vascular resistance and regional blood flow (Sato and Sato 1995; Scremin and Jenden 1996). Moreover, several studies suggest that deficits in cortical cholinergic vasodilation may play a role in the

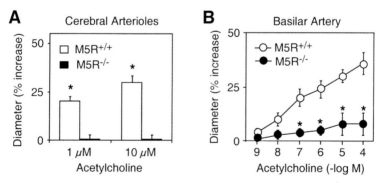

Fig. 3A, B Loss of ACh-mediated dilation of cerebral blood vessels from M5R$^{-/-}$ mice. Effect of ACh on the diameter of (**A**) cerebral (pial) arterioles (in vivo) and (**B**) basilar artery preparations (in vitro) from M5R$^{-/-}$ mice and their WT littermates. Experiments were carried out with adult female mice, as described by Yamada et al. (2001b). Basilar artery preparations were precontracted submaximally with the thromboxane mimetic, U-46619. Results are given as mean±SEM (n=7 or 8 per dose/concentration and genotype; data were taken from Yamada et al. 2001b). *p<0.05 (compared to WT)

pathophysiology of Alzheimer's disease (Geaney et al. 1990; Tong and Hamel 1999) and that cholinergic vasodilator fibers may play a protective role during focal cerebral ischemia (Kano et al. 1991; Scremin and Jenden 1996). Based on these findings, the M_5 mAChR may therefore represent a potential novel target for the treatment of various cerebrovascular disorders.

6.3
M5R$^{-/-}$ Mice Show Reduced Sensitivity to the Rewarding Effects of Morphine

Receptor localization studies (Vilaro et al. 1990) have shown that the M_5 receptor is the predominant mAChR subtype expressed by the dopamine-containing neurons of the ventral tegmental area (VTA) which innervate the nucleus accumbens and other limbic areas. This mesolimbic dopaminergic pathway is known to play a key role in mediating the rewarding effects of opiates and other drugs of abuse (Wise 1996; Koob et al. 1998).

Interestingly, Forster et al. (2002) recently reported that the sustained increase in dopamine levels in the nucleus accumbens observed after electrical stimulation of the laterodorsal tegmental nucleus (LDT) is absent in M5R$^{-/-}$ mice. LDT neurons represent the major source of cholinergic input to the dopamine-containing neurons of the VTA (Oakman et al. 1995; Blaha et al. 1996). It is therefore likely that activation of M_5 receptors expressed by VTA neurons is responsible for the prolonged efflux of dopamine following LDT stimulation.

On the basis of these findings, we recently tested the hypothesis that the lack of M_5 receptors might be associated with changes in drug-seeking behavior. In an initial set of experiments, we studied the behavioral and biochemical manifestations of morphine reward and withdrawal (Basile et al. 2002). We found that the rewarding effects of morphine, as studied in the conditioned place preference paradigm, were substantially reduced in M5R$^{-/-}$ mice. Furthermore, both the somatic and affective components of naloxone-induced morphine withdrawal symptoms were significantly attenuated in the absence of M_5 receptors (Basile et al. 2002). On the other hand, the analgesic efficacy of morphine and the degree of tolerance that mice developed to the analgesic effects of morphine were similar in WT and M5R$^{-/-}$ mice. Blockade of central M_5 receptors by selective muscarinic antagonists may therefore represent a new strategy for the treatment of addiction to opiates and, perhaps, other drugs of abuse.

6.4
Other Phenotypes Displayed by M5R$^{-/-}$ Mice

Takeuchi et al. (2002) recently reported that mAChR-mediated salivation was slightly impaired in M5R$^{-/-}$ mice. Whereas WT and M5R$^{-/-}$ mice showed similar salivary flow during the first 15 min after pilocarpine administration (1 mg/ kg, s.c.), a slight reduction (by ~10%–20%) in salivary output became apparent between 20 and 60 min after application of the drug. These findings raise the possibility that glandular M_5 receptors contribute to ACh-mediated salivary secretion.

Takeuchi et al. (2002) also found that $M5R^{-/-}$ mice drank more than twice as much water than WT mice following an extended period (18 h) of food and water deprivation. The specific mechanisms underlying this behavioral phenotype are not clear at present.

7
Conclusions

The data summarized in this chapter indicate that the recently generated M_1–M_5 mAChR-mutant mice represent powerful new research tools for delineating the physiological and pathophysiological roles of the individual mAChR subtypes. These new findings should be highly useful for directing the design of novel muscarinic drugs useful for the treatment of a variety of important pathophysiological conditions, including Alzheimer's and Parkinson's disease, pain, and drug dependence.

Acknowledgements. This work was supported by the JSPS Research Fellowship Program (M.Y.) and by a CRADA between the Eli Lilly Research Laboratories and the NIDDK. We thank all individuals who are not listed as coauthors but who contributed to various aspects of the work summarized in this chapter.

References

Basile AS, Fedorova I, Zapata A, Liu X, Shippenberg T, Duttaroy A, Yamada M, Wess J (2002) Deletion of the M_5 muscarinic acetylcholine receptor attenuates morphine reinforcement and withdrawal but not morphine analgesia. Proc Natl Acad Sci USA 99:11452–11457.

Bayer L, Risold PY, Griffoond B, Fellmann D (1999) Rat diencephalic neurons producing melanin-concentrating hormone are influenced by ascending cholinergic projections. Neuroscience 91:1087–1101

Berkeley JL, Gomeza J, Wess J, Hamilton SE, Nathanson NM, Levey AI (2001) M_1 Muscarinic acetylcholine receptors activate extracellular signal-regulated kinase in CA1 pyramidal neurons in mouse hippocampal slices. Mol. Cell Neurosci 18:512–524.

Bernard V, Normand E, Bloch B (1992 Phenotypical characterization of the rat striatal neurons expressing muscarinic receptor genes.) J Neurosci 12:3591–3600

Bernardini N, Sauer SK, Haberberger R, Fischer MJM, Reeh PW (2001a) Excitatory nicotinic and desensitizing muscarinic (M2) effects on C-nociceptors in isolated rat skin. J Neurosci 21:3295–3302

Bernardini N, Reeh PW, Sauer SK (2001b) M2 Receptors inhibit heat-induced CGRP release from isolated rat skin, in vitro. Neuroreport 12:2457–2460

Bernardini N, Roza C, Sauer SK, Gomeza J, Wess J, Reeh PW (2002) Muscarinic M2 receptors on peripheral nerve endings: a molecular target of nociception. J Neurosci 22:RC229, 1–5

Blaha CD, Allen LF, Das S, Inglis WL, Latimer MP, Vincent SR, Winn P (1996) Modulation of dopamine efflux in the nucleus accumbens after cholinergic stimulation of the ventral tegmental area in intact, pedunculopontine tegmental nucleus-lesioned, and laterodorsal tegmental nucleus-lesioned rats. J Neurosci 16:714–722

Bonner TI, Young AC, Brann MR, Buckley NJ (1988) Cloning and expression of the human and rat m5 muscarinic acetylcholine receptor genes. Neuron 1:403–410.

Boschero AC, Szpak-Glasman M, Carneiro EM, Bordin S, Paul I, Rojas E, Atwater I (1995) Oxotremorine-m potentiation of glucose-induced insulin release from rat islets involves M_3 muscarinic receptors. Am J Physiol 268:E336-E342

Brodde OE and Michel MC (1999) Adrenergic and muscarinic receptors in the human heart. Pharmacol Rev 51 651–690

Buchly R, Ndoye A, Rodriguez J G, Zia S, Webber RJ, Grando SA (1999) Human skin fibroblasts express m2, m4, and m5 subtypes of muscarinic acetylcholine receptors. J Cell Biochem 74:264–277

Bymaster FP, Shannon HE, Rasmussen K, DeLapp NW, Ward JS, Calligaro DO, Mitch CH, Whitesitt C, Ludvigsen TS, Sheardown M, Swedberg M, Rasmussen T, Olesen PH, Jeppesen L, Sauerberg P, Fink-Jensen A (1999) Potential role of muscarinic receptors in schizophrenia. Life Sci 64:527–534

Caulfield MP (1993) Muscarinic receptors—characterization, coupling and function. Pharmacol Ther 58:319–379

Caulfield MP, Birdsall NJM (1998) International Union of Pharmacology. XVII. Classification of muscarinic acetylcholine receptors. Pharmacol Rev 1998; 50:279–290

Cole AE, Nicoll RA (1984) The pharmacology of cholinergic excitatory responses in hippocampal pyramidal cells. Brain Res 305:283–290

Coyle JT, Price DL, DeLong MR (1983) Alzheimer's disease: a disorder of cortical cholinergic innervation. Science 219:1184–1190

Deng C, Wynshaw-Boris A, Zhou F, Kuo A, Leder P (1996) Fibroblast growth factor receptor 3 is a negative regulator of bone growth. Cell 84:911–921

Di Chiara G, Morelli M, Consolo S (1994) Modulatory functions of neurotransmitters in the striatum: ACh/dopamine/NMDA interactions. Trends Neurosci 17:228–233

Duttaroy A, Gomeza J, Gan JW, Siddiqui N, Basile AS, Harman WD, Smith PI, Felder CC, Levey AI, Wess J (2002) Evaluation of muscarinic agonist-Induced analgesia in muscarinic acetylcholine receptor knockout mice. Mol Pharmacol, 62:1084–1093

Eglen RM, Nahorski SR (2000) The muscarinic M_5 receptor: a silent or emerging subtype? Br J Pharmacol 130:13–21

Eglen RM, Hegde SS, Watson N (1996) Muscarinic receptor subtypes and smooth muscle function. Pharmacol Rev 48:531–565

Eglen RM, Choppin A, Dillon MP, Hegde S (1999) Muscarinic receptor ligands and their therapeutic potential. Curr Opin Chem Biol 3:426–432

Elhusseiny A, Cohen Z, Olivier A, Stanimirovic DB, Hamel E (1999) Functional acetylcholine muscarinic receptor subtypes in human brain microcirculation: identification and cellular localization. J Cereb Blood Flow Metab 19:794–802

Elmquist JK, Elias CF, Saper CB (1999) From lesions to leptin: hypothalamic control of food intake and body weight. Neuron 22:221–232

Faraci FM, Sigmund CD (1999) Vascular biology in genetically altered mice: smaller vessels, bigger insight. Circ Res 85:1214–1225

Felder CC, Bymaster FP, Ward J, DeLapp N (2000) Therapeutic opportunities for muscarinic receptors in the central nervous system. J Med Chem 43:4333–4353

Fisahn A, Yamada M, Duttaroy A, Gan JW, Deng CX, McBain CJ, Wess J (2002) Muscarinic induction of hippocampal gamma oscillations requires coupling of the M_1 receptor to two mixed cation channels. Neuron 33:615–624

Fisher A, Heldman E, Gurwitz D, Haring R, Karton Y, Meshulam H, Pittel Z, Marciano D, Brandeis R, Sadot E, Barg Y, Pinkas-Kramarski R, Vogel Z, Ginzburg I, Treves TA, Verchovsky R, Klimowsky S, Korczyn AD (1996) M1 agonists for the treatment of Alzheimer's disease. Novel properties and clinical update. Ann N Y Acad Sci 777:189–196.

Forster GL, Yeomans JS, Takeuchi J, Blaha CD (2002) M5 muscarinic receptors are required for prolonged accumbal dopamine release after electrical stimulation of the pons in mice. J Neurosci 22:RC190

Fuder H, Muscholl E (1995) Heteroreceptor-mediated modulation of noradrenaline and acetylcholine release from peripheral nerves. Rev Physiol Biochem Pharmacol 126:265–412

Furchgott RF, Zawadzki JV (1980) The obligatory role of endothelial cells in the relaxation of arterial smooth muscle by acetylcholine. Nature 288:373–376

Geaney D, Soper N, Shepstone BJ, Cowen PJ (1990) Effect of central cholinergic stimulation on regional cerebral blood flow in Alzheimer disease. Lancet 335:1484–1487

Gerber DJ, Sotnikova TD, Gainetdinov RR, Huang SY, Caron MG, Tonegawa S (2001) Hyperactivity, elevated dopaminergic transmission, and response to amphetamine in M1 muscarinic acetylcholine receptor-deficient mice. Proc Natl Acad Sci USA 98:15312–15317

Gomeza J, Shannon H, Kostenis E, Felder C, Zhang L, Brodkin J, Grinberg A, Sheng H, Wess J (1999a) Pronounced pharmacologic deficits in M2 muscarinic acetylcholine receptor knockout mice. Proc Natl Acad Sci USA 96:1692–1697

Gomeza J, Zhang L, Kostenis E, Felder C, Bymaster F, Brodkin J, Shannon H, Xia B, Deng C, Wess J (1999b) Enhancement of D1 dopamine receptor-mediated locomotor stimulation in M_4 muscarinic acetylcholine receptor knockout mice. Proc Natl Acad Sci USA 96:10483–10488

Grando SA, Kist DA, Qi M, Dahl MV (1993) Human keratinocytes synthesize, secrete and degrade acetylcholine. J Invest Dermatol 101:32–36

Green PG, Kitchen I (1986) Antinociception opioids and the cholinergic system. Prog Neurobiol 26:119–146

Greene SJ, Felder CC, Hamilton SE, Nathanson NM, Gannon KS (2001) Analyses of spatial learning and activity in muscarinic M1 receptor knockout mice: Evidence for a cognitive deficit. Soc Neurosci Abstr 27 prg # 79.12

Hagan JJ, Jansen JH, Broekkamp CL (1987) Blockade of spatial learning by the M1 muscarinic antagonist pirenzepine. Psychopharmacology 93:470–476

Hamilton SE, Loose MD, Qi M, Levey AI, Hille B, McKnight GS, Idzerda RL, Nathanson NM (1997) Disruption of the m1 receptor gene ablates muscarinic receptor-dependent M current regulation and seizure activity in mice. Proc Natl Acad Sci USA 94:13311–13316

Hamilton SE, Nathanson NM (2001) The M_1 receptor is required for muscarinic activation of mitogen-activated protein (MAP) kinase in murine cerebral cortical neurons. J Biol Chem 276:15850–15853

Hardouin SN, Richmond KN, Zimmerman A, Hamilton SE, Feigl EO, Nathanson NM (2002) Altered cardiovascular responses in mice lacking the M_1 muscarinic acetylcholine receptor. J Pharmacol Exp Ther 301:129–137

Hartvig P, Gillberg PG, Gordh T, Jr, Post C (1989) Cholinergic mechanisms in pain and analgesia. Trends Pharmacol Sci 10 (Suppl.):75–79

Hemrick-Luecke SK, Bymaster FP, Evans DC, Wess J, Felder CC (2002) Muscarinic agonist-mediated increases in serum corticosterone levels are abolished in M_2 muscarinic acetylcholine receptor knockout mice. J Pharmacol Exp Ther, 303:99–103

Hersch SM, Gutekunst CA, Rees HD, Heilman CJ, Levey AI (1994) Distribution of m1-m4 muscarinic receptor proteins in the rat striatum: light and electron microscopic immunocytochemistry using subtype-specific antibodies. J Neurosci 14:3351–3363

Horst WD, Pool WR, Spiegel HE (1973) Correlation between brain dopamine levels and l-dopa activity in anti-Parkinson tests. Eur J Pharmacol 21:337–342

Huang PL, Huang Z, Mashimo H, Bloch KD, Moskowitz MA, Bevan JA, Fishman MC (1995) Hypertension in mice lacking the gene for endothelial nitric oxide synthase. Nature 377:239–242

Ince E, Ciliax BJ, Levey AI (1997) Differential expression of D1 and D2 dopamine and m4 muscarinic acetylcholine receptor proteins in identified striatonigral neurons. Synapse 27:357–366

Iwamoto ET, Marion L (1993) Characterization of the antinociception produced by intrathecally administered muscarinic agonists in rats. J Pharmacol Exp Ther 266:329–338

Iversen SD (1997) Behavioural evaluation of cholinergic drugs. Life Sci 1997; 60:1145–52.

Janowsky DS, Overstreet DH, Nurnberger JI Jr (1994) Is cholinergic sensitivity a genetic marker for the affective disorders? Am J Med Genet 54:335–344

Kano M, Moskowitz MA, Yokota M (1991) Parasympathetic denervation of rat pial vessels significantly increases infarction volume following middle cerebral artery occlusion. J Cereb Blood Flow Metab 11:628–637

Kilbinger H (1984) Presynaptic muscarinic receptors modulating acetylcholine release. Trends Pharmacol Sci 7:103–105

Kleiber M (1975) The Fire of Life, 2nd edn. R. E. Krieger Publishing Company, Huntington, New York

Koob GF, Sanna PP, Bloom FE (1998) Neuroscience of addiction. Neuron 21:467–76.

Korczyn AD and Eshel Y (1979) Abolition of oxotremorine effects by L-DOPA pretreatment. Neuropharmacology 18:601–603

Lehmann J, Langer SZ (1982) Muscarinic receptors on dopamine terminals in the cat caudate nucleus: neuromodulation of [^{3}H]dopamine release in vitro by endogenous acetylcholine. Brain Res 248:61–69

Levey AI, Edmunds SM, Heilman CJ, Desmond TJ, Frey KA (1994) Localization of muscarinic m3 receptor protein and M3 receptor binding in rat brain. Neuroscience 63:207–221

Levey AI, Kitt CA, Simonds WF, Price DL, Brann MR (1991) Identification and localization of muscarinic acetylcholine receptor proteins in brain with subtype-specific antibodies. J Neurosci 11:3218–3226

Levey AI (1993) Immunological localization of m1-m5 muscarinic acetylcholine receptors in peripheral tissues and brain. Life Sci 52:441–448

Levine RR, Birdsall NJM, Nathanson NM, eds (1999) Proceedings of the Eight International Symposium on Subtypes of Muscarinic Receptors. Life Sci 64:355–593

Levine RR, Birdsall NJM, Nathanson NM, eds (2001) Proceedings of the Ninth International Symposium on Subtypes of Muscarinic Receptors. Life Sci 68:2449–2642

Matsui M, Motomura D, Karasawa H, Fujikawa T, Jiang J, Komiya Y, Takahashi S, Taketo MM (2000) Multiple functional defects in peripheral autonomic organs in mice lacking muscarinic acetylcholine receptor gene for the M_3 subtype. Proc Natl Acad Sci USA 97:9579–9584

Miyakawa T, Yamada M, Duttaroy A, Wess J (2001) Hyperactivity and intact hippocampus-dependent learning in mice lacking the M_1 muscarinic acetylcholine receptor. J Neurosci 21:5239–5250

Myers RD (1980) Hypothalamic control of thermoregulation: neurochemical mechanisms. In: Morgane PJ, Panksepp J (eds) Handbook of the Hypothalamus (Part A) vol. 3. Marcel Dekker, New York, p 83

Oakman SA, Faris PL, Kerr PE, Cozzari C, Hartman BK (1995) Distribution of pontomesencephalic cholinergic neurons projecting to substantia nigra differs significantly from those projecting to ventral tegmental area. J Neurosci 15:5859–5869

Olianas MC, Adem A, Karlsson E, Onali P (1996) Rat striatal muscarinic receptors coupled to the inhibition of adenylyl cyclase activity: potent block by the selective m4 ligand muscarinic toxin 3 (MT3). Br J Pharmacol 118:283–288

Paule MG, Rowland AS, Ferguson SA, Chelonis JJ, Tannock R, Swanson JM, Castellanos FX (2000) Attention deficit/hyperactivity disorder: characteristics, interventions and models. Neurotoxicol Teratol 22:631–651

Phillips JK, Vidovic M, Hill CE (1997) Variation in mRNA expression of alpha-adrenergic, neurokinin and muscarinic receptors amongst four arteries of the rat. J Auton Nerv Syst 62:85–93

Porter AC, Bymaster FP, DeLapp NW, Yamada M, Wess J, Hamilton SE, Nathanson NM, Felder CC (2002) M1 muscarinic receptor signaling in mouse hippocampus and cortex. Brain Res 944:82–89

Quirion R, Aubert I, Lapchak PA, Schaum RP, Teolis S, Gauthier S, Araujo DM (1989) Muscarinic receptor subtypes in human neurodegenerative disorders: focus on Alzheimer's disease. Trends Pharmacol Sci 10 (Suppl):80–84

Quock RM, Lucas TS (1983) Potentiation by naloxone of the anti-oxotremorine effect of L-DOPA. Eur J Pharmacol 95:193–198

Raiteri M, Leardi R, Marchi M (1984) Heterogeneity of presynaptic muscarinic receptors regulating neurotransmitter release in the rat brain. J Pharmacol Exp Ther 228:209–214

Ringdahl B, Roch M, Jenden DJ (1988) Tertiary 3- and 4-haloalkylamine analogues of oxotremorine as prodrugs of potent muscarinic agonists. J Med Chem 31 160–164

Rosenblum WI (1986) Endothelial dependent relaxation demonstrated in vivo in cerebral arterioles. Stroke 17:494–497

Rouse ST, Hamilton SE, Potter LT, Nathanson NM, Conn PJ (2000) Muscarinic-induced modulation of potassium conductances is unchanged in mouse hippocampal pyramidal cells that lack functional M_1 receptors. Neurosci Lett 278:61–64

Sanchez C, Meier E (1993) Central and peripheral mediation of hypothermia, tremor and salivation induced by muscarinic agonists in mice. Pharmacol Toxicol 72 262–267

Sato A, Sato Y (1995) Cholinergic neural regulation of regional cerebral blood flow. Alzheimer Dis Assoc Disord 9:28–38

Schwartz MW, Woods SC, Porte D Jr, Seeley RJ, Baskin DG (2000) Central nervous system control of food intake. Nature 404:661–671

Scremin OU, Jenden DJ (1996) Cholinergic control of cerebral blood flow in stroke, trauma and aging. Life Sci 5:2011–18

Shapiro MS, Loose MD, Hamilton SE, Nathanson NM, Gomeza J, Wess J, Hille B (1999) Assignment of muscarinic receptor subtypes mediating G-protein modulation of Ca^{2+} channels by using knockout mice. Proc Natl Acad Sci USA 96:10899–10904

Shimada M, Tritos NA, Lowell BB, Flier JS, Maratos-Flier E (1998) Mice lacking melanin-concentrating hormone are hypophagic and lean. Nature 396:670–674

Starke K, Gothert M, Kilbinger H (1989) Modulation of neurotransmitter release by presynaptic autoreceptors. Pharmacol Rev 69:864–989

Stengel PW, Cohen ML (2002) Muscarinic receptor knockout mice: role of muscarinic acetylcholine receptors M_2, M_3, and M_4 in carbamylcholine-induced gallbladder contractility. J Pharmacol Exp Ther 301:643–650

Stengel PW, Gomeza J, Wess J, Cohen ML (2000) M_2 and M_4 receptor knockout mice: muscarinic receptor function in cardiac and smooth muscle in vitro. J Pharmacol Exp Ther 292:877–885

Stengel PW, Yamada M, Wess J, Cohen ML (2002) M_3-receptor knockout mice: muscarinic receptor function in atria, stomach fundus, urinary bladder, and trachea. Am J Physiol Regul Integr Comp Physiol 282:R1443–1449

Swedberg MD, Sheardown MJ, Sauerberg P, Olesen PH, Suzdak PD, Hansen KT, Bymaster FP, Ward JS, Mitch CH, Calligaro DO, Delapp NW, Shannon HE (1997) Butylthio[2.2.2] (NNC 11–1053/LY297802): an orally active muscarinic agonist analgesic. J Pharmacol Exp Ther 281:876–883

Takeuchi J, Fulton J, Jia Z, Abramov-Newerly W, Jamot L, Sud M, Coward D, Ralph M, Roder J, Yeomans J (2002) Increased drinking in mutant mice with truncated M5 muscarinic receptor genes. Pharmacol Biochem Behav 72:117–123

Tong XK, Hamel E (1999) Regional cholinergic denervation of cortical microvessels and nitric oxide synthase-containing neurons in Alzheimer's disease. Neuroscience 92:163–175

Trendelenburg AU, Gomeza J, Klebroff W, Zhou H, Wess J (2002) Heterogeneity of pre-synaptic muscarinic receptors mediating inhibition of sympathetic transmitter re-lease: a study with M_2- and M_4-receptor-deficient mice. Br J Pharmacol, 138:469–480

Vilaro MT, Palacios JM, Mengod G (1990) Localization of m5 muscarinic receptor mRNA in rat brain examined by in situ hybridization histochemistry. Neurosci Lett 114:154–159

Vilaro MT, Mengod G, Palacios JM (1993) Advances and limitations of the molecular neu-roanatomy of cholinergic receptors: the example of multiple muscarinic receptors. Prog Brain Res 98:95–101

Wall SJ, Yasuda RP, Hory F, Flagg S, Martin BM, Ginns EI, Wolfe BB (1991) Mol Pharma-col 39:643–649

Weiner DM, Levey AI, Brann MR (1990) Expression of muscarinic acetylcholine and do-pamine receptor mRNAs in rat basal ganglia. Proc Natl Acad Sci USA 87:7050–7054

Wess J (1996) Molecular biology of muscarinic acetylcholine receptors. Crit Rev Neuro-biol 10:69–99

Wess J, Buhl T, Lambrecht G, Mutschler E (1990) Cholinergic receptors. In: Emmett EC (ed) Comprehensive Medicinal Chemistry, vol. 3. Pergamon Press, Oxford, p 423

Widman M, Tucker S, Brase DA, Dewey WL (1985) Cholinergic agents: antinociception without morphine type dependence in rats. Life Sci 36:2007–2015

Wise RA (1996) Neurobiology of addiction. Curr Opin Neurobiol 6:243–251

Wolfe BB and Yasuda RP (1995) Development of selective antisera for muscarinic cholin-ergic receptor subtypes. Ann N Y Acad Sci 757:186–193

Yaksh TL, Dirksen R, Harty GJ (1985) Antinociceptive effects of intrathecally injected cholinomimetic drugs in the rat and cat. Eur J Pharmacol 117:81–88

Yamada M, Miyakawa T, Duttaroy A, Yamanaka A, Moriguchi T, Makita R, Ogawa M, Chou CJ Xia B, Crawley JN, Felder CC, Deng CX, Wess J (2001a) Mice lacking the M3 muscarinic acetylcholine receptor are hypophagic and lean. Nature 410:207–212

Yamada M, Lamping KG, Duttaroy A, Zhang W, Cui Y, Bymaster FP, McKinzie DL, Felder CC, Deng CX, Faraci FM, Wess J (2001b) Cholinergic dilation of cerebral blood ves-sels is abolished in M_5 muscarinic acetylcholine receptor knockout mice. Proc Natl Acad Sci USA 98:14096–14101

Zhang W, Basile AS, Gomeza J, Volpicelli LA, Levey AI, Wess J (2002a) Characterization of central inhibitory muscarinic autoreceptors by the use of muscarinic acetylcholine receptor knock-out mice. J Neurosci 22:1709–1717

Zhang W, Yamada M, Gomeza J, Basile AS, Wess J (2002b) Multiple muscarinic acetylcho-line receptor subtypes modulate striatal dopamine release, as studied with M_1-M_5 muscarinic receptor knock-out mice. J Neurosci 22:6347–6352

Zhou H, Meyer A, Starke K, Gomeza J, Wess J, Trendelenburg AU (2002) Heterogeneity of release-inhibiting muscarinic autoreceptors in heart atria and urinary bladder: a study with M_2- and M_4-receptor-deficient mice. Naunyn Schmiedebergs Arch Phar-macol 365:112–22

Mouse Models of NO/Natriuretic Peptide/cGMP Kinase Signaling

F. Hofmann[1] · M. Biel[2] · R. Feil[1] · T. Kleppisch[1]

[1] Institut für Pharmakologie und Toxikologie, Technische Universität München,
Biedersteiner Str. 29, 80802 München, Germany
e-mail: Hofmann@ipt.med.tu-muenchen.de

[2] Department Pharmazie, Zentrum für Pharmaforschung,
Lehrstuhl Pharmakologie für Naturwissenschaftler, Ludwig-Maximilians-Universität,
Butenandtstraße 5, 81377 München, Germany

Abstract NO-generating drugs (e.g., glyceryl trinitrate) and natriuretic peptides have been long known to exert beneficial effects on cardiovascular function. Both NO and natriuretic peptides activate guanylyl cyclases which generate the second messenger cGMP. Intracellular targets for cGMP are cyclic nucleotide-regulated cation channels, phosphodiesterases and cGMP-dependent protein kinases. Here, we review the phenotypes of transgenic mice which lack or overexpress proteins involved in NO/natriuretic peptide/cGMP signaling. The analysis of these mouse models confirms existing ideas and provides new concepts on the (patho-)physiological roles of this signaling system in sensory neurons, the CNS, the cardiovascular system, and some other organs. Based on these recent findings, novel therapeutic strategies might be developed to treat human diseases.

Keywords Nitric oxide · ANP · Guanylyl cyclase · CNG · PDE · cGMP kinase · Nervous system · Cardiovascular system · Gene targeting · Transgenic mice

1
Introduction

NO-generating drugs (e.g., glyceryl trinitrate or sodium nitroprusside) have been used to treat cardiovascular diseases in humans for more than 100 years. Twenty three years ago, Furchtgott and Zawadzki (1980) reported that acetylcholine relaxed blood vessels by a factor generated in the endothelium (EDRF). Seven years later, EDRF was identified as the gas NO (Ignarro et al. 1987; Palmer et al. 1987). Since then, a plethora of pharmacological studies with NO-donor compounds and NO synthase (NOS) inhibitors underscored the importance of NO for almost all tissues including the nervous, cardiovascular, gastrointestinal, endocrine, and immune system. NO is generated by three different isozymes, the constitutively expressed neuronal and endothelial NO synthase (nNOS/NOS1 and eNOS/NOS3) and the inducible NO synthase (iNOS or NOS2). In many cells, NO activates the soluble guanylyl cyclase (sGC) and thereby increases the concentration of cyclic guanosine monophosphate (cGMP) (Fig. 1). cGMP is also generated by membrane-bound particulate guanylyl cyclases (pGCs, e.g., GC-A, GC-B, and GC-C). GC-A and GC-B are major receptors for a family of natriuretic peptides released from the heart, like atrio-natriuretic peptide (ANP), brain-natriuretic peptide (BNP), and C-type natriuretic peptide (CNP), whereas GC-C is the receptor for guanylin, an intestinal peptide involved in intestinal fluid regulation (Garbers 1992). Further analysis of the cGMP system identified a number of intracellular targets for cGMP (Fig. 1). For example, cGMP binds to cyclic adenosine monophosphate (cAMP)-specific phosphodiesterases (PDEs) and thereby modulates the concentration of cAMP. cGMP and cAMP activate cyclic nucleotide-gated (CNG) cation channels that are an important part of the signal transduction pathway in the visual and olfactory system. Most cells contain at least one of three cGMP-dependent protein kinases (cGKs): cGKIα, cGKIβ, or cGKII (Pfeifer et al. 1998; Hofmann et al. 2000). The two iso-

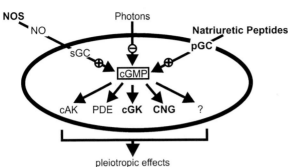

Fig. 1 NO/natriuretic peptide/cGMP signaling pathways. Shown are the signaling pathways, their components, and functional effects which will be reviewed in this chapter. Genes for which transgenic mouse models will be discussed are indicated in *bold*. For abbreviations see text. Please note that photons decrease cGMP levels (−) by a signaling cascade involving rhodopsin, transducin, and PDE6

zymes of cGKI are predominantly expressed in smooth muscle, platelets, and a subset of neurons, whereas cGKII is mainly expressed in intestinal epithelium and brain. The three cGKs are targeted by their amino termini to distinct substrates and are involved in the regulation of different cellular functions.

1.1
Scope and Limitations

Genetic modification (global and tissue-specific overexpression or deletion) and phenotype analysis of following genes have been reported: nNOS, eNOS, iNOS, the pGC GC-A, GC-C and GC-E, the natriuretic peptides ANP, BNP, CNP and the NPR3, the cGKI and cGKII. The editors requested that this chapter reviews all of these animals. Naturally this is an impossible task considering the limited space available. We will concentrate on the effects of the modification of CNG channel, NOS, pGC, ANP, and cGK genes for the sensory, nervous, cardiovascular, and intestinal system. We apologize to all those colleagues who do not find their results dealt with adequately. We would also like to point out that deletion or overexpression of a specific gene can produce phenotypes unrelated to the gene of interest. Furthermore, phenotypes can be affected severely by the genetic background of the animals and by the expression or lack of the gene product in cells not considered at all by the analysis. Thus, as is known also for other techniques, genetic modification may produce artifacts and controversial phenotypes.

The reader should keep in mind that NO signals not only through the cGMP pathway but has several effects that are independent of cGMP elevation. NO gives rise to reactive oxygen radicals (Stamler et al. 1997) and increases ADP ribosylation (Zhang et al. 1994) and nitrosylation (Xu et al. 1998; Jaffrey et al. 2001) of a number of proteins. Deletion of a NOS gene should affect all functions of NO. Therefore, it is mandatory to show which effects are mediated by cGMP, i.e., by analysis of sGC gene modifications. Analysis of mice with modification of these genes is very limited, because deletion of the sGC genes, a major target of NO, has not been reported so far. The same cautions are necessary for the effects of cGMP, because again cGMP has several effectors that may be used simultaneous in various tissues (Fig. 1). Furthermore, cGMP might activate directly or indirectly cAMP-dependent protein kinases. However, the analysis in this area is more advanced, since mice have been described with deletion of the genes encoding the CNG channels or the cGKs.

2
Cyclic Nucleotide Signaling in Sensory Neurons

2.1
Visual Transduction

Vision in vertebrates is conferred by the concerted action of two phototransduction pathways, the rod and the cone photoreceptor system. Rods are responsible for vision at low light intensities, whereas color vision and vision at high light intensities are provided by cones. In both types of photoreceptors, signal transduction is mediated by a cGMP-dependent cascade that controls the activity of a CNG channel in the surface membrane of the outer segment (Yau and Baylor 1989). In the dark, high cGMP levels activate the CNG channel, allowing a depolarizing current ("dark current") to flow into the outer segment. Light absorption by opsins initiates a G protein-mediated signaling cascade which leads to activation of a cGMP phosphodiesterase, hydrolysis of cGMP, and a fall in cytosolic cGMP levels. As a consequence, the CNG channel closes, hyperpolarizing the cell and turning off transmitter release. By closing the CNG channel, light also decreases the cellular calcium concentration, which initiates the recovery from the light response by stimulating the synthesis of new cGMP molecules by the guanylyl cyclase (Dizhoor and Hurley 1999).

The CNG channel family comprises six homologous subunits. Based on phylogenetic relationship these proteins are classified as A subunits (CNGA1-A4) and B subunits (CNGB1, and CNGB3) (Biel et al. 1999b; bradley et al. 2001a). Native CNG channels are heterotetramers composed of both types of subunits. The rod channel is composed of CNGA1 (Kaupp et al. 1989) and a long splice variant of CNGB1 (CNGB1a) (Körschen et al. 1995) whereas CNGA3 (Bönigk et al. 1993) and CNGB3 (Gerstner et al. 2000) assemble to form the cone channel. The unique role of the CNGA3 subunit for cone function was demonstrated by a gene targeting approach (Biel et al. 1999a) (Table 1). Mice lacking the CNGA3 subunit reveal a complete loss of the cone-mediated photoresponse, whereas rods function normally in these mice. The impairment of cone function correlates with a progressive degeneration of cone photoreceptors but not of other retinal cell types. The retinal phenotype of CNGA3-deficient mice is very similar to human total colorblindness (achromatopsia). Indeed, patients suffering from this disease

Table 1 Sensory neuron phenotypes of transgenic mice with genetic alterations of cyclic nucleotide signaling

Cell type	Gene	Mouse model	Phenotypes	Reference(s)
Photoreceptors	CNGA3	Null mutation	Achromatopsia	Biel et al. 1999a
			Slow degeneration of cone photoreceptors	Biel et al. 1999a
			Normal rod morphology and function	Biel et al. 1999a
	CNGA1	Overexpression of antisense RNA	Degeneration of photoreceptor and bipolar cells	Leconte and Barnstable 2000
	GC-E	Null mutation	Cone dystrophy and loss of cone function	Yang et al. 1999a
			Normal rod morphology	Yang et al. 1999a
			Paradoxical rod behavior	Yang et al. 1999a
	PDE-6γ	Null mutation	Loss of PDE function	Tsang et al. 1996
			Rapid photoreceptor degeneration	Tsang et al. 1996
Olfactory neurons	CNGA2	Null mutation	General anosmia	Brunet et al. 1996
			Impaired development of olfactory epithelium and olfactory bulb	Baker et al. 1999
			Reduced survival of olfactory neurons	Zhao and Reed 2001
			Diminished LTP on theta burst stimulation in hippocampal CA1 region	Parent et al. 1998
			Impaired axonal pathfinding in a subset of olfactory neurons	Zheng et al. 2000
	CNGA4	Null mutation	Decelerated adaptation of olfactory neurons to odor stimulation	Munger et al. 2001

have mutations in the CNGA3 gene (Kohl et al. 1998). The role of the rod CNGA1 subunit was studied by overexpressing an antisense CNGA1 RNA in a transgenic mouse model (Leconte and Barnstable 2000). These mice reveal an approximately 50% reduction of retinal CNGA1 mRNA levels and develop a degeneration of photoreceptors and bipolar cells. In agreement with this finding, mutations in the human CNGA1 gene were linked to autosomal recessive retinitis pigmentosa (RP), a heterogenous group of genetic diseases that are characterized by a progressive retinal degeneration leading to blindness (Dryja et al. 1995).

The cGMP concentration in photoreceptor outer segments is regulated by the action of pGCs and a cGMP-specific PDE. Two types of transmembrane GCs have been found in photoreceptors, GC-E and GC-F (Shyjan et al. 1992; Yang et al. 1995). Unlike the structurally related GC-A, GC-B, and GC-C, retinal GCs are not regulated by extracellular ligands but by intracellular Ca^{2+}-sensitive guanylyl cyclase-activating proteins (GCAPs) (Dizhoor et al. 1995; Gorczyca et al. 1995). GC-E-deficient mice exhibit a severe reduction in cone function within the first post-natal month and a complete loss of cone function after the first

2 months (Yang et al. 1999a). Like CNGA3 knockout mice, GC-E knockouts reveal a degeneration of cones. The morphology of GC-E-deficient rods is normal compared with wild-type mice. This finding suggests that GC-E may be the major or the only GC in cones, whereas another cyclase, possibly GC-F, is supporting rod function. Mutations in the human GC-E gene have been linked to certain cases of two inherited retinal dystrophies, Leber's congenital amaurosis (Perrault et al. 1996), and cone-rod dystrophy (Kelsell et al. 1998). The retinal phosphodiesterase (PDE-6) is an $\alpha\beta\gamma_2$ heterotetramer. The α and β subunits contain sites for cGMP hydrolysis, whereas the γ subunits serve as a protein inhibitor of the enzyme. Visual excitation of photoreceptors enables the activated GTP-bound form of the G protein transducin to remove the inhibitory action of the γ subunit, thereby triggering PDE-6 activation. Loss-of-function mutations in the catalytic α and β subunits of PDE-6 account for about 5% of RP cases (Shastry 1997). Unexpectedly, mice lacking the inhibitory PDEγ subunit (Tsang et al. 1996) reveal a reduced rather than an increased PDE activity and develop a phenotype that is similar to RP. This finding indicates that the interaction between the inhibitory PDEγ subunit and the PDE catalytic core may be critical for the proper action of the enzyme, as well as for the proper folding or conformation of the catalytic sites of the PDE$\alpha\beta$ core.

2.2
Olfaction

Olfactory receptor neurons (ORNs) respond to odorant stimulation with a receptor-mediated increase in intracellular cAMP, which directly activates a CNG channel in the plasma membrane and thereby produces a depolarization of the cell (Nakamura and GOLD 1987). Calcium ions entering through the open channel, in addition to contributing to the receptor potential, mediate cellular adaptation by reducing the cAMP sensitivity of the CNG channel and by stimulating the activity of olfactory PDE (Menini 1999; Frings 2001). The olfactory CNG channel is a tetramer composed of three different subunits, CNGA2 (Dhallan et al. 1990; Ludwig et al. 1990), CNGA4 (Bradley et al. 1994; Liman and Buck 1994), and a short splice variant of CNGB1 (CNGB1b) (Sautter et al. 1998; Bönigk et al. 1999). The physiological role of two of these subunits, CNGA2 and CNGA4, has been investigated in mouse models (Table 1).

Mice lacking the CNGA2 subunit exhibit no detectable responses to odorants, i.e., suffer from general anosmia (Brunet et al. 1996). This finding demonstrates that (1) CNGA4 and CNGB1b are modulatory subunits which in the absence of CNGA2 cannot form a functional channel and that (2) the CNG channel is required for olfactory signaling in response to many, if not all odorant stimuli. Clearly, the finding challenges the physiological relevance of alternative signaling pathways that have been proposed in the past (e.g., IP$_3$-mediated olfaction) (Boekhoff et al. 1990). The disruption of the CNGA2 gene has also morphological consequences. CNGA2-deficient mice display a thinner olfactory epithelium and a smaller olfactory bulb than wild-type mice (Baker et al. 1999). A possible explanation for this observation is that the loss of odorant-evoked depolarizations may activate apoptotic processes and thereby reduce the survival of CNGA2-deficient neurons (Zhao and Reed 2001). Finally, under theta-burst stimulation, CNGA2-deficient mice display a reduced hippocampal long-term potentiation (LTP) suggesting that the olfactory CNG channel may be involved in the control of synaptic plasticity (Parent et al. 1998).

Deletion of the CNGA4 subunit in mice produces a more subtle phenotype (Munger et al. 2001). Unlike the ORNs of CNGA2-deficient mice, ORNs of CNGA4-deficient mice respond to odorants and contain a cAMP-activated current. However, the cAMP affinity of the mutant channel is reduced by about tenfold compared with the native channel, indicating that CNGA4 is required to confer high cAMP affinity in the olfactory CNG channel. In addition, adaptation kinetics during prolonged odorant exposure is much slower in CNGA4-deficient mice than in wild-type littermates. Previous studies indicated that the principal mechanism underlying odorant adaptation is by Ca^{2+}-calmodulin (Ca^{2+}-CaM) feedback inhibition on the CNG channel (Kurahashi and Menini 1997). A high-affinity binding site for Ca^{2+}-CaM is localized in the N-terminus of the CNGA2 subunit (Liu et al. 1994). However, because Ca^{2+}-CaM binds much better to a closed rather than open CNGA2 channel, its inhibitory effect would be of little use during odorant stimulation. High-affinity binding to the open channel state requires the presence of the CNGA4 subunit (Bradley et al. 2001b; Munger et al. 2001). Thus, this subunit is needed to facilitate fast odorant adaptation.

3
NO/cGMP Signaling in the Nervous System

NO has been linked to a variety of functions in the CNS where its principal source is nNOS. This isoform is expressed ubiquitously and abundantly in the CNS. Endothelial NOS is also found in neurons, e.g., in hippocampal pyramidal cells (O'Dell et al. 1994). In contrast to these two constitutive forms of NOS, iNOS is normally not detectable in the CNS, but is upregulated after toxic stimuli within several hours. Knockout mice lacking NO synthases display diverse neuronal phenotypes characterized by an impairment in synaptic plasticity, behavior, nociception, motor function, neurotoxicity, or neurodegeneration (Table 2). Mice deficient for different NOS isozymes show divergent phenotypes, emphasizing that the function of NO largely depends on the source and localization of its generation. Note that the nNOS knockout mice referred to below carry a deletion of exon 2 which eliminates the dominant splice variant nNOSα (which accounts for ≈95% of the overall catalytic activity in the brain), but that two alternative splice variants (nNOSβ and nNOSγ) which lack exon 2 are still expressed and may represent a significant portion of total NOS in particular brain regions of these mice (Eliasson et al. 1997). This might alleviate neuronal phenotypes and, in general, complicates the interpretation of the data obtained with nNOS knockout mice. Mice lacking cGKs exhibit subtle phenotypes in the CNS.

3.1
Development of the Nervous System

Several reports suggested that pathfinding in various areas of the developing brain is affected by cGMP (Song et al. 1998; Polleux et al. 2000). A defective or aberrant guidance of nerve axons or dendrites has not been described to occur in NOS knockout mice, suggesting that NO is not involved in nerve fiber guidance. However, it was reported that the number of bifurcations in the dendritic tree of motor neurons, a useful model for studying activity-dependent synaptic development, was significantly less in nNOS-deficient than in wild-type mice (Inglis et al. 1998). In addition, it was recently demonstrated that branching of sensory nerve fibers in the entry zone of the dorsal root is defective in cGKI-null embryos leading to a decreased sensory transmission in newborn mice (Schmidt et al. 2002). Dorsal root ganglia express cGKIα, suggesting that this isozyme modifies pain perception.

3.2
Synaptic Plasticity and Learning

Cerebellar long-term depression (LTD) represents a potential cellular mechanism underlying motor learning. Fitting well with high expression of nNOS in cerebellar granule cells, LTD is abolished in the parallel fiber pathway of nNOS-mutant mice (Lev-Ram et al. 1997). Although exogenous NO and cGMP normally restore LTD blocked by inhibitors of nNOS and sGC, respectively, both failed to rescue LTD in nNOS-deficient animals (Lev-Ram et al. 1997). Most likely, the lack of nNOS induced atrophy of the signaling pathway distal from NOS in these mice. Cerebellar Purkinje cells contain high concentrations of cGKIα. Purkinje cell-specific deletion of the cGKI gene abolished cerebellar LTD, demonstrating that the NO/cGMP/cGKI signaling pathway regulates the cerebellar output (R. Feil et al., submitted). Interestingly, neither nNOS-deficient nor cGKI-deficient mice are grossly defective in motor functions (Nelson et al. 1995; R. Feil et al., submitted).

Contrary to cerebellar LTD, LTP in the CA1 region of the hippocampus is normal in nNOS-deficient mice (O'Dell et al. 1994). The brain of nNOS mutants retains significant NOS activity, possibly reflecting the function of the remaining isoform, eNOS. LTP in eNOS-deficient mice was reported to be markedly reduced (Wilson et al. 1999) or only marginally affected (Son et al. 1996). However, compound nNOS/eNOS knockout mice exhibit a strong impairment of LTP (Son et al. 1996), suggesting that NO produced by either NOS isozyme contributes to the induction of LTP. eNOS-deficient mice have also been reported to show defective LTP in other areas such as the mossy fiber pathway (Doreulee et al. 2001) and the neocortex (Haul et al. 1999). The signaling pathway of NO in CA1 LTP induction is unclear. LTP is normal in young (age below 4 weeks) conventional knockout mice lacking cGKI, cGKII, or both (Kleppisch et al. 1999). In hippocampus-specific cGKI knockout mice, LTP is normal in young animals

Table 2 CNS phenotypes of transgenic mice with genetic alterations of NO/cGMP signaling

Gene	Mouse model	Phenotypes	Reference(s)
nNOSα	Null mutation	Impairment in the development of spinal motor neurons (reduction of dendritic bifurcations)	Inglis et al. 1998
		Impaired LTD in parallel fiber synapses in the cerebellum	Lev-Ram et al. 1997
		Normal LTP in hippocampal CA1 region	O'Dell et al. 1994
		Increased aggression in male mice	Nelson et al. 1995
		Defects in maternal aggression	Gammie and Nelson 1999
		Lack of cocaine-induced locomotor sensitization and conditional place preference for the drug-paired compartment of the cage	Itzhak et al. 1998a;
		Lack of phencyclidine-induced hyperlocomotion and stereotyped turning	Itzhak et al. 1998c
		Lack of Δ^9-THC induced decrease of body temperature and ocomotor activity	Bird et al. 2001
		NOS inhibitors fail to potentiate the analgesic effect of morphine	Azad et al. 2001
		NOS inhibitors fail to block formalin-induced nociceptive behavior (e.g., licking), while the response is normal in the absence of NOS inhibitors	Li and Clark 2001
		NOS inhibitors fail to reduce the anesthesia threshold, while the threshold is normal in the absence of NOS inhibitors	Crosby et al. 1995
		Resistance to methamphetamine-induced dopaminergic neurotoxicity	Ichinose et al. 1995
		Reduction of malonate-induced striatal lesions	Itzhak et al. 1998b
		Increased resistance to cerebral ischemia	Schulz et al. 1996
		Impairment of balance/coordination selectively during night-time	Huang et al. 1994
		Defective LTP in hippocampal CA1 region	Kriegsfeld et al. 1999
eNOS	Null mutation	Defective hippocampal mossy fiber LTP	Wilson et al. 1999
		Impaired LTP in cerebral cortex	Doreulee et al. 2001
		Normal performance in radial maze learning test	Haul et al. 1999
		Improved spatial learning in water maze and increased anxiety in elevated plus-maze	Dere et al. 2001
		Lack of aggressive behavior in male mice	Frisch et al. 2000
		Normal maternal aggression	Demas et al. 1999
		Enhanced sensitivity to cerebral ischemia	Gammie et al. 2000
		Normal circadian organization in male mice	Huang et al. 1996
			Kriegsfeld et al. 2001

Table 2 (continued)

Gene	Mouse model	Phenotypes	Reference(s)
eNOS +nNOSα	Null mutation	Defective LTP in stratum radiatum of hippocampal CA1 region (but not in stratum oriens)	Son et al. 1996
iNOS	Null mutation	Decreased methamphetamine-induced hyperthermia, while methamphetamine-induced behavioral sensitization is unaffected	Itzhak et al. 1999
		Reduced zymosan-induced spinal heat sensitization	Guhring et al. 2000
		Reduction of methamphetamine-induced, but not MPTP-induced dopaminergic neurodegeneration	Itzhak et al. 1999
		Diminished MPTP-induced dopaminergic neurodegeneration	Liberatore et al. 1999
		Deficit in Morris water maze performance after traumatic brain injury, but not in control	Sinz et al. 1999
cGKI	Null mutation	Normal synaptic plasticity in the hippocampal CA1 region	Kleppisch et al. 1999
cGKII	Null mutation	Normal synaptic plasticity in the hippocampal CA1 region	Kleppisch et al. 1999
cGKI +cGKII	Null mutation	Normal synaptic plasticity in the hippocampal CA1 region	Kleppisch et al. 1999
cGKI	Hippocampus-specific mutation	Normal LTP in young animals, reduced LTP in adult animals in CA1 region	Kleppisch et al. 2002

but, interestingly, is reduced in older (age 12 weeks) mutants (Kleppisch et al. 2003). These results suggest a very intricate signaling pathway for NO/cGMP modulation of LTP in the CA1 region.

Spatial learning and memory have been associated with the induction of hippocampal LTP. However, the performance of eNOS-deficient mice is normal in a radial maze (Dere et al. 2001) and even superior in the Morris water maze (Frisch et al. 2000). The water maze performance of hippocampus-specific cGKI knockout mice is not grossly altered (Kleppisch et al. 2003).

3.3
Behavior

NOS-deficient mice attracted considerable attention due to a striking and overt behavioral phenotype. Male mice lacking nNOS exhibit extreme aggressiveness and distorted sexual behavior (Nelson et al. 1995). The importance of the genetic background for this phenotype has been reported recently (Le Roy et al. 2000). Increased aggressiveness of male mutants cannot be explained by increased levels of male sex hormones (Nelson et al. 1995). Nevertheless, excessive aggressive behavior in the mutant requires testosterone (Kriegsfeld et al. 1997). Recently, Chiavegetto et al. (2001) reported that 5-HT precursors and specific 5-HT_{1A} and 5-HT_{1B} receptor agonists diminish elevated aggression of male nNOS knockout mice, supporting the view that the phenotype is caused by selective decline in 5-HT turnover and deficient 5-HT_{1A} and 5-HT_{1B} receptor function in brain regions regulating emotion. This suggests a role for NO in normal brain 5-HT function.

Endothelial NOS appears to serve the opposite function in aggressive behavior, as mice lacking this isoform display many fewer attacks and a largely increased latency to attack the stimulus male in the resident-intruder paradigm compared to wild-type mice (Demas et al. 1999). The deletion of nNOS did not result in defects in routine behavior of females (Nelson et al. 1995), but it affected maternal aggression. Gammie and Nelson (1999) reported that the percentage of lactating nNOS-deficient females displaying aggression, the average number of their attacks against a male intruder, and the total time they spent during these attacks is significantly reduced compared to lactating wild-type mice. Following an aggressive encounter with a male intruder, the strongest increase in citrulline immunoreactivity was detected in the medial preoptical area, the suprachiasmatic nucleus, and the supraventricular zone. Surprisingly, this effect was most prominent in lactating nNOS mutant females (Gammie and Nelson 1999). In contrast to nNOS-deficient females, lactating eNOS knockout mice show normal maternal aggression (Gammie et al. 2000).

Other studies in nNOS-deficient mice have documented a specific role of this isoform in behavioral responses to psychotropics, e.g., cocaine, phencyclidine, methamphetamine (METH) and tetrahydrocannabinol (Δ^9-THC). Mice lacking nNOS were reported to be resistant to conditional place preference for the drug-paired compartment and to the progressive increase in locomotor activity induced by repeated administration of cocaine (Itzhak et al. 1998a,c). Similarly, METH failed to induce a sensitized locomotor response in these animals (Itzhak et al. 1998b), and phencyclidine-injected nNOS knockout mice displayed significantly less locomotion and stereotyped turning behavior as the corresponding wild-type animals (Bird et al. 2001). In contrast, iNOS deficiency did not affect METH-induced locomotor sensitization (Itzhak et al. 1999). Furthermore, nNOS-deficient animals lack the cannabinoid-induced decrease in locomotor activity and body temperature, while the analgesic effect of Δ^9-THC is preserved (Azad et al. 2001). Similarly, hyperthermia induced by METH was missing in mice lacking nNOS or iNOS (Itzhak et al. 1998b, 1999). These findings indicate a role for nNOS in behavioral responses including rewarding, locomotor activity, and stereotyped behavior, while nNOS and iNOS appear to be involved in thermoregulation. The signaling pathway for these behavioral phenotypes is unclear. cGKII knockout mice show a slightly enhanced fear perception in the elevated maze and an abnormal alcohol preference during a first encounter but not in later test sessions (Werner et al. 2000). No defects in other behavioral tests were reported in cGKI or cGKII mutants.

3.4
Nociception and Anesthesia

In a model of thermal hyperalgesia, mice lacking iNOS exhibited a significant delay in thermal sensitization (Guhring et al. 2000). In wild-type mice, spinal prostaglandin production rises after peripheral nociceptive stimulation. In contrast, iNOS-deficient mice did not show this response. Treatment with the NO donor RE-2047 restored both the thermal hyperalgesia and nociception-dependent stimulation of the prostaglandin production in these mice. These findings clearly demonstrate a functional role for iNOS-derived NO in spinal processing of nociceptive information. These effects are probably mediated by cGKIα (see Sect. 3.1).

The spinal analgesic effect of morphine is thought to be reduced due to activation of NOS by the drug itself. In line with this idea, the NOS inhibitor L-NAME facilitated morphine analgesia examined in a hot plate test in wild-type mice. However, L-NAME did not potentiate the analgesic action of morphine in mice lacking nNOS and morphine-induced stimulation of cGMP production was selectively absent in spinal cord slices from these mice (Li and Clark 2001). According to another study, formalin-induced nociceptive behavior (licking) is normal in mice lacking nNOS (Crosby et al. 1995). These data indicate a specific role of nNOS-derived NO for the modulation of acute analgesic actions of morphine.

NOS might negatively regulate the action of anesthetics (Johns et al. 1992). To further evaluate the role of NOS, the alveolar isoflurane concentration (EC_{50}) needed to induce anesthesia and loss of righting reflex was examined in wild-type and nNOS-deficient mice (Ichinose et al. 1995). Isoflurane concentrations required for these effects were the same in the two genotypes. However, NOS inhibitors reduced isoflurane requirement only in wild-type mice and had no effect in nNOS mutant animals, indicating that anesthetic action may be modulated by nNOS.

3.5
Neurotoxicity

Effects of NOS inhibitors imply a functional role of NO in various forms of neurotoxicity. METH and 1-methyl-4-phenyl-1,2,3,6-tetrahydropyridine (MPTP) are utilized in well-established models of dopaminergic neurotoxicity. Doses of METH causing profound depletion of dopamine and its metabolites had no effect in mice lacking nNOS (Itzhak et al. 1998b) or iNOS (Itzhak et al. 1999). Similarly, malonate-induced lesions are attenuated in nNOS knockout mice (Schulz et al. 1996). Depending on the authors, iNOS deficiency protected or did not protect against METH-induced neurotoxicity (Itzhak et al. 1999; Liberatore et al. 1999). A possible explanation for neuroprotection selectively from METH but not MPTP might give the additional lack of METH-induced hyperthermia in the iNOS-deficient mice. Taken together, these findings indicate that both nNOS and iNOS can facilitate neurotoxicity and that inhibitors of these isoforms may provide benefit in the treatment of neurodegenerative diseases.

Oppositely, a beneficial role for iNOS in traumatic brain injury (TBI) has been suggested by Sinz et al. (1999). Deletion of iNOS exaggerated the negative cognitive performance after TBI. These data correlate well with an increased loss of neurons in the CA1 and CA3 region of the hippocampus after TBI in rats treated with iNOS inhibitors (Sinz et al. 1999).

nNOS and eNOS appear to serve opposite functions in neurotoxicity following cerebral ischemia. Huang et al. (1994) have reported that basal levels of NO and cGMP are significantly reduced in the brain of nNOS mutants compared with wild-type mice and do not rise following cerebral ischemia (but see also Wei et al. 1999). In line with these findings, nNOS deficiency protects from ischemic toxicity as the magnitude of infarcts developing in various models of ischemia was substantially reduced in nNOS knockout mice (Huang et al. 1994; Hara et al. 1996; Panahian et al. 1996). There are no vascular anatomic or functional differences between nNOS-deficient and wild-type mice leading to the conclusion that, indeed, nNOS contributes to toxicity following cerebral ischemia. In contrast, eNOS is protective in cerebral ischemia: infarcts developing after cerebral ischemia are enlarged in mice lacking eNOS (Huang et al. 1996). Hemodynamic mechanisms are likely to underlie protection from cerebral ischemia by eNOS (see Sect. 4.1).

4
NO/Natriuretic Peptide/cGMP Signaling in the Cardiovascular System

4.1
NO Signaling

Since the demonstration that the endothelium-derived relaxing factor, EDRF (Furchgott and Zawadzki 1980), which mediates vasorelaxation in response to acetylcholine is NO (Ignarro et al. 1987; Palmer et al. 1987), a plethora of pharmacological studies with NO-donor compounds and NOS inhibitors underscored the importance of NO for cardiovascular function in health and disease. These experiments suggested that endogenous NO not only relaxes vascular smooth muscle cells (VSMCs), thereby, leading to vasodilatation. In addition, NO appears to modulate other important aspects of cardiovascular homeostasis, including VSMC proliferation, platelet aggregation, and cardiac contractility (Kelly et al. 1996; Lloyd-Jones and Bloch 1996). A condition of decreased bioavailability of endothelium-derived NO, termed endothelial dysfunction, may be associated with the development of hypertension and atherosclerosis. The following sections describe the major cardiovascular phenotypes observed in transgenic mice which lack or overexpress eNOS and iNOS (Table 3).

4.1.1
Blood Pressure and Hemostasis

The prominent phenotype of eNOS knockout mice is an impaired endothelium-dependent vasodilator response to acetylcholine associated with an elevated systemic blood pressure ($\approx$20%–30% higher compared to wild-type mice) both in anesthetized and awake animals (Huang et al. 1995; Shesely et al. 1996). Furthermore, eNOS knockout mice have mild pulmonary hypertension (Steudel et al. 1997). In contrast, blood pressure is normal in iNOS-deficient (Macmicking et al. 1995) and nNOS-deficient (Huang et al. 1993) mice. These findings are in line with the postulated role of endothelium-derived NO for the maintenance of normal blood pressure. The anti-hypertensive effect of eNOS-derived NO may involve direct relaxation of VSMCs and/or modulation of the baroreceptor set point (Huang et al. 1995). Although eNOS-deficient animals develop systemic hypertension, flow-induced dilation of distinct vascular beds is maintained (see Godecke and Schrader 2000, and refs. therein). These studies indicated that the loss of eNOS can be partially compensated by upregulation of nNOS and soluble guanylyl cyclase activity, as well as by mechanisms that do not require the generation of NO. Surprisingly, eNOS-null mutants showed a paradoxical decrease in blood pressure in response to the non-specific NOS inhibitor L-nitroarginine (Huang et al. 1995). This result suggests that non-eNOS isoforms are involved in the maintenance of blood pressure in these mice or, alternatively, that L-nitroarginine has effects in addition to NOS inhibition.

Table 3 Cardiovascular phenotypes of transgenic mice with genetic alterations of NO/natriuretic peptide/cGMP signaling

Gene	Mouse model	Phenotypes	Reference(s)
NO signaling eNOS	Null mutation	Systemic hypertension	Huang et al. 1995; Shesely et al. 1996
		Pulmonary hypertension	Steudel et al. 1997
		Increased leukocyte-endothelial cell interactions	Lefer et al. 1999
		Increased endotoxin-induced platelet-endothelial cell adhesion	Cerwinka et al. 2002
		Decreased bleeding time	Freedman et al. 1999
		Exaggerated response to vascular injury	Moroi et al. 1998; Rudic et al. 1998; Yogo et al. 2000
		Enhanced atherosclerosis on ApoE$^{-/-}$ background	Knowles et al. 2000; Chen et al. 2001; Kuhlencordt et al. 2001b
		Impaired angiogenesis	Murohara et al. 1998; Lee et al. 1999; Fukumura et al. 2001
		Cardiac hypertrophy (age-related)	Yang et al. 1999b; Barouch et al. 2002
		Increased infarct size after myocardial infarction	Jones et al. 1999
		Exacerbated cardiac remodeling after myocardial infarction	Scherrer-Crosbie et al. 2001
	Overexpression (endothelial)	Hypotension	Ohashi et al. 1998
iNOS	Null mutation	Reduced response to vascular njury	Chyu et al. 1999; Tolbert et al. 2001
		Reduced atherosclerosis on ApoE$^{-/-}$ background	Detmers et al. 2000; Kuhlencordt et al. 2001a
		Increased transplant atherosclerosis	Koglin et al. 1998
		Reduced pathological neovascularization in the ischemic retina	Sennlaub et al. 2001
		Improved contractile function after myocardial infarction	Sam et al. 2001
		Reduced cardioprotection after ischemic preconditioning	Guo et al. 1999
	Overexpression (cardiomyocytes)	Normal cardiac function	Heger et al. 2002
		Heart block and sudden death	Mungrue et al. 2002
nNOS	Null mutation	Suppressed beta-adrenergic inotropic responses	Barouch et al. 2002
		Cardiac hypertrophy (age-related)	Barouch et al. 2002

Table 3 (continued)

Gene	Mouse model	Phenotypes	Reference(s)
Natriuretic peptide signaling			
ANP	Null mutation	Systemic hypertension (salt-sensitive)	John et al. 1995
		Pulmonary hypertension	Klinger et al. 1999
		Cardiac hypertrophy	John et al. 1995
	Overexpression (liver)	Hypotension	Steinhelper et al. 1990
		Reduced heart weight	Barbee et al. 1994
		Blunted hypertrophic response to pulmonary hypertension	Klinger et al. 1993
BNP	Null mutation	Cardiac fibrosis	Tamura et al. 2000
	Overexpression (liver)	Hypotension	Ogawa et al. 1994
GC-A	Null mutation	Systemic hypertension (salt-resistant)	Lopez et al. 1995; Oliver et al. 1997
		Cardiac hypertrophy and fibrosis	Lopez et al. 1995; Oliver et al. 1997; Knowles et al. 2001
		Decreased infarct size after myocardial infarction	Izumi et al. 2001
	Overexpression	Hypotension	Oliver et al. 1998
NPR-C	Null mutation	Hypotension and diuresis	Matsukawa et al. 1999
cGK signaling			
cGKI	Null mutation	Systemic hypertension	Pfeifer et al. 1998
		Enhanced platelet activation	Massberg et al. 1999
	Cardiomyocyte-specific mutation	Blunted negative inotropic response to cGMP	Wegener et al. 2002

Transgenic mice overexpressing eNOS in the endothelium had a lowered blood pressure associated with reduced basal vascular tone (Ohashi et al. 1998) confirming the importance of eNOS for blood pressure regulation. Interestingly, eNOS transgenic mice displayed reduced vascular reactivity to NO, a phenomenon clinically known as nitrate tolerance. This observation suggests that chronic release of relatively high amounts of endothelial NO may induce undesirable side effects, and thus has implications for efforts to increase eNOS expression in humans to treat cardiovascular diseases.

In addition to blood pressure regulation, NO may control hemostasis and limit ischemia/reperfusion injury and thrombus formation by inhibiting vascular cell–cell interactions including platelet aggregation. Supporting this view, eNOS knockout mice showed increased leukocyte–endothelial cell interactions (Lefer et al. 1999) and platelet–endothelial cell adhesion (Cerwinka et al. 2002) as well as decreased bleeding times (Freedman et al. 1999). The roles of NOS isoforms in cerebral infarction are described above (Sect. 3.5).

4.1.2
Vascular Remodeling

Many groups have investigated the effects of NOS gene disruption on the development of vascular disorders using either models of mechanical vascular injury or the hyperlipidemic ApoE-deficient mouse model which develops diet-induced atherosclerotic lesions closely resembling the human disease (Plump et al. 1992; Zhang et al. 1992). Following mechanical vessel injury, eNOS knockout mice showed exaggerated vascular remodeling with increased neointima formation (Moroi et al. 1998; Rudic et al. 1998) which was not related to the elevated blood pressure of these mice (Yogo et al. 2000). Likewise, the development of atherosclerotic lesions on an ApoE-deficient background was accelerated in eNOS mutant animals (Knowles et al. 2000; Chen et al. 2001), eventually leading to ischemic heart disease (Kuhlencordt et al. 2001b). The increased proliferative response of the vessel wall in the absence of eNOS suggests that eNOS-derived NO may directly inhibit VSMC proliferation in response to vascular injury. However, it is not clear whether (Knowles et al. 2000) or not (Chen et al. 2001) the hypertension of eNOS knockout mice contributed to the atherogenic effects of eNOS deficiency.

In sharp contrast to the findings with eNOS mutants, iNOS knockout mice showed decreased neointimal thickening after arterial wall injury (Chyu et al. 1999; Tolbert et al. 2001) as well as reduced atherosclerosis on an ApoE-deficient background (Detmers et al. 2000; Kuhlencordt et al. 2001a). However, in a model of transplant atherosclerosis (which is initiated by immune injury), iNOS deficiency resulted in accelerated lesion formation (Koglin et al. 1998). Taken together, these findings indicate that the effects of NO on vascular remodeling are complex. In a given pathophysiologic setting, NO may both inhibit and stimulate vascular cell proliferation depending on the magnitude and spatiotemporal profile of NO synthesis. In general, it appears that eNOS-derived NO is vasoprotective, whereas iNOS-derived NO promotes vascular injury. This potential double-edged role of vascular NO may limit the usefulness of NO-based therapies for vascular disorders. Indeed, to date there is no evidence from clinical studies that treatment with NO-generating drugs has a beneficial effect on the development of atherosclerosis in humans.

Female animals were less vulnerable to vascular injury compared with male animals independent of the absence or presence of eNOS (Moroi et al. 1998) or iNOS (Tolbert et al. 2001). These results do not support the hypothesis that the vasoprotective effect of female gender is solely related to an estrogen-induced modulation of NO levels in the vascular wall. Interestingly, after removal of gonads, blood pressure and atherosclerotic lesion size were decreased in eNOS/ ApoE-deficient mice but not in ApoE-deficient mice (Hodgin et al. 2002). These unexpected findings suggest that the hypertensive and atherogenic effects of eNOS deficiency depend on the presence of endogenous sex hormones. In other words, endogenous sex hormones may in fact cause vascular damage in the absence of eNOS.

Another process which involves vascular remodeling is angiogenesis. Mice lacking eNOS showed impaired re-vascularization in response to hindlimb ischemia and this defect could not be rescued by administration of vascular endothelial growth factor (VEGF) (Murohara et al. 1998). Further studies confirmed and extended these findings showing that eNOS facilitates wound repair (Lee et al. 1999) and is involved in the increase in vascular permeability in response to VEGF (Fukumura et al. 2001). Thus, eNOS-derived NO may be an essential downstream messenger of VEGF-induced angiogenesis in adult mice and may indeed stimulate proliferative processes in the vascular system. Inducible NOS-derived NO could play a pathophysiological role in ischemic retinopathy since pathological neovascularization in the ischemic retina was reduced in iNOS-deficient mice (Sennlaub et al. 2001).

4.1.3
Cardiac Function and Remodeling

Many previous studies suggested that NO is an important regulator of cardiac muscle function (Kelly et al. 1996). However, baseline cardiac contractility was normal in eNOS knockout mice (Gyurko et al. 2000). Additional studies with eNOS-deficient mice led to inconsistent results concerning the role of eNOS for the autonomic control of cardiac function. For example, the positive inotropic response to beta-adrenergic agonists was either potentiated (Gyurko et al. 2000; Varghese et al. 2000; Godecke et al. 2001) or unaltered (Vandecasteele et al. 1999), and the anti-adrenergic effect of muscarinic agonists was either absent (Han et al. 1998) or preserved (Vandecasteele et al. 1999; Godecke et al. 2001). Furthermore, transgenic mice overexpressing eNOS in cardiomyocytes showed normal responses of the heart to acetylcholine (Brunner et al. 2001). Thus, it is not clear whether or not eNOS-derived NO modulates neurohormonal control of myocardial contractility. Mice lacking nNOS demonstrate suppressed beta-adrenergic inotropic responses, indicating that nNOS facilitates myocardial contractile reserve (Barouch et al. 2002). Interestingly, both eNOS- and nNOS-deficient mice develop cardiac hypertrophy with increasing age, and this age-related phenotype is exacerbated in compound eNOS/nNOS knockout mice supporting independent roles for each NOS isoform in maintaining normal cardiac structure (Yang et al. 1999b; Barouch et al. 2002).

The role of NOS isoforms for cardiac remodeling was studied using mouse models of myocardial infarction. After ischemia/reperfusion, infarct size was either increased (Jones et al. 1999) or unaltered (Yang et al. 1999b; Scherrer-Crosbie et al. 2001) in eNOS knockout mice. In one study, eNOS deficiency was associated with exacerbated left ventricular remodeling and dysfunction and increased mortality after myocardial infarction, and this phenotype was not affected by normalization of blood pressure (Scherrer-Crosbie et al. 2001). It was concluded that eNOS-derived NO limits the deleterious effects of myocardial ischemia by an afterload-independent mechanism, possibly by increasing capillary density and/or by decreasing myocyte hypertrophy in the remote myocardium. Mice lacking iNOS displayed improved contractile function associated with reduced myocyte apoptosis and mortality during the late phase after myocardial infarction (Sam et al. 2001). However, iNOS-deficient mice lack the protective effect of ischemic preconditioning on infarct size (Guo et al. 1999). These results suggest a protective role for eNOS after myocardial infarction, whereas iNOS can be a detrimental or beneficial depending on the specific setting of myocardial ischemia. Cardiac-specific overexpression of iNOS did not result in severe cardiac dysfunction (Heger et al. 2002) or led to a high incidence of sudden cardiac death due to bradyarrhythmia (Mungrue et al. 2002). Thus, the view that iNOS-derived NO is causally involved in the pathomechanism leading to heart failure is controversial.

In conclusion, the analysis of NOS-deficient mice not only confirmed old ideas but yielded many unexpected results leading to new concepts on the (patho-)physiological role of NO in the cardiovascular system. In many cases, eNOS- and iNOS-derived NO may have opposite effects on the structure and function of the vessel wall and heart. However, the general view that eNOS protects from and iNOS promotes cardiovascular disorders may be oversimplified. eNOS is also important for the control of glucose and lipid homeostasis, providing a link between cardiovascular and metabolic disease (Duplain et al. 2001).

4.2
Natriuretic Peptide Signaling

It has been long known that acute administration of ANP exerts diverse effects on cardiovascular and renal function including reduction of blood pressure and promotion of salt excretion (Brenner et al. 1990), but the (patho-)physiological role of endogenous natriuretic peptides and their receptors has only recently been dissected using transgenic mice (Table 3).

4.2.1
Blood Pressure and Fluid-Electrolyte Balance

Mouse null mutants for ANP (John et al. 1995) or its receptor GC-A (Lopez et al. 1995; Oliver et al. 1997) had an elevated systemic blood pressure ($\approx$10%–30% higher compared to wild-type mice). In addition, pulmonary hypertension was reported for ANP knockout mice (Klinger et al. 1999). Conversely, overexpression of ANP (Steinhelper et al. 1990) or GC-A (Oliver et al. 1998), the receptor for ANP, resulted in hypotension. ANP transgenic mice showed decreased sensitivity to ANP- and acetylcholine-dependent vasorelaxation (Ku et al. 1996), indicating that chronic ANP administration may induce tolerance. Neither ANP overexpressing mice nor GC-A knockout mice showed a significant change of blood pressure on a high-salt diet (Steinhelper et al. 1990; Lopez et al. 1995; Oliver et al. 1997). The appropriate handling of salt in these mice implies that neither ANP nor GC-A plays a critical role for normal kidney function. Taken together, these phenotypes demonstrate the physiological importance of ANP/GC-A signaling for chronic blood pressure regulation and suggest a model whereby activation of GC-A by ANP lowers blood pressure predominantly via induction of vasorelaxation but not natriuresis/diuresis. The vasodilator effect of ANP may at least in part be mediated by attenuation of vascular sympathetic tone (Melo et al. 1999).

In contrast to the findings in ANP-overexpressing and GC-A-null mice, the blood pressure of ANP-null mice was increased on a high-salt diet, pointing to a role for ANP in the regulation of kidney function. However, disruption of the ANP gene also eliminated the ANP-containing granules in the heart that may contain additional natriuretic factors (John et al. 1995). Thus, an explanation for the development of salt-sensitive hypertension in ANP but not GC-A knockout mice might be that, in the granule-deficient ANP mutant, a natriuretic factor other than ANP was lost which normally induces natriuresis/diuresis via activation of a receptor other than GC-A. Consistent with a general role for endogenous natriuretic peptides in cardiovascular/renal function, mice deficient for the NPR-C receptor which is thought to act as clearance receptor for natriuretic peptides displayed mild hypotension and diuresis (Matsukawa et al. 1999). It is unlikely that BNP is involved in the regulation of blood pressure and fluid-electrolyte balance under physiological conditions, since BNP knockout mice are normotensive on a standard-salt or high-salt diet (Tamura et al. 2000). However, BNP-overexpressing mice which show a 10- to 100-fold increase in plasma BNP are hypotensive (Ogawa et al. 1994). This result suggests that BNP may affect blood pressure if present in very high concentrations. Similar to ANP, this blood pressure-lowering effect of high BNP concentrations appears to be mediated through GC-A, whereas CNP may act through another receptor (Lopez et al. 1997).

4.2.2
Cardiac Function and Remodeling

Baseline cardiac function is not grossly affected in mice with genetic alterations of ANP, BNP, or GC-A. However, overexpression of ANP caused a reduced heart weight (Barbee et al. 1994) and prevented right ventricular hypertrophy induced by pulmonary hypertension (Klinger et al. 1993). Both ANP-deficient and GC-A-deficient mice had an increased heart-to-body weight ratio under basal conditions (John et al. 1995; Oliver et al. 1997). Further analysis revealed that cardiac hypertrophy in GC-A-null mutants is not caused by hypertension, but is exaggerated by pressure-induced overload (Knowles et al. 2001). Unexpectedly, the cardiac hypertrophy of GC-A knockout mice could not be rescued by cardiomyocyte-specific overexpression of GC-A (Kishimoto et al. 2001). Thus, the stimulation of GC-A, presumably by ANP, appears to exert an antihypertrophic effect on the heart independent of its function in blood pressure control, but it is not clear whether or not this action is mediated by the GC-A of cardiomyocytes. Interestingly, BNP knockout mice showed cardiac fibrosis in the absence of cardiac hypertrophy (Tamura et al. 2000). Cardiac fibrosis has also been reported for GC-A-deficient (Oliver et al. 1997) but not in ANP-deficient mice. Therefore, it is tempting to speculate that ANP and BNP stimulate GC-A to produce an antihypertrophic and antifibrotic effect, respectively. This model would imply important functional differences between local ANP/GC-A and BNP/GC-A signaling in the heart. Surprisingly, infarct size after myocardial ischemia/reperfusion was smaller in GC-A-deficient mice than in wild-type mice, suggesting that natriuretic peptide/GC-A signaling may contribute to pathological myocardial remodeling, possibly via the potentiation of NF-κB-mediated inflammatory processes (Izumi et al. 2001).

Taken together, the analysis of mice with genetic alterations of the natriuretic peptide system has uncovered a marked complexity of signaling via ANP, BNP, and their receptor, GC-A, in the cardiovascular system. It appears that under physiological conditions ANP/GC-A control blood pressure on the level of the vasculature and protect from cardiac hypertrophy, whereas BNP/GC-A limit cardiac fibrosis. However, in cardiovascular disease states which are associated with high levels of circulating natriuretic peptides, both ANP/GC-A and BNP/GC-A may contribute to the modulation of blood pressure and cardiac growth and may indeed be detrimental in specific pathophysiological settings like myocardial infarction.

4.3
cGK Signaling

As described in the previous sections, both NO and natriuretic peptide signaling play important roles for the maintenance of cardiovascular homeostasis. The effects of both NO and natriuretic peptides are mediated, at least in part, by activation of guanylyl cyclases and intracellular synthesis of the second messenger cGMP. cGKI is a major cGMP receptor in the cardiovascular system (Pfeifer et al. 1999; Lincoln et al. 2001) and might therefore mediate many effects of NO and natriuretic peptides.

Indeed, cGKI knockout mice (Table 3) show impaired NO/cGMP-dependent vasorelaxation and hypertension (Pfeifer et al. 1998; Sausbier et al. 2000). Furthermore, cGKI-deficient platelets display increased adhesion and aggregation during ischemia/reperfusion of the microcirculation (Massberg et al. 1999). Thus, cGKI may at least in part mediate the antihypertensive effects of NO and ANP as well as the hemostatic action of NO. In addition, cGKI improved vascular remodeling in an ischemia model (Yamahara et al. 2003). Recently, the role of cGKI in the heart has been investigated using myocardial preparations from cGKI-null mutants and from cardiomyocyte-specific cGKI knockout mice (Wegener et al. 2002). In both cGKI-deficient mouse models, the negative inotropic effect of cGMP but not carbachol was lost. These findings indicate that certain effects of NO and natriuretic peptides on cardiac function might involve cGMP and cGKI. However, it is unlikely that these pathways contribute to the anti-adrenergic action of acetylcholine.

It is important to note that with increasing age cGKI-deficient animals develop additional phenotypes including gastrointestinal dysfunction and inflammation associated with an apparent "normalization" of blood pressure and a low viability (Pfeifer et al. 1998) (Werner et al. 2001). In contrast, eNOS-, ANP-, or GC-A-null mutants are hypertensive throughout life in the absence of other severe defects and have a normal life span. These findings suggest that the apparent blood pressure "normalization" in older cGKI-deficient mice is due to the progressive pathophysiology in these mice. The fact that cGKI knockout mice develop several phenotypes that are not observed in either eNOS, ANP, or GC-A single mutants indicates that cGKI may have functions independent of these signaling systems.

5
NO/Natriuretic Peptide/cGMP Signaling in Some Other Organs

It is well established that organs like the intestine and the penis are innervated by neurons that do not release catecholamines or acetylcholine. These non-adrenergic non-cholinergic (NANC) neurons synthesize NO and usually release it together with a peptide transmitter such as aso-intestinal peptide (VIP) (Sanders and Ward 1992; Andersson 2001) In general, the effects of deletion of NOS isozymes as well as natriuretic peptides or their receptors on the function of the gastrointestinal and urogenital system have not been analyzed in detail. However, disruption of cGK genes has shown that these enzymes are important regulators in these organs (Table 4).

Table 4 Phenotypes in selected organs of transgenic mice with genetic alterations of NO/natriuretic peptide/cGMP signaling

Organ	Gene	Mouse model	Phenotypes	Reference(s)
Kidney	GC-A	Null mutation	Decreased water excretion	Dubois et al. 2000
	eNOS	Null mutation	Decreased renin secretion	Wagner et al. 2000
	cGKII	Null mutation	Increased renin secretion	Wagner et al. 1998
Bladder	cGKI	Null mutation	Decreased relaxation and rhythmic activity	Persson et al. 2000
Intestine	nNOS	Null mutation	Pylorus stenosis	Huang et al. 1993
	cGKI	Null mutation	Severe motility defects	Pfeifer et al. 1998
	cGKII	Null mutation	Decreased anion and water secretion response to STa in small intestine	Pfeifer et al. 1996; Vaandrager et al. 2000
	GC-C	Null mutation	Decreased anion and water secretion response to STa in small intestine	Schulz et al. 1997
Penis	eNOS	Null mutation	Reduced papaverine-induced penile erection	Hurt et al. 2002
	cGKI	Null mutation	Dysfunction in penile erection	Hedlund et al. 2000
Bone	cGKII	Null mutation	Short bones, defect in endo-chondral ossification	Pfeifer et al. 1996; Miyazawa et al. 2002
	BNP	Overexpression (liver)	Skeletal overgrowth	Suda et al. 1998
	CNP	Null mutation	Short bones, defect in endo-chondral ossification	Chusho et al. 2001
	NPR-C	Null mutation	Skeletal overgrowth	Matsukawa et al. 1999

5.1
Kidney and Bladder Function

NO and natriuretic peptides may affect blood pressure and other functions by modulating renin release and salt secretion. Deletion of the ANP receptor GC-A (Lopez et al. 1995; Oliver et al. 1997) resulted in elevated basal blood pressure that was not increased by a high-salt diet (salt-resistant hypertension) and a marked cardiac hypertrophy (see Sect. 4.2). Further studies showed that, in contrast to expectation, GC-A is not involved in the acute regulation of sodium excretion, but is involved in water disposal after acute expansion of the blood volume (Dubois et al. 2000).

NO appears to enhance and inhibit renin secretion. Analysis of eNOS- and nNOS-deficient mice suggested that eNOS-derived NO enhances renin release (Wagner et al. 2000) by cGMP-dependent inhibition of PDE-3 activity which results in an increase of the cAMP level (Kurtz et al. 1998). Deletion of the cGKI gene had no overt effect on salt retention or renin secretion. In contrast, disruption of the cGKII gene increased renin secretion by alleviating the inhibitory effect of NO on renin release (Wagner et al. 1998). However, this regulation is of minor importance since cGKII knockout mice do not develop high blood pressure.

cGKI has a significant effect on the motility of the urinary duct and the bladder. cGKI-deficient mice show diminished relaxation of the duct smooth muscle, reduced rhythmic contractility of the bladder, and an increased bladder volume (Persson et al. 2000).

5.2
Gastrointestinal Function

NO has been invoked in the regulation of intestinal motility, because the intestine is innervated by NANC (non-adrenergic non-cholinergic) neurons (Sanders and Ward 1992). Deletion of the nNOS had no major impact on the overall intestinal motility (Huang et al. 1993). In line with the pathology of human pylorus stenosis (Vanderwinden et al. 1992) the emptying of the stomach was slowed due to a spasm of the pylorus muscle. Relaxation of this muscle is induced in part by NANC neurons that release NO and VIP. Apparently, the lack of nNOS in these neurons decreased the release of VIP, a peptide relaxing the smooth muscle of pylorus. In contrast to these mild phenotype, deletion of cGKI resulted in severe intestinal motility defects (Pfeifer et al. 1998). Relaxation of intestinal smooth muscle by cAMP analogues was unaffected, whereas that induced by cGMP analogues was abolished. This motility defect led to an extensive increase in the passage time and may contribute to malabsorption and gastrointestinal infections.

Guanylin and the *Escherichia coli* heat-stable toxin STa increase water secretion in the small intestine through activation of GC-C. Deletion of cGKII which is expressed in the secretory epithelium of the small intestine, as well as GC-C, prevents basal and STa-induced anion and water secretion (Pfeifer et al. 1996; Schulz et al. 1997). cGKII phosphorylates the cystic fibrosis transmembrane conductance regulator (CFTR) ion channel (Vaandrager et al. 1998) which results in a stimulation of chloride and water secretion. The secretory function of cGKII is restricted to the small intestine, whereas cGMP affects water balance in the colon through modulation of PDE-3 activity and cAMP levels (Vaandrager et al. 2000).

5.3
Penile Erection

It has been well established that penile erection is mediated by NANC neurons that release NO upon excitation (Andersson 2001). It was therefore surprising that mice deficient for nNOS or eNOS bred normal and had no apparent defect in penile erection (Huang et al. 1993; Shesely et al. 1996). Presumably, deletion of one NOS gene was compensated by the other NOS enzyme. A role for eNOS in penile erection was suggested by recent work showing that pharmacologically elicited erection was associated with Akt-dependent phosphorylation and activation of eNOS, and was diminished markedly in eNOS-deficient mice (Hurt et al. 2002). Regulation of erectile function by NO is most likely mediated by cGMP and cGKI, since cGKI knockout mice demonstrate a pronounced reduction in reproductive capacity in the absence of any functional defects of cGKI-deficient sperm (Hedlund et al. 2000). cGKII-mutant mice breed normal suggesting that cGKII is not involved in mouse fertility.

5.4
Bone Growth

Deletion of cGKII resulted in mice with short bones (Pfeifer et al. 1996). Analysis of this phenotype showed that cGKII is necessary for normal endochondral ossification at the endochondral plate. Overexpression of BNP increased bone size (Suda et al. 1998). Further analyses indicated that the physiological peptide regulating bone growth is CNP acting through GC-B (Chusho et al. 2001; Miyazawa et al. 2002). Mice in which the NPR-C gene (NPR-C or NPR3 is the so-called clearance receptor for natriuretic peptides which is not coupled to cGMP production) has been inactivated by either gene targeting (Matsukawa et al. 1999) or spontaneous mutation (Jaubert et al. 1999) have locally elevated concentrations of natriuretic peptides and show skeletal overgrowth. These findings support the concept that CNP acts on endochondral ossification. The growth retardation of cGKII-deficient mice cannot be rescued by overexpression of CNP, indicating that cGKII is absolutely required for CNP-mediated regulation of endochondral bone growth (Miyazawa et al. 2002).

5.5
cGK and Phosphodiesterase

cGMP is hydrolyzed by a number of phosphodiesterases, the major enzyme being PDE-5 (Soderling and Beavo 2000). PDE-5 binds cGMP at an allosteric site which allows phosphorylation of the enzyme at Ser-92. Phosphorylation increases the activity of the enzyme and allows reduction of elevated cGMP levels (Wyatt et al. 1998; Mullershausen et al. 2001). Comparison of wild-type and cGKI knockout smooth muscle cells showed that PDE-5 is phosphorylated by cGKI in intact smooth muscle (Rybalkin et al. 2002). Phosphorylation approximately doubled the activity of PDE-5. These results suggest that cGKI controls the concentration of its activator cGMP by a classical feedback regulation. However analysis of NO-stimulated smooth muscle cells showed that cGMP levels increase to the same level in wild-type and knockout cells (Sausbier et al. 2000), suggesting that the speed of hydrolysis of cGMP was similar in each cell type. This result seems to be in line with the finding that the PDE-5 inhibitor sildenafil has strong effects on penile erection but minimal effects on vascular muscle tone. Presumably, cGMP hydrolysis is regulated also by other PDEs in vascular smooth muscle.

References

Andersson KE (2001) Pharmacology of penile erection. Pharmacol Rev 53:417–450

Azad SC, Marsicano G, Eberlein I, Putzke J, Zieglgänsberger W, Spanagel R, Lutz B (2001) Differential role of the nitric oxide pathway on delta(9)-THC-induced central nervous system effects in the mouse. Eur J Neurosci 13:561–568

Baker H, Cummings DM, Munger SD, Margolis JW, Franzen L, Reed RR, Margolis FL (1999) Targeted deletion of a cyclic nucleotide-gated channel subunit (OCNC1): biochemical and morphological consequences in adult mice. J Neurosci 19:9313–9321

Barbee RW, Perry BD, Re RN, Murgo JP, Field LJ (1994) Hemodynamics in transgenic mice with overexpression of atrial natriuretic factor. Circ Res 74:747–751

Barouch LA, Harrison RW, Skaf MW, Rosas GO, Cappola TP, Kobeissi ZA, Hobai IA, Lemmon CA, Burnett AL, O'Rourke B, Rodriguez ER, Huang PL, Lima JA, Berkowitz DE, Hare JM (2002) Nitric oxide regulates the heart by spatial confinement of nitric oxide synthase isoforms. Nature 416:337–339

Biel M, Seeliger M, Pfeifer A, Kohler K, Gerstner A, Ludwig A, Jaissle G, Fauser S, Zrenner E, Hofmann F (1999a) Selective loss of cone function in mice lacking the cyclic nucleotide- gated channel CNG3. Proc Natl Acad Sci USA 96:7553–7557

Biel M, Zong X, Ludwig A, Sautter A, Hofmann F (1999b) Structure and function of cyclic nucleotide-gated channels. Rev Physiol Biochem Pharmacol 135:151–171

Bird DC, Bujas-Bobanovic M, Robertson HA, Dursun SM (2001) Lack of phencyclidine-induced effects in mice with reduced neuronal nitric oxide synthase. Psychopharmacology (Berl) 155:299–309

Boekhoff I, Tareilus E, Strotmann J, Breer H (1990) Rapid activation of alternative second messenger pathways in olfactory cilia from rats by different odorants. Embo J 9:2453–2458

Bönigk W, Altenhofen W, Müller F, Dose A, Illing M, Molday RS, Kaupp UB (1993) Rod and cone photoreceptor cells express distinct genes for cGMP-gated channels. Neuron 10:865–877

Bönigk W, Bradley J, Müller F, Sesti F, Boekhoff I, Ronnett GV, Kaupp UB, Frings S (1999) The native rat olfactory cyclic nucleotide-gated channel is composed of three distinct subunits. J Neurosci 19:5332–5347

Bradley J, Frings S, Yau KW, Reed R (2001a) Nomenclature for ion channel subunits. Science 294:2095–2096

Bradley J, Li J, Davidson N, Lester HA, Zinn K (1994) Heteromeric olfactory cyclic nucleotide-gated channels: a subunit that confers increased sensitivity to cAMP. Proc Natl Acad Sci USA 91:8890–8894

Bradley J, Reuter D, Frings S (2001b) Facilitation of calmodulin-mediated odor adaptation by cAMP-gated channel subunits. Science 294:2176–2178

Brenner BM, Ballermann BJ, Gunning ME, Zeidel ML (1990) Diverse biological actions of atrial natriuretic peptide. Physiol Rev 70:665–699

Brunet LJ, Gold GH, Ngai J (1996) General anosmia caused by a targeted disruption of the mouse olfactory cyclic nucleotide-gated cation channel. Neuron 17:681–693

Brunner F, Andrew P, Wolkart G, Zechner R, Mayer B (2001) Myocardial contractile function and heart rate in mice with myocyte- specific overexpression of endothelial nitric oxide synthase. Circulation 104:3097–3102

Cerwinka WH, Cooper D, Krieglstein CF, Feelisch M, Granger DN (2002) Nitric oxide modulates endotoxin-induced platelet-endothelial cell adhesion in intestinal venules. Am J Physiol Heart Circ Physiol 282: H1111–1117

Chen J, Kuhlencordt PJ, Astern J, Gyurko R, Huang PL (2001) Hypertension does not account for the accelerated atherosclerosis and development of aneurysms in male apolipoprotein e/endothelial nitric oxide synthase double knockout mice. Circulation 104:2391–2394

Chusho H, Tamura N, Ogawa Y, Yasoda A, Suda M, Miyazawa T, Nakamura K, Nakao K, Kurihara T, Komatsu Y, Itoh H, Tanaka K, Saito Y, Katsuki M (2001) Dwarfism and early death in mice lacking C-type natriuretic peptide. Proc Natl Acad Sci USA 98:4016–4021

Chyu KY, Dimayuga P, Zhu J, Nilsson J, Kaul S, Shah PK, Cercek B (1999) Decreased neointimal thickening after arterial wall injury in inducible nitric oxide synthase knockout mice. Circ Res 85:1192–1198

Crosby G, Marota JJ, Huang PL (1995) Intact nociception-induced neuroplasticity in transgenic mice deficient in neuronal nitric oxide synthase. Neuroscience 69:1013–1017

Demas GE, Kriegsfeld LJ, Blackshaw S, Huang P, Gammie SC, Nelson RJ, Snyder SH (1999) Elimination of aggressive behavior in male mice lacking endothelial nitric oxide synthase. J Neurosci 19: RC30

Dere E, Frisch C, De Souza Silva MA, Godecke A, Schrader J, Huston JP (2001) Unaltered radial maze performance and brain acetylcholine of the endothelial nitric oxide synthase knockout mouse. Neuroscience 107:561–570

Detmers PA, Hernandez M, Mudgett J, Hassing H, Burton C, Mundt S, Chun S, Fletcher D, Card DJ, Lisnock J, Weikel R, Bergstrom JD, Shevell DE, Hermanowski-Vosatka A, Sparrow CP, Chao YS, Rader DJ, Wright SD, Pure E (2000) Deficiency in inducible nitric oxide synthase results in reduced atherosclerosis in apolipoprotein E-deficient mice. J Immunol 165:3430–3435

Dhallan RS, Yau KW, Schrader KA, Reed RR (1990) Primary structure and functional expression of a cyclic nucleotide- activated channel from olfactory neurons. Nature 347:184–187

Dizhoor AM, Hurley JB (1999) Regulation of photoreceptor membrane guanylyl cyclases by guanylyl cyclase activator proteins. Methods 19.521–531

Dizhoor AM, Olshevskaya EV, Henzel WJ, Wong SC, Stults JT, Ankoudinova I, Hurley JB (1995) Cloning, sequencing, and expression of a 24-kDa Ca(2+)-binding protein activating photoreceptor guanylyl cyclase. J Biol Chem 270:25200–25206

Doreulee N, Brown RE, Yanovsky Y, Godecke A, Schrader J, Haas HL (2001) Defective hippocampal mossy fiber long-term potentiation in endothelial nitric oxide synthase knockout mice. Synapse 41:191–194

Dryja TP, Finn JT, Peng YW, McGee TL, Berson EL, Yau KW (1995) Mutations in the gene encoding the alpha subunit of the rod cGMP-gated channel in autosomal recessive retinitis pigmentosa. Proc Natl Acad Sci USA 92:10177–10181

Dubois SK, Kishimoto I, Lillis TO, Garbers DL (2000) A genetic model defines the importance of the atrial natriuretic peptide receptor (guanylyl cyclase-A) in the regulation of kidney function. Proc Natl Acad Sci USA 97:4369–4373

Duplain H, Burcelin R, Sartori C, Cook S, Egli M, Lepori M, Vollenweider P, Pedrazzini T, Nicod P, Thorens B, Scherrer U (2001) Insulin resistance, hyperlipidemia, and hypertension in mice lacking endothelial nitric oxide synthase. Circulation 104:342–345

Eliasson MJ, Blackshaw S, Schell MJ, Snyder SH (1997) Neuronal nitric oxide synthase alternatively spliced forms: prominent functional localizations in the brain. Proc Natl Acad Sci USA 94:3396–3401

Freedman JE, Sauter R, Battinelli EM, Ault K, Knowles C, Huang PL, Loscalzo J (1999) Deficient platelet-derived nitric oxide and enhanced hemostasis in mice lacking the NOSIII gene. Circ Res 84:1416–1421

Frings S (2001) Chemoelectrical signal transduction in olfactory sensory neurons of airbreathing vertebrates. Cell Mol Life Sci 58:510–519

Frisch C, Dere E, Silva MA, Godecke A, Schrader J, Huston JP (2000) Superior water maze performance and increase in fear-related behavior in the endothelial nitric oxide synthase-deficient mouse together with monoamine changes in cerebellum and ventral striatum. J Neurosci 20:6694–6700

Fukumura D, Gohongi T, Kadambi A, Izumi Y, Ang J, Yun CO, Buerk DG, Huang PL, Jain RK (2001) Predominant role of endothelial nitric oxide synthase in vascular endothelial growth factor-induced angiogenesis and vascular permeability. Proc Natl Acad Sci USA 98:2604–2609

Furchgott RF, Zawadzki JV (1980) The obligatory role of endothelial cells in the relaxation of arterial smooth muscle by acetylcholine. Nature 288:373–376

Gammie SC, Huang PL, Nelson RJ (2000) Maternal aggression in endothelial nitric oxide synthase-deficient mice. Horm Behav 38:13–20

Gammie SC, Nelson RJ (1999) Maternal aggression is reduced in neuronal nitric oxide synthase- deficient mice. J Neurosci 19:8027–8035

Garbers DL (1992) Guanylyl cyclase receptors and their endocrine, paracrine, and autocrine ligands. Cell 71:1-4

Gerstner A, Zong X, Hofmann F, Biel M (2000) Molecular cloning and functional characterization of a new modulatory cyclic nucleotide-gated channel subunit from mouse retina. J Neurosci 20:1324–1332

Godecke A, Heinicke T, Kamkin A, Kiseleva I, Strasser RH, Decking UK, Stumpe T, Isenberg G, Schrader J (2001) Inotropic response to beta-adrenergic receptor stimulation and anti- adrenergic effect of ACh in endothelial NO synthase-deficient mouse hearts. J Physiol 532:195–204

Godecke A, Schrader J (2000) Adaptive mechanisms of the cardiovascular system in transgenic mice– lessons from eNOS and myoglobin knockout mice. Basic Res Cardiol 95:492–498

Gorczyca WA, Polans AS, Surgucheva IG, Subbaraya I, Baehr W, Palczewski K (1995) Guanylyl cyclase activating protein. A calcium-sensitive regulator of phototransduction. J Biol Chem 270:22029–22036

Guhring H, Gorig M, Ates M, Coste O, Zeilhofer HU, Pahl A, Rehse K, Brune K (2000) Suppressed injury-induced rise in spinal prostaglandin E2 production and reduced early thermal hyperalgesia in iNOS-deficient mice. J Neurosci 20:6714–6720

Guo Y, Jones WK, Xuan YT, Tang XL, Bao W, Wu WJ, Han H, Laubach VE, Ping P, Yang Z, Qiu Y, Bolli R (1999) The late phase of ischemic preconditioning is abrogated by targeted disruption of the inducible NO synthase gene. Proc Natl Acad Sci USA 96:11507–11512

Gyurko R, Kuhlencordt P, Fishman MC, Huang PL (2000) Modulation of mouse cardiac function in vivo by eNOS and ANP. Am J Physiol Heart Circ Physiol 278: H971–981

Han X, Kubota I, Feron O, Opel DJ, Arstall MA, Zhao YY, Huang P, Fishman MC, Michel T, Kelly RA (1998) Muscarinic cholinergic regulation of cardiac myocyte ICa-L is absent in mice with targeted disruption of endothelial nitric oxide synthase. Proc Natl Acad Sci USA 95:6510–6515

Hara H, Huang PL, Panahian N, Fishman MC, Moskowitz MA (1996) Reduced brain edema and infarction volume in mice lacking the neuronal isoform of nitric oxide synthase after transient MCA occlusion. J Cereb Blood Flow Metab 16:605–611

Haul S, Godecke A, Schrader J, Haas HL, Luhmann HJ (1999) Impairment of neocortical long-term potentiation in mice deficient of endothelial nitric oxide synthase. J Neurophysiol 81:494–497

Hedlund P, Aszodi A, Pfeifer A, Alm P, Hofmann F, Ahmad M, Fassler R, Andersson KE (2000) Erectile dysfunction in cyclic GMP-dependent kinase I-deficient mice. Proc Natl Acad Sci USA 97:2349–2354

Heger J, Godecke A, Flogel U, Merx MW, Molojavyi A, Kuhn-Velten WN, Schrader J (2002) Cardiac-specific overexpression of inducible nitric oxide synthase does not result in severe cardiac dysfunction. Circ Res 90:93–99

Hodgin JB, Knowles JW, Kim HS, Smithies O, Maeda N (2002) Interactions between endothelial nitric oxide synthase and sex hormones in vascular protection in mice. J Clin Invest 109:541–548

Hofmann F, Ammendola A, Schlossmann J (2000) Rising behind NO: cGMP-dependent protein kinases. J Cell Sci 113:1671–1676

Huang PL, Dawson TM, Bredt DS, Snyder SH, Fishman MC (1993) Targeted disruption of the neuronal nitric oxide synthase gene. Cell 75:1273–1286

Huang PL, Huang Z, Mashimo H, Bloch KD, Moskowitz MA, Bevan JA, Fishman MC (1995) Hypertension in mice lacking the gene for endothelial nitric oxide synthase. Nature 377:239–242

Huang Z, Huang PL, Ma J, Meng W, Ayata C, Fishman MC, Moskowitz MA (1996) Enlarged infarcts in endothelial nitric oxide synthase knockout mice are attenuated by nitro-L-arginine. J Cereb Blood Flow Metab 16:981–987

Huang Z, Huang PL, Panahian N, Dalkara T, Fishman MC, Moskowitz MA (1994) Effects of cerebral ischemia in mice deficient in neuronal nitric oxide synthase. Science 265:1883–1885

Hurt KJ, Musicki B, Palese MA, Crone JK, Becker RE, Moriarity JL, Snyder SH, Burnett AL (2002) Akt-dependent phosphorylation of endothelial nitric-oxide synthase mediates penile erection. Proc Natl Acad Sci USA 99:4061–4066

Ichinose F, Huang PL, Zapol WM (1995) Effects of targeted neuronal nitric oxide synthase gene disruption and nitroG-L-arginine methylester on the threshold for isoflurane anesthesia. Anesthesiology 83:101–108

Ignarro LJ, Buga GM, Wood KS, Byrns RE, Chaudhuri G (1987) Endothelium-derived relaxing factor produced and released from artery and vein is nitric oxide. Proc Natl Acad Sci USA 84:9265–9269

Inglis FM, Furia F, Zuckerman KE, Strittmatter SM, Kalb RG (1998) The role of nitric oxide and NMDA receptors in the development of motor neuron dendrites. J Neurosci 18:10493–10501

Itzhak Y, Ali SF, Martin JL, Black MD, Huang PL (1998a) Resistance of neuronal nitric oxide synthase-deficient mice to cocaine- induced locomotor sensitization. Psychopharmacology (Berl) 140:378–386

Itzhak Y, Gandia C, Huang PL, Ali SF (1998b) Resistance of neuronal nitric oxide synthase-deficient mice to methamphetamine-induced dopaminergic neurotoxicity. J Pharmacol Exp Ther 284:1040–1047

Itzhak Y, Martin JL, Ali SF (1999) Methamphetamine- and 1-methyl-4-phenyl- 1,2,3, 6-tetrahydropyridine- induced dopaminergic neurotoxicity in inducible nitric oxide synthase- deficient mice. Synapse 34:305–312

Itzhak Y, Martin JL, Black MD, Huang PL (1998c) The role of neuronal nitric oxide synthase in cocaine-induced conditioned place preference. Neuroreport 9:2485–2488

Izumi T, Saito Y, Kishimoto I, Harada M, Kuwahara K, Hamanaka I, Takahashi N, Kawakami R, Li Y, Takemura G, Fujiwara H, Garbers DL, Mochizuki S, Nakao K (2001) Blockade of the natriuretic peptide receptor guanylyl cyclase-A inhibits NF-kappaB activation and alleviates myocardial ischemia/reperfusion injury. J Clin Invest 108:203–213

Jaffrey SR, Erdjument-Bromage H, Ferris CD, Tempst P, Snyder SH (2001) Protein S-nitrosylation: a physiological signal for neuronal nitric oxide. Nat Cell Biol 3:193–197

Jaubert J, Jaubert F, Martin N, Washburn LL, Lee BK, Eicher EM, Guenet JL (1999) Three new allelic mouse mutations that cause skeletal overgrowth involve the natriuretic peptide receptor C gene (Npr3). Proc Natl Acad Sci USA 96:10278–10283

John SW, Krege JH, Oliver PM, Hagaman JR, Hodgin JB, Pang SC, Flynn TG, Smithies O (1995) Genetic decreases in atrial natriuretic peptide and salt-sensitive hypertension. Science 267:679–681

Johns RA, Moscicki JC, DiFazio CA (1992) Nitric oxide synthase inhibitor dose-dependently and reversibly reduces the threshold for halothane anesthesia. A role for nitric oxide in mediating consciousness? Anesthesiology 77:779–784

Jones SP, Girod WG, Palazzo AJ, Granger DN, Grisham MB, Jourd'Heuil D, Huang PL, Lefer DJ (1999) Myocardial ischemia-reperfusion injury is exacerbated in absence of endothelial cell nitric oxide synthase. Am J Physiol 276: H1567–1573

Kaupp UB, Niidome T, Tanabe T, Terada S, Bönigk W, Stühmer W, Cook NJ, Kangawa K, Matsuo H, Hirose T, et al. (1989) Primary structure and functional expression from complementary DNA of the rod photoreceptor cyclic GMP-gated channel. Nature 342:762–766

Kelly RA, Balligand JL, Smith TW (1996) Nitric oxide and cardiac function. Circ Res 79:363–380

Kelsell RE, Gregory-Evans K, Payne AM, Perrault I, Kaplan J, Yang RB, Garbers DL, Bird AC, Moore AT, Hunt DM (1998) Mutations in the retinal guanylate cyclase (RETGC-1) gene in dominant cone-rod dystrophy. Hum Mol Genet 7:1179–1184

Kishimoto I, Rossi K, Garbers DL (2001) A genetic model provides evidence that the receptor for atrial natriuretic peptide (guanylyl cyclase-A) inhibits cardiac ventricular myocyte hypertrophy. Proc Natl Acad Sci USA 98:2703–2706

Kleppisch T, Pfeifer A, Klatt P, Ruth P, Montkowski A, Fassler R, Hofmann F (1999) Long-term potentiation in the hippocampal CA1 region of mice lacking cGMP-dependent kinases is normal and susceptible to inhibition of nitric oxide synthase. J Neurosci 19:48–55

Kleppisch T, Wolfsgruber W, Feil S, Allmann R, Wotjak CT, Goebbels S, Nave K-A, Hofmann F, Feil R (2003) Hippocampal cyclic GMP-dependent protein kinase I supports an age- and protein synthesis-dependent component of long-term potentiation but is not essential for spatial reference and contextual memory. J Neurosci (in press)

Klinger JR, Petit RD, Curtin LA, Warburton RR, Wrenn DS, Steinhelper ME, Field LJ, Hill NS (1993) Cardiopulmonary responses to chronic hypoxia in transgenic mice that overexpress ANP. J Appl Physiol 75:198–205

Klinger JR, Warburton RR, Pietras LA, Smithies O, Swift R, Hill NS (1999) Genetic disruption of atrial natriuretic peptide causes pulmonary hypertension in normoxic and hypoxic mice. Am J Physiol 276: L868–874

Knowles JW, Esposito G, Mao L, Hagaman JR, Fox JE, Smithies O, Rockman HA, Maeda N (2001) Pressure-independent enhancement of cardiac hypertrophy in natriuretic peptide receptor A-deficient mice. J Clin Invest 107:975–984

Knowles JW, Reddick RL, Jennette JC, Shesely EG, Smithies O, Maeda N (2000) Enhanced atherosclerosis and kidney dysfunction in eNOS(-/-)Apoe(-/-) mice are ameliorated by enalapril treatment. J Clin Invest 105:451–458

Koglin J, Glysing-Jensen T, Mudgett JS, Russell ME (1998) Exacerbated transplant arteriosclerosis in inducible nitric oxide- deficient mice. Circulation 97:2059–2065

Kohl S, Marx T, Giddings I, Jägle H, Jacobson SG, Apfelstedt-Sylla E, Zrenner E, Sharpe LT, Wissinger B (1998) Total colourblindness is caused by mutations in the gene encoding the alpha-subunit of the cone photoreceptor cGMP-gated cation channel. Nat Genet 19:257–259

Körschen HG, Illing M, Seifert R, Sesti F, Williams A, Gotzes S, Colville C, Müller F, Dosé A, Godde M, et al. (1995) A 240 kDa protein represents the complete beta subunit of the cyclic nucleotide-gated channel from rod photoreceptor. Neuron 15:627–636

Kriegsfeld LJ, Dawson TM, Dawson VL, Nelson RJ, Snyder SH (1997) Aggressive behavior in male mice lacking the gene for neuronal nitric oxide synthase requires testosterone. Brain Res 769:66–70

Kriegsfeld LJ, Drazen DL, Nelson RJ (2001) Circadian organization in male mice lacking the gene for endothelial nitric oxide synthase (eNOS-/-). J Biol Rhythms 16:142–148

Kriegsfeld LJ, Eliasson MJ, Demas GE, Blackshaw S, Dawson TM, Nelson RJ, Snyder SH (1999) Nocturnal motor coordination deficits in neuronal nitric oxide synthase knock-out mice. Neuroscience 89:311–315

Ku DD, Guo L, Dai J, Acuff CG, Steinhelper ME (1996) Coronary vascular and endothelial reactivity changes in transgenic mice overexpressing atrial natriuretic factor. Am J Physiol 271: H2368–2376

Kuhlencordt PJ, Chen J, Han F, Astern J, Huang PL (2001a) Genetic deficiency of inducible nitric oxide synthase reduces atherosclerosis and lowers plasma lipid peroxides in apolipoprotein E- knockout mice. Circulation 103:3099–3104

Kuhlencordt PJ, Gyurko R, Han F, Scherrer-Crosbie M, Aretz TH, Hajjar R, Picard MH, Huang PL (2001b) Accelerated atherosclerosis, aortic aneurysm formation, and ischemic heart disease in apolipoprotein E/endothelial nitric oxide synthase double-knockout mice. Circulation 104:448–454

Kurahashi T, Menini A (1997) Mechanism of odorant adaptation in the olfactory receptor cell. Nature 385:725–729

Kurtz A, Gotz KH, Hamann M, Wagner C (1998) Stimulation of renin secretion by nitric oxide is mediated by phosphodiesterase 3. Proc Natl Acad Sci USA 95:4743–4747

Le Roy I, Pothion S, Mortaud S, Chabert C, Nicolas L, Cherfouh A, Roubertoux PL (2000) Loss of aggression, after transfer onto a C57BL/6 J background, in mice carrying a targeted disruption of the neuronal nitric oxide synthase gene. Behav Genet 30:367–373

Leconte L, Barnstable CJ (2000) Impairment of rod cGMP-gated channel alpha-subunit expression leads to photoreceptor and bipolar cell degeneration. Invest Ophthalmol Vis Sci 41:917–926

Lee PC, Salyapongse AN, Bragdon GA, Shears LL, 2nd, Watkins SC, Edington HD, Billiar TR (1999) Impaired wound healing and angiogenesis in eNOS-deficient mice. Am J Physiol 277:H1600–1608

Lefer DJ, Jones SP, Girod WG, Baines A, Grisham MB, Cockrell AS, Huang PL, Scalia R (1999) Leukocyte-endothelial cell interactions in nitric oxide synthase- deficient mice. Am J Physiol 276: H1943–1950

Lev-Ram V, Nebyelul Z, Ellisman MH, Huang PL, Tsien RY (1997) Absence of cerebellar long-term depression in mice lacking neuronal nitric oxide synthase. Learn Mem 4:169–177

Li X, Clark JD (2001) Spinal cord nitric oxide synthase and heme oxygenase limit morphine induced analgesia. Brain Res Mol Brain Res 95:96–102

Liberatore GT, Jackson-Lewis V, Vukosavic S, Mandir AS, Vila M, McAuliffe WG, Dawson VL, Dawson TM, Przedborski S (1999) Inducible nitric oxide synthase stimulates dopaminergic neurodegeneration in the MPTP model of Parkinson disease. Nat Med 5:1403–1409

Liman ER, Buck LB (1994) A second subunit of the olfactory cyclic nucleotide-gated channel confers high sensitivity to cAMP. Neuron 13:611–621

Lincoln TM, Dey N, Sellak H (2001) Invited Review: cGMP-dependent protein kinase signaling mechanisms in smooth muscle: from the regulation of tone to gene expression. J Appl Physiol 91:1421–1430

Liu M, Chen TY, Ahamed B, Li J, Yau KW (1994) Calcium-calmodulin modulation of the olfactory cyclic nucleotide-gated cation channel. Science 266:1348–1354

Lloyd-Jones DM, Bloch KD (1996) The vascular biology of nitric oxide and its role in atherogenesis. Annu Rev Med 47:365–375

Lopez MJ, Garbers DL, Kuhn M (1997) The guanylyl cyclase-deficient mouse defines differential pathways of natriuretic peptide signaling. J Biol Chem 272:23064–23068

Lopez MJ, Wong SK, Kishimoto I, Dubois S, Mach V, Friesen J, Garbers DL, Beuve A (1995) Salt-resistant hypertension in mice lacking the guanylyl cyclase-A receptor for atrial natriuretic peptide. Nature 378:65–68

Ludwig J, Margalit T, Eismann E, Lancet D, Kaupp UB (1990) Primary structure of cAMP-gated channel from bovine olfactory epithelium. FEBS Lett 270:24–29

MacMicking JD, Nathan C, Hom G, Chartrain N, Fletcher DS, Trumbauer M, Stevens K, Xie QW, Sokol K, Hutchinson N, et al. (1995) Altered responses to bacterial infection and endotoxic shock in mice lacking inducible nitric oxide synthase. Cell 81:641–650

Massberg S, Sausbier M, Klatt P, Bauer M, Pfeifer A, Siess W, Fassler R, Ruth P, Krombach F, Hofmann F (1999) Increased adhesion and aggregation of platelets lacking cyclic guanosine 3',5'-monophosphate kinase I. J Exp Med 189:1255–1264

Matsukawa N, Grzesik WJ, Takahashi N, Pandey KN, Pang S, Yamauchi M, Smithies O (1999) The natriuretic peptide clearance receptor locally modulates the physiological effects of the natriuretic peptide system. Proc Natl Acad Sci USA 96:7403–7408

Melo LG, Veress AT, Ackermann U, Steinhelper ME, Pang SC, Tse Y, Sonnenberg H (1999) Chronic regulation of arterial blood pressure in ANP transgenic and knockout mice: role of cardiovascular sympathetic tone. Cardiovasc Res 43:437–444

Menini A (1999) Calcium signalling and regulation in olfactory neurons. Curr Opin Neurobiol 9:419–426

Miyazawa T, Ogawa Y, Chusho H, Yasoda A, Tamura N, Komatsu Y, Pfeifer A, Hofmann F, Nakao K (2002) Cyclic GMP-dependent protein kinase ii plays a critical role in c-type natriuretic peptide-mediated endochondral ossification. Endocrinology 143:3604–3610

Moroi M, Zhang L, Yasuda T, Virmani R, Gold HK, Fishman MC, Huang PL (1998) Interaction of genetic deficiency of endothelial nitric oxide, gender, and pregnancy in vascular response to injury in mice. J Clin Invest 101:1225–1232

Mullershausen F, Russwurm M, Thompson WJ, Liu L, Koesling D, Friebe A (2001) Rapid nitric oxide-induced desensitization of the cGMP response is caused by increased activity of phosphodiesterase type 5 paralleled by phosphorylation of the enzyme. J Cell Biol 155:271–278

Munger SD, Lane AP, Zhong H, Leinders-Zufall T, Yau KW, Zufall F, Reed RR (2001) Central role of the CNGA4 channel subunit in Ca2+-calmodulin-dependent odor adaptation. Science 294:2172–2175

Mungrue IN, Gros R, You X, Pirani A, Azad A, Csont T, Schulz R, Butany J, Stewart DJ, Husain M (2002) Cardiomyocyte overexpression of iNOS in mice results in peroxynitrite generation, heart block, and sudden death. J Clin Invest 109:735–743

Murohara T, Asahara T, Silver M, Bauters C, Masuda H, Kalka C, Kearney M, Chen D, Symes JF, Fishman MC, Huang PL, Isner JM (1998) Nitric oxide synthase modulates angiogenesis in response to tissue ischemia. J Clin Invest 101:2567–2578

Nakamura T, Gold GH (1987) A cyclic nucleotide-gated conductance in olfactory receptor cilia. Nature 325:442–444

Nelson RJ, Demas GE, Huang PL, Fishman MC, Dawson VL, Dawson TM, Snyder SH (1995) Behavioural abnormalities in male mice lacking neuronal nitric oxide synthase. Nature 378:383–386

O'Dell TJ, Huang PL, Dawson TM, Dinerman JL, Snyder SH, Kandel ER, Fishman MC (1994) Endothelial NOS and the blockade of LTP by NOS inhibitors in mice lacking neuronal NOS. Science 265:542–546

Ogawa Y, Itoh H, Tamura N, Suga S, Yoshimasa T, Uehira M, Matsuda S, Shiono S, Nishimoto H, Nakao K (1994) Molecular cloning of the complementary DNA and gene that encode mouse brain natriuretic peptide and generation of transgenic mice that overexpress the brain natriuretic peptide gene. J Clin Invest 93:1911–1921

Ohashi Y, Kawashima S, Hirata K, Yamashita T, Ishida T, Inoue N, Sakoda T, Kurihara H, Yazaki Y, Yokoyama M (1998) Hypotension and reduced nitric oxide-elicited vasorelaxation in transgenic mice overexpressing endothelial nitric oxide synthase. J Clin Invest 102:2061–2071

Oliver PM, Fox JE, Kim R, Rockman HA, Kim HS, Reddick RL, Pandey KN, Milgram SL, Smithies O, Maeda N (1997) Hypertension, cardiac hypertrophy, and sudden death in mice lacking natriuretic peptide receptor A. Proc Natl Acad Sci USA 94:14730–14735

Oliver PM, John SW, Purdy KE, Kim R, Maeda N, Goy MF, Smithies O (1998) Natriuretic peptide receptor 1 expression influences blood pressures of mice in a dose-dependent manner. Proc Natl Acad Sci USA 95:2547–2551

Palmer RM, Ferrige AG, Moncada S (1987) Nitric oxide release accounts for the biological activity of endothelium-derived relaxing factor. Nature 327:524–526

Panahian N, Yoshida T, Huang PL, Hedley-Whyte ET, Dalkara T, Fishman MC, Moskowitz MA (1996) Attenuated hippocampal damage after global cerebral ischemia in mice mutant in neuronal nitric oxide synthase. Neuroscience 72:343–354

Parent A, Schrader K, Munger SD, Reed RR, Linden DJ, Ronnett GV (1998) Synaptic transmission and hippocampal long-term potentiation in olfactory cyclic nucleotide-gated channel type 1 null mouse. J Neurophysiol 79:3295–3301

Perrault I, Rozet JM, Calvas P, Gerber S, Camuzat A, Dollfus H, Chatelin S, Souied E, Ghazi I, Leowski C, Bonnemaison M, Le Paslier D, Frezal J, Dufier JL, Pittler S, Munnich A, Kaplan J (1996) Retinal-specific guanylate cyclase gene mutations in Leber's congenital amaurosis. Nat Genet 14:461–464

Persson K, Pandita RK, Aszodi A, Ahmad M, Pfeifer A, Fassler R, Andersson KE (2000) Functional characteristics of urinary tract smooth muscles in mice lacking cGMP protein kinase type I. Am J Physiol Regul Integr Comp Physiol 279: R1112–1120

Pfeifer A, Aszodi A, Seidler U, Ruth P, Hofmann F, Fassler R (1996) Intestinal secretory defects and dwarfism in mice lacking cGMP- dependent protein kinase II. Science 274:2082–2086

Pfeifer A, Klatt P, Massberg S, Ny L, Sausbier M, Hirneiss C, Wang GX, Korth M, Aszodi A, Andersson KE, Krombach F, Mayerhofer A, Ruth P, Fassler R, Hofmann F (1998) Defective smooth muscle regulation in cGMP kinase I-deficient mice. Embo J 17:3045–3051

Pfeifer A, Ruth P, Dostmann W, Sausbier M, Klatt P, Hofmann F (1999) Structure and function of cGMP-dependent protein kinases. Rev Physiol Biochem Pharmacol 135:105–149

Plump AS, Smith JD, Hayek T, Aalto-Setala K, Walsh A, Verstuyft JG, Rubin EM, Breslow JL (1992) Severe hypercholesterolemia and atherosclerosis in apolipoprotein E-deficient mice created by homologous recombination in ES cells. Cell 71:343–353

Polleux F, Morrow T, Ghosh A (2000) Semaphorin 3A is a chemoattractant for cortical apical dendrites. Nature 404:567–573

Rudic RD, Shesely EG, Maeda N, Smithies O, Segal SS, Sessa WC (1998) Direct evidence for the importance of endothelium-derived nitric oxide in vascular remodeling. J Clin Invest 101:731–736

Rybalkin SD, Rybalkina IG, Feil R, Hofmann F, Beavo JA (2002) Regulation of cGMP-specific phosphodiesterase (PDE5) phosphorylation in smooth muscle cells. J Biol Chem 277:3310–3317

Sam F, Sawyer DB, Xie Z, Chang DL, Ngoy S, Brenner DA, Siwik DA, Singh K, Apstein CS, Colucci WS (2001) Mice lacking inducible nitric oxide synthase have improved left ventricular contractile function and reduced apoptotic cell death late after myocardial infarction. Circ Res 89:351–356

Sanders KM, Ward SM (1992) Nitric oxide as a mediator of nonadrenergic noncholinergic neurotransmission. Am J Physiol 262: G379–392

Sausbier M, Schubert R, Voigt V, Hirneiss C, Pfeifer A, Korth M, Kleppisch T, Ruth P, Hofmann F (2000) Mechanisms of NO/cGMP-dependent vasorelaxation. Circ Res 87:825–830

Sautter A, Zong X, Hofmann F, Biel M (1998) An isoform of the rod photoreceptor cyclic nucleotide-gated channel beta subunit expressed in olfactory neurons. Proc Natl Acad Sci USA 95:4696–4701

Scherrer-Crosbie M, Ullrich R, Bloch KD, Nakajima H, Nasseri B, Aretz HT, Lindsey ML, Vancon AC, Huang PL, Lee RT, Zapol WM, Picard MH (2001) Endothelial nitric oxide synthase limits left ventricular remodeling after myocardial infarction in mice. Circulation 104:1286–1291

Schmidt H, Werner M, Heppenstall PA, Henning M, Moré MI, Kühbandner S, Lewin GR, Hofmann F, Feil R, Rathjen FG (2002) cGMP-mediated signaling via cGKIα is required for the guidance and connectivity of sensory axons. J Cell Biol 159:489–498

Schulz JB, Huang PL, Matthews RT, Passov D, Fishman MC, Beal MF (1996) Striatal malonate lesions are attenuated in neuronal nitric oxide synthase knockout mice. J Neurochem 67:430–433

Schulz S, Lopez MJ, Kuhn M, Garbers DL (1997) Disruption of the guanylyl cyclase-C gene leads to a paradoxical phenotype of viable but heat-stable enterotoxin-resistant mice. J Clin Invest 100:1590–1595

Sennlaub F, Courtois Y, Goureau O (2001) Inducible nitric oxide synthase mediates the change from retinal to vitreal neovascularization in ischemic retinopathy. J Clin Invest 107:717–725

Shastry BS (1997) Signal transduction in the retina and inherited retinopathies. Cell Mol Life Sci 53:419–429

Shesely EG, Maeda N, Kim HS, Desai KM, Krege JH, Laubach VE, Sherman PA, Sessa WC, Smithies O (1996) Elevated blood pressures in mice lacking endothelial nitric oxide synthase. Proc Natl Acad Sci USA 93:13176–13181

Shyjan AW, de Sauvage FJ, Gillett NA, Goeddel DV, Lowe DG (1992) Molecular cloning of a retina-specific membrane guanylyl cyclase. Neuron 9:727–737

Sinz EH, Kochanek PM, Dixon CE, Clark RS, Carcillo JA, Schiding JK, Chen M, Wisniewski SR, Carlos TM, Williams D, DeKosky ST, Watkins SC, Marion DW, Billiar TR (1999) Inducible nitric oxide synthase is an endogenous neuroprotectant after traumatic brain injury in rats and mice. J Clin Invest 104:647–656

Soderling SH, Beavo JA (2000) Regulation of cAMP and cGMP signaling: new phosphodiesterases and new functions. Curr Opin Cell Biol 12:174–179

Son H, Hawkins RD, Martin K, Kiebler M, Huang PL, Fishman MC, Kandel ER (1996) Long-term potentiation is reduced in mice that are doubly mutant in endothelial and neuronal nitric oxide synthase. Cell 87:1015–1023

Song H, Ming G, He Z, Lehmann M, McKerracher L, Tessier-Lavigne M, Poo M (1998) Conversion of neuronal growth cone responses from repulsion to attraction by cyclic nucleotides. Science 281:1515–1518

Stamler JS, Toone EJ, Lipton SA, Sucher NJ (1997) (S)NO signals: translocation, regulation, and a consensus motif. Neuron 18:691–696

Steinhelper ME, Cochrane KL, Field LJ (1990) Hypotension in transgenic mice expressing atrial natriuretic factor fusion genes. Hypertension 16:301–307

Steudel W, Ichinose F, Huang PL, Hurford WE, Jones RC, Bevan JA, Fishman MC, Zapol WM (1997) Pulmonary vasoconstriction and hypertension in mice with targeted disruption of the endothelial nitric oxide synthase (NOS 3) gene. Circ Res 81:34–41

Suda M, Ogawa Y, Tanaka K, Tamura N, Yasoda A, Takigawa T, Uehira M, Nishimoto H, Itoh H, Saito Y, Shiota K, Nakao K (1998) Skeletal overgrowth in transgenic mice that overexpress brain natriuretic peptide. Proc Natl Acad Sci USA 95:2337–2342

Tamura N, Ogawa Y, Chusho H, Nakamura K, Nakao K, Suda M, Kasahara M, Hashimoto R, Katsuura G, Mukoyama M, Itoh H, Saito Y, Tanaka I, Otani H, Katsuki M (2000) Cardiac fibrosis in mice lacking brain natriuretic peptide. Proc Natl Acad Sci USA 97:4239–4244

Tolbert T, Thompson JA, Bouchard P, Oparil S (2001) Estrogen-induced vasoprotection is independent of inducible nitric oxide synthase expression: evidence from the mouse carotid artery ligation model. Circulation 104:2740–2745

Tsang SH, Gouras P, Yamashita CK, Kjeldbye H, Fisher J, Farber DB, Goff SP (1996) Retinal degeneration in mice lacking the gamma subunit of the rod cGMP phosphodiesterase. Science 272:1026–1029

Vaandrager AB, Bot AG, Ruth P, Pfeifer A, Hofmann F, De Jonge HR (2000) Differential role of cyclic GMP-dependent protein kinase II in ion transport in murine small intestine and colon. Gastroenterology 118:108–114

Vaandrager AB, Smolenski A, Tilly BC, Houtsmuller AB, Ehlert EM, Bot AG, Edixhoven M, Boomaars WE, Lohmann SM, de Jonge HR (1998) Membrane targeting of cGMP-dependent protein kinase is required for cystic fibrosis transmembrane conductance regulator Cl- channel activation. Proc Natl Acad Sci USA 95:1466–1471

Vandecasteele G, Eschenhagen T, Scholz H, Stein B, Verde I, Fischmeister R (1999) Muscarinic and beta-adrenergic regulation of heart rate, force of contraction and calcium current is preserved in mice lacking endothelial nitric oxide synthase. Nat Med 5:331–334

Vanderwinden JM, Mailleux P, Schiffmann SN, Vanderhaeghen JJ, De Laet MH (1992) Nitric oxide synthase activity in infantile hypertrophic pyloric stenosis. N Engl J Med 327:511–515

Varghese P, Harrison RW, Lofthouse RA, Georgakopoulos D, Berkowitz DE, Hare JM (2000) beta(3)-adrenoceptor deficiency blocks nitric oxide-dependent inhibition of myocardial contractility. J Clin Invest 106:697–703

Wagner C, Godecke A, Ford M, Schnermann J, Schrader J, Kurtz A (2000) Regulation of renin gene expression in kidneys of eNOS- and nNOS- deficient mice. Pflugers Arch 439:567–572

Wagner C, Pfeifer A, Ruth P, Hofmann F, Kurtz A (1998) Role of cGMP-kinase II in the control of renin secretion and renin expression. J Clin Invest 102:1576–1582

Wegener JW, Nawrath H, Wolfsgruber W, Kuhbandner S, Werner C, Hofmann F, Feil R (2002) cGMP-dependent protein kinase I mediates the negative inotropic effect of cGMP in the murine myocardium. Circ Res 90:18–20

Wei G, Dawson VL, Zweier JL (1999) Role of neuronal and endothelial nitric oxide synthase in nitric oxide generation in the brain following cerebral ischemia. Biochim Biophys Acta 1455:23–34

Werner C, Pryzwansky KB, Hofmann F (2001) Cyclic GMP kinase I affects murine neutrophil migration and superoxide production. Naunyn-Schmiedebergś Arch Pharmacol 363: R81

Werner C, Sillaber I, Spanagel R, Hofmann F (2000) Reduced ethanol sensitivity and enhanced ethanol consumption in cGMP-kinase 2 deficient mice. Naunyn-Schmiedeberg's Arch Pharmacol 361: R105

Wilson RI, Godecke A, Brown RE, Schrader J, Haas HL (1999) Mice deficient in endothelial nitric oxide synthase exhibit a selective deficit in hippocampal long-term potentiation. Neuroscience 90:1157–1165

Wyatt TA, Naftilan AJ, Francis SH, Corbin JD (1998) ANF elicits phosphorylation of the cGMP phosphodiesterase in vascular smooth muscle cells. Am J Physiol 274: H448–455

Xu L, Eu JP, Meissner G, Stamler JS (1998) Activation of the cardiac calcium release channel (ryanodine receptor) by poly-S-nitrosylation. Science 279:234–237

Yamahara K, Itoh H, Chun T-H, Ogawa Y, Yamashita J, Sawada N, Fukunaga Y, Sone M, Yurugi-Kobayashi T, Miyashita K, Tsujimoto H, Kook H, Feil R, Garbers DL, Hofmann F, Nakao K (2003) Significance and therapeutic potential of natriuretic peptides/cGMP/cGMP-dependent protein kinase pathway in vascular regeneration. Proc Natl Acad Sci USA 100:3404–3409

Yang RB, Foster DC, Garbers DL, Fülle HJ (1995) Two membrane forms of guanylyl cyclase found in the eye. Proc Natl Acad Sci USA 92:602–606

Yang RB, Robinson SW, Xiong WH, Yau KW, Birch DG, Garbers DL (1999a) Disruption of a retinal guanylyl cyclase gene leads to cone-specific dystrophy and paradoxical rod behavior. J Neurosci 19:5889–5897

Yang XP, Liu YH, Shesely EG, Bulagannawar M, Liu F, Carretero OA (1999b) Endothelial nitric oxide gene knockout mice: cardiac phenotypes and the effect of angiotensin-converting enzyme inhibitor on myocardial ischemia/reperfusion injury. Hypertension 34:24–30

Yau KW, Baylor DA (1989) Cyclic GMP-activated conductance of retinal photoreceptor cells. Annu Rev Neurosci 12:289–327

Yogo K, Shimokawa H, Funakoshi H, Kandabashi T, Miyata K, Okamoto S, Egashira K, Huang P, Akaike T, Takeshita A (2000) Different vasculoprotective roles of NO synthase isoforms in vascular lesion formation in mice. Arterioscler Thromb Vasc Biol 20: E96-E100

Zhang J, Dawson VL, Dawson TM, Snyder SH (1994) Nitric oxide activation of poly(ADP-ribose) synthetase in neurotoxicity. Science 263:687–689

Zhang SH, Reddick RL, Piedrahita JA, Maeda N (1992) Spontaneous hypercholesterolemia and arterial lesions in mice lacking apolipoprotein E. Science 258:468–471

Zhao H, Reed RR (2001) X inactivation of the OCNC1 channel gene reveals a role for activity- dependent competition in the olfactory system. Cell 104:651–660

Zheng C, Feinstein P, Bozza T, Rodriguez I, Mombaerts P (2000) Peripheral olfactory projections are differentially affected in mice deficient in a cyclic nucleotide-gated channel subunit. Neuron 26:81–91

Transgenic Models for the Study of Protein Kinase A-Regulated Signal Transduction

C. M. Niswender · G. S. McKnight

Department of Pharmacology, University of Washington,
K-540B HSB, Box 357750, Seattle, WA 98195, USA
e-mail: mcknight@u.washington.edu

Abstract Protein kinase A (PKA) is a ubiquitous serine–threonine kinase involved in the transduction of cellular signals through the second messenger cyclic adenosine monophosphate (cAMP). Knockout and transgenic manipulation of PKA subunits has resulted in the generation of mice with deficits in developmental processes, neuronal signaling, metabolic regulation, cardiovascular parameters, and reproductive function. These observations indicate that targeting the PKA system may be of therapeutic value in a myriad of human diseases. This review will provide a comprehensive compilation of PKA mouse mutants generated to date and discuss future directions within this complex signaling system that are amenable to pharmacological manipulation.

Keywords cAMP · Protein kinase A · Mouse genetics · Phenotype

1
Introduction

The development of transgenic models to study intracellular signal transduction has provided clues regarding the roles that distinct proteins play within the context of multi-component cascades. The cyclic adenosine monophosphate (cAMP) signaling system is one of the best-characterized signal transduction pathways and a number of animal models have been generated to study specific aspects of this cascade. These include animals with manipulations in G protein subunits, adenylyl cyclase isoforms, protein kinase A (PKA) regulatory and catalytic subunits, and phosphodiesterases. This review will focus on genetic strategies that target the PKA system, highlighting those which provide models particularly relevant to pharmacological study. We will also address issues and caveats relevant to the use of gene manipulation strategies in the study of a major signaling cascade, such as the development of compensation, the potential need for tissue-specific alterations, and the emerging role for the coupling of genetics and pharmacology.

2
Brief Overview of Cellular cAMP Signaling

The classical pathway for eliciting the cellular cAMP signal begins with the stimulation of surface receptors linked to specific heterotrimeric guanosine triphosphate (GTP)-binding proteins (G proteins) (Fig. 1). G proteins critical for regulation of cAMP include those of the stimulatory (G_s) and inhibitory ($G_{i/o}$) families. Upon agonist-receptor G protein coupling, these G proteins hydrolyze GTP and either activate (G_s) or inhibit ($G_{i/o}$), the effector adenylyl cyclase. When stimulated, adenylyl cyclases convert ATP into cAMP and pyrophosphate. One of the major described functions of cAMP is the activation of PKA; cAMP has also been shown to modify the activity of cyclic nucleotide gated ion channels and several guanine nucleotide exchange factors (reviewed in Antoni 2000). PKA is a ubiquitous serine/threonine protein kinase that phosphorylates pro-

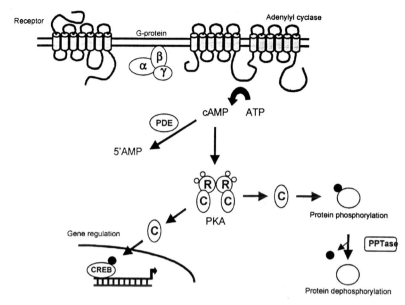

Fig. 1 Signal transduction through the PKA pathway. Agonist occupation of receptors linked to G$_s$ heterotrimeric GTP-binding proteins stimulate the conversion of ATP to cAMP by adenylyl cyclases. cAMP occupies binding sites on the PKA regulatory subunits which result in the release of the catalytic proteins. PKA phosphorylates cytoplasmic proteins which can be dephosphorylated by protein phosphatases. cAMP-mediated activation of PKA holoenzymes also results in translocation of the C subunit into the nucleus with corresponding phosphorylation of nuclear components such as the transcription factor CREB. The cAMP signal is terminated by the action of phosphodiesterases which degrade cAMP into AMP

teins at the consensus sequence RRXS/T, resulting in the direct regulation of protein function and the induction of gene transcription by the phosphorylation of transcription factors, most classically CREB (cAMP-response element binding protein). PKA-mediated phosphorylation is balanced by the activity of cellular phosphatases and phosphodiesterases, which terminate the signal by either dephosphorylation of PKA targets or degradation of cAMP, respectively.

3
General Overview of PKA Holoenzyme Characteristics

In mice, there are two PKA catalytic subunits termed Cα and Cβ. mRNAs encoding each of these proteins are produced from single genes using alternate exons and transcriptional start sites, resulting in the expression of two (Cα1 and Cα2) (Desseyn et al. 2000; Reinton et al. 2000) or three (Cβ1, Cβ2, and Cβ3) (Guthrie et al. 1997) splice variants. Four regulatory subunits, termed RIα, RIIα, RIβ, and RIIβ, complement the catalytic proteins. The various subunits exhibit distinct but often overlapping expression patterns. In general, the α subunits show widespread expression whereas the β isoforms are expressed in a more re-

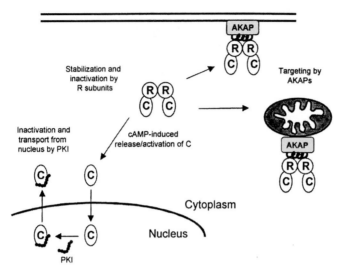

Fig. 2 Mechanisms of PKA regulation. Binding of C subunits to R subunits results in inactivation of catalytic activity and a retention of C subunit in the cytoplasm. When complexed as holoenzyme, both C and R subunit proteins are stabilized. The holoenzyme complex is anchored to specific sites within the cell by AKAPs, which bind with high affinity to R subunits through an amphipathic helix region. C subunits in the nucleus are further regulated by the activity of PKI, which inhibits C subunit activity by two mechanisms: occupying the substrate binding site and translocating C subunit from the nucleus

stricted fashion (reviewed in McKnight et al. 1996). The PKA holoenzyme is composed of two catalytic and two regulatory subunits; in the absence of cAMP, the enzyme is inactive. Cyclic AMP binding to two sites on each regulatory subunit results in the release of the catalytically active C subunits. One major source of regulation of the levels of PKA within a cell involves the stabilization of both catalytic and regulatory subunits induced by R–C interaction. For example, the half-life of the RIα protein rises four- to fivefold when complexed into a holoenzyme form (Amieux et al. 1997).

In addition to regulation induced by differences in tissue expression and R–C interactions, tetrameric PKA holoenzyme can be "anchored" in specific locations within the cell by A-kinase anchoring proteins, or AKAPs (Fig. 2). This large family of cellular scaffolding proteins are quite divergent in sequence, but all share a common amphipathic helix region which interacts with the dimerized amino terminus of the RII subunits, localizing type II PKA holoenzymes to subcellular structures such as the plasma membrane, the mitochondria, or the endoplasmic reticulum (reviewed in Feliciello et al. 2001; Michel and Scott 2002). While the majority of AKAPs preferentially bind to RII subunits, S-AKAP84/D-AKAP-1 has been shown to bind with similar affinity to both RI and RII subunits (Huang et al. 1997; Reinton et al. 2000). These distinct preferences in R subunit–AKAP interaction as well as the growing number of identified AKAPs suggest that there are distinct localizations and, potentially, unique signaling ca-

Table 1 PKA system knockout mice. PKA subunit knockout mice that have been generated to date are listed with a brief phenotypic description, a qualitative assessment of PKA activity levels, a description of subunits that have been observed to increase in a compensatory manner in tissues from a given knockout line, and the corresponding reference(s)

Gene	Phenotype	PKA activity Region	Basal	cAMP-stim	Protein compensation	Reference(s)
Cα1/2	Increased neonatal mortality, growth retardation, sperm dysfunction	Many	Decreased	Decreased	Increased Cβ1/2/3 (brain) Increased Cβ1 (kidney)	Skalhegg et al. 2002
Cα2	In progress					
Cβ1	Defects in hippocampal synaptic plasticity	Brain	No change	No change	None	Qi et al. 1995; Huang et al. 1995
Cβall	Impaired cued fear conditioning (background dependent)	Amygdala/Hipp	Decreased	No change	Increased Cα (amygdala, hipp)	Howe et al. 2002
RIα	Embryonic lethality by day 10.5; defective mesoderm migration and lack of heart tube formation	Embryo	Increased	Decreased	None	Amieux et al. 2002
RIβ	Defects in hippocampal synaptic plasticity Impaired nociception Impaired plasticity in visual cortex	Brain	No change	No change	Increased RIα	Brandon et al. 1995; Huang et al. 1995 Malmberg et al. 1997 Hensch et al. 1998
RIIα	None apparent	Sk. muscle	No change	Decreased	Increased RIα	Burton et al. 1997
		Testes	Not reported	Not reported	Increased RIα	Burton et al. 1999
RIIβ	Leanness; resistance to diet-induced obesity	BAT	Increased	No change	Increased RIα	Cummings et al. 1996
	Resistance to diet-induced diabetes	WAT	Increased	Decreased	Increased RIα	Planas et al. 1999 Schreyer et al. 2001
	Impaired rotorod performance Impaired gene regulation induced by dopaminergic drugs Increased ethanol self-admin	Striatum	Decreased	Decreased	Increased RIα/RIβ	Brandon et al. 1998 Adams et al. 1997 Thiele et al. 2000

Table 1 (continued)

Gene	Phenotype	PKA activity			Protein compensation	Reference(s)
		Region	Basal	cAMP-stim		
$C\alpha^{-/-}/C\beta^{-/-}$	Embryonic lethality (after implantation)		Not reported	Not reported	Not reported	Huang et al. 2002
$C\alpha^{+/-}/C\beta^{-/-}$	Spina bifida (100%)		Not reported	Not reported	Not reported	Huang et al. 2002
$C\alpha^{-/-}/C\beta^{+/-}$	Spina bifida (100%) Exencephaly (25%)		Not reported	Not reported	Not reported	Huang et al. 2002
PKIα	Defective gene regulation	Sk. muscle	Decreased	No change	Increased RIα	Gangolli et al. 2000
PKIβ	None apparent		Not reported	Not reported	Not reported	Belyamani et al. 2001

BAT, brown adipose tissue; hipp, hippocampus; LTD, long-term depression; LTP, long-term potentiation; sk, skeletal; WAT, white adipose tissue.

pacities of different holoenzymes within the cell (Feliciello et al. 2001; Michel and Scott 2002).

PKA catalytic subunits are also regulated in an inhibitory fashion by members of the protein kinase inhibitor (PKI) family (Fig. 2) (Walsh et al. 1971). These 70–75 amino acid proteins bind within the C subunit substrate binding site and "lock" the catalytic subunit into a closed and inactive conformation. Amino acids 5–24 of the PKI peptide are sufficient for inhibitory activity and this PKI-derived peptide has been used extensively as a tool to dissect the contribution of PKA to kinase activity observed in vitro (Scott et al. 1985a,b). There are three known PKI isoforms, α, β, and γ, which are encoded by distinct genes and show unique tissue expression (Walsh et al. 1971; Beale et al. 1977; Van Patten et al. 1992; Collins and Uhler 1997). Full length PKI proteins also contain a leucine-rich nuclear export signal (NES) that promotes PKI-mediated transport of C subunits from the nucleus to the cytoplasm in transfected cells (Fantozzi et al. 1992, 1994; Wiley et al. 1999). It has been hypothesized that the in vivo role of PKI might be to terminate the activity of C subunit in the nucleus, thereby decreasing levels of PKA-mediated gene transcription when present. However, recent mouse knockout experiments that have eliminated PKIα and/or PKIβ have led to the opposite effect, suggesting that the PKI system may have a more complex role in the nuclear actions of PKA (Gangolli et al. 2000).

It was anticipated, due to the widespread expression and pivotal role of PKA in the transduction of major cellular signals, that disruption or overexpression of the various PKA subunit genes would produce significant alterations in a variety of biological processes. This has indeed been the case, with PKA mutations affecting developmental, neural, metabolic, cardiovascular, and reproductive functions. Genes encoding each of the PKA subunits have now been separately disrupted within the mouse genome (Table 1). The majority of mice that lack one PKA subunit appear healthy and fertile; only two deletions, Cα and RIα, have produced severe effects on growth and development. The phenotypes resulting from all of these deletions will be grouped into physiological categories and discussed in detail in this review. Additionally, studies describing the use of transgenic technology to overexpress wild-type or mutant PKA subunits will also be described (Table 2). A common theme of these studies is the remarkable compensation that can occur within the PKA system, suggesting that tight control of PKA activity represents a critical homeostatic mechanism.

4
Developmental Phenotypes

4.1
Embryonic Lethality of Mice Lacking RIα

Despite the ubiquitous expression of the α forms of the PKA catalytic and regulatory subunits, the only knockout that results in embryonic lethality is that of RIα. It has been observed that RIα (and, in the brain, RIβ) can compensate for

Table 2 PKA system transgenic mice. PKA subunit transgenic mice that have been generated to date are listed with the promoter used to drive transgene expression, the tissues in which expression of the transgene was observed, a brief phenotypic description, a qualitative assessment of PKA activity levels, and the corresponding reference

Gene	Promoter	Area of expression	Phenotype	PKA activity			Reference
				Region	Basal	cAMP-stim	
R(AB)	CaM Kinase IIα	Hippocampus, striatum, amygdala, cortex	Defects in synaptic plasticity, learning and memory tasks	CA-1	Decreased	Decreased	Abel et al. 1997
R(AB)	Wnt-1 enhancer	CNS	"Ventralization" of dorsal regions of CNS		Not reported	Not reported	Epstein et al. 1996
Cα	α-Myosin Heavy chain	Cardiomyocytes	Dilated cardiomyopathy Arrhythmias Edema Increased mortality	Heart	Increased	Not reported	Antos et al. 2001

CNS, central nervous system.

the loss of the remaining regulatory subunits (Brandon et al. 1995; Amieux et al. 1997) and it has been postulated that RIα acts as a physiological "buffer" against inappropriate levels of PKA activity (Amieux et al. 1997; Amieux and McKnight 2002).

Knockout of the RIα gene results in embryonic lethality at approximately day 10.5, although phenotypic abnormalities are noted earlier than this time point (Amieux et al. 2002). For example, at day 9.5, the embryos lack a defined heart tube and show deficits in the normal formation of tissues derived from mesoderm (Amieux et al. 2002). Even at day 6.5, it is noted that mesodermal cell formation is greatly reduced and that there is a failure of the remaining cells to migrate normally from the primitive streak. These observations suggest that a defect has occurred during the gastrulation process and that the embryo has failed to undergo the normal epithelial to mesenchymal transition necessary to form mesodermal tissue (Hogan et al. 1994). Tissue extracts from embryos at day 8.5 reveal a three- to fourfold increase in basal PKA activity coupled with a 40% decrease in cAMP-stimulated, or total, PKA activity. These results indicate that there is a lack of compensation for the missing RIα protein and that the abnormally high basal level of activity might be affecting cell fate. To confirm this hypothesis, RI$\alpha^{+/-}$-mutant mice were crossed with animals carrying a disruption for the Cα allele. Interbreeding of these animals resulted in mice with graded levels of Cα activity upon the RI$\alpha^{-/-}$ background. Decreasing basal PKA levels resulted in a corresponding rescue of the RI$\alpha^{-/-}$ phenotype, with C$\alpha^{-/-}$ RI$\alpha^{-/-}$ embryos appearing similar to wild-type littermates. This rescue is still incomplete, however, as these embryos do not survive to term (Amieux et al. 2002).

How might increases in basal PKA activity affect gastrulation and, ultimately, the formation of mesodermal tissue? Examination of other mouse mutants resembling RI$\alpha^{-/-}$ embryos indicates that mice with manipulations in the fibroblast growth factor (FGF) signaling cascade show similarities to many phenotypes seen in RIα mutants (Yamaguchi et al. 1994; Ciruna et al. 1997; Sun et al. 1999; Ciruna and Rossant 2001). These observations suggest that PKA, which can inhibit signaling by growth factor tyrosine kinase receptors, might be functioning to inhibit FGF-dependent mesodermal migration from the primitive streak. Alternatively, increased basal PKA activity might be affecting the function of members of the integrin family as embryos lacking focal adhesion kinase and fibronectin also show deficits in heart formation and other mesodermal lineages (Furuta et al. 1995; Ilic et al. 1995; Georges-Labouesse et al. 1996).

4.2
Catalytic Subunit Distinctions: Growth Retardation in Mice Lacking Cα but Normal Development of Cβ Knockouts

Due to the widespread use of the cAMP signaling cascade and the ubiquitous expression of PKA, it was hypothesized that loss of either of the two catalytic subunits might also result in embryonic lethality. This has not been the case. Simultaneous knockout of all three isoforms of Cβ generates animals with only subtle defects in neurological function (Howe et al. 2002). Deletion of the Cα gene generates a much more severe phenotype, with a large percentage of pups dying in the early postnatal period (Skålhegg et al. 2002). Approximately 25% of the knockout animals do survive for longer periods, however, and this is particularly evident on a mixed 129 SvJ/C57Bl6 background. These surviving animals are runted and the majority of pups attain only 60% of the size of their wild-type and heterozygous littermates (Skålhegg et al. 2002). The phenotype is not dependent upon defects in growth hormone but does correlate with decreases in insulin-like growth factor (IGF)-1 in the liver, suggesting that IGF-1 function may be abnormal in these animals. PKA activity assays reveal that all tissues examined show dramatic reductions in total PKA activity and Western analyses show that Cβ1 only compensates for the loss of Cα in a small subset of tissues, particularly in the brain. Protein levels of the R subunits are also decreased in most regions, suggesting that Cα is a predominant binding and stabilizing partner for these proteins in most tissues (Skålhegg et al. 2002).

The very mild phenotype of Cβ knockouts, coupled with the ability of a subset of animals to survive without Cα, has prompted an examination of the consequences of the loss of three or four C subunit alleles. In these studies, C$\alpha^{+/-}$ mice and Cβ1$^{+/-}$ animals were crossed and the progeny were examined for the consequences of a progressive loss of PKA activity (Huang et al. 2002). Mice completely lacking both Cα and Cβ1 die after implantation but prior to the completion of gastrulation. Mice that lack three C subunit alleles exhibit an inappropriate expansion of the neural tube and a lack of vertebral arch closure, resulting in spina bifida (Huang et al. 2002). The defective area is exquisitely specific to the thoracic to sacral region of the neural tube and occurs with 100% penetrance. Additionally, exencephaly is seen in 25% of the animals with one remaining Cβ allele; embryos containing one remaining Cα allele do not develop exencephaly (Huang et al. 2002).

PKA is known to be a negative regulator of the Sonic hedgehog (Shh) pathway (Fan et al. 1995; Hynes et al. 1995; Epstein et al. 1996; Hammerschmidt et al. 1996), a critical signal transduction cascade necessary for pattern formation in the CNS. In the PKA-deficient embryos described above, Shh and several proteins transcriptionally regulated by the Shh cascade are inappropriately expressed only in the phenotypically affected regions of the neural tube (Huang et al. 2002). For example, Shh and Hnf3β, which are normally expressed only in the floor plate, were expanded dorsally. The role of Shh in neural tube patterning is to produce a concentration gradient of signal that induces or represses a series of genes which then define the dorsal/ventral neural tube axis (Roelink et al. 1995; Chiang et al. 1996; Ericson et al. 1997; Briscoe et al. 1999). C deficiency leads to an inappropriately "ventralized" identity only within the affected region of the neural tube. This altered cell fate phenotype indicates that precise levels of PKA activity are necessary for patterning specific regions of the central nervous system.

4.3
Dominant-Negative RIα Subunit Expression in the CNS

Within the R subunits, there are two binding sites for cAMP termed the A and B sites. While these two sites share high amino acid homology and bind cAMP in a positively cooperative fashion, they exhibit distinct cAMP dissociation kinetics and preference for cAMP analogs (Doskeland 1978; Rannels and Corbin 1980; Corbin et al. 1982). Clones of RIα subunits that act in a dominant negative fashion have been identified by phenotypic analysis of S49 lymphoma cells and subsequent sequencing and expression in mammalian cells (Clegg et al. 1987). Substitution of a glutamic acid for a glycine at position 200 within the A site results in the generation of a stable holoenzyme with a fourfold higher K_a for cAMP (Woodford et al. 1989). Mutation of position 324 (glycine to aspartic acid) within the B site drastically reduces the affinity of the R subunit to more than 5 μM cAMP.

The double mutant form of this RIα subunit (G200E and G324D) is termed R(AB) and has been used in a variety of in vivo systems to create a dominant-negative holoenzyme (Concordet et al. 1996; Epstein et al. 1996; Hammerschmidt et al. 1996). Epstein et al. expressed the R(AB) subunit in mouse embryos under control of the *Wnt-1* enhancer (Epstein et al. 1996). Expression of this transgene in dorsal regions of the mouse CNS results in the ectopic expression of Shh as well as the Shh targets Hnf3β, Patched, and Gli 1 (Epstein et al. 1996). This inappropriate Shh pathway signaling again induces ventral cell types in dorsal areas of the CNS. While these studies indicate that PKA normally functions to antagonize Shh signaling in dorsal regions of the CNS, the exact mechanism for this inhibition is unknown. Since decreasing PKA activity results in ectopic expression of Shh itself, PKA's major role may be to simply repress Shh expression. If this hypothesis is correct, then crossing the PKA-deficient mice described by Huang et al. to Shh$^{-/-}$ animals should result in embryos with corrected dorsal/ventral patterning. There are many other points along the Shh pathway where PKA may be functioning, however, as a number of Shh cascade components such as Smoothened and members of the Gli family of transcriptional activators/repressors are phosphorylated by PKA (Alcedo et al. 2000; Wang et al. 2000). It also remains formally possible that PKA functions in a parallel but independent pathway to Shh and that the ectopic expression of Shh is a byproduct of manipulation of this second pathway.

5
Neural Phenotypes

5.1
The Involvement of Cβ1 and RIβ in Synaptic Plasticity

The involvement of cAMP in neuronal processes such as learning and memory, reward behaviors, and pain perception has previously been demonstrated in mice using pharmacological techniques. All of the PKA subunits are expressed in the brain with very high expression in neurons (Cadd and McKnight 1989; Guthrie et al. 1997), suggesting that manipulations of PKA subunits in the brain should affect basic neuronal function. This has indeed been the case; several subunit deletions result in defects in measurements of synaptic plasticity and in learning paradigms. Additionally, mice with alterations in PKA activity show changes in neuronal gene induction patterns, indicating that neurons employ isoform-specific transduction of cellular signals.

Mice lacking either the Cβ1 or RIβ PKA subunits show deficits in synaptic plasticity that have been hypothesized to provide a mechanism for learning and memory (long-term potentiation [LTP] and long-term depression [LTD]) (Brandon et al. 1995; Huang et al. 1995; Qi et al. 1996; Hensch et al. 1998). Animals initially designed to lack the Cβ protein were generated prior to the knowledge that three distinct isoforms, termed Cβ1, Cβ2, and Cβ3, could be produced from the Cβ gene by alternative promoter usage (Guthrie et al. 1997). Therefore, because of the recombination strategy used, these original mice lacked only the Cβ1 isoform. Both the Cβ1 and RIβ proteins are expressed at high levels in the cortex and hippocampus, prompting analysis of learning and memory paradigms in these knockouts. Cβ1-mutant mice are deficient in their ability to sustain the late phase of Schaffer collateral/CA1 LTP (Huang et al. 1995; Qi et al. 1996). These observations correlate with previous findings that the late phase of LTP, in contrast to the early phase, is cAMP-dependent and requires PKA-mediated gene transcription (Frey et al. 1993; Matthies and Reymann 1993; Huang and Kandel 1994). Both Cβ1 and RIβ animals are also deficient in their ability to induce LTD within the Schaffer Collateral pathway (Brandon et al. 1995; Qi et al. 1996), suggesting that these specific subunits are critical for the manifestation of LTD in these neurons. Despite specific defects in LTP and LTD within hippocampal pathways, the RIβ and Cβ1 knockout mice behave normally in a number of learning tasks (Huang et al. 1995), dissociating the electrophysiological parameters from observed deficits at the behavioral level.

5.2
The Involvement of Cβ2 and Cβ3 in Learning and Memory

Messenger RNA and protein for the Cβ2 and Cβ3 isoforms are expressed specifically in the brain (Guthrie et al. 1997), suggesting that these enzymes play important roles in neural function. As a result of alternative mRNA splicing, the Cβ2 and 3 proteins lack the necessary consensus sequence for myristoylation (an N-terminal glycine residue). This post-translation modification is postulated to affect protein stability (Yonemoto et al. 1993) or membrane tethering of the catalytic protein (Gangal et al. 1999). Cβ2 mRNA is highly expressed within the amygdala and hippocampus and other limbic structures while Cβ3 is expressed at a very low level in many brain areas (Guthrie et al. 1997). Mice have now been generated that lack all three forms of Cβ, termed Cβall$^{-/-}$ (Howe et al. 2002). The high level of expression of Cβ2 in limbic areas, coupled with pharmacological evidence that memory formation or consolidation in the hippocampus and amygdala is dependent upon PKA (Bourtchouladze et al. 1998; Schafe et al. 1999; Goosens et al. 2000; Schafe and LeDoux 2000), suggested that examination of the ability of $C\beta all^{-/-}$ mice to perform in learning and memory paradigms might be informative. As discussed above, previous studies have shown that loss of $C\beta1$ does not affect learning tasks such as contextual and cued fear conditioning (Huang et al. 1995). In contrast, when mated onto certain genetic backgrounds, $C\beta all^{-/-}$ mice are deficient in their ability to acquire cued fear conditioning. $C\beta all^{-/-}$ animals perform normally in other models of learning and memory such as contextual fear conditioning (a hippocampal-dependent task) and conditioned taste aversion (an amygdala-dominant learning paradigm). It is important to note that PKA activity levels in brain regions from these mice are not different from wild-type animals, and Western analyses reveal a compensatory increase in the level of $C\alpha$ protein (Howe et al. 2002). This suggests that $C\alpha$ can compensate for most, but not all, of the functions of $C\beta$ in the brain.

5.3
Dominant-Negative RIα Subunit Expression in Neurons

The physiological effect of decreasing PKA activity in neurons has also been studied using transgenic mice that express the dominant-negative R(AB) transgene under control of the calcium-calmodulin dependent protein kinase IIα promoter (Abel et al. 1997). In these studies, high levels of transgene expression are observed in the hippocampus, amygdala, striatum, and cortex, and the authors show that both basal and cAMP-stimulated PKA activity were reduced in the CA-1 hippocampal region of these mice by 50% and 25%, respectively (Abel et al. 1997). These mice show electrophysiological deficits within the late, but not the early, phase of LTP. The animals also exhibit a significant decrement in spatial memory and long-term contextual fear conditioning (Abel et al. 1997). The authors conclude that PKA is essential for the consolidation of short-term memory and long-term storage.

There are a number of explanations that might account for the behavioral differences between the R(AB) transgenics and the several PKA knockouts generated to date. It is possible that R(AB) hippocampal neurons have lower overall levels of PKA activity (compared with $C\beta1^{-/-}$ or $C\beta all^{-/-}$ neurons, for example) due to the ability of this dominant-negative R subunit to interact with both $C\alpha$ and $C\beta$ proteins. If so, it remains possible that *either* $C\alpha$ or $C\beta$ is capable of transmitting the cellular signals necessary for the manifestation of contextual fear conditioning. On the other hand, these discrepancies may indicate that $C\alpha$ plays a more important role in the type of learning represented by the contextual fear conditioning paradigm, since $C\beta all^{-/-}$ mice do not show deficits in contextual fear conditioning. A tissue-specific knockout of $C\alpha$ in neurons would be of value in determining if the two catalytic subunits of PKA are distinct in their ability to regulate the type of memory characteristic of the contextual fear conditioning paradigm.

The idea that there are distinct combinations of R and C subunits that are responsible for different responses to neuronal stimulation is supported by the work of Woo et al. (2000). These authors studied the role of PKA in LTP induced by two distinct paradigms differing in their timing and intensity of stimulation. R(AB) mice responded normally when the signal was compressed but abnormally when stimulation was administered in a regular, spaced pattern (Woo et al. 2000). In contrast, both forms of synaptic plasticity were inhibited by infusion of the PKA inhibitor Rp-cAMPS. The authors conclude that these different forms of LTP recruit distinct PKA holoenzymes, only some of which are inhibited by the R(AB) protein.

5.4
Role for RIβ in the Manifestation of Nociceptive Pain

PKA has been implicated in the central and peripheral processing of pain. For example, increasing cAMP levels or injecting C subunit into dorsal horn neurons potentiates their response to glutamatergic ion channel stimulation (Cerne et al. 1992; Cerne et al. 1993). The localization of RIβ to the CNS prompted an examination of nociceptive responses in mice lacking this regulatory subunit (Malmberg et al. 1997). When injected with 2% formalin into the paw, wild-type mice exhibit responses that occur in two phases. The first phase is dependent upon an acute transmission by primary afferent pain neurons while the second, prolonged, phase reflects an inflammatory response. RIβ-mutant mice exhibit a significant decrease in the second phase response with a corresponding decrease in the amount of swelling of the injected paw. As a measurement of the sensory neuron activity, *c-fos* immunoreactivity was assessed and found to be significantly lower in the RI$\beta^{-/-}$ mice. In another model of tissue injury, produced by injection of capsaicin into the paw, RI$\beta^{-/-}$ mice are also less sensitive than wild-type animals. These results indicate that RIβ is required for the inflammatory and subsequent pain response evoked by tissue injury, possibly by influencing PKA-mediated phosphorylation of ion channels (Malmberg et al. 1997).

5.5
The Involvement of RIIβ in Dopaminergic Signal Transduction

The RIIβ regulatory subunit is also highly expressed in the brain, particularly in the striatum, and loss of this subunit leads to a significant ($\sim$75%) decrease in total PKA activity in this brain region (Brandon et al. 1998). Acute motor effects mediated by the dopamine system appear to be intact in these mice, but the mice display motor learning defects as assessed by impaired performance on an accelerating rotorod. The induction of genes by agonists or antagonists of D_1 and D_2 dopamine receptors is also affected by the loss of RIIβ. For example, basal dynorphin mRNA expression, mediated by dopamine signaling through

D_1 receptors, is decreased in the mutants (Brandon et al. 1998). Administration of haloperidol, a D_2 receptor antagonist, failed to induce the normal increase in expression of *c-fos* and neurotensin in the striatum of RIIβ knockouts, and the mice do not succumb to the haloperidol-induced catalepsy characteristic of wild-type mice (Adams et al. 1997). These results suggest that the PKA activity mediated by RIIβ-containing holoenzyme is essential for dopaminergic gene induction in these neurons.

5.6
RIIβ and the Response to Drugs of Abuse

The cAMP/PKA system has been implicated in the response to drugs of abuse such as psychostimulants and ethanol. Gene induction mediated by amphetamine, as assessed by measurement of *c-fos* mRNA, has been shown to be blunted in RIIβ$^{-/-}$ mice and these animals are more sensitive to amphetamine sensitization (Brandon et al. 1998). Ethanol has been shown in several studies to affect the activity of PKA both in vivo and in vitro (Ortiz et al. 1995; Dohrman et al. 1996; Diamond and Gordon 1997). RIIβ$^{-/-}$ animals show increased voluntary ethanol consumption and are less sensitive to the sedative effects of ethanol when compared to wild-type mice (Thiele et al. 2000). While it is currently unknown which area of the brain mediates the effects of ethanol in these mice, regions of the brain considered to be ethanol targets such as the nucleus accumbens, the hippocampus, the amygdala, and the hypothalamus (Ryabinin et al. 1997) all show reductions in cAMP-stimulated PKA activity in RIIβ knockouts. The regulation of PKA activity in the RIIβ$^{-/-}$ brain is complex; in contrast to other tissues, there is incomplete compensation by RIα in RIIβ$^{-/-}$ brain. Due to the instability and increased degradation of C protein that is not bound to R subunits, total PKA activity in mutant brain is greatly reduced. The basal/total ratio, however, is predicted to be higher than normal due to an R/C subunit imbalance. Therefore, despite lowered cAMP-stimulated PKA activity, it is postulated that an altered basal/total ratio may lead to chronic PKA activation and mediate the increased ethanol-consumption phenotype characteristic of these animals (Thiele et al. 2000).

It will be of interest to determine the brain area responsible for RIIβ-regulated ethanol consumption. Toward this goal, our laboratory has generated mice that employ the Cre-*lox* recombination system to "re-express" normal levels of RIIβ in specific tissues while maintaining the "knockout" genotype in all other areas (M. A. Sikorski and G.S. McKnight, unpublished). These animals encode a silent RIIβ gene in which protein expression is regulated by *loxP* sequences; in the presence of the bacterial enzyme Cre recombinase, RIIβ is re-expressed in the tissue of choice. The widespread use of viral vectors expressing Cre recombinase indicates that it will be possible to "turn on" RIIβ in very specific brain areas and neurons to define locations important for PKA-regulated ethanol consumption. Once identified, it may then be possible to target drugs to receptors expressed on these neurons to alter PKA activity in a desirable direction.

6
Metabolic Phenotypes

6.1
Leanness and Resistance to Diet-Induced Obesity in Mice Lacking RIIβ

Adipose tissue expresses a subset of PKA subunits, namely $C\alpha$, $C\beta 1$, RIα, and RIIβ. Normally, the PKA holoenzyme found in fat cells consists primarily of type II kinase (McKnight et al. 1998) suggesting that RIIβ plays a pivotal role in the regulation of PKA activity in this tissue. Knockout of RIIβ protein generates mice that are lean compared to their wild-type littermates (Cummings et al. 1996). In both brown (BAT) and white adipose tissue (WAT), loss of RIIβ causes a holoenzyme switch from type II to type I kinase due to a compensatory increase in RIα protein (Cummings et al. 1996; Amieux et al. 1997; Planas et al. 1999). This is significant since the type I kinase activates at a lower threshold concentration of cAMP, resulting in higher levels of basal PKA activity in both WAT and BAT. In BAT, there is a noted stabilization of uncoupling protein (UCP)-1 (Cummings et al. 1996), a mitochondrial protein specialized for thermogenesis by "uncoupling" the proton gradient across the mitochondrial membrane from ATP production. RII$\beta^{-/-}$ mice have been noted to exhibit an increased metabolic rate, and this has lead to the hypothesis that the lean phenotype of these animals is related to the increase in UCP-1 levels in BAT (Cummings et al. 1996). Mating of the RII$\beta^{-/-}$ mice to UCP-1$^{-/-}$ animals is currently ongoing in the laboratory (M. Nolan and G.S. McKnight, unpublished) to determine the involvement of PKA's regulation of UCP as a mechanism of leanness. In preliminary results, the combined double knockout mice (RIIβ/UCP1) remain significantly leaner than wild-type littermate controls. This suggests that although changes in BAT may account for some of the metabolic alterations in RIIβ knockouts, these BAT-dependent effects are not essential for the lean phenotype.

RII$\beta^{-/-}$ animals show deficits in white adipose stores, which are decreased by approximately 60% compared to wild-type littermates (Cummings et al. 1996; Planas et al. 1999). The number of adipocytes is approximately the same but triglyceride storage and size of each adipocyte is considerably smaller in the RIIβ mice (Cummings et al. 1996). The major role of PKA in the triglyceride storage/breakdown balance is to promote triglyceride breakdown by affecting the levels and activity of lipolytic enzymes such as hormone-sensitive lipase (HSL) and lipoprotein lipase. In this regard, PKA activation in WAT, produced mainly by stimulation of the sympathetic nervous system and subsequent activation of β_3-adrenergic receptors, opposes the fat-storing activity of insulin. RII$\beta^{-/-}$ mice show enhanced levels of basal but blunted levels of agonist-stimulated lipolysis both in vivo and from WAT pads extracted and examined in vitro (Planas et al. 1999). The observation of increased basal but decreased total PKA activity correlates with the observed incomplete compensation by RIα in WAT, resulting in reduced total holoenzyme levels. Examination of the levels of mRNAs postulated to be regulated by PKA in WAT, such as lipoprotein lipase (Antras et al. 1991), acetyl-CoA carboxylase (Kim et al. 1989; Foufelle et al. 1994), and GLUT4 (Kaestner et al. 1991) revealed normal levels of all RNA transcripts examined (Planas et al. 1999). This suggests that the changes in lipolysis arise from alterations in PKA-mediated phosphorylation of cytoplasmic proteins rather than changes in PKA-dependent transcription. Although it has not yet been directly examined, it remains a strong possibility that PKA changes in WAT affect the phosphorylation status of perilipins, proteins which coat lipid droplets and "protect" them from the hydrolyzing activity of HSL (Londos et al. 1995, 1999; Souza et al. 1998; Martinez-Botas et al. 2000). PKA phosphorylation of perilipin on multiple sites results in the movement of perilipin from fat droplets to the cytoplasm, allowing HSL access to the fat droplet (Londos et al. 1999; Clifford et al. 2000). Interestingly, knockout of the perilipin gene generates animals with a strikingly similar phenotype to that seen in RII$\beta^{-/-}$ mice (Martinez-Botas et al. 2000; Tansey et al. 2001).

Mice lacking RIIβ have also been studied for their ability to resist the development of diet-induced obesity (Cummings et al. 1996) and diet-induced diabetes (Schreyer et al. 2001). When fed a high-fat diet, RII$\beta^{-/-}$ mice do not become overweight or develop the fatty liver characteristic of their wild-type littermates (Cummings et al. 1996). In an expansion of these findings, RII$\beta^{-/-}$ mice were fed a diabetogenic diet, consisting of 35% fat and 37% carbohydrate, for 15 weeks (Schreyer et al. 2001). While both groups of mice gained weight on this diet, RII$\beta^{-/-}$ mice did so more slowly than controls and remained leaner as assessed by fat pad weight. Despite elevated serum glucose levels in both groups subjected to this diet, RII$\beta^{-/-}$ mice had lower levels of serum insulin than wild-types and exhibited significantly better glucose tolerance when challenged with an acute intraperitoneal bolus of glucose. Loss of RIIβ was also beneficial in terms of lipid profile; RII$\beta^{-/-}$ mice were protected from the dyslipidemia characteristic of diet-induced diabetes (Schreyer et al. 2001).

As yet, it is unclear if there is a single tissue that is responsible for RII$\beta^{-/-}$ leanness. Since RIIβ is expressed in BAT, WAT, and the brain, it remains possible that any of these tissues, or a combination of them, is involved in the lean phenotype of these animals. While adipose tissue is an attractive target, RIIβ is also highly expressed within feeding centers in the hypothalamus. RII$\beta^{-/-}$ mice do not show differences in food intake when compared to their wild-type littermates on a normal chow diet (Cummings et al. 1996). When fed a diabetogenic diet, RIIβ mice do consume a larger number of calories per body weight compared to wild-type animals, but this is because they are lean and weigh less; hyperphagia on a per mouse basis is not seen (Schreyer et al. 2001). Consistent with their reduced adiposity, RIIβ mice also have lower levels of circulating leptin. Coupled with the observation that they are not hyperphagic, these findings suggest that RII$\beta^{-/-}$ mice may be more leptin-sensitive at the level of the hypothalamus.

As described above, mice have been produced in our laboratory that use the Cre-*lox* recombination system to re-express normal levels of RIIβ in a tissue of choice while maintaining the knockout genotype elsewhere (M.A. Sikorski and G.S. McKnight, unpublished). It is anticipated that the availability of mice expressing the Cre enzyme specifically in adipose tissue or in the brain will help localize the tissue responsible for PKA-mediated leanness. Once identified, it may be possible to design pharmacological agents to mimic this phenotype.

6.2
Defective Metabolic Gene Regulation in PKIα Knockouts

PKA activity is inhibited by a variety of mechanisms including C–R interactions and the activity of the PKI family of inhibitory peptides. After injection of PKA into the cytoplasm of tissue culture cells, free C subunit can translocate into the nucleus while C protein complexed as holoenzyme is retained in the cytoplasm. PKIs can diffuse freely into the nucleus and participate in the export of free C subunit back into the cytoplasm (Fantozzi et al. 1992, 1994). A leucine-rich nuclear export signal has been identified on PKI (Wen et al. 1994). This chaperone function, as well as the direct ability of PKI to inhibit C subunit activity by occupying the substrate binding site, has been postulated to control levels of PKA activity in the nucleus (Wiley et al. 1999). The high expression of the PKIα isoform in skeletal muscle indicates that loss of this inhibitor peptide might result in enhanced nuclear activity of PKA, increasing the transcription of genes regulated by CREB and other PKA-regulated transcription factors. In skeletal muscle, transcription of the RNA for the gluconeogenic enzyme PEPCK is elevated by increases in cAMP (Snell and Duff 1979; Beebe et al. 1987; Hanson and Reshef 1997), suggesting that deletion of PKIα might alter PEPCK levels in these mice. In PKIα$^{-/-}$ animals, PKA activity assays indicate that there is a loss of PKI inhibitory function in skeletal muscle extracts and that there is no compensation by the β and γ forms of PKI (Gangolli et al. 2000). Surprisingly, both basal and cAMP-induced transcription of PEPCK mRNA is actually decreased in skeletal muscle from these mice. These tissue extracts also show deficits in phospho-CREB levels that correlate with blunted gene induction. While basal PKA activity is decreased by approximately 40%, cAMP-stimulated activity levels are comparable to wild-type skeletal muscle. Western analyses confirm that the mechanism responsible for this discrepancy is a compensation by RIα subunits, which preserve overall kinase levels but serve to sequester C subunit in the cytoplasm and decrease basal kinase activity. It is interesting to note that PEPCK mRNA levels are decreased in both the basal and cAMP-stimulated states even though the amount of total kinase activity measured in vitro is not altered. It is possible that R subunits are more effective than PKI in inhibiting gene induction due to differences in cellular location. Alternatively, PKI may be serving an additional, positive, role in the regulation of gene transcription that is lost when the peptide is missing.

6.2.1
Cardiovascular Phenotypes

It is widely accepted that patients with heart failure show impairments in β_1- and β_2- adrenergic receptor function (Bristow et al. 1982; Brodde et al. 1989; Ungerer et al. 1993; Engelhardt et al. 1996), resulting in defects in the ionotropic and chronotropic control of cardiomyocytes. Within this cascade, cAMP and PKA play critical roles in the transduction of signals from β receptors. PKA is activated by both β_1 and β_2 receptor stimulation and, in cardiomyocytes, phosphorylates several target substrates such as phospholamban, L-type calcium channels, ryanodine receptors, and β_2 receptors themselves (reviewed in Lohse and Engelhardt 2001). The majority of transgenic models produced thus far indicate that overexpression of components of the β_1 receptor pathway, be it the receptor itself (Engelhardt et al. 1999; Bisognano et al. 2000), a $G\alpha_s$ GTP-binding protein subunit (Iwase et al. 1996), or the PKA target phospholamban (Haghighi et al. 2001), are detrimental to heart function and contribute to heart failure. In contrast, overexpression of a sarcoplasmic reticulum Ca^{2+} ATPase, normally inhibited by PKA-mediated phosphorylation of phospholamban, improves cardiac contractility (del Monte et al. 2001). Several models, however, including those that have achieved overexpression of either the type VI or type VIII forms of adenylyl cyclase (AC), indicate that enhanced signaling through some aspects of the cAMP system does not result in heart failure and can actually improve heart function when heart failure has been established (Gao et al. 1999; Roth et al. 1999; Lipskaia et al. 2000). Antos et al. have extended these findings by overexpressing the $C\alpha$ subunit of PKA specifically in cardiomyocytes using an α-myosin heavy chain promoter-driven transgene (Antos et al. 2001). Hearts from founder animals exhibit two- to eightfold higher levels of basal PKA activity. These animals develop cardiac hypertrophy, arrhythmias, and decreased heart contractility, and 100% of the transgenic animals die by 20 weeks of age. Substrates known to be phosphorylated by PKA in the heart, such as the ryanodine receptor and phospholamban, show increased levels of phosphorylation in these mice. The authors postulate that the major effect of PKA overactivity is a hyperphosphorylation of the ryanodine receptor, which alters the calcium conductance of these channels and enhances their activity at low calcium concentrations (Marx et al. 2000). The hyperphosphorylation of phospholamban, which should protect against inappropriate calcium fluxes by increasing calcium removal from the sarcoplasm (Neyses et al. 1985; Hawkins et al. 1994; Reddy et al. 1996; Antos et al. 2001), does not appear to dominate over the negative effects of enhanced PKA phosphorylation of the ryanodine receptor (Antos et al. 2001). Interestingly, increased phosphorylation of ryanodine receptors is also seen in human patients with heart failure, and improving heart function results in decreased phosphorylation of this protein (Marx et al. 2000). These results suggest that PKA activity in the failing heart is a potential site for pharmacological intervention and that mice overexpressing PKA may serve as an appropriate model amenable to drug testing.

It is notable that there appear to be several dichotomies within the β-adrenergic/cAMP signaling pathway in the heart that have been identified using mouse genetics, suggesting previously unrecognized complexity within this signal transduction cascade. Two groups have reported that heart-specific overexpression of either of the type VI or type VIII isoforms of adenylyl cyclase does not deleteriously affect heart function (Gao et al. 1999; Lipskaia et al. 2000). In the case of overexpression of the calcium-regulated type VIII AC, mice show improved contractility but no adverse consequences in cardiac function despite a fourfold elevation of basal PKA activity (Lipskaia et al. 2000). Overexpression of the calcium-inhibited type VI AC using a similar strategy resulted in normal basal cAMP levels but an enhancement in agonist-stimulated cAMP production (Gao et al. 1999). In addition, overexpression of the type VI AC improves cardiac function in a mouse model of heart failure (Roth et al. 1999). The discrepancy between the phenotypes of the AC mutants and the other transgenic models described above may be due to a number of possibilities (reviewed in Lohse and Engelhardt 2001; Patel et al. 2001), but an attractive hypothesis involves subcellular localization of signaling components. For example, PKA isoforms interact with unique AKAPs in different tissues (Feliciello et al. 2001; Michel and Scott 2002). AKAP binding is predicted to localize PKA isoforms to distinct areas within the cell, presumably creating local "pockets" of PKA near important membrane signaling components, such as receptors and specific AC isoforms. When PKA itself is overexpressed, localization of all membrane pools is presumably altered. In contrast, the expression of more than one AC isoform in the heart (predominantly type V and type VI) suggests that the manipulations produced within the type VI and VIII isoforms thus far may not have altered the same PKA pool as that responsible for previously described heart phenotypes.

7
Reproductive Phenotypes

7.1
Defective Sperm Motility and Infertility in Cα Knockouts

PKA lies downstream of receptors for luteinizing hormone (LH) and follicle stimulating hormone (FSH), suggesting that manipulations within the PKA system might affect the fertility of both males and females and possibly point to a novel direction for contraception. We have focused on male reproduction in several lines of mutant mice due to the high expression of Cα2 and RIIα in both testis and sperm. Cβ1 and RIα are also expressed in testes, although at much lower levels. Treatment of sperm with cAMP analogues or phosphodiesterase inhibitors has been shown to enhance sperm motility (Brandt and Hoskins 1980; Garbers and Kopf 1980; Tash and Means 1983; Lindemann and Kanous 1989). PKA has also been implicated in the process of capacitation, a phenomenon that normally occurs in the female reproductive tract and is necessary for fertilization (Visconti et al. 1995).

In wild-type sperm, Cα2 and RIIα are found primarily within the midpiece and the principal piece of the flagellum (Lieberman et al. 1988; Pariset et al. 1989; Vijayaraghavan et al. 1997). Based upon fractionation experiments that separate membrane and cytosolic fractions of sperm, RIIα-containing holoenzyme is thought to be tightly anchored to the flagella of mature sperm by AKAPs (Horowitz et al. 1984). In bovine sperm, motility can be decreased using peptides that block AKAP interaction with RII subunits (Vijayaraghavan et al. 1997). These findings, coupled with the high expression of Cα and RIIα in sperm, has prompted an examination of mice with deletions in these subunit genes for potential changes in sperm function and fertility.

Mice have been generated in our laboratory that lack both the Cα1 and Cα2 isoforms. In terms of male reproductive physiology, Cα2 mRNA and protein are produced only in male germ cells starting at the mid-pachytene stage (Desseyn et al. 2000; Reinton et al. 2000). Cα1, however, is also found in supporting cells of the testis such as Leydig and Sertoli cells as well as in all other tissues in the mouse. As previously described, Cα knockout mice show severe growth retardation and increased neonatal death; those few males that survive past puberty produce sperm that completely lack forward motility. These mice show almost no kinase activity in extracts derived from either testis or mature sperm (Skålhegg et al. 2002). There is no observable compensation by Cβ1, which is normally expressed at low levels in testis. Levels of the regulatory subunits RIα and RIIα are also extremely low, as they are no longer stabilized in the absence of Cα. Despite a dramatic loss of PKA activity, all sperm stages are present in testes derived from these animals although a substantial percentage of mature sperm appear morphologically abnormal (Skålhegg et al. 2002). One conclusion from these results is that PKA activity is not required in male germ cells for sperm development, since mature sperm were found in these mice. However, it may be the residual (presumably Cβ-1 mediated) PKA activity within testicular support cells that is sufficient to maintain PKA-dependent Leydig and Sertoli cell functions and permit progression through the spermatogenic stages (Skålhegg et al. 2002).

We have recently produced a specific knockout of the Cα2 isoform which leaves the Cα1 variant intact (M. Nolan and G.S. McKnight, unpublished). Unlike C$\alpha^{-/-}$ mice, these animals are healthy with no growth retardation. This will permit a direct examination of fertility and mating behaviors of these animals without the confounding phenotypes seen in mice lacking Cα1. Preliminary results indicate that Cα2-null sperm undergo normal spermatogenesis but lack the ability to capacitate and initiate the forward motility that is required for fertility. These results point to an essential role for PKA activity in the process of capacitation but demonstrate that at least from mid-pachytene stages onward, PKA does not play an essential role in germ cell development.

7.2
Lack of Sperm Dysfunction Despite Altered PKA Localization in RIIα Knockouts

Animals lacking the RIIα regulatory subunit have also been examined for defects in sperm function. Mature sperm express both RIIα and RIα, although RIIα-containing enzyme represents the predominant form (Conti et al. 1983). Sperm also express at least two distinct AKAPs called S-AKAP84, localized to mitochondria, and AKAP82, localized to the sperm fibrous sheath (Carrera et al. 1994; Lin et al. 1995). S-AKAP84 binds with 25-fold higher affinity to RIIα versus RIα, while AKAP82 may bind both subunits in vivo due to distinct RI versus RII binding sites (Huang et al. 1997; Miki and Eddy 1998). Due to the high expression and distinct localization of RIIα in sperm, it was hypothesized that removal of RIIα would change the localization of PKA. This prediction, in conjunction with previous observations in bovine sperm indicating that disruption of RII-AKAP binding decreases sperm motility (Vijayaraghavan et al. 1997), suggested that mice lacking RIIα would have defects in sperm function. Surprisingly, knockout of RIIα appears to have no effect on sperm differentiation, production, motility, or fertilization (Burton et al. 1999). A dramatic upregulation of RIα was observed in these mutant sperm, and immunolocalization studies show that the remaining PKA holoenzyme is now redistributed to the cytosol (Burton et al. 1999). This observation reveals two important points: (1) that anchoring of PKA does not appear to be essential for sperm function and (2) that RIα does not appear to bind to the same AKAPs as the RIIα subunit in sperm. By contrast, in this same line of RII$\alpha^{-/-}$ mice, colocalization of PKA with L-type calcium channels was preserved in skeletal muscle (Burton et al. 1997). It has previously been shown that skeletal muscle L-type calcium channels, located at the membrane, require anchored PKA for enhanced activation (Sculptoreanu et al. 1993; Johnson et al. 1994; Wang and Kotlikoff 1996). Activity of these channels in RII$\alpha^{-/-}$ skeletal muscle was observed to be unaltered, suggesting that RIα-containing holoenzyme can be anchored in certain tissues (Burton et al. 1997).

7.3
Lack of Sperm Dysfunction in PKIβ Knockouts

PKIβ is expressed predominantly within the germ cells of the testes, with a low level of expression in the brain (Seasholtz et al. 1995; Van Patten et al. 1992, 1997). Due to the relatively selective expression of PKIβ in male germ cells, it was hypothesized that manipulation of PKIβ levels might affect sperm PKA function and could provide a new direction for male contraceptives. Disruption of the PKIβ gene, however, does not result in observable changes in reproductive function (Belyamani et al. 2001). Creation of double knockout animals, lacking both PKIα and β, also revealed no defects in fertility, although these mice should be missing PKI activity in testicular support cells as well as sperm itself (Belyamani et al. 2001). PKI$\beta^{-/-}$ mice also show normal regulation of genes thought to be regulated by PKA in the testes, such as protamine 1. These results indicate that either PKI activity is not critical for spermatogenesis and sperm function or that the remaining PKI isoform, PKIγ, is capable of substituting for the other family members. In summary, while the results from the Cα knockout point to a clear role for PKA activity in sperm function, anchoring of type II holoenzyme, as well as PKI-mediated inhibition, does not appear to be necessary for fertility.

8
Tissue-Specific Manipulations

The ability to manipulate genes only in specific tissues has opened new avenues of research for mouse geneticists. Due to the widespread expression of PKA isoforms and the severe phenotypes produced by the deletion of several subunits, we have begun to employ the Cre-*loxP* recombination system to alter PKA subunit genes in restricted tissues. Cre recombinase is an enzyme derived from bacteria that recognizes 34 base pair, palindromic sequences termed *loxP* sites and catalyzes a recombination event between them (reviewed in Le and Sauer 2000; Sauer 1998). Depending upon the orientation of the *lox* sequences, DNA between the sites can be removed (if the sites are in the same orientation) or reversed (if the sites are in opposite directions).

The Cre/lox system has been used most often to delete genes in specific tissues. In these types of strategies, *lox* sites are inserted flanking exonic regions of a gene. In cell types where Cre is expressed, recombination between the *lox* sequences occurs and deletes a coding portion of the gene to generate a null allele. The tissue specificity possible with this system is generated by the use of mice expressing Cre recombinase under the control of a specific promoter, either as a transgene or when the Cre coding sequence has been directly inserted into a specific locus. In the case of the PKA system, it will be of value to create tissue-specific knockouts of several of the subunits, most notably Cα, RIα, and RIIβ. Due to the severe phenotypes produced when the Cα or RIα proteins are deleted, it has been particularly difficult to study the roles of these subunits in distinct tissues.

Another potential use for a tissue-specific knockout of RIα revolves around the hypothesized role of RIα as a tumor suppressor. In patients with a disorder termed the Carney complex, characterized by a number of neuroendocrine neoplasias, one copy of the RIα gene is mutated such that no functional protein is produced from this allele (Casey et al. 2000; Kirschner et al. 2000). Loss of heterozygosity occurs in a somatic cell that then stimulates a proliferative response and tumor formation (Kirschner et al. 2000; Stratakis et al. 2001). Based on studies of RI$\alpha^{-/-}$ mice, it is predicted that tissues lacking both copies of RIα would have an increase in unregulated PKA activity and alterations in growth factor-mediated proliferation and cellular adhesion. Use of an animal with a tissue-specific deletion of RIα may prove useful in determining the involvement of RIα in cancer development or spread and provide a model to study the effectiveness of blocking PKA activity in the types of tumors characteristic of this syndrome.

We are currently using the Cre recombinase system to introduce "knock-in" PKA mutations into the mouse germline. As previously described for RIIβ, this strategy involves "silencing" a PKA allele by introduction of a stop cassette. This silent allele can then be activated in specific tissues when Cre recombinase is present. We have now used this strategy to successfully regulate two mutant PKA subunits (C.M. Niswender, B.S. Willis, and G.S. McKnight, unpublished). The first line of animals encodes an allele of Cα that produces a protein with reduced affinity for R subunits, resulting in a holoenzyme that activates at a lower concentration of cAMP compared to the wild-type enzyme. The second line encodes an RIα subunit with a mutation in the "B" cAMP binding site, producing an RIα subunit with reduced affinity for cAMP and which functions in a dominant-negative fashion. One copy of each of these alleles, in silent form, has been introduced into the mouse germline, and mice have been generated which are phenotypically normal Cα or RIα heterozygotes. Using mice expressing Cre recombinase, mutant protein from these alleles can be produced in a tissue-specific fashion and results in the expected changes in PKA activity (C.M. Niswender, B.S. Willis, and G.S. McKnight, unpublished). Due to the widespread expression of Cα and RIα, these mice will prove invaluable for the study of PKA function in a variety of in vivo situations.

9
The Coupling of Genetic and Pharmacologic Approaches

The development of knockout and transgenic animals has been invaluable in the identification of areas where manipulations of PKA activity may represent new treatments for diseases such as heart failure, fertility, cancer, and obesity. One inherent disadvantage to the genetic approach, however, is the compensation that may occur when a protein is missing from the onset of embryonic development and this is certainly an issue within the PKA system. The use of pharmacological inhibitors or activators represents another method useful in the control of protein function. The major limitation with this approach, however, involves the inherent lack of specificity of drugs for their desired target. The emergence of a novel method termed "chemical genetics" (Mitchison 1994) couples the power of genetic techniques with the temporal aspects of drug therapy, thereby limiting potential compensation and greatly improving specificity. This approach has now been used to manipulate the function of a number of protein kinases, providing an exquisitely sensitive way to selectively inhibit a single cellular protein kinase (reviewed in Bishop et al. 2000). We have now employed this method to study the function of the catalytic proteins of PKA (Niswender et al. 2002) and plan to extend these findings to the in vivo setting.

The ATP binding sites of eukaryotic protein kinases are highly conserved and all kinases identified to date contain a bulky, hydrophobic amino acid at a key position within the binding pocket (Bishop et al. 2001). In the case of the PKA subunits $C\alpha$ and $C\beta$, this residue corresponds to methionine 120. When the analogous position within other kinases such as Src and Cdc28 is mutated to a smaller amino acid (Shah et al. 1997; Bishop et al. 2000), the modified kinases will now accept unique inhibitors that do not bind the to wild-type proteins. When position 120 of PKA is mutated to an alanine or glycine, certain structural members of a series of C-3 derivatized pyrazolo [3,4-d] pyrimidine-based inhibitors are able to bind and inhibit transcription induced by the mutant kinases (Niswender et al. 2002). It should now be possible to generate mice that express this "inhibitable" kinase. Ideally, in the absence of drug, the enzyme will function normally; when drug is administered, the mutant kinase will be specifically inhibited. This approach should allow a measurement of the acute role of the PKA catalytic subunits in the transmission of cellular signals in either the whole animal or in tissues derived from these mice. Obviously, people do not express these mutant variants of PKA, but this approach represents a strategy to conclusively define or identify previously unknown targets of PKA that are linked to disease processes. It is hoped that a better understanding of these substrates will open new avenues for drug treatment in disorders that involve inappropriate PKA activity or that might be treated by manipulation of the PKA system.

Acknowledgements. This work was supported by NIH grants DK10005–03 (C.M.N.) and GM32875 (G.S.M.). The authors would like to thank Dr. Paul Amieux, Dr. Douglas Howe, Dr. Ama Sikorski, Dr. Yong-Zhao Huang, Brandon Willis, and Michael Nolan for review of this manuscript and for providing unpublished information.

References

Abel T, Nguyen PV, Barad M, Deuel TA, Kandel ER, and Bourtchouladze R (1997) Genetic demonstration of a role for PKA in the late phase of LTP and in hippocampus-based long-term memory. Cell 88:615–626

Adams MR, Brandon EP, Chartoff EH, Idzerda RL, Dorsa DM, and McKnight GS (1997) Loss of haloperidol induced gene expression and catalepsy in protein kinase A-deficient mice. Proc Natl Acad Sci U S A 94:12157–12161

Alcedo J, Zou Y, and Noll M (2000) Posttranscriptional regulation of smoothened is part of a self- correcting mechanism in the Hedgehog signaling system. Mol Cell 6:457–465

Amieux P, and McKnight GS (2002) The essential role of $RI\alpha$ in the maintenance of regulated PKA activity. Annals of the New York Academy of Sciences 968:75–95

Amieux PS, Cummings DE, Motamed K, Brandon EP, Wailes LA, Le K, Idzerda RL, and McKnight GS (1997) Compensatory regulation of RIalpha protein levels in protein kinase A mutant mice. J Biol Chem 272:3993–3998

Amieux PS, Howe D, Knickerbocker H, Lee DL, Su T, Idzerda RL, and McKnight GS (2002) Increased basal PKA activity inhibits the formation of mesoderm-derived structures in the developing mouse embryo. Journal of Biological Chemistry online

Anthonsen MW, Ronnstrand L, Wernstedt C, Degerman E, and Holm C (1998) Identification of novel phosphorylation sites in hormone-sensitive lipase that are phosphorylated in response to isoproterenol and govern activation properties in vitro. J Biol Chem 273:215–221

Antos CL, Frey N, Marx SO, Reiken S, Gaburjakova M, Richardson JA, Marks AR, and Olson EN (2001) Dilated cardiomyopathy and sudden death resulting from constitutive activation of protein kinase A. Circ Res 89:997–1004

Antras J, Lasnier F, and Pairault J (1991) Beta-adrenergic-cyclic AMP signalling pathway modulates cell function at the transcriptional level in 3T3-F442A adipocytes. Mol Cell Endocrinol 82:183–190

Beale EG, Dedman JR, and Means AR (1977) Isolation and characterization of a protein from rat testis which inhibits cAMP dependent protein kinase and phosphodiesterase. J Biol Chem 252:6322–6327

Beebe SJ, Koch SR, Chu DT, Corbin JD, and Granner DK (1987) Regulation of phosphoenolpyruvate carboxykinase gene transcription in H4IIE hepatoma cells: evidence for a primary role of the catalytic subunit of 3',5'-cyclic adenosine monophosphate-dependent protein kinase. Mol Endocrinol 1:639–647

Belyamani M, Gangolli EA, and Idzerda RL (2001) Reproductive function in protein kinase inhibitor-deficient mice. Mol Cell Biol 21:3959–3963

Bishop A, Buzko O, Heyeck-Dumas S, Jung I, Kraybill B, Liu Y, Shah K, Ulrich S, Witucki L, Yang F, Zhang C, and Shokat KM (2000) Unnatural ligands for engineered proteins: new tools for chemical genetics. Annu Rev Biophys Biomol Struct 29:577–606

Bishop AC, Buzko O, and Shokat KM (2001) Magic bullets for protein kinases. Trends Cell Biol 11:167–172

Bishop AC, Ubersax JA, Petsch DT, Matheos DP, Gray NS, Blethrow J, Shimizu E, Tsien JZ, Schultz PG, Rose MD, Wood JL, Morgan DO, and Shokat KM (2000) A chemical switch for inhibitor-sensitive alleles of any protein kinase. Nature 407:395–401

Bisognano JD, Weinberger HD, Bohlmeyer TJ, Pende A, Raynolds MV, Sastravaha A, Roden R, Asano K, Blaxall BC, Wu SC, Communal C, Singh K, Colucci W, Bristow MR, and Port DJ (2000) Myocardial-directed overexpression of the human beta(1)-adrenergic receptor in transgenic mice. J Mol Cell Cardiol 32:817–830

Bourtchouladze R, Abel T, Berman N, Gordon R, Lapidus K, and Kandel ER (1998) Different training procedures recruit either one or two critical periods for contextual memory consolidation, each of which requires protein synthesis and PKA. Learn Mem 5:365–374

Brandon EP, Logue SF, Adams MR, Qi M, Sullivan SP, Matsumoto AM, Dorsa DM, Wehner JM, McKnight GS, and Idzerda RL (1998) Defective motor behavior and neural gene expression in RIIbeta-protein kinase A mutant mice. J Neurosci 18:3639–3649

Brandon EP, Zhuo M, Huang YY, Qi M, Gerhold KA, Burton KA, Kandel ER, McKnight GS, and Idzerda RL (1995) Hippocampal long-term depression and depotentiation are defective in mice carrying a targeted disruption of the gene encoding the RI beta subunit of cAMP-dependent protein kinase. Proc Natl Acad Sci U S A 92:8851–8855

Brandt H, and Hoskins DD (1980) A cAMP-dependent phosphorylated motility protein in bovine epididymal sperm. J Biol Chem 255:982–987

Briscoe J, Sussel L, Serup P, Hartigan-O'Connor D, Jessell TM, Rubenstein JL, and Ericson J (1999) Homeobox gene Nkx2.2 and specification of neuronal identity by graded Sonic hedgehog signalling. Nature 398:622–627

Bristow MR, Ginsburg R, Minobe W, Cubicciotti RS, Sageman WS, Lurie K, Billingham ME, Harrison DC, and Stinson EB (1982) Decreased catecholamine sensitivity and B-adrenergic-receptor density in failing human hearts. N. Engl. J. Med. 307:205–211

Brodde OE, Zerkowski HR, Doetsch N, Motomura S, Khamssi M, and Michel MC (1989) Myocardial beta-adrenoceptor changes in heart failure: concomitant reduction in beta 1- and beta 2-adrenoceptor function related to the degree of heart failure in patients with mitral valve disease. J Am Coll Cardiol 14:323–331

Burton KA, Johnson BD, Hausken ZE, Westenbroek RE, Idzerda RL, Scheuer T, Scott JD, Catterall WA, and McKnight GS (1997) Type II regulatory subunits are not required for the anchoring- dependent modulation of Ca2+ channel activity by cAMP-dependent protein kinase. Proc Natl Acad Sci U S A 94:11067–11072

Burton KA, Treash-Osio B, Muller CH, Dunphy EL, and McKnight GS (1999) Deletion of type IIalpha regulatory subunit delocalizes protein kinase A in mouse sperm without affecting motility or fertilization. J Biol Chem 274:24131–24136

Cadd G, and McKnight GS (1989) Distinct patterns of cAMP-dependent protein kinase gene expression in mouse brain. Neuron 3:71–79

Carrera A, Gerton GL, and Moss SB (1994) The major fibrous sheath polypeptide of mouse sperm: structural and functional similarities to the A-kinase anchoring proteins. Dev Biol 165:272–284

Casey M, Vaughan CJ, He J, Hatcher CJ, Winter JM, Weremowicz S, Montgomery K, Kucherlapati R, Morton CC, and Basson CT (2000) Mutations in the protein kinase A R1alpha regulatory subunit cause familial cardiac myxomas and Carney complex. J Clin Invest 106:R31–38

Cerne R, Jiang M, and Randic M (1992) Cyclic adenosine 3'5'-monophosphate potentiates excitatory amino acid and synaptic responses of rat spinal dorsal horn neurons. Brain Res 596:111–123

Cerne R, Rusin KI, and Randic M (1993) Enhancement of the N-methyl-D-aspartate response in spinal dorsal horn neurons by cAMP-dependent protein kinase. Neurosci Lett 161:124–128

Chiang C, Litingtung Y, Lee E, Young KE, Corden JL, Westphal H, and Beachy PA (1996) Cyclopia and defective axial patterning in mice lacking Sonic hedgehog gene function. Nature 383:407–413

Ciruna B, and Rossant J (2001) FGF signaling regulates mesoderm cell fate specification and morphogenetic movement at the primitive streak. Dev Cell 1:37–49

Ciruna BG, Schwartz L, Harpal K, Yamaguchi TP, and Rossant J (1997) Chimeric analysis of fibroblast growth factor receptor-1 (Fgfr1) function: a role for FGFR1 in morphogenetic movement through the primitive streak. Development 124:2829–2841

Clegg CH, Correll LA, Cadd GG, and McKnight GS (1987) Inhibition of intracellular cAMP-dependent protein kinase using mutant genes of the regulatory type I subunit. J Biol Chem 262:13111–13119

Clifford GM, Londos C, Kraemer FB, Vernon RG, and Yeaman SJ (2000) Translocation of hormone-sensitive lipase and perilipin upon lipolytic stimulation of rat adipocytes. J Biol Chem 275:5011–5015

Collins SP, and Uhler MD (1997) Characterization of PKIgamma, a novel isoform of the protein kinase inhibitor of cAMP-dependent protein kinase. J Biol Chem 272:18169–18178

Concordet J-P, Lewis K, Moore J, Goodrich LV, Johnson RL, Scoot MP, and Ingham PW (1996) Spatial regulation of a zebrafish Patched homologue reflects the roles of Sonic hedgehog and protein kinase A in neural tube and somite patterning. Development 122:2835–2846

Conti M, Adamo S, Geremia R, and Monesi V (1983) Developmental changes of cyclic adenosine monophosphate-dependent protein kinase activity during spermatogenesis in the mouse. Biol Reprod 28:860–869

Corbin JD, Rannels SR, Flockhart DA, Robinson-Steiner AM, Tigani MC, Doskeland SO, Suva RH, Suva R, and Miller JP (1982) Effect of cyclic nucleotide analogs on intrachain site I of protein kinase isozymes. Eur J Biochem 125:259–266

Cummings DE, Brandon EP, Planas JV, Motamed K, Idzerda RL, and McKnight GS (1996) Genetically lean mice result from targeted disruption of the RII beta subunit of protein kinase A. Nature 382:622–626

del Monte F, Williams E, Lebeche D, Schmidt U, Rosenzweig A, Gwathmey JK, Lewandowski ED, and Hajjar RJ (2001) Improvement in survival and cardiac metabolism after gene transfer of sarcoplasmic reticulum Ca2+ ATPase in a rat model of heart failure. Circulation 104:1424–1429

Desseyn JL, Burton KA, and McKnight GS (2000) Expression of a nonmyristylated variant of the catalytic subunit of protein kinase A during male germ-cell development. Proc Natl Acad Sci U S A 97:6433–6438

Diamond I, and Gordon AS (1997) Cellular and molecular neuroscience of alcoholism. Physiol Rev 77:1–20

Dohrman DP, Diamond I, and Gordon AS (1996) Ethanol causes translocation of cAMP-dependent protein kinase catalytic subunit to the nucleus. Proc Natl Acad Sci U S A 93:10217–10221

Doskeland SO (1978) Evidence that rabbit muscle protein kinase has two kinetically distinct binding sites for adenosine 3' ; 5'-cyclic monophosphate. Biochem Biophys Res Commun 83:542–549

Engelhardt S, Bohm M, Erdmann E, and Lohse MJ (1996) Analysis of beta-adrenergic receptor mRNA levels in human ventricular biopsy specimens by quantitative polymerase chain reactions: progressive reduction of beta 1-adrenergic receptor mRNA in heart failure. J Am Coll Cardiol 27:146–154

Engelhardt S, Hein L, Wiesmann F, and Lohse MJ (1999) Progressive hypertrophy and heart failure in beta1-adrenergic receptor transgenic mice. Proc Natl Acad Sci U S A 96:7059–7064

Epstein DJ, Marti E, Scott MP, and McMahon AP (1996) Antagonizing cAMP-dependent protein kinase A in the dorsal CNS activates a conserved Sonic hedgehog signaling pathway. Development 122:2885–2894

Ericson J, Rashbass P, Schedl A, Brenner-Morton S, Kawakami A, van Heyningen V, Jessell TM, and Briscoe J (1997) Pax6 controls progenitor cell identity and neuronal fate in response to graded Shh signaling. Cell 90:169–180

Fan CM, Porter JA, Chiang C, Chang DT, Beachy PA, and Tessier-Lavigne M (1995) Long-range sclerotome induction by sonic hedgehog: direct role of the amino-terminal cleavage product and modulation by the cyclic AMP signaling pathway. Cell 81:457–465

Fantozzi DA, Harootunian AT, Wen W, Taylor SS, Feramisco JR, Tsien RY, and Meinkoth JL (1994) Thermostable inhibitor of cAMP-dependent protein kinase enhances the rate of export of the kinase catalytic subunit from the nucleus. J Biol Chem 269:2676–2686

Fantozzi DA, Taylor SS, Howard PW, Maurer RA, Feramisco JR, and Meinkoth JL (1992) Effect of the thermostable protein kinase inhibitor on intracellular localization of the catalytic subunit of cAMP-dependent protein kinase. J Biol Chem 267:16824–16828

Feliciello A, Gottesman ME, and Avvedimento EV (2001) The biological functions of A-kinase anchor proteins. J Mol Biol 308:99–114

Foufelle F, Gouhot B, Perdereau D, Girard J, and Ferre P (1994) Regulation of lipogenic enzyme and phosphoenolpyruvate carboxykinase gene expression in cultured white adipose tissue. Glucose and insulin effects are antagonized by cAMP. Eur J Biochem 223:893–900

Frey U, Huang YY, and Kandel ER (1993) Effects of cAMP simulate a late stage of LTP in hippocampal CA1 neurons. Science 260:1661–1664

Furuta Y, Ilic D, Kanazawa S, Takeda N, Yamamoto T, and Aizawa S (1995) Mesodermal defect in late phase of gastrulation by a targeted mutation of focal adhesion kinase, FAK. Oncogene 11:1989–1995

Gangal M, Clifford T, Deich J, Cheng X, Taylor SS, and Johnson DA (1999) Mobilization of the A-kinase N-myristate through an isoform-specific intermolecular switch. Proc Natl Acad Sci U S A 96:12394–12399

Gangolli EA, Belyamani M, Muchinsky S, Narula A, Burton KA, McKnight GS, Uhler MD, and Idzerda RL (2000) Deficient gene expression in protein kinase inhibitor alpha Null mutant mice. Mol Cell Biol 20:3442–3448

Gao MH, Lai NC, Roth DM, Zhou J, Zhu J, Anzai T, Dalton N, and Hammond HK (1999) Adenylylcyclase increases responsiveness to catecholamine stimulation in transgenic mice. Circulation 99:1618–1622

Garbers DL, and Kopf GS (1980) The regulation of spermatozoa by calcium cyclic nucleotides. Adv Cyclic Nucleotide Res 13:251–306

Georges-Labouesse EN, George EL, Rayburn H, and Hynes RO (1996) Mesodermal development in mouse embryos mutant for fibronectin. Dev Dyn 207:145–156

Goosens KA, Holt W, and Maren S (2000) A role for amygdaloid PKA and PKC in the acquisition of long-term conditional fear memories in rats. Behav Brain Res 114:145–152

Guthrie CR, Skalhegg BS, and McKnight GS (1997) Two novel brain-specific splice variants of the murine Cbeta gene of cAMP-dependent protein kinase. J Biol Chem 272:29560–29565

Haghighi K, Schmidt AG, Hoit BD, Brittsan AG, Yatani A, Lester JW, Zhai J, Kimura Y, G.W. D, MacLennan DH, and Kranias EG (2001) Super-inhibition of sarcoplasmi reticulum function by phospholamban induces cardiac contractile failure. J. Biol. Chem. 276:24145–24152

Hammerschmidt M, Bitgood MJ, and McMahon AP (1996) Protein kinase A is a common negative regulator of Hedgehog signaling in the vertebrate embryo. Genes Dev 10:647–658

Hanson RW, and Reshef L (1997) Regulation of phosphoenolpyruvate carboxykinase (GTP) gene expression. Annu Rev Biochem 66:581–611

Hawkins C, Xu A, and Narayanan N (1994) Sarcoplasmic reticulum calcium pump in cardiac and slow twitch skeletal muscle but not fast twitch skeletal muscle undergoes phosphorylation by endogenous and exogenous Ca2+/calmodulin-dependent protein kinase. Characterization of optimal conditions for calcium pump phosphorylation. J Biol Chem 269:31198–31206

Hensch T, Gordon J, Brandon E, McKnight G, Idzerda R, Stryker M (1998) Comparison of plasticity in vivo and in vitro in the developing visual cortex of normal and protein kinase A RIbeta-deficient mice. J Neurosci 18:2108–2117

Hogan B, Beddington R, Costantini F, and Lacy E. (1994). Manipulating the Mouse Embryo, 2nd edition (New York, NY: Cold Spring Harbor Laboratory Press).

Horowitz JA, Toeg H, and Orr GA (1984) Characterization and localization of cAMP-dependent protein kinases in rat caudal epididymal sperm. J Biol Chem 259:832–838

Howe DG, Wiley JC, and McKnight GS (2002) Molecular and behavioral effects of a null mutation in all PKA Cβ isoforms. Molecular and Cellular Neuroscience 20:515–524

Huang LJ, Durick K, Weiner JA, Chun J, and Taylor SS (1997) Identification of a novel protein kinase A anchoring protein that binds both type I and type II regulatory subunits. J Biol Chem 272:8057–8064

Huang Y, Roelink H, and McKnight GS (2002) Protein kinase A deficiency causes axially localized neural tube defects in mice. J Biol Chem 8:19889–19896

Huang YY, and Kandel ER (1994) Recruitment of long-lasting and protein kinase A-dependent long-term potentiation in the CA1 region of hippocampus requires repeated tetanization. Learn Mem 1:74–82

Huang YY, Kandel ER, Varshavsky L, Brandon EP, Qi M, Idzerda RL, McKnight GS, and Bourtchouladze R (1995) A genetic test of the effects of mutations in PKA on mossy fiber LTP and its relation to spatial and contextual learning. Cell 83:1211–1222

Hynes M, Porter JA, Chiang C, Chang D, Tessier-Lavigne M, Beachy PA, and Rosenthal A (1995) Induction of midbrain dopaminergic neurons by Sonic hedgehog. Neuron 15:35–44

Ilic D, Furuta Y, Kanazawa S, Takeda N, Sobue K, Nakatsuji N, Nomura S, Fujimoto J, Okada M, and Yamamoto T (1995) Reduced cell motility and enhanced focal adhesion contact formation in cells from FAK-deficient mice. Nature 377:539–544

Iwase M, Bishop SP, Uechi M, Vatner DE, Shannon RP, Kudej RK, Wight DC, Wagner TE, Ishikawa Y, Homcy CJ, and Vatner SF (1996) Adverse effects of chronic endogenous sympathetic drive induced by cardiac GS alpha overexpression. Circ Res 78:517–524

Johnson BD, Scheuer T, and Catterall WA (1994) Voltage-dependent potentiation of L-type Ca2+ channels in skeletal muscle cells requires anchored cAMP-dependent protein kinase. Proc Natl Acad Sci U S A 91:11492–11496

Kaestner KH, Flores-Riveros JR, McLenithan JC, Janicot M, and Lane MD (1991) Transcriptional repression of the mouse insulin-responsive glucose transporter (GLUT4) gene by cAMP. Proc Natl Acad Sci U S A 88:1933–1937

Kim KH, Lopez-Casillas F, Bai DH, Luo X, and Pape ME (1989) Role of reversible phosphorylation of acetyl-CoA carboxylase in long- chain fatty acid synthesis. Faseb J 3:2250–2256

Kirschner LS, Carney JA, Pack SD, Taymans SE, Giatzakis C, Cho YS, Cho-Chung YS, and Stratakis CA (2000) Mutations of the gene encoding the protein kinase A type I-alpha regulatory subunit in patients with the Carney complex. Nat Genet 26:89–92

Le Y, and Sauer B (2000) Conditional gene knockout using cre recombinase. Methods Mol Biol 136:477–485

Lieberman SJ, Wasco W, MacLeod J, Satir P, and Orr GA (1988) Immunogold localization of the regulatory subunit of a type II cAMP- dependent protein kinase tightly associated with mammalian sperm flagella. J Cell Biol 107:1809–1816

Lin RY, Moss SB, and Rubin CS (1995) Characterization of S-AKAP84, a novel developmentally regulated A kinase anchor protein of male germ cells. J Biol Chem 270:27804

Lindemann CB, and Kanous KS (1989) Regulation of mammalian sperm motility. Arch Androl 23:1–22

Lipskaia L, Defer N, Esposito G, Hajar I, Garel MC, Rockman HA, and Hanoune J (2000) Enhanced cardiac function in transgenic mice expressing a Ca(2+)- stimulated adenylyl cyclase. Circ Res 86:795–801

Lohse MJ, and Engelhardt S (2001) Protein kinase A transgenes: the many faces of cAMP. Circ Res 89:938–940

Londos C, Brasaemle DL, Gruia-Gray J, Servetnick DA, Schultz CJ, Levin DM, and Kimmel AR (1995) Perilipin: unique proteins associated with intracellular neutral lipid droplets in adipocytes and steroidogenic cells. Biochem Soc Trans 23:611–615

Londos C, Brasaemle DL, Schultz CJ, Segrest JP, and Kimmel AR (1999) Perilipins, ADRP, and other proteins that associate with intracellular neutral lipid droplets in animal cells. Semin Cell Dev Biol 10:51–58

Malmberg AB, Brandon EP, Idzerda RL, Liu H, McKnight GS, and Basbaum AI (1997) Diminished inflammation and nociceptive pain with preservation of neuropathic pain in mice with a targeted mutation of the type I regulatory subunit of cAMP-dependent protein kinase. J Neurosci 17:7462–7470

Martinez-Botas J, Anderson JB, Tessier D, Lapillonne A, Chang BH, Quast MJ, Gorenstein D, Chen KH, and Chan L (2000) Absence of perilipin results in leanness and reverses obesity in Lepr(db/db) mice. Nat Genet 26:474–479

Marx SO, Reiken S, Hisamatsu Y, Jayaraman T, Burkhoff D, Rosemblit N, and Marks AR (2000) PKA phosphorylation dissociates FKBP12.6 from the calcium release channel (ryanodine receptor): defective regulation in failing hearts. Cell 101:365–376

Matthies H, and Reymann KG (1993) Protein kinase A inhibitors prevent the maintenance of hippocampal long- term potentiation. Neuroreport 4:712–714

McKnight GS, Cummings DE, Amieux PS, Sikorski MA, Brandon EP, Planas JV, Motamed K, and Idzerda RL (1998) Cyclic AMP, PKA, and the physiological regulation of adiposity. Recent Prog Horm Res 53:139–159

McKnight GS, Idzerda RL, Kandel ER, Brandon EP, Zhuo M, Wi M, Bourtchouladze R, Huang Y, Burton KA, Skalhegg BS, Cummings DE, Varshavsky L, Planas JV, Motamed

K, Gerhold KA, Amieux PS, Guthrie CR, Millet KM, Belyamani M, and Su T (1996) 9th European Testis Workshop, Geilo, Norway

Michel JJ, and Scott JD (2002) Akap mediated signal transduction. Annu Rev Pharmacol Toxicol 42:235–257

Miki K, and Eddy EM (1998) Identification of tethering domains for protein kinase A type Ialpha regulatory subunits on sperm fibrous sheath protein FSC1. J Biol Chem 273:34384–34390

Mitchison TJ (1994) Towards a pharmacological genetics. Chem Biol 1:3–6

Neyses L, Reinlib L, and Carafoli E (1985) Phosphorylation of the Ca2+-pumping ATPase of heart sarcolemma and erythrocyte plasma membrane by the cAMP-dependent protein kinase. J Biol Chem 260:10283–10287

Niswender CM, Ishihara RW, Judge LM, Zhang C, Shokat KM, and McKnight GS (2002) Protein engineering of Protein Kinase A catalytic subunits results in the acquisition of novel inhibitor sensitivity. J Biol Chem online, May 28

Ortiz J, Fitzgerald LW, Charlton M, Lane S, Trevisan L, Guitart X, Shoemaker W, Duman RS, and Nestler EJ (1995) Biochemical actions of chronic ethanol exposure in the mesolimbic dopamine system. Synapse 21:289–298

Pariset C, Feinberg J, Dacheux JL, Oyen O, Jahnsen T, and Weinman S (1989) Differential expression and subcellular localization for subunits of cAMP-dependent protein kinase during ram spermatogenesis. J Cell Biol 109:1195–1205

Patel TB, Du Z, Pierre S, Cartin L, and Scholich K (2001) Molecular biological approaches to unravel adenylyl cyclase signaling and function. Gene 269:13–25

Planas JV, Cummings DE, Idzerda RL, and McKnight GS (1999) Mutation of the RIIbeta subunit of protein kinase A differentially affects lipolysis but not gene induction in white adipose tissue. J Biol Chem 274:36281–36287

Qi M, Zhuo M, Skalhegg BS, Brandon EP, Kandel ER, McKnight GS, and Idzerda RL (1996) Impaired hippocampal plasticity in mice lacking the Cbeta1 catalytic subunit of cAMP-dependent protein kinase. Proc Natl Acad Sci U S A 93:1571–1576.

Rannels SR, and Corbin JD (1980) Studies of functional domains of the regulatory subunit from cAMP- dependent protein kinase isozyme I. J Cyclic Nucleotide Res 6:201–215

Reddy LG, Jones LR, Pace RC, and Stokes DL (1996) Purified, reconstituted cardiac Ca2+-ATPase is regulated by phospholamban but not by direct phosphorylation with Ca2+/calmodulin- dependent protein kinase. J Biol Chem 271:14964–14970

Reinton N, Collas P, Haugen TB, Skalhegg BS, Hanson V, Jahnsen T, and Tasken K (2000) Localization of a novel human A-kinase-anchoring protein, hAKAP220, during spermatogenesis. Dev Biol 223:194–204

Reinton N, Orstavik S, Haugen TB, Jahnsen T, Tasken K, and Skalhegg BS (2000) A novel isoform of human cyclic 3',5'-adenosine monophosphate-dependent protein kinase, c alpha-s, localizes to sperm midpiece. Biol Reprod 63:607–611

Roelink H, Porter JA, Chiang C, Tanabe Y, Chang DT, Beachy PA, and Jessell TM (1995) Floor plate and motor neuron induction by different concentrations of the amino-terminal cleavage product of sonic hedgehog autoproteolysis. Cell 81:445–455

Roth DM, Gao MH, Lai NC, Drumm J, Dalton N, Zhou JY, Zhu J, Entrikin D, and Hammond HK (1999) Cardiac-directed adenylyl cyclase expression improves heart function in murine cardiomyopathy. Circulation 99:3099–3102

Ryabinin AE, Criado JR, Henriksen SJ, Bloom FE, and Wilson MC (1997) Differential sensitivity of c-Fos expression in hippocampus and other brain regions to moderate and low doses of alcohol. Mol Psychiatry 2:32–43

Sauer B (1998) Inducible gene targeting in mice using the Cre/lox system. Methods 14:381–392

Schafe GE, and LeDoux JE (2000) Memory consolidation of auditory pavlovian fear conditioning requires protein synthesis and protein kinase A in the amygdala. J Neurosci 20:RC96

Schafe GE, Nadel NV, Sullivan GM, Harris A, and LeDoux JE (1999) Memory consolidation for contextual and auditory fear conditioning is dependent on protein synthesis, PKA, and MAP kinase. Learn Mem 6:97–110

Schreyer SA, Cummings DE, McKnight GS, and LeBoeuf RC (2001) Mutation of the RI-Ibeta subunit of protein kinase A prevents diet- induced insulin resistance and dyslipidemia in mice. Diabetes 50:2555–2562

Scott JD, Fischer EH, Demaille JG, and Krebs EG (1985a) Identification of an inhibitory region of the heat-stable protein inhibitor of the cAMP-dependent protein kinase. Proc Natl Acad Sci U S A 82:4379–4383

Scott JD, Fischer EH, Takio K, Demaille JG, and Krebs EG (1985b) Amino acid sequence of the heat-stable inhibitor of the cAMP-dependent protein kinase from rabbit skeletal muscle. Proc Natl Acad Sci U S A 82:5732–5736

Sculptoreanu A, Scheuer T, and Catterall WA (1993) Voltage-dependent potentiation of L-type Ca2+ channels due to phosphorylation by cAMP-dependent protein kinase. Nature 364:240–243

Seasholtz AF, Gamm DM, Ballestero RP, Scarpetta MA, and Uhler MD (1995) Differential expression of mRNAs for protein kinase inhibitor isoforms in mouse brain. Proc Natl Acad Sci U S A 92:1734–1738

Shah K, Liu Y, Deirmengian C, and Shokat KM (1997) Engineering unnatural nucleotide specificity for Rous sarcoma virus tyrosine kinase to uniquely label its direct substrates. Proc Natl Acad Sci U S A 94:3565–3570

Skalhegg BS, Huang Y, Su T, Idzerda RL, McKnight GS, and Burton KA (2002) Mutation of the Ca subunit of PKA leads to growth retardation and sperm dysfunction. Mol Endo 16

Snell K, and Duff DA (1979) Muscle phosphoenolpyruvate carboxykinase activity and alanine release in progressively starved rats. Int J Biochem 10:423–426

Souza SC, de Vargas LM, Yamamoto MT, Lien P, Franciosa MD, Moss LG, and Greenberg AS (1998) Overexpression of perilipin A and B blocks the ability of tumor necrosis factor alpha to increase lipolysis in 3T3-L1 adipocytes. J Biol Chem 273:24665–24669

Stralfors P, and Belfrage P (1983) Phosphorylation of hormone-sensitive lipase by cyclic AMP-dependent protein kinase. J Biol Chem 258:15146–15152

Stralfors P, Bjorgell P, and Belfrage P (1984) Hormonal regulation of hormone-sensitive lipase in intact adipocytes: identification of phosphorylated sites and effects on the phosphorylation by lipolytic hormones and insulin. Proc Natl Acad Sci U S A 81:3317–3321

Stratakis CA, Kirschner LS, and Carney JA (2001) Clinical and molecular features of the Carney complex: diagnostic criteria and recommendations for patient evaluation. J. Clin. Endocrinol. Metab. 86:4041–4046

Sun X, Meyers EN, Lewandoski M, and Martin GR (1999) Targeted disruption of Fgf8 causes failure of cell migration in the gastrulating mouse embryo. Genes Dev 13:1834–1846

Tansey JT, Sztalryd C, Gruia-Gray J, Roush DL, Zee JV, Gavrilova O, Reitman ML, Deng CX, Li C, Kimmel AR, and Londos C (2001) Perilipin ablation results in a lean mouse with aberrant adipocyte lipolysis, enhanced leptin production, and resistance to diet-induced obesity. Proc Natl Acad Sci U S A 98:6494–6499

Tash JS, and Means AR (1983) Cyclic adenosine 3',5' monophosphate, calcium and protein phosphorylation in flagellar motility. Biol Reprod 28:75–104

Thiele TE, Willis B, Stadler J, Reynolds JG, Bernstein IL, and McKnight GS (2000) High ethanol consupmtion and low sensitivity to ethanol-induced sedation in protein kinase A-mutant mice. J Neurosci 20:RC75

Ungerer M, Bohm M, Elce JS, Erdmann E, and Lohse MJ (1993) Altered expression of beta-adrenergic receptor kinase and beta 1- adrenergic receptors in the failing human heart. Circulation 87:454–463

Van Patten SM, Donaldson LF, McGuinness MP, Kumar P, Alizadeh A, Griswold MD, and Walsh DA (1997) Specific testicular cellular localization and hormonal regulation of the PKIalpha and PKIbeta isoforms of the inhibitor protein of the cAMP- dependent protein kinase. J Biol Chem 272:20021–20029

Van Patten SM, Howard P, Walsh DA, and Maurer RA (1992) The alpha- and beta-isoforms of the inhibitor protein of the 3',5'- cyclic adenosine monophosphate-dependent protein kinase: characteristics and tissue- and developmental-specific expression. Mol Endocrinol 6:2114–2122

Vijayaraghavan S, Goueli SA, Davey MP, and Carr DW (1997) Protein kinase A-anchoring inhibitor peptides arrest mammalian sperm motility. J Biol Chem 272:4747–4752

Vijayaraghavan S, Olson GE, NagDas S, Winfrey VP, and Carr DW (1997) Subcellular localization of the regulatory subunits of cyclic adenosine 3',5'-monophosphate-dependent protein kinase in bovine spermatozoa. Biol Reprod 57:1517–1523

Visconti PE, Moore GD, Bailey JL, Leclerc P, Connors SA, Pan D, Olds-Clarke P, and Kopf GS (1995) Capacitation of mouse spermatozoa. II. Protein tyrosine phosphorylation and capacitation are regulated by a cAMP-dependent pathway. Development 121:1139–1150

Walsh DA, C.D. A, Gonzalez C, Calkins D, Fischer EH, and Krebs EG (1971) Purification and characterization of a protein kinase inhibitor of adenosine 3', 5' monophosphate-dependent protein kinases. J Biol Chem 246:1977–1985

Wang B, Fallon JF, and Beachy PA (2000) Hedgehog-regulated processing of Gli3 produces an anterior/posterior repressor gradient in the developing vertebrate limb. Cell 100:423–434

Wang ZW, and Kotlikoff MI (1996) Activation of KCa channels in airway smooth muscle cells by endogenous protein kinase A. Am J Physiol 271:L100–105

Wen W, Harootunian AT, Adams SR, Feramisco J, Tsien RY, Meinkoth JL, and Taylor SS (1994) Heat-stable inhibitors of cAMP-dependent protein kinase carry a nuclear export signal. J Biol Chem 269:32214–32220

Wiley JC, Wailes LA, Idzerda RL, and McKnight GS (1999) Role of regulatory subunits and protein kinase inhibitor (PKI) in determining nuclear localization and activity of the catalytic subunit of protein kinase A. J Biol Chem 274:6381–6387

Woo NH, Duffy SN, Abel T, and Nguyen PV (2000) Genetic and pharmacological demonstration of differential recruitment of cAMP-dependent protein kinases by synaptic activity. J Neurophysiol 84:2739–2745

Woodford TA, Correll LA, McKnight GS, and Corbin JD (1989) Expression and characterization of mutant forms of the type I regulatory subunit of cAMP-dependent protein kinase. The effect of defective cAMP binding on holoenzyme activation. J Biol Chem 264:13321–13328

Yakar S, Liu JL, Stannard B, Butler A, Accili D, Sauer B, and LeRoith D (1999) Normal growth and development in the absence of hepatic insulin-like growth factor I. Proc Natl Acad Sci U S A 96:7324–7329

Yamaguchi TP, Harpal K, Henkemeyer M, and Rossant J (1994) fgfr-1 is required for embryonic growth and mesodermal patterning during mouse gastrulation. Genes Dev 8:3032–3044

Yonemoto W, McGlone ML, and Taylor SS (1993) N-myristylation of the catalytic subunit of cAMP-dependent protein kinase conveys structural stability. J Biol Chem 268:2348–2352.

G Protein-Mediated Signalling Pathways

S. Offermanns

Pharmakologisches Institut, Universität Heidelberg, Im Neuenheimer Feld 366,
69120 Heidelberg, Germany
e-mail: stefan.offermanns@urz.uni-heidelberg.de

Abstract The G protein-mediated signalling system operates in all mammalian cells and is involved in many physiological and pathological processes. This review summarizes some general aspects of G protein-mediated signalling and focuses on recent data especially from studies in mutant mice, which have elucidated some of the cellular and biological functions of signalling pathways mediated by heterotrimeric G proteins.

Keywords G protein · Gene targeting · Transgenic animals · Effector · Transmembrane signalling

1
Introduction

G protein-mediated signalling has evolved as the most widely used transmembrane signalling mechanism in the mammalian organism. All cells of the mammalian organism express G protein-coupled receptors as well as several types of heterotrimeric G proteins and effectors. G proteins consist of α, β and γ subunits and couple activated receptors to effector proteins. The receptor-activated heterotrimeric G protein dissociates into the α subunit and the $\beta\gamma$-complex which both regulate effectors. The main properties of individual G proteins appear to be determined by the identity of the α subunit. More than 20 G protein α subunits have been described in the mammalian system, and they can be divided into four subfamilies based on structural and functional homologies (Table 1) (Simon et al. 1991). Five G protein β subunits and 11 γ subunits which form the $\beta\gamma$-complex have been found so far in the mammalian system. G protein-mediated signalling is involved in many physiological and pathological processes. Most of the information about the function of G proteins and their effectors has been derived from in vitro cell culture studies. Transgenic and gene targeting techniques have recently allowed us to generate mice lacking individual G protein α subunits and G protein-regulated effectors or carrying additional copies of their genes (see Tables 1, 2, 3 and 4). Analysis of these mouse models shows how G protein-mediated signalling processes are involved in a wide variety of biological processes. This review summarises major findings in mouse lines carrying mutant genes of G protein α subunits and of G protein effectors.

2
Nervous System

Most neurotransmitters of the central nervous system (CNS) act on G protein-coupled receptors to modulate neuronal activity. The receptors are found pre- and postsynaptically and mediate relatively slow responses. Inhibitory modulation is mostly mediated by coupling of receptors to members of the $G_{i/o}$ family whereas G_q and G_s family members are primarily involved in excitatory responses.

Table 1 Phenotypical changes in mice lacking α subunits of heterotrimeric G proteins

Family	Type	Gene	Expression	Effectors	Phenotype	Reference(s)
$G\alpha_s$	$G\alpha_s$[a]	Gnas	Ubiquitous	AC (all types)↑	Embryonic Lethal[d]	Yu et al. 1998
	$G\alpha_{olf}$	Gnal	olf. Epithelium, brain	AC ↑	Anosmia, hyperactivity	Belluscio et al. 1998
$G\alpha_{i/o}$	$G\alpha_{i1}$	Gnai1	Widely distributed	AC ↓[e]; GIRK[f] ↑	No obvious phenotype seen so far	L. Birnbaumer, M. Jiang, G. Boulay, K. Spicher[j]
	$G\alpha_{i2}$	Gnai2	Ubiquitous	GIRK[f] ↑	Inflammatory bowel disease	Rudolph et al. 1995
	$G\alpha_{i3}$	Gnai3	Widely distributed	GIRK[f] ↑	No obvious phenotype seen so far	L. Birnbaumer, M. Jiang, G. Boulay, K. Spicher[j]
	$G\alpha_o$[b]	Gnao	Neuronal, neuroendocr.	VDCC ↓[9]; GIRK[f] ↑	Various CNS defects	Valenzuela et al. 1997; Jiang et al. 1998
	$G\alpha_z$	Gnaz	Neuronal, platelets	AC ↓; ?	Mild platelet/CNS defects	Hendry et al. 2000; Yang et al. 2000
	$G\alpha_{gust}$	Gnat3	Taste cells, brush cells	?	Impaired bitter and sweet sensation	Wong et al. 1996
	$G\alpha_{t-r}$	Gnat1	Retinal rods, taste cells	cGMP PDE ↑	Mild retinal degeneration	Calvert et al. 2000
	$G\alpha_{t-c}$	Gnat2	Retinal cones	cGMP PDE ↑	No mouse mutant available	–
	$G\alpha_{i1}+G\alpha_{i3}$				No obvious phenotype seen so far	L. Birnbaumer, M. Jiang, G. Boulay, K. Spicher[j]
	$G\alpha_{i2}+G\alpha_{i3}$				Lethal	L. Birnbaumer, M. Jiang, G. Boulay, K. Spicher[j]

Table 1 (continued)

Family	Type	Gene	Expression	Effectors	Phenotype	Reference(s)
$G\alpha_q$	$G\alpha_q$	Gnaq	Ubiquitous	PLC-β ↑[h]	Ataxia, defective platelet activation	Offermanns et al. 1997a,c
	$G\alpha_{11}$	Gna11	Almost ubiquitous	PLC-β ↑[h]	No obvious phenotype seen so far	Offermanns et al. 1998
	$G\alpha_{14}$	Gna14	Kidney, lung, cells	PLC-β ↑[h]	No obvious phenotype seen so far	Davignon et al. 2000
	$G\alpha_q+G\alpha_{11}$				Myocardial ypoplasia (lethal e11)	Offermanns et al. 1998
					Cardiomyocyte-restricted: pressure overload induced hypertrophy ↓	Wettschureck et al. 2001
	$G\alpha_q+G\alpha_{15}$				Like $G\alpha_q$ (−/−)	
$G\alpha_{12}$	$G\alpha_{12}$	Gna-12	Ubiquitous	?	No obvious phenotype seen so far	Davignon et al. 2000
						Gu et al. 2002
$G\alpha_{13}$	$G\alpha_{13}$	Gna-13	Ubiquitous	?[i]	Defective angiogenesis (lethal e9.5)	Offermanns et al. 1997b
$G\alpha_{12}+G\text{-}\alpha_{13}$	$G\alpha_{12}+G\text{-}\alpha_{13}$				Embryonic lethal (e8.5)	Gu et al. 2002

AC, adenylyl cyclase; cGMP-PDE, cGMP-phosphodiesterase; PLC-β, β-isoforms of phospholipase C; VDCC, voltage-dependent Ca^{2+}-channel.

a Several splice variants.
b Two splice variants.
c Mouse form ($G\alpha_{16}$, human counterpart).
d Parent of origin specific defects in heterozygotes.
e Adenylyl cyclase types I, V, VI.
f GIRK1-GIRK4 (Kir3.1-Kir3.4), effector is regulated through $\beta\gamma$ subunits.
g N-,P/Q-,R-type ($Ca_V2.1$-$Ca_V2.3$), effector is regulated through $\beta\gamma$ subunits.
h $\beta_4; \beta_3 \geq \beta_1 >> \beta_2$.
i RhoGEF proteins (p115RhoGEF).
j Personal communication.

Table 2 Phenotypical changes in mice lacking functional G protein-regulated effectors and G protein regulators

Effector	Subtype	Gene	Expression	G Protein	Phenotype	Reference(s)
AC	I	Adcy1	Brain, adrenal gland	$G\alpha_s(\uparrow)$; $G\alpha_{i/o}$ $G\beta\gamma(\downarrow)$	Altered behaviour, LTP and somatosensory cortex patterning	Wu et al. 1995; Abdel-Majid et al. 1998; Storm et al. 1998; Villacres et al. 1998
	III	Adcy3	Brain, heart, olfactory epith.	$G\alpha_s\uparrow G\alpha_{i/o}\downarrow$	Anosmia	Wong et al. 2000
	VIII	Adcy8	Brain, lung, pancreas	$G\alpha_s\uparrow G\alpha_{i/o}\downarrow$	Altered stress-induced anxiety	Schaefer et al. 2000
	I+VIII				Loss of late phase LTP/long-term memory	Wong et al. 1999
PDE	6γ	Pdeg	Retinal rods	$G\alpha_{t-r}$	Retinal degeneration	Tsang et al. 1996
PLC	β1	Plcb1	Brain	$G\alpha_{q/11}(\uparrow)$	Epilepsy	Kim et al. 1997
	β2	Plcb2	Hematopoietic cells	$G\alpha_{q/11},G\beta\gamma$ $(\uparrow)$	Chemotactic responses ↑	Jiang et al. 1997
	β3	Plcb3	Ubiquitous	$G\alpha_{q/11},G\beta\gamma$ $(\uparrow)$	Viable	Xie et al. 1999
	β4	Plcb4	Brain	$G\alpha_{q/11}(\uparrow)$	Cerebellar ataxia	Kim et al. 1997; Kano et al. 1998
	β2+β3				Defective leukocyte activation	Li et al. 2000
GIRK	Kir3.2	Kcnj6	Brain, testis, pancreas	$G\beta\gamma\uparrow$	Seizure susceptibility ↑	Signorini et al. 1997
	Kir3.4	Kcnj5	Brain, heart	$G\beta\gamma(\uparrow)$	Vagal mediated heart rate slowing ↓	Wickman et al. 1998
VDCC	$Ca_v2.1$	Cacna1a	Brain, cochlea	$G\beta\gamma\downarrow$	Ataxia, dystonia, death <4 weeks	Jun et al. 1999
	$Ca_v2.2$	Cacna1b	Neuronal	$G\beta\gamma\downarrow$	Heart rate/blood pressure↑	Ino et al. 2001
	$Ca_v2.3$	Cacna1e	Brain, heart etina	$G\beta\gamma\downarrow$	Inflammatory pain response↑	Saegusa et al. 2000
PI-3-K	PI-3-Kγ	Pik3cg	Widely	$G\beta\gamma\uparrow$	Defective eukocyte activation	Li et al. 2000; Hirsch et al. 2000; Sasaki et al. 2000; Hirsch et al. 2001
GRK	GRK2	Adrbk1	Brain, skeletal muscle, spleen	$G\beta\gamma\uparrow$	Embryonic lethal	Jaber et al. 1996
	GRK3	Adrbk2	Brain, heart, kidney, olf. epith.	$G\beta\gamma\uparrow$	Baroreflex ↑, airway response to methacholine ↓	Peppel et al. 1997
RhoGEF	lsc	Arhgef1	Haematopoietic cells	$G\alpha_{12/13}$ $(\uparrow)$	Altered marginal zone B cell homeostasis	Girkontaite et al. 2001
RGS	RGS2	Rgs2	Widely	$G\alpha_{q11}$	T cell activation ↓, male aggression ↓, anxiety ↑	Oliveira-Dos-Santos et al. 2000
	RGS9	Rgs9	Brain, retina, pineal gland	$G\beta_5G\alpha_{t-r}$	Retinal rod photoresponse recovery ↓	Chen et al. 2000

AC, adenylyl cyclase; epith., epithelium; GIRK, G protein-regulated inward rectifier potassium channel; GRK, G protein-regulated kinase; olf., olfactory; PI-3-K, phospho-inositide-3-kinase; PLC, phospholipase C; RGS, regulator of G protein signalling; VDCC, voltage-dependent Ca^{2+}-channel.

Table 3 Genetically engineered mice with transgenic expression of wild-type or mutant G protein α subunits

Transgene	Promoter	Tissue	Phenotype	Reference(s)
Gα_s (wt)	α-MHC	Cardiomyocytes	Increased inotropic and chronotropic responses to catecholamines; cardiomyopathy	Gaudin et al. 1995; Iwase et al. 1996, 1997
Gα_s(R201H) (const. active)	Thyroglobulin	Thyrocytes	Hyperfunctioning thyroid adenoma	Michiels et al. 1994
Gα_s(R201C) (const. active)	Insulin	Pancreatic β-cells	Normal glucose homeostasis increased glucose tolerance in the presence of IBMX	Ma et al. 1994
Gα_s(Q227L) (const. active)	PEPCK	Liver, fat cells, skeletal muscle	Decreased glucose tolerance	Huang et al. 2002
Gα_{i2}(Q205L) (const. active)	PEPCK	Liver, fat cells, skeletal muscle	Increased glucose tolerance; reduced fasting blood glucose levels	Chen et al. 1997; Guo et al. 1998; Zheng et al. 1998
Gα_{t-c}(Q204L) (const. active)	Rhodopsin	Retinal cones	Downregulation of PDE α- and β subunits	Raport et al. 1994
Gα_q (wt)	α-MHC	Cardiomyocytes	Cardiac hypertrophy, cardiomyopathy	D'Angelo et al. 1997; Adams et al. 1998
Gα_q(Q209L) (const. active)	α-MHC	Cardiomyocytes	Cardiac hypertrophy and dilatation	Mende et al. 1998
Gα_q-peptide (305–359)	α-MHC	Cardiomyocytes	Pressure overload induced ventricular hypertrophy ↓	Akhter et al. 1998

Const. active, constitutively active mutant; IBMX, isobutyl-methyl-xanthine; MHC, myosin heavy chain; PDE, phosphodiesterase; PEPCK, phosphoenolpyruvate carboxykinase; wt, wild type form.

2.1
The Role of G$_o$ in Central Nervous System Function

The G protein G$_o$ is highly abundant in the mammalian nervous system. On a cellular level, G$_o$ has been demonstrated to mediate inhibitory effects by inhibition of neuronal (N-, P/Q-, R-type) Ca^{2+} channels and activation of inward-rectifier K$^+$ channels (GIRK). Regulation of these channels occurs through direct interaction of G$\beta\gamma$ and the channel protein (Catterall 2000; Mark and Herlitze 2000). This regulation has been implicated in the pre- and postsynaptic inhibitory modulation of neuronal activity. Gα_o-deficient mice are clearly impaired, being smaller and weaker than their littermates and showing greatly reduced postnatal survival rates (Valenzuela et al. 1997; Jiang et al. 1998). Gα_o-deficient mice suffer from tremors and have occasional seizures. A severely abnormal motor behaviour can be observed in Gα_o-deficient mice, which show an elevated level of motoric activity and an extreme turning behaviour (http://www.anes.ucla.edu/~lutzb/realmice.htm). In addition, Gα_o-deficient mice appear to be hyperalgesic when tested in the hot plate assay (Jiang et al. 1998). The hyperalgesia

Table 4 Phenotypical changes in mice transgenically expressing G protein-regulated effectors or G protein regulators

Transgene	Promoter	Tissue	Phenotype	Reference
AC V	α-MHC	Cardiomyocyte	Increased basal but not βAR-mediated signalling	Tepe et al. 1999
AC VI	α-MHC	Cardiomyocyte	Increases responsiveness to catecholamine	Gao et al. 1999
			Improves heart function in cardiomyopathy	Roth et al. 1999
AC VIII	α-MHC	Cardiomyocyte	Enhanced cardiac function	Lipskaia et al. 2000
GRK2	α-MHC	Cardiomyocyte	β-AR-mediated stimulation of cardiac function $\downarrow$	Koch et al. 1995
GRK2	SM22α	VSM	Increases resting blood pressure	Eckhart et al. 2002
GRK3	α-MHC	Cardiomyocyte	Mild alterations	Iaccarino et al. 1998
GRK2^{ct*}	α-MHC	Cardiomyocyte	Left ventricular contractility $\uparrow$	
			Response to isoproterenol $\uparrow$	Koch et al. 1995
RGS4	α-MHC	Cardiomyocyte	Increased mortality and reduced cardiac hypertrophy in response to pressure overload	Rogers et al. 1999

*C-terminal 194 amino acids of GRK2 (G$\beta\gamma$-binding pleckstrin homology domain-containing portion).

may at least in part be due to a reduction of opioid-induced Ca^{2+} channel inhibition in cells of dorsal root ganglia from $G\alpha_o^{(-/-)}$ mice (Jiang et al. 1998). Electrophysiological analysis of various neuronal cells from $G\alpha_o$-deficient mice showed that modulation of GIRK channels and of voltage-dependent Ca^{2+} channels through G protein-coupled receptors did not have an absolute requirement for G_o (Jiang et al. 1998; Greif et al. 2000). This indicates that other G proteins, most likely G_i-type G proteins, can contribute to the regulation of these ion channels via their $\beta\gamma$-complexes. The neurological defects observed in $G\alpha_o$-deficient mice indicate that $G\alpha_o$ plays an important functional role in the central nervous system, while it is obviously not crucially involved in the morphogenesis of the CNS.

2.2
G$\beta\gamma$-Regulated K$^+$ and Ca^{2+} Channels of the Central Nervous System

Mice lacking the α_1 subunit of G$\beta\gamma$-inhibited P/Q-, N- and R-type voltage-dependent Ca^{2+} channels ($Ca_v2.1$, $Ca_v2.2$ and $Ca_v2.3$) have recently been generated and show various defects. The α_1 subunit of P/Q-type Ca^{2+} channels ($Ca_v2.1$) is the most abundant in the CNS, and mice deficient in $Ca_v2.1$ develop ataxia, dystonia and absent seizures, resulting in death within a few weeks postnatally (Jun et al. 1999). Mice lacking $Ca_v2.2$, the α_1 subunit of N-type Ca^{2+} channels, which has been involved in regulation of transmitter release in the central as well as the peripheral nervous system show a less severe phenotype. These mice showed a defective function of sympathetic neurons resulting, e.g. in a marked reduction of the baroreceptor reflex (Ino et al. 2001). Defects were also observed in the nociceptive system where these animals showed altered nociceptive responses (Hatakeyama et al. 2001; Kim et al. 2001; Saegusa et al. 2001). Altered nociception was also observed in mice deficient in the α_1 subunit of R-type Ca^{2+} channels ($Ca_v2.3$), which showed a decreased response to somatic inflammatory pain stimuli (Saegusa et al. 2000).

Of the $G\beta\gamma$-activated GIRK channels (Mark and Herlitze 2000) expressed in the brain the gene of the GIRK2 subform has been inactivated in mice resulting in increased susceptibility to seizures (Signorini et al. 1997). Only subtle changes in central nervous system functions were observed in animals lacking GIRK4 (Wickman et al. 2000).

2.3
G_z Function in the Nervous System

G_z, a member of the $G_{i/o}$ family of G proteins, shares with G_{i1}, G_{i2} and G_{i3} the ability to inhibit adenylyl cyclases and is found in brain, adrenal medulla and platelets (Fields and Casey 1997; Ho and Wong 1998). Mice which lack $G\alpha_z$ are viable and do not show any obvious neurological defects. However, $G\alpha_z$-deficient mice exhibit altered responses to a variety of psychoactive drugs. Cocaine-induced increases in locomotor activity were much more pronounced in these animals compared to wild-type mice, and short-term antinociceptive effects of morphine were found to be slightly reduced (Yang et al. 2000). However, Hendry et al. (2000), using a different strain and a different experimental protocol, did not observe an alteration in the acute effect of morphine, while tolerance to the antinociceptive effects after chronic morphine administration was increased. Most strikingly, it was found that behavioural effects of catecholamine reuptake inhibitors like reboxetine and desipramine were abolished in $G\alpha_z$-deficient mice (Yang et al. 2000). The receptors involved in the various effects of psychoactive drugs are not always clearly defined. Nevertheless, the results of these studies clearly indicate that G_z is involved in signalling processes regulated by various neurotransmitters.

2.4
The Role of G_{olf} in Striatal Signalling

$G\alpha_{olf}$, a member of the $G\alpha_s$ family, has been shown to be expressed in olfactory sensory neurons as well as in the basal ganglia, olfactory tubercle, the hippocampus and the Purkinje cells of the cerebellar cortex (Herve et al. 1993; Zhuang et al. 2000). Most of these brain regions also express $G\alpha_s$. However, $G\alpha_{olf}$ expression levels clearly exceed those of $G\alpha_s$ in the nucleus accumbens, the olfactory tubercle and in the striatum (Belluscio et al. 1998; Zhuang et al. 2000). Apart from olfactory defects (see below), surviving $G\alpha_{olf}$-deficient mice exhibit clear motoric abnormalities like hypermotoric behavior (Belluscio et al. 1998). Similar phenotypical changes have been observed in mice lacking the dopamine D_1 receptor (Xu et al. 1994) which has been found to be coexpressed with $G\alpha_{olf}$ in striatal neurons (Herve et al. 1995), and recent data indicate that G_{olf} is critically involved in dopamin (D_1) and adenosine (A_{2A}) receptor-mediated effects in the striatum (Zhuang et al. 2000; Herve et al. 2001). Functional data as well as regional coexpression suggest the existence of a signalling cascade consisting of the D_1 receptors, G_{olf} and adenylyl cyclase type 5 in the nigrostriatal pathway (Zhuang et al. 2000). Thus, the function of G_{olf} is not restricted to olfactory sensory cells but obviously plays a defined role also in other areas of the CNS.

2.5
$G_{q/11}$-Mediated Signalling in the Cerebellar Cortex

The two main members of the G_q family, G_q and G_{11}, are widely expressed in the central nervous system and couple numerous receptors to β-isoforms of phospholipase C. Usually, levels of $G\alpha_q$ exceed those of $G\alpha_{11}$ several fold in the CNS. Mice lacking $G\alpha_q$ develop an ataxia with clear signs of motor coordination deficits, and functional defects could be observed in the cerebellar cortex of $G\alpha_q$-deficient mice (Offermanns et al. 1997a). While excitatory synaptic transmission from parallel fibres (PFs) to cerebellar Purkinje cells (PCs) and from climbing fibres (CFs) to PCs was functional; about 40% of adult $G\alpha_q$-deficient PCs remained multiply innervated by CFs due to a defect in regression of supernumerary CFs in the third postnatal week, which most likely resulted from a functional defect at the PF-PC-synapse. A defect in the modulation of the PF-PC synapse in mice lacking $G\alpha_q$ is also suggested by the fact that long-term depression (LTD) of the PF–PC synapse was deficient in $G\alpha_q^{(-/-)}$ mice (M. Kano et al., unpublished). Very similar phenotypes have been described in mice lacking the $G_{q/11}$-coupled metabotropic glutamate type 1 receptor (GluR1) (Aiba et al. 1995; Kano et al. 1997) as well as in mice deficient in the $\beta 4$-isoform of phospholipase C, which shows predominant expression in Purkinje cells of the rostral cerebellum (Kano et al. 1998; Miyata et al. 2001). The mGluR1, $G\alpha_q$ and PLC$\beta 4$ are colocalised in dendritic spines of PCs (Kano et al. 1998; Watanabe et al. 1998; Tanaka et al. 2000), suggesting that a defined signalling cascade in the postsynaptic membrane of PF–PC synapses is involved in the postnatal elimination of multiple CF innervation as well as in cerebellar LTD (Fig. 1).

2.6
Barrel Formation in the Somatosensory Cortex

The primary somatosensory cortex shows distinct cytoarchitectonic features called barrels. Each barrel consists of a group of neurons representing one facial vibrissal hair and is innervated by a bundle of axons from the ventral posterial complex of the thalamus. The postnatal development of barrels on the somatosensory cortex is induced by thalamic axons which grow up in the cortex and organise themselves into bundles which determine the pattern of barrels in the

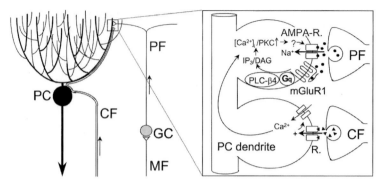

Fig. 1 Main neuronal connections of the cerebellar cortex and some of the putative mechanisms of cerebellar LTD. The cerebellar cortex has basically one output, the Purkinje cell (*PC*) axon, and two inputs, one in form of climbing fibres (*CFs*) which directly synapse on PCs and one in form of Mossy fibres (*MFs*) which synapse on granule cells (*GCs*). GCs send their bifurcating axon (parallel fibres) into the outer layer of the cerebellar cortex where they form multiple synaptic contacts with PCs. Long-term depression (*LTD*) of the parallel fibre (PF)–PC synapse requires conjunctive stimulation of PFs and CFs innervating the same PC. It results from a long-lasting depression of the α-amino-3-hydroxy-5-methyl-4-isoxazolepropionic acid (*AMPA*) receptor-mediated current which is induced by a long increase in the Ca^{2+} concentration in PC dendrites as well as the activation of metabotropic glutamate type 1 receptors (*mGluR1*) which signal through G_q. PLC-$\beta4$, $\beta4$-isoform of phospholipase C; *IP$_3$*, inositol-1,4,5-trisphosphate; *DAG*, diacyl glycerol; *PKC*, protein kinase C; *AMPA-R.*, ionotropic non-*N*-methyl-d-aspartate glutamate receptor

cortex. Mice lacking the metabotropic glutamate type 5 receptor (mGluR5) fail to form cortical barrels and show only partial segregation of thalamic efferent neurons (Hannan et al. 2001). The $G_{q/11}$-coupled mGluR5 receptor regulates β-isoforms of phospholipase C, leading to increases in the intracellular calcium concentration. Interestingly, mice lacking the $\beta1$-subtype of phospholipase C do not form cortical barrels, while the segregation of thalamocortical neurons occurs normally (Hannan et al. 2001). This shows that bundling of thalamic neurons is necessary but not sufficient for the formation of the barrel cortex. Glutamate-induced, mGluR5-mediated phospholipase Cβ-1 activation appears to be required for differentiation of cortical neurons into barrel-like structures. Mice lacking the type 1 isoform of adenylyl cyclase lack barrels in the somatosensory cortex and show a complete failure of thalamic axons to segregate (Abdel-Majid 1998). Since type 1 adenylyl cyclase is activated by calcium, it could be regulated through mGluR5 receptors. The difference in phenotype of mice lacking PLCβ-1 and adenylyl cyclase type 1, however, suggests that PLC$\beta1$-mediated signalling is not necessarily upstream of adenylyl cyclase type 1.

3
Development

3.1
G$_{13}$-Mediated Signalling in Embryonic Angiogenesis

The inactivation of some Gα genes leads to phenotypes which are manifest during mouse development. G$_{12}$ and G$_{13}$ constitute the G$_{12}$ family and are expressed ubiquitously. Both G proteins have been shown to induce cytoskeletal rearrangements in a Rho-dependent manner (Buhl et al. 1995; Sah et al. 2000). Lack of Gα_{13} in mice results in embryonic lethality at about mid-gestation. At this stage, mouse embryos express both Gα_{12} and Gα_{13}. Analysis of Gα_{13}-deficient mouse embryos revealed that loss of Gα_{13} leads to a defective organisation of the vascular system which is most prominent in the yolk sac and in the head mesenchyme (Offermanns et al. 1997b). Vasculogenic blood vessel formation through the differentiation of progenitor cells into endothelial cells was not affected by the loss of Gα_{13}. However, angiogenesis which include sprouting, growth, migration and remodelling of existing endothelial cells (Risau 1997) was severely disturbed in G$\alpha_{13}^{(-/-)}$ embryos. Chemokinetic effects of thrombin were completely abrogated in fibroblasts lacking Gα_{13}, indicating that Gα_{13} is required for full migratory responses of cells to certain stimuli. The defects observed in Gα_{13}-deficient embryos and cells occurred in the presence of Gα_{12}, and loss of Gα_{12} did not result in any obvious defects. Interestingly, Gα_{12}-deficient mice which carry only one intact Gα_{13} allele also die in utero (Gu et al. 2002). This genetic evidence indicates that Gα_{13} and its closest relative, Gα_{12}, fulfil at least partially non-overlapping cellular and biological functions which are required for proper development.

3.2
The G$_{q/11}$-Mediated Pathway Is Required for Embryonic Myocardial Growth

The Gα_q/Gα_{11}-mediated signalling pathway appears to play a pivotal role in the regulation of physiological myocardial growth during embryogenesis. This is demonstrated by the phenotype of Gα_q/Gα_{11}-double-deficient mice which die at embryonic day 11 due to a severe thinning of the myocardial layer of the heart (Offermanns et al. 1998). Both the trabecular ventricular myocardium as well as the subepicardial layer appeared to be underdeveloped. The G$_q$/G$_{11}$-coupled receptors involved in the regulation of cardiac growth at mid-gestation are currently unknown. Inactivation of the gene encoding the G$_{q/11}$-coupled serotonin 5-HT$_{2B}$ receptors in mice resulted in cardiomyopathy with a loss of ventricular mass due to a reduction in number and size of cardiomyocytes (Nebigil et al. 2001); and lack of both endothelin A (ET$_A$) and B (ET$_B$) receptors, which can signal through G$_{q/11}$, resulted in mid-gestational cardiac failure (Yanagisawa et al. 1998). There is most likely some degree of signalling redundancy with several inputs into the G$_{q/11}$ pathway, and only deletion of both the Gα_q and the Gα_{11}

genes results in severe phenotypic defects during early heart development. Interestingly, one intact allele of the $G\alpha_q$ or $G\alpha_{11}$ gene was obviously sufficient to overcome the early developmental block in heart development. However, $G\alpha_q{}^{(-/-)};G\alpha_{11}{}^{(-/+)}$, and to a lesser degree $G\alpha_q{}^{(-/+)};G\alpha_{11}{}^{(-/-)}$, pups showed an increased incidence of cardiac defects ranging from septal defects to univentricular hearts (Offermanns et al. 1998).

3.3
Neural Crest

Apart from the role of $G_{q/11}$ in heart development, signalling through G_q class members has also been implicated in the proliferation and/or migration of neural crest cells. Endothelin-1 and the $G_{q/11}$-coupled ET_A receptor are essential for normal function of craniofacial and cardiac neural crest. Endothelin-1 and ET_A receptor-deficient mice die shortly after birth due to respiratory failure (Kurihara et al. 1994, 1995; Clouthier et al. 1998). Severe skeletal abnormalities could be observed in their craniofacial region, including retarded mandibular bones, aberrant zygomatic and temporal bones, and absence of auditory ossicles and tympanic ring. A milder form of the endothelin-1/ET_A-receptor $(-/-)$ craniofacial phenotype was observed in $G\alpha_q{}^{(-/-)};G\alpha_{11}{}^{(-/+)}$ mice (Offermanns et al. 1998). In contrast, $G\alpha_q{}^{(-/+)};G\alpha_{11}{}^{(-/-)}$ mice did not show craniofacial abnormalities, suggesting that ET_A receptor-mediated neural crest development involves primarily $G\alpha_q$. It is also possible that a certain amount of $G\alpha_q/G\alpha_{11}$ is required for endothelin-1-dependent craniofacial development, and that this is only provided by one intact allele of the $G\alpha_q$ gene but not of the $G\alpha_{11}$ gene.

4
Immune System

4.1
Function of G_i-Type G Proteins in the Immune System

The first transgenic experiment to study the function of $G\alpha_{i/o}$ family members in vivo was done by expression of the S1 subunit of pertussis toxin (PTX) under the control of the lck promoter in mouse thymocytes which express $G\alpha_{i2}$ and $G\alpha_{i3}$ (Chaffin et al. 1990). PTX, the main exotoxin of *Bordetella pertussis*, specifically ADP-ribosylates a cysteine residue close to the C terminus of $G_{i/o}$ α subunits, which leads to uncoupling of the G proteins from their receptors. PTX expression in thymocytes did not affect activation of cells by mitogenic stimuli. However, the distribution of T-lineage cells among lymphoid compartments of transgenic mice was drastically changed. Whereas peripheral organs contained greatly reduced levels of T cells, abnormally large levels of mature T cells were found in the thymi, indicating that a G_i-mediated pathway is involved in T lymphocyte emigration and/or homing (Chaffin and Perlmutter 1991). The large family of chemokines and their respective receptors which couple to G proteins of the $G_{i/o}$ family are likely to be involved in these trafficking processes (Baggiolini 1998).

4.1.1
Inflammatory Bowel Disease in Mice Lacking $G\alpha_{i2}$

While transgenic expression of the catalytic subunit of PTX is basically an elegant way to inactivate $G_{i/o}$-mediated signalling in vivo, lack of subtype selectivity as well as usually incomplete inactivation of $G_{i/o}$ by PTX are clear drawbacks of this approach. Mouse lines are now available which carry inactivating mutations of each of the three $G\alpha_i$-subtypes. Mice lacking $G\alpha_{i2}$ develop a T_H1-mediated diffuse inflammatory colitis which resembles in many aspects ulcerative colitis in humans (Rudolph et al. 1995; Hörnquist et al. 1997). The penetrance of this phenotype was greatly affected by the genetic background of the mice homozygous for the mutation. Marked increases in proinflammatory T_H1-type cytokines and of interleukin (IL)-12 were found in the inflamed colon of $G\alpha_{i2}$-deficient mice (Hörnquist et al. 1997), and antigen-presenting cells like $CD8\alpha^+$ dendritic cells from $G\alpha_{i2}$-deficient mice showed a highly increased basal production of IL-12 (He et al. 2000). This indicates that the production of proinflammatory cytokines is constitutively suppressed through a G_i-mediated pathway. Dysregulation of the immune system in the intestinal mucosa clearly precedes the histopathological and clinical onset of bowel inflammation, further supporting a role of immunological abnormalities in the pathogenesis of colitis in the $G\alpha_{i2}$-deficient mice (Öhman et al. 2000). In addition to the colitis, many $G\alpha_{i2}$-deficient mice develop colonic adenocarcinomas. Cytogenetic examination of normal non-inflamed mucosa and inflamed mucosa in $G\alpha_{i2}$-deficient mice suggest that hyperplasia and dysplasia were secondary to colonic inflammation (Broaddus et al. 1998).

4.1.2
G_i-Mediated Signalling Pathways Induce Chemotactic Responses and O_2^--Production in Neutrophils

Phagocytic cells of the immune system are able to move along concentration gradients of chemical attractants. This directional motility called chemotaxis is governed by chemoattractants such as N-formyl-Met-Leu-Phe (fMLP). Activated chemoattractant receptors coupled to G proteins of the G_i family result in the release of $\beta\gamma$ subunits of G proteins. Neutrophils lacking $G\alpha_{i2}$ show a reduced chemotactic response to fMLP (Spicher et al. 2002). Two main effectors regulated by $\beta\gamma$ subunits released from activated G_i-type G proteins in neutrophils are the β-isoforms 2 and 3 of phospholipase C , as well as the γ-isoform of the phosphoinositide 3-kinase (PI-3-kinase). The intracellular messengers generated by these enzymes are believed to initiate a cascade of events resulting in cellular responses namely production of superoxide anions (O_2^-) and chemotaxis. In neutrophils of mice lacking the γ-isoform of PI-3-kinase, the production of

PtdIns(3,4,5)P$_3$ (PIP$_3$) through chemoattractant receptors is abrogated while an elevation of cytosolic calcium concentrations can still be induced. The absence of PI-3-kinase-mediated PIP$_3$ production results in strongly reduced neutrophil migration and chemotaxis and blocks the chemoattractant-induced O$_2^-$-formation (Hirsch et al. 2000; Li et al. 2000; Sasaki et al. 2000). In contrast, neutrophils from mice lacking both the β2- and the β3-isoform of phospholipase C show still full chemotactic responses which in some cases are even enhanced, whereas chemoattractant-induced O$_2^-$-production is abrogated (Li et al. 2000). Greatly impaired chemotactic responses of myeloid cells could also be demonstrated in various in vivo models using PI-3-kinase-γ-deficient, but not PLCβ2/β3-deficient, mice. These data clearly show that receptor-mediated activation of PLCβ2/β3, which leads to increases of intracellular calcium and PKC activation, is not required for chemotactic responses to chemoattractants but that this pathway is involved in the generation of O$_2^-$ through activation of nicotinamide adenine dinucleotide phosphate, reduced (NADPH) oxidase. In contrast, PI-3-kinase-γ-mediated PIP$_3$ formation is required for both chemotactic responses as well as NADPH oxidase-dependent O$_2^-$-formation (Wu et al. 2000; Wymann et al. 2000).

4.2
Lsc Is Essential for Marginal Zone B Cell Homeostasis: A Potential Role for G$_{13}$

Cellular motility is an important property of many cells in the immune system, and small guanosine triphosphate (GTP)ases of the Rho family have been shown to play important roles in these motile responses (Ridley 2001). The Rho-specific guanine-nucleotide-exchange-factor (GEF) Lsc (p115RhoGEF) is expressed exclusively in haematopoietic cells and couples Gα_{13} to the activation of RhoA (Hart et al. 1998). In lymphocytes lacking Lsc, actin polymerisations and motility in response to thromboxane A$_2$ A$_2$ or lysophosphatidic acid (LPA) was greatly reduced, whereas responses to chemokines were not affected (Girkontaite et al. 2001). Lsc-deficient mice show various immunological defects. In addition, Lsc-deficient mice demonstrate altered trafficking of T lymphocytes to secondary lymphoid organs. Most prominently, they lack marginal zone B cells in the spleen, a subset of B cells essentially involved in the humoral immune response. Interestingly, mice lacking the tyrosine kinase Pyk-2 show the same phenotype (Guinamard et al. 2000). This suggests that Lsc and Pyk-2 are functioning in a G protein-mediated signalling pathway which is involved in the proper migration or homing of marginal zone B cells. The G protein-coupled receptors, which are upstream of the signalling cascade, are currently not known.

5
Heart

5.1
G Protein-Mediated Signalling in the Sympathetic Control of Heart Function

Sympathetic activation of the heart through β-adrenergic receptor-mediated G_s activation results in G_s-dependent activation of adenylyl cyclase and subsequent cyclic adenosine monophosphate (cAMP) production. If the expression of the short form of $G\alpha_s$ ($G\alpha_{s-S}$) was raised about threefold in the murine heart, no effect on basal or stimulated adenylyl cyclase activity was observed. However, a slightly increased rate of adenylyl cyclase activation through $G\alpha_s$ as well as an increased number of β-adrenergic receptors in the high-affinity state could be observed in cardiac membranes from these transgenic animals (Gaudin et al. 1995). Under in vivo conditions, cardiac overexpression of $G\alpha_s$ had no apparent effect on basal cardiac function but clearly enhanced the efficacy of β-adreno- ceptor G_s signalling, resulting in increased chronotropic and inotropic respons- es to catecholamine infusion (Iwase et al. 1996). Older mice overexpressing $G\alpha_s$ in the heart develop a clinical and pathological picture of cardiomyopathy (Iwase et al. 1997), supporting the concept that chronic sympathetic stimulation over an extended period of time results in cardiomyopathy. The pathogenetic processes leading to cardiomyopathy in these mice are not clear, but the lack of normal heart rate variability as well as of protective desensitisation mechanisms in hearts overexpressing $G\alpha_s$ may be a contributing mechanism (Uechi et al. 1998; Vatner et al. 1998).

5.2
G protein-Mediated Signalling in the Parasympathetic Control of Heart Function

$G_{i/o}$-coupled muscarinic acetylcholine (M_2) receptors mediate the parasympa- thetic regulation of the heart. One of the major $M_2/G_{i/o}$-regulated effectors in the atrium are inward rectifier I_{K-Ach} potassium channels consisting of Kir3.1 (GIRK1) and Kir3.4 (GIRK4) subunits which are activated by $\beta\gamma$ subunits re- leased from activated $G_{i/o}$. In mice lacking GIRK4, I_{K-Ach} is absent (Wickman et al. 1998). These animals have normal basal heart rates but show reduced vagal and adenosine-mediated slowing of heart rate as well as markedly reduced heart rate variability, which is thought to be determined by the vagal tone. The in- volvement of $G\beta\gamma$-complexes in this regulation could also be demonstrated in a mouse model in which the amount of functional $G\beta\gamma$ protein was reduced by more than 50% in cardiomyocytes. These animals showed also an impaired parasympathetic heart rate control (Gehrmann et al. 2002). Muscarinic regula- tion of heart function also involves inhibition of voltage-dependent L-type Ca^{2+} channels through an unknown mechanism. Although $G\alpha_o$ represents only a mi- nor fraction of all G proteins in the heart, it was shown that the inhibitory mus- carinic regulation of cardiac L-type Ca^{2+} channels in the heart was completely

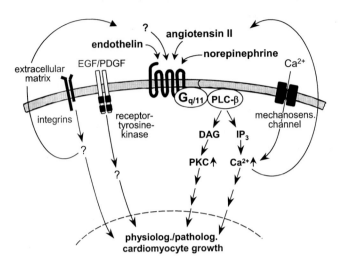

Fig. 2 Potential signalling pathways leading to physiological or pathological cardiomyocyte growth. The primary transformation of a mechanical stimulus caused by an increased hemodynamic load into a growth signal may be mediated by integrins, receptor tyrosine kinases or mechanically activated ion channels. These mechanosensitive processes result in the release of auto-/paracrine factors which are crucially involved in the induction of growth by activating the Gq/G11-mediated pathway through specific G protein-coupled receptors. *PLC-β*, β-isoforms of phospholipase C; *IP₃*, inositol-1,4,5-trisphosphate; *DAG*, diacyl glycerol; *PKC*, protein kinase C

abrogated in the $G\alpha_o^{(-/-)}$ mice (Valenzuela et al. 1997). Subsequent studies showed that also $G\alpha_{i2}$ was absolutely required for inhibition of L-type Ca^{2+} channels in the heart through muscarinic M_2 receptors (Nagata et al. 2000; Chen et al. 2001). These unexpected findings suggest that both G proteins regulate cardiac L-type Ca^{2+} channels in a complex fashion.

5.3
The Role of G_q/G_{11}-Mediated Signalling Pathways in Myocardial Hypertrophy

Adult cardiomyocytes are terminally differentiated postmitotic cells which respond to stimulatory signals with cell growth rather than proliferation. There is increasing evidence that the G_q/G_{11}-mediated pathway is also involved in myocardial hypertrophy in the adult heart following mechanical stress. In line with this, transgenic expression of wild-type $G\alpha_q$ or of a constitutively active mutant of $G\alpha_q$ in the heart (D'Angelo et al. 1997; Mende et al. 1998) results in cardiac hypertrophy. To prove that G_q/G_{11} are required for the induction of cardiac hypertrophy, two genetic approaches were used. G_q/G_{11}-mediated signalling was inhibited by transgenic expression of a short fragment of the $G\alpha_q$ C terminus (Akhter et al. 1998), which resulted in a reduced hypertrophic response. In a different approach, the G_q/G_{11}-mediated pathway was completely abrogated by conditional cardiomyocyte-specific inactivation of the $G\alpha_q/G\alpha_{11}$ genes

(Wettschureck et al. 2001). Mice with cardiomyocyte-specific $G\alpha_q/G\alpha_{11}$ double deficiency showed no ventricular hypertrophy in response to pressure overload. This strongly supports the concept that G_q/G_{11}-mediated phospholipase C activation is critically involved in the development of mechanical stress-induced cardiac hypertrophy by coupling receptors of various paracrine and autocrine factors to the induction of a genetic program which results in the growth of cardiomyocytes (Fig. 2).

6
Endocrine System and Metabolism

6.1
Parent of Origin-Specific Defects in Mice Lacking One Allele of the $G\alpha_s$ Gene

Stimulatory regulation of adenylyl cyclases through G protein-coupled receptors involves G proteins of the G_s family, of which two main members are known, G_s and G_{olf}. The ubiquitously expressed $G\alpha_s$ gene gives rise to several splice variants. $G\alpha_s$ is the only member of its subfamily expressed in most, if not all, mammalian cells; and the complete loss of $G\alpha_s$ in mice homozygous for an inactivating $G\alpha_s$ mutation leads to embryonic lethality during early postimplantation development (Yu et al. 1998). Heterozygotes which inherited the intact allele from their fathers [$G\alpha_s$(m−/p+)] or from their mothers [$G\alpha_s$(m+/p−)] have distinct phenotypical manifestations which lead to early postnatal death in the majority of animals (Yu et al. 1998). Adult $G\alpha_s$(m−/p+) animals develop obesity, have lower resting metabolic rates and are resistant to parathyroid hormone (PTH). Heterozygous mice which have inherited one intact $G\alpha_s$ allele from their mothers [$G\alpha_s$(m+/p−)] are lean, hypermetabolic and have no PTH resistance (Yu et al. 2000). These phenotypical differences are most likely due the fact that the $G\alpha_s$ gene is paternally imprinted (i.e. only the maternal allele is expressed) in a tissue-specific manner. In contrast to the maternally inherited allele, the paternal allele is not expressed in white and brown adipose tissue as well as in the proximal tubulus of the kidney (Yu et al. 1998). Similar phenotypes have been observed in humans carrying a mutation in one of the $G\alpha_s$ alleles (Weinstein et al. 2001).

6.2
Modulation of Insulin Sensitivity Through G_s and G_i

Despite the differences in fat mass and resting metabolic rates, both $G\alpha_s$(m−/p+) and $G\alpha_s$(m+/p−) animals exhibit an increased sensitivity to insulin with increased insulin-dependent glucose uptake into the skeletal muscle (Yu et al. 2001). In skeletal muscle, the $G\alpha_s$ gene is not imprinted, suggesting that the observed effects are caused by genetic haploinsufficiency. Based on studies in skeletal muscle of heterozygotes, it has been proposed that $G\alpha_s$ has a direct inhibitory effect on glucose utilisation by skeletal muscle, which appears to be independent of counterregulatory hormones like glucagon or catecholamines (Yu et al. 2001). This is supported by the finding that transgenic expression of a constitutively active mutant of $G\alpha_s$ ($G\alpha_sQ227L$) in fat, liver and skeletal muscle decreases glucose tolerance (Huang et al. 2002), while mice expressing a constitutively active mutant of $G\alpha_{i2}$ ($G\alpha_{i2}Q205L$) in fat, liver and skeletal muscle cells had reduced fasting blood glucose levels and increased glucose tolerance (Chen et al. 1997). In addition, mice in which $G\alpha_{i2}$ has been downregulated in liver and adipose tissue using an antisense RNA approach show insulin resistance with hyperinsulinaemia and decreased glucose tolerance (Moxham and Malbon 1996). These data indicate that regulation of glucose metabolism by insulin is antagonistically regulated through G_s- and G_i-mediated pathways. Regulation may occur on the level of the insulin receptor or by influencing downstream signalling events (Tao et al. 2001; Song et al. 2001).

7
Sensory Systems

Signal transduction of many sensory stimuli involves heterotrimeric G proteins. Odours, light and most tastants act directly on G protein-coupled receptors.

7.1
Olfactory System

The G protein G_{olf} is centrally involved in the transduction of odorant stimuli, and $G\alpha_{olf}$-deficient mice exhibit dramatically reduced electrophysiological responses to all odours tested (Belluscio et al. 1998) supporting the idea that G_{olf} mediates the activation of seven transmembrane domain receptors for odorants in the olfactory cilia (Ronnett and Moon 2002). Since nursing and mothering behaviour in rodents is mediated to a great deal by the olfactory system, most $G\alpha_{olf}$-deficient pups die a few days after birth due to insufficient feeding, and rare surviving mothers exhibit inadequate maternal behaviour, resulting in the death of all pups born to $G\alpha_{olf}$-deficient mothers (Belluscio et al. 1998). Both, $G\alpha_{olf}$ and adenylyl cyclase type III (ACIII) colocalise in olfactory cilia, suggesting that they form a pathway which links olfactory receptors to cAMP production. This is supported by the phenotype of ACIII-deficient mice in which odorant-induced responses are absent and which show impaired odour-dependent learning (Wong et al. 2000). In contrast to the olfactory epithelium, the vomeronasal organ which responds to pheromones expresses receptors which are coupled to $G_{i/o}$. Absence of $G\alpha_o$ results in apoptotic death of receptor cells which usually express $G\alpha_o$, indicating that cell survival in these cells requires G_o-mediated signalling (Tanaka et al. 1999).

7.2
Visual System

Rod-transducin (G_{t-r}) and cone-transducin (G_{t-c}) play well-established roles in the phototransduction cascade in the outer segments of retinal rods and cones where they couple light receptors to cyclic guanosine monophosphate (cGMP)-phosphodiesterase (PDE). Activation of PDE lowers cytosolic cGMP levels, leading to decreased open probability of cGMP-regulated cation channels in the plasma membrane which eventually results in hyperpolarisation of rods/cones (Arshavsky et al. 2002). In mice lacking $G\alpha_{t-r}$, the majority of retinal rods does not respond to light anymore, and these animals develop mild retinal degeneration with age (Calvert et al. 2000). Efficient termination of transducin-mediated signalling is required for adequate time resolution of the light signal. At least three proteins are involved in the rapid deactivation of transducin by increasing its GTPase activity, RGS9 and $G\beta 5L$ which form a complex, as well as the γ subunit of the transducin effector, cGMP-PDE (Arshavsky et al. 2002). In mice lacking RGS9, rod- and cone-derived light responses increase in their half time of recovery (Chen et al. 2000; Lyubarsky et al. 2001). Similarly, mice in which the PDE γ subunit was replaced by a mutant form with highly reduced affinity for transducin exhibited an increased recovery time of rod responses (Tang et al. 1998).

The light response is transferred from the receptor cell to ON bipolar cells of the retina. ON bipolar cells are inhibited by glutamate released from rods and cones through metabotropic glutamate type 6 receptors (mGluR6). Light-induced hyperpolarisation of rods and cones results in decreased glutamate release and disinhibition of ON bipolar cells. In mice lacking mGluR6 or $G\alpha_o$, modulation of ON bipolar cells in response to light is abrogated (Masu et al. 1995; Dhingra et al. 2000), indicating that mGluR6/G_o are critically involved in the tonic inhibition of these cells which occurs in the absence of light.

7.3
Gustatory System

Unlike the perception of odorants and light, gustatory stimuli are only in part transduced through G protein-mediated mechanisms. Among the four taste qualities, sweet, bitter, sour and salty, bitter and sweet tastes appear to signal through heterotrimeric G proteins. Gustducin is a G protein mainly expressed in taste cells. $G\alpha_{gust}$-deficient mice show impaired electrophysiological and behavioural responses to bitter and sweet agents, while responses to sour and salty stimuli were indistinguishable from those of wild-type mice (Wong et al. 1996). The residual bitter and sweet taste responsiveness of $G\alpha_{gust}$-deficient mice could be further diminished by a dominant-negative mutant of gustducin-α, suggesting the involvement of other G proteins related to $G\alpha_{gust}$ (Ruiz-Avila et al. 2001; Margolskee 2002).

8
Platelets

Platelets are discoid cell fragments which under physiological conditions become activated at sites of vascular injury. Activated platelets immediately undergo a shape-change reaction during which they become spherical and extrude pseudopodia-like structures. Full platelet activation includes secretion of granule contents as well as inside-out activation of the fibrinogen receptor, integrin $\alpha_{IIb}\beta_3$, resulting in platelet aggregation. Most of the physiological activators of platelets, such as thrombin, thromboxane A_2 or ADP, act through G protein-coupled receptors which in turn activate G_i, G_q, G_{12} and G_{13} (Offermanns et al. 2000). Platelets from $G\alpha_q$-deficient mice did not aggregate and secrete their granule contents in response to thromboxane A_2, ADP, thrombin, as well as to low concentrations of collagen (Offermanns et al. 1997c). Similarly, thromboxane A_2, ADP and thrombin failed to induce production of inositol-1,4,5-trisphosphate and transient increases in the free cytosolic Ca^{2+}-concentration in $G\alpha_q$-deficient platelets, indicating that $G\alpha_q$-mediated activation of phospholipase C is the central pathway through which various physiological platelet activators signal in order to induce full activation of mouse platelets. G protein $\beta\gamma$ subunits released from other G proteins are obviously not able to compensate the loss of $G\alpha_q$. Lack of $G\alpha_q$-mediated phospholipase C activation did not interfere with the ability of thromboxane A_2 and thrombin to induce platelet shape change. Thus, induction of platelet shape change through receptors of different platelet stimuli is mediated by G proteins other than G_q. Studies employing $G\alpha_q$-deficient platelets indicate that the G proteins G_{12}/G_{13}, but not G_i, are critically involved in the receptor-mediated shape-change response in platelets, and the G_{12}/G_{13}-mediated shape change involves a Rho/Rho kinase-mediated pathway, resulting in the phosphorylation of the myosin light chain (Klages et al. 1999). The defective activation of $G\alpha_q$-deficient platelets results in a primary hemostasis defect. In addition, $G\alpha_q^{(-/-)}$ mice are protected against platelet-dependent thromboembolism.

The role of G proteins of the $G_{i/o}$ family in platelet activation has recently been elucidated. Platelets contain at least three members of this class, G_{i2}, G_{i3} and G_z. ADP, which is released from activated platelets and functions as a positive-feedback mediator during platelet activation, induces full platelet activation by activating at least two receptors, the G_q-coupled P2Y1 receptor as well as the G_i-coupled P2Y12 purinergic receptor. The importance of the G_i-mediated pathway is indicated by the fact that responses to ADP or thrombin were markedly reduced in platelets lacking $G\alpha_{i2}$ (Jantzen et al. 2001). In contrast to ADP or thrombin, epinephrine is not a full platelet activator per se in murine platelets. However, it is able to potentiate the effect of other platelet stimuli. In platelets from $G\alpha_z$-deficient mice, inhibition of adenylyl cyclase by epinephrine as well as epinephrine's potentiating effects were clearly impaired, while the effects of other platelet activators appeared to be unaffected by the lack of $G\alpha_z$ (Yang et al. 2000). One of the potential downstream effectors of G_i-type G proteins involved

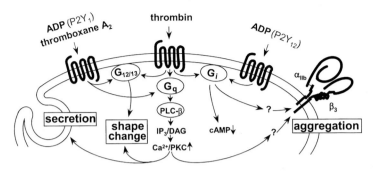

Fig. 3 Involvement of heterotrimeric G proteins in platelet activation. Various platelet stimuli, like ADP, thromboxane A$_2$ or thrombin, function through heptahelical transmembrane receptors which couple to G proteins of the G$_i$, G$_q$ and G$_{12}$ families. These heterotrimeric G proteins mediate signalling pathways which eventually lead to platelet responses like shape change, secretion and aggregation. *PLC*, phospholipase C ; *IP$_3$*, inositol 1,4,5 trisphosphate; *DAG*, diacylglycerol; *PKC*, protein kinase C. For details, see text

in platelet activation may be the $\beta\gamma$-activated γ-isoform of PI-3 kinase, the absence of which in platelets results in decreased responses to ADP (Hirsch et al. 2001). Thus, G$_q$, G$_{12}$ as well as G$_{i/o}$ family members are involved in processes leading to full platelet activation (see Fig. 3).

9
Conclusions

During recent years, gene targeting techniques have been used to delete almost all known genes encoding G protein α subunits as well as variety of G protein effectors in mice. These studies have led to considerable advances in the understanding of G protein-mediated signalling processes. However, only a minor fraction of the wide-ranged biological functions of G protein-mediated signalling processes have probably been elucidated by targeted inactivation of components of the G protein-mediated signalling pathway so far. Many functions remain difficult to analyse because of functional redundancy of closely related G proteins or because a loss of function mutation results in early death or induces compensatory processes. To reduce this problem, researchers have started to generate mice with tissue-restricted or inducible gene deletions. These approaches will advance our understanding of how G protein-mediated signalling pathways function in vivo.

Acknowledgements. The authors own research was supported by the Deutsche Forschungsgemneinschaft.

References

Abdel-Majid RM, Leong WL, Schalkwyk LC, Smallman DS, Wong ST, Storm DR, Fine A, Dobson MJ, Guernsey DL, Neumann PE (1998) Loss of adenylyl cyclase I activity disrupts patterning of mouse somatosensory cortex. Nat Genet 19:289–291

Adams JW, Sakata Y, Davis MG, Sah VP, Wang Y, Liggett SB, Chien KR, Brown JH, Dorn GW 2nd (1998) Enhanced Galphaq signaling: a common pathway mediates cardiac hypertrophy and apoptotic heart failure. Proc Natl Acad Sci U S A 95:10140–10145

Aiba A, Kano M, Chen C, Stanton ME, Fox GD, Herrup K, Zwingman TA, Tonegawa S (1994) Deficient cerebellar long-term depression and impaired motor learning in mGluR1 mutant mice. Cell 79:377–388

Akhter SA, Luttrell LM, Rockman HA, Iaccarino G, Lefkowitz RJ, Koch WJ (1998) Targeting the receptor-Gq interface to inhibit in vivo pressure overload myocardial hypertrophy. Science 280:574–577

Arshavsky VY, Lamb TD, Pugh EN Jr (2002) G proteins and phototransduction. Annu Rev Physiol 64:153–187

Baggiolini M (1998) Chemokines and leukocyte traffic. Nature 392:565–568

Belluscio L, Gold GH, Nemes A, Axel R (1998) Mice deficient in G(olf) are anosmic. Neuron 20:69–81

Broaddus R, Dinh M, Finegold M (1998) Flow cytometric DNA analysis of colonic mucosa from Gα_{i2}-deficient mice. FASEB J. 12:A736

Buhl AM, Johnson ML, Dhanasekaran N, Johnson G (1995) G alpha 12 and G alpha 13 stimulate Rho-dependent stress fiber formation and focal adhesion assembly. J Biol Chem 270:24631–24634

Calvert PD, Krasnoperova NV, Lyubarsky AL, Isayama T, Nicolo M, Kosaras B, Wong G, Gannon KS, Margolskee RF, Sidman RL, Pugh EN Jr, Makino CL, Lem J (2000) Phototransduction in transgenic mice after targeted deletion of the rod transducin alpha -subunit. Proc Natl Acad Sci U S A 97:13913–13918

Catterall WA (2000) Structure and regulation of voltage-gated Ca2+ channels. Annu Rev Cell Dev Biol 16:521–555

Chaffin KE, Beals CR, Wilkie TM, Forbush KA, Simon MI, Perlmutter RM (1990) Dissection of thymocyte signaling pathways by in vivo expression of pertussis toxin ADP-ribosyltransferase EMBO J 9:3821–3829

Chaffin KE, Perlmutter RM (1991) A pertussis toxin-sensitive process controls thymocyte emigration. Eur J Immunol 21:2565–2573

Chen JF, Guo JH, Moxham CM, Wang HY, Malbon CC (1997) Conditional, tissue-specific expression of Q205L Gαi2 in vivo mimics insulin action. J Mol Med 75:283–289

Chen CK, Burns ME, He W, Wensel TG, Baylor DA, Simon MI (2000) Slowed recovery of rod photoresponse in mice lacking the GTPase accelerating protein RGS9–1. Nature 403:557–560

Chen F, Spicher K, Jiang M, Birnbaumer L, Wetzel GT (2001) Lack of muscarinic regulation of Ca(2+) channels in G(i2)alpha gene knockout mouse hearts. Am J Physiol 280, H1989–1995

Clouthier DE, Hosoda K, Richardson JA, Williams SC, Yanagisawa H, Kuwaki T, Kumada M, Hammer RE, Yanagisawa M (1998) Cranial and cardiac neural crest defects in endothelin-A receptor-deficient mice. Development 125:813–824

D'Angelo DD, Sakata Y, Lorenz JN, Boivin GP, Walsh RA, Ligget SB, Dorn, GW (1997) Transgenic Galphaq overexpression induces cardiac contractile failure in mice. Proc Natl Acad Sci USA 94:8121–8126

Davignon I, Catalina MD, Smith D, Montgomery J, Swantek J, Croy J, Siegelman M, Wilkie TM (2000) Normal hematopoiesis and inflammatory responses despite discrete signaling defects in Galpha15 knockout mice. Mol Cell Biol 20:797–804

Dhingra A, Lyubarsky A, Jiang M, Pugh EN Jr, Birnbaumer L, Sterling P, Vardi N (2000) The light response of ON bipolar neurons requires G[alpha]o. J Neurosci 20:9053–9058

Eckhart AD, Ozaki T, Tevaearai H, Rockman HA, Koch WJ (2002) Vascular-targeted overexpression of G protein-coupled receptor kinase-2 in transgenic mice attenuates beta-adrenergic receptor signaling and increases resting blood pressure. Mol Pharmacol 61:749–758

Fields TA, Casey PJ (1997) Signalling functions and biochemical properties of pertussis toxin-resistant G-proteins. Biochem J 321:561–571

Gao MH, Lai NC, Roth DM, Zhou J, Zhu J, Anzai T, Dalton N, Hammond HK. (1999) Adenylylcyclase increases responsiveness to catecholamine stimulation in transgenic mice. Circulation 99:1618–1622

Gaudin C, Ishikawa Y, Wight DC, Mahdavi V, Nadal-Ginard B, Wagner TE, Vatner DE, Homcy CJ (1995) Overexpression of Gsα protein in the hearts of transgenic mice. J Clin Invest 95:1676–1683

Gehrmann J, Meister M, Maguire CT, Martins DC, Hammer PE, Neer EJ, Berul CI, Mende U (2002) Impaired parasympathetic heart rate control in mice with a reduction of functional G protein betagamma-subunits. Am J Physiol Heart Circ Physiol 282:H445–456

Girkontaite I, Missy K, Sakk V, Harenberg A, Tedford K, Potzel T, Pfeffer K, Fischer KD (2001) Lsc is required for marginal zone B cells, regulation of lymphocyte motility and immune responses. Nat Immunol 2:855–862

Greif GJ, Sodickson DL, Bean BP, Neer EJ, Mende U (2000) Altered regulation of potassium and calcium channels by GABA(B) and adenosine receptors in hippocampal neurons from mice lacking Galpha(o). J Neurophysiol 83:1010–1018

Gu JL, Müller S, Mancino V, Offermanns S, Simon MI (2002) Interaction of Gα_{12} with Gα_{13} and Gα_q signaling pathways. Proc. Natl. Acad. Sci. USA 99, 9352–9357

Guinamard R, Okigaki M, Schlessinger J, Ravetch JV (2000) Absence of marginal zone B cells in Pyk-2-deficient mice defines their role in the humoral response. Nat Immunol 1:31–36

Hannan AJ, Blakemore C, Katsnelson A, Vitalis T, Huber KM, Bear M, Roder J, Kim D, Shin HS, Kind PC (2001) PLC-beta1, activated via mGluRs, mediates activity-dependent differentiation in cerebral cortex. Nat Neurosci 4:282–288

Hart MJ, Jiang X, Kozasa T, Roscoe W, Singer WD, Gilman AG, Sternweis PC, Bollag G (1998) Direct stimulation of the guanine nucleotide exchange activity of p115 Rho-GEF by Galpha13. Science 280:2112–2114

Hatakeyama S, Wakamori M, Ino M, Miyamoto N, Takahashi E, Yoshinaga T, Sawada K, Imoto K, Tanaka I, Yoshizawa T, Nishizawa Y, Mori Y, Niidome T, Shoji S (2001) Differential nociceptive responses in mice lacking the alpha(1B) subunit of N-type Ca(2+) channels. Neuroreport 12:2423–2427

He J, Gurunathan S, Iwasaki A, Ash-Shaheed B, Kelsall BL (2000) Primary role for Gi protein signaling in the regulation of interleukin 12 production and the induction of T helper cell type 1 responses. J Exp Med 191:1605–1610

Hendry IA, Kelleher KL, Bartlett SE, Leck KJ, Reynolds AJ, Heydon K, Mellick A, Megirian D, Matthaei KI (2000) Hypertolerance to morphine in G(z alpha)-deficient mice. Brain Res 870:10–19

Herve D, Levi-Strauss M, Marey-Semper I, Verney C, Tassin JP, Glowinski J, Girault JA (1993) G(olf) and Gs in rat basal ganglia: possible involvement of G(olf) in the coupling of dopamine D1 receptor with adenylyl cyclase. Neurosci 13:2237–2248

Herve D, Rogard M, Levi-Strauss M (1995) Molecular analysis of the multiple Golf alpha subunit mRNAs in the rat brain. Brain Res Mol Brain Res 32:125–134

Herve D, Le Moine C, Corvol JC, Belluscio L, Ledent C, Fienberg AA, Jaber M, Studler JM, Girault JA (2001) Galpha(olf) levels are regulated by receptor usage and control dopamine and adenosine action in the striatum. J Neurosci 21:4390–4399

Hirsch E, Katanaev VL, Garlanda C, Azzolino O, Pirola L, Silengo L, Sozzani S, Mantovani A, Altruda F, Wymann MP (2000) Central role for G protein-coupled phosphoinositide 3-kinase gamma in inflammation. Science 287:1049–1053

Hirsch E, Bosco O, Tropel P, Laffargue M, Calvez R, Altruda F, Wymann M, Montrucchio G (2001) Resistance to thromboembolism in PI3Kgamma-deficient mice. FASEB J 15:2019–2021

Ho MK, Wong YH (1998) Structure and function of the pertussis-toxin-insensitive Gz protein. Biol Signals Recept 7:80–89

Hornquist CE, Lu X, Rogers-Fani PM, Rudolph U, Shappell S, Birnbaumer L, Harriman GR (1997) G(alpha)i2-deficient mice with colitis exhibit a local increase in memory CD4+ T cells and proinflammatory Th1-type cytokines. J Immunol 158:1068–1077

Huang XP, Song X, Wang HY, Malbon CC (2002) Targeted expression of activated Q227L G(alpha)(s) in vivo. Am J Physiol 283:C386–395

Iaccarino G, Rockman HA, Shotwell KF, Tomhave ED, Koch WJ (1998) Myocardial overexpression of GRK3 in transgenic mice: evidence for in vivo selectivity of GRKs. Am J Physiol 275:H1298–306

Ino M, Yoshinaga T, Wakamori M, Miyamoto N, Takahashi E, Sonoda J, Kagaya T, Oki T, Nagasu T, Nishizawa Y, Tanaka I, Imoto K, Aizawa S, Koch S, Schwartz A, Niidome T, Sawada K, Mori Y (2001)Functional disorders of the sympathetic nervous system in mice lacking the alpha 1B subunit (Cav 2.2) of N-type calcium channels. Proc Natl Acad Sci 98:5323–5328

Iwase M, Bishop SP, Uechi M, Vatner DE, Shannon RP, Kudej RK, Wight DC, Wagner TE, Ishikawa Y, Homcy CJ, Vatner SF (1996) Adverse effects of chronic endogenous sympathetic drive induced by cardiac Gsα overexpression. Circ Res 78:517–524

Iwase M, Uechi M, Vatner DE, Asai K, Shannon RP, Kudej RK, Wagner TE, Wight DC, Patrick TA, Ishikawa Y, Homcy CJ, Vatner SF (1997) Cardiomyopathy induced by cardiac $G_{s\alpha}$ overexpression. Am J Physiol 272:H585-H589

Jantzen HM, Milstone DS, Gousset L, Conley PB, Mortensen RM (2001) Impaired activation of murine platelets lacking G alpha(i2). J Clin Invest 108:477–483

Jiang M, Gold MS, Boulay G, Spicher K, Peyton M, Brabet P, Srinivasan Y, Rudolph U, Ellison G, Birnbaumer L (1998) Multiple neurological abnormalities in mice deficient in the G protein Go. Proc Natl Acad Sci U S A 95:3269–3274

Jun K, Piedras-Renteria ES, Smith SM, Wheeler DB, Lee SB, Lee TG, Chin H, Adams ME, Scheller RH, Tsien RW, Shin HS (1999) Ablation of P/Q-type Ca(2+) channel currents, altered synaptic transmission, and progressive ataxia in mice lacking the alpha(1A)-subunit. Proc Natl Acad Sci U S A 96:15245–15250

Kano M, Hashimoto K, Kurihara H, Watanabe M, Inoue Y, Aiba A, Tonegawa S (1997) Persistent multiple climbing fiber innervation of cerebellar Purkinje cells in mice lacking mGluR1. Neuron 18:71–79

Kano M, Hashimoto K, Watanabe M, Kurihara H, Offermanns S, Jiang H, Wu Y, Jun K, Shin HS, Inoue Y, Simon MI, Wu D (1998) Phospholipase cbeta4 is specifically involved in climbing fiber synapse elimination in the developing cerebellum. Proc Natl Acad Sci U S A 95:15724–15729

Kim C, Jun K, Lee T, Kim SS, McEnery MW, Chin H, Kim HL, Park JM, Kim DK, Jung SJ, Kim J, Shin HS (2001) Altered nociceptive response in mice deficient in the alpha(1B) subunit of the voltage-dependent calcium channel. Mol Cell Neurosci 18:235–245

Klages B, Brandt U, Simon MI, Schultz G, Offermanns S (1999) Activation of G12/G13 results in shape change and Rho/Rho-kinase-mediated myosin light chain phosphorylation in mouse platelets. J Cell Biol 144:745–754

Kleppisch T, Voigt V, Allmann R, Offermanns S (2001) $G\alpha_q$-deficient mice lack metabotropic glutamate receptor-dependent long-term depression but show normal long-term potentiation in the hippocampal CA1 region. J Neurosci 21:4943–4948

Kurihara Y, Kurihara H, Suzuki H, Kodama T, Maemura K, Nagai R, Oda H, Kuwaki T, Cao WH, Kamada N, Jishage N, Ouchi Y, Azuma S, Toyoda Y, Ishikawa T, Kumada M,

Yazaki Y (1994) Elevated blood pressure and craniofacial abnormalities in mice deficient in endothelin-1. Nature 368:703–710

Kurihara Y, Kurihara H, Oda H, Maemura K, Nagai R, Ishikawa T, Yazaki Y (1995) Aortic arch malformations and ventricular septal defect in mice deficient in endothelin-1. J Clin Invest 96:293–300

Li Z, Jiang H, Xie W, Zhang Z, Smrcka AV, Wu D (2000) Roles of PLC-beta2 and -beta3 and PI3Kgamma in chemoattractant-mediated signal transduction. Science 287:1046–1049

Lipskaia L, Defer N, Esposito G, Hajar I, Garel MC, Rockman HA, Hanoune J (2000) Enhanced cardiac function in transgenic mice expressing a Ca(2+)-stimulated adenylyl cyclase. Circ Res 86:795–801

Lyubarsky AL, Naarendorp F, Zhang X, Wensel T, Simon MI, Pugh EN Jr (2001) RGS9-1 is required for normal inactivation of mouse cone phototransduction. Mol Vis 7:71–78

Ma YH, Landis C, Tchao N, Wang J, Rodd G, Hanahan D, Bourne HR, Grodsky GM (1994) Constitutively active stimulatory G-protein αs in β-cells of transgenic mice causes counterregulation of the increased adenosine 3',5'-monophosphate and insulin secretion. Endocrinology 134:42–47

Margolskee RF (2002) Molecular mechanisms of bitter and sweet taste transduction. J Biol Chem 277:1–4

Mark MD, Herlitze S (2000) G-protein mediated gating of inward-rectifier K+ channels. Eur J Biochem 267:5830–5836

Masu M, Iwakabe H, Tagawa Y, Miyoshi T, Yamashita M, Fukuda Y, Sasaki H, Hiroi K, Nakamura Y, Shigemoto R, et al (1995) Specific deficit of the ON response in visual transmission by targeted disruption of the mGluR6 gene. Cell 80:757–765

Mende U, Kagen A, Cohen A, Aramburu J, Schoen FJ, Neer EJ (1998) Transient cardiac expression of constitutively active Galphaq leads to hypertrophy and dilated cardiomyopathy by calcineurin-dependent and independent pathways. Proc Natl Acad Sci U S A 95:13893–13898

Michiels FM, Caillou B, Talbot M, Dessarps-Freichey F, Maunoury MT, Schlumberger M, Mercken L, Monier R, Feunteun J (1994) Oncogenic potential of guanine nucleotide stimulatory factor α subunit in thyroid glands of transgenic mice. Proc Natl Acad Sci U S A 91:10488–10492

Miyata M, Kim HT, Hashimoto K, Lee TK, Cho SY, Jiang H, Wu Y, Jun K, Wu D, Kano M, Shin HS (2001) Deficient long-term synaptic depression in the rostral cerebellum correlated with impaired motor learning in phospholipase C beta4 mutant mice. Eur J Neurosci 13:1945–1954

Moxham CM, Malbon CC (1996) Insulin action impaired by deficiency of the G-protein subunit $G_{i\alpha2}$. Nature 379:840–844

Nagata K, Ye C, Jain M, Milstone DS, Liao R, Mortensen RM (2000) Galpha(i2) but not Galpha(i3) is required for muscarinic inhibition of contractility and calcium currents in adult cardiomyocytes. Circ Res 87:903–909

Nebigil CG, Choi DS, Dierich A, Hickel P, Le Meur M, Messaddeq N, Launay JM, Maroteaux L (2000) Serotonin 2B receptor is required for heart development. Proc Natl Acad Sci U S A 97:9508–9513

Offermanns S (2000) The role of heterotrimeric G-proteins in platelet activation. Biol Chem 381:389–396

Offermanns S, Hashimoto K, Watanabe M, Sun W, Kurihara H, Thompson RF, Inoue Y, Kano M, Simon MI (1997a) Impaired motor coordination and persistent multiple climbing fiber innervation of cerebellar Purkinje cells in mice lacking Galphaq. Proc Natl Acad Sci U S A 94:14089–14094

Offermanns S, Mancino V, Revel JP, Simon MI (1997b) Vascular system defects and impaired cell chemokinesis as a result of Galpha13 deficiency. Science 275:533–536

Offermanns S, Toombs CF, Hu YH, Simon MI (1997c) Defective platelet activation in G alpha(q)-deficient mice. Nature 389:183–186

Offermanns S, Zhao L-P, Gohla A, Sarosi I, Simon MI, Wilkie TM (1998) Embryonic cardiomyocyte hypoplasia and craniofacial defects in G alpha q/G alpha 11-mutant mice. EMBO J 17:4304–4312

Ohman L, Franzen L, Rudolph U, Harriman GR, Hultgren Hornquist E (2000) Immune activation in the intestinal mucosa before the onset of colitis in Galphai2-deficient mice. Scand J Immunol 52:80–90

Raport CJ, Lem J, Makino C, Chen CK, Fitch CL, Hobson A, Baylor D, Simon MI, Hurley JB (1994) Downregulation of cGMP phosphodiesterase induced by expression of GTPase-deficient cone transducin in mouse rod photoreceptors. Invest Ophthalmol Vis Sci 35:2932–2947

Ridley AJ (2001) Rho proteins, PI 3-kinases, and monocyte/macrophage motility. FEBS Lett 498:168–171

Risau W (1997) Mechanisms of angiogenesis. Nature 386:671–674

Rogers JH, Tamirisa P, Kovacs A, Weinheimer C, Courtois M, Blumer KJ, Kelly DP, Muslin AJ (1999) RGS4 causes increased mortality and reduced cardiac hypertrophy in response to pressure overload. J Clin Invest 104:567–576

Ronnett GV, Moon C (2002) G proteins and olfactory signal transduction. Annu Rev Physiol 64:189–222

Roth DM, Gao MH, Lai NC, Drumm J, Dalton N, Zhou JY, Zhu J, Entrikin D, Hammond HK (1999) Cardiac-directed adenylyl cyclase expression improves heart function in murine cardiomyopathy. Circulation 99:3099–3102

Rudolph U, Finegold MJ, Rich SS, Harriman GR, Srinivasan Y, Brabet P, Boulay G, Bradley A, Birnbaumer L (1995) Ulcerative colitis and adenocarcinoma of the colon in G alpha i2-deficient mice. Nat Genet 10:143–150

Ruiz-Avila L, Wong GT, Damak S, Margolskee RF (2001) Dominant loss of responsiveness to sweet and bitter compounds caused by a single mutation in alpha -gustducin. Proc Natl Acad Sci U S A 98:8868–8873

Saegusa H, Kurihara T, Zong S, Minowa O, Kazuno A, Han W, Matsuda Y, Yamanaka H, Osanai M, Noda T, Tanabe T ((2000) Altered pain responses in mice lacking alpha 1E subunit of the voltage-dependent Ca2+ channel. Proc Natl Acad Sci U S A 97:6132–6137

Saegusa H, Kurihara T, Zong S, Kazuno A, Matsuda Y, Nonaka T, Han W, Toriyama H, Tanabe T (2001) Suppression of inflammatory and neuropathic pain symptoms in mice lacking the N-type Ca2+ channel. EMBO J 20:2349–2356

Sah VP, Seasholtz TM, Sagi SA, Brown JH (2000) The role of Rho in G protein-coupled receptor signal transduction. Annu Rev Pharmacol Toxicol 40:459–489

Sasaki T, Irie-Sasaki J, Jones RG, Oliveira-dos-Santos AJ, Stanford WL, Bolon B, Wakeham A, Itie A, Bouchard D, Kozieradzki I, Joza N, Mak TW, Ohashi PS, Suzuki A, Penninger JM (2000) Function of PI3Kgamma in thymocyte development, T cell activation, and neutrophil migration. Science 287:1040–1046

Signorini S, Liao YJ, Duncan SA, Jan LY, Stoffel M (1997) Normal cerebellar development but susceptibility to seizures in mice lacking G protein-coupled, inwardly rectifying K+ channel GIRK2. Proc Natl Acad Sci U S A 94:923–927

Simon MI, Strathmann MP, Gautam N (1991) Diversity of G proteins in signal transduction. Science 252:802–808.

Song X, Zheng X, Malbon CC, Wang H (2001) Galpha i2 enhances in vivo activation of and insulin signaling to GLUT4. J Biol Chem 276:34651–34658

Spicher K, Rudolph U, Brandt U, Jiang M, Boulay G, Nüsse O, Nürnberg B, Schultz G, Birnbaumer L (2002) Targeted inactivation of G-protein ai-subunits affects neutrophil function. Naunyn-Schmiedeberg's Arch Pharmacol 365:R46

Tanaka M, Treloar H, Kalb RG, Greer CA, Strittmatter SM (1999) G(o) protein-dependent survival of primary accessory olfactory neurons. Proc Natl Acad Sci U S A 96:14106–14111

Tanaka J, Nakagawa S, Kushiya E, Yamasaki M, Fukaya M, Iwanaga T, Simon MI, Sakimura K, Kano M, Watanabe M (2000) Gq protein alpha subunits Galphaq and Galpha11 are localized at postsynaptic extra-junctional membrane of cerebellar Purkinje cells and hippocampal pyramidal cells. Eur J Neurosci 12:781–792

Tao J, Malbon CC, Wang HY (2001) Galpha(i2) enhances insulin signaling via suppression of protein-tyrosine phosphatase 1B. J Biol Chem 276:39705–39712

Tepe NM, Lorenz JN, Yatani A, Dash R, Kranias EG, Dorn GW 2nd, Liggett SB (1999) Altering the receptor-effector ratio by transgenic overexpression of type V adenylyl cyclase: enhanced basal catalytic activity and function without increased cardiomyocyte beta-adrenergic signalling. Biochemistry 38:16706–16713

Tsang SH, Gouras P, Yamashita CK, Kjeldbye H, Fisher J, Farber DB, Goff SP (1996) Retinal degeneration in mice lacking the gamma subunit of the rod cGMP phosphodiesterase. Science 272:1026–1029

Tsang SH, Burns ME, Calvert PD, Gouras P, Baylor DA, Goff SP, Arshavsky VY (1998) Role for the target enzyme in deactivation of photoreceptor G protein in vivo. Science 282:117–121

Uechi M, Asai K, Osaka M, Smith A, Sato N, Wagner TE, Ishikawa Y, Hayakawa H, Vatner DE, Shannon RP, Homcy CJ, Vatner SF (1998) Depressed heart rate variability and arterial baroreflex in conscious transgenic mice with overexpression of cardiac Gsα. Circ Res 82:416–423

Valenzuela D, Han X, Mende U, Fankhauser C, Mashimo H, Huang P, Pfeffer J, Neer EJ, Fishman MC (1997) G alpha(o) is necessary for muscarinic regulation of Ca2+ channels in mouse heart. Proc Natl Acad Sci U S A 94:1727–1732

Vatner DE, Asai K, Iwase M, Ishikawa Y, Wagner TE, Shannon RP, Homcy CJ, Vatner SF (1998) Overexpression of myocardial Gsα prevents full expression of catecholamine desensitization despite increased β-adrenergic receptor kinase. J Clin Invest 101:1916–1922

Watanabe M, Nakamura M, Sato K, Kano M, Simon MI, Inoue Y (1998) Patterns of expression for the mRNA corresponding to the four isoforms of phospholipase Cbeta in mouse brain. Eur J Neurosci 10:2016–2025

Weinstein LS, Yu S, Warner DR, Liu J (2001) Endocrine manifestations of stimulatory G protein alpha-subunit mutations and the role of genomic imprinting. Endocr Rev 22:675–705

Wettschureck N, Rutten H, Zywietz A, Gehring D, Wilkie TM, Chen J, Chien KR, Offermanns S (2001) Absence of pressure overload induced myocardial hypertrophy after conditional inactivation of Galphaq/Galpha11 in cardiomyocytes. Nat Med 7:1236–1240

Wickman K, Nemec J, Gendler SJ, Clapham DE (1998) Abnormal heart rate regulation in GIRK4 knockout mice. Neuron 20:103–114

Wickman K, Karschin C, Karschin A, Picciotto MR, Clapham DE (2000) Brain localization and behavioral impact of the G-protein-gated K+ channel subunit GIRK4. J Neurosci 20:5608–5615

Wong GT, Gannon KS, Margolskee RF (1996) Transduction of bitter and sweet taste by gustducin. Nature 381:796–800

Wong ST, Trinh K, Hacker B, Chan GC, Lowe G, Gaggar A, Xia Z, Gold GH, Storm DR (2000) Disruption of the type III adenylyl cyclase gene leads to peripheral and behavioral anosmia in transgenic mice. Neuron 27:487–497

Wu D, Huang CK, Jiang H (2000) Roles of phospholipid signaling in chemoattractant-induced responses. J Cell Sci 113 (Pt 17):2935–2940

Wymann MP, Sozzani S, Altruda F, Mantovani A, Hirsch E (2000) Lipids on the move: phosphoinositide 3-kinases in leukocyte function. Immunol Today 21:260–264

Xie W, Samoriski GM, McLaughlin JP, Romoser VA, Smrcka A, Hinkle PM, Bidlack JM, Gross RA, Jiang H, Wu D (2000) Genetic alteration of phospholipase C beta3 expression modulates behavioral and cellular responses to mu opioids. Proc Natl Acad Sci U S A 96:10385–10390

Xu M, Moratalla R, Gold LH, Hiroi N, Koob GF, Graybiel AM, Tonegawa S (1994) Dopamine D1 receptor mutant mice are deficient in striatal expression of dynorphin and in dopamine-mediated behavioral responses. Cell 79:729–742

Yanagisawa H, Yanagisawa M, Kapur RP, Richardson JA, Williams SC, Clouthier DE, deWit D, Emoto N, Hammer RE (1998) Dual genetic pathways of endothelin-mediated intercellular signaling revealed by targeted disruption of endothelin converting enzyme-1 gene. Development 125:825–836

Yang J, Wu J, Kowalska MA, Dalvi A, Prevost N, O'Brien PJ, Manning D, Poncz M, Lucki I, Blendy JA, Brass LF (2000) Loss of signaling through the G protein, Gz, results in abnormal platelet activation and altered responses to psychoactive drugs. Proc Natl Acad Sci USA 97:9984–9989

Yu S, Yu D, Lee E, Eckhaus M, Lee R, Corria Z, Accili D, Westphal H, Weinstein LS (1998) Variable and tissue-specific hormone resistance in heterotrimeric Gs protein alpha-subunit (Gsalpha) knockout mice is due to tissue-specific imprinting of the gsalpha gene. Proc Natl Acad Sci U S A 95:8715–8720

Yu S, Gavrilova O, Chen H, Lee R, Liu J, Pacak K, Parlow AF, Quon MJ, Reitman ML, Weinstein LD (2000) Paternal versus maternal transmission of a stimulatory G-protein alpha subunit knockout produces opposite effects on energy metabolism. J Clin Invest 105:615–623

Yu S, Castle A, Chen M, Lee R, Takeda K, Weinstein LS (2001) Increased insulin sensitivity in Gsalpha knockout mice. J Biol Chem 276:19994–19998

Zheng XL, Guo J, Wang Hy, Malbon CC (1998) Expression of constitutively activated $G_{i\alpha2}$ in vivo ameliorates streptozotocin-induced diabetes. J Biol Chem 273:23649–23651

Zhuang X, Belluscio L, Hen R (2000) GOLFalpha Mediates Dopamine D1 Receptor Signaling J Neurosci 20:1–5

Analysis of Integrin Function by Gene Targeting in Mice

O. Brandau · R. Fässler

Department for Molecular Medicine, Max Planck Institute of Biochemistry,
Am Klopferspitz 18a, 82152 Martinsried, Germany
e-mail: brandau@biochem.mpg.de

Abstract Integrins are dimeric cell-surface receptors whose extracellular domain can interact with extracellular matrix (ECM) molecules and cellular receptors, while the intracellular domain binds directly or indirectly to the actin cytoskeleton. Thus, integrins link the cytoskeleton to the ECM and occupy a central position in the regulation of many essential cell functions, such as cell–cell contacts, adhesion to the ECM, or migration. Dimerization of 18 α- and 8 β-integrin subunits results in at least 24 different heterodimers, with distinct ligand binding and signaling properties. The generation of mice deficient for specific integrin subunits has significantly contributed to our knowledge of integrin function in vivo. The analysis of recently generated conditional gene-targeted mice and knock-ins will allow researchers to investigate integrin subunits, which upon constitutive deletion show an embryonic lethal phenotype, and to dissect integrin signaling in vivo. In this review, the results of the analysis of mice deficient for specific integrins are discussed in the context of functional systems or organs of the mouse and compared with phenotypes of mice lacking known integrin ligands.

Keywords Integrin · Knockout · Extracellular matrix

1
Introduction

Integrins are heterodimeric transmembrane glycoproteins that are involved in a wide range of biological processes including cell migration, tissue organization, growth, differentiation, and cell survival. Integrins are composed of non-covalently linked α and β subunits. So far, 24 integrin receptors, assembled from various combinations of 18 α- and 8 β-chains, have been identified (Fig. 1). The diversity of integrin receptors is further increased by alternative mRNA splicing of genes encoding for α and β subunits, affecting intracellular and extracellular domains.

The extracellular domains of integrins can bind different extracellular matrix (ECM) ligands such as collagens, fibronectins, laminins, and cellular receptors including vascular cell adhesion molecule (VCAM)-1 and the intercellular cell adhesion molecule (ICAM) family (Plow et al. 2000). One integrin can often bind different ligands, while one ligand might be recognized by different integrin receptors. The cytoplasmic domain is indirectly linked to the actin cytoskeleton. Extracellular ligand binding is followed by recruitment of cytoskeletal

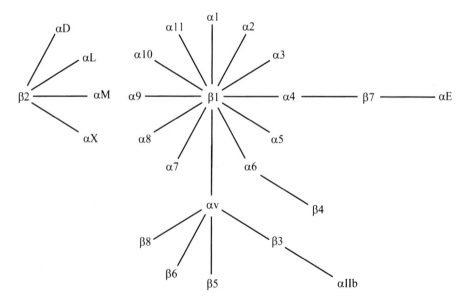

Fig. 1 Integrin family. The β- and α-integrin subunits heterodimerize to 24 different integrin receptors

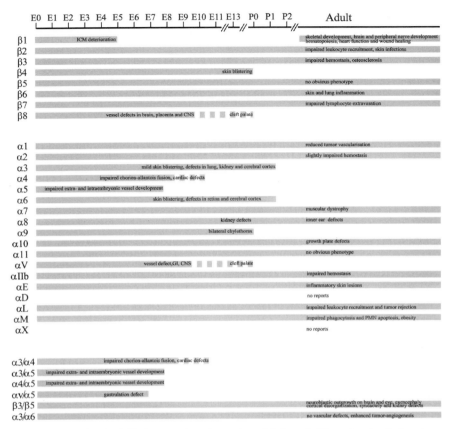

Fig. 2 Integrin-null mice. With the exception of α_X and α_D, deletions of all integrin subunits have been performed by conventional gene-targeting techniques. Conditional knockout studies have been published for the β_1 integrin subunit, allowing the analysis of β_1 function in adult mice. In addition, several double knockout mouse models have been analyzed to test for compensation of different integrin subunits. Lifespan of embryos is marked by *gray bars*. If only a portion of the embryos die, surviving animals are indicated by *interrupted gray bars* and the phenotypes are indicated for both groups. All listed mouse strains are described and cited in the text

proteins and signaling proteins to the cytoplasmic part of the integrin and initiation of signaling cascades that modulate cell behavior and gene transcription (Hynes 1992; Giancotti 2000). Intracellular signals, on the other hand, can change the affinity of integrins for their extracellular ligands, which is called "inside-out signaling" (Schwartz et al. 1995; Dedhar and Hannigan 1996). In addition, integrin clustering at the cell membrane can be regulated by extracellular and intracellular signals. Modulation of integrin affinity changes the adhesive properties of cells and is, for example, important for the aggregation of platelets (Shattil et al. 1998). The analysis of mutations in man has documented the importance of integrins for the development and hemostasis of different tissues and organs and for disease-related processes such as hemostasis, inflammation, or skin blistering (McEver et al. 1980; Arnaout et al. 1984; Beatty et al. 1984; Dana et al. 1984, Vidal et al. 1995; Pulkkinen et al. 1997; Pulkkinen and Uitto 1999).

Experimental data on integrin function have been mainly obtained by using in vitro cell culture systems. Gene targeting technology has permitted the generation of mice that lack specific integrins in a constitutive, inducible, or cell type-specific manner. The analysis of these mice demonstrates how integrin-mediated adhesion and signal transduction affects development and maintenance of tissues and additionally provides insights into integrin function in specific tissues and disease processes in adult mice (Fig. 2).

2
Proliferation, Differentiation, and Cell Survival

Integrin-mediated signals modulate migration, proliferation, survival, and differentiation of cells (Giancotti and Ruoslahti. 1999; Brakebusch et al. 2002). These processes are rather well understood from studies of cell lines in vitro. The analysis of integrin-mutant mice confirmed an in vivo role of integrins in these processes.

Mice lacking β_1 integrin in keratinocytes have less proliferating hair matrix cells and display a reduced proliferation of basal keratinocytes (Brakebusch et al. 2000; Raghavan et al. 2000). Reduced proliferation was also observed in β_1-deficient chondrocytes, which had an additional perturbation in differentiation (Aszódi et al. 2003). In a dominant-negative approach, the cytoplasmic and transmembrane domains of β_1 integrin were fused to the extracellular domain of CD4 and expressed in transgenic mice. Such a dominant-negative protein interferes with endogenous β_1 integrin function, and its expression in the mammary gland results in decreased proliferation, increased apoptosis, and impaired differentiation of the mammary epithelial cells (Faraldo et al. 1998). Although overall organization of the mammary tissue was not altered, an abnormal co-localization of β_4 integrin with laminin has been observed to the lateral surface of luminal epithelial cells (Faraldo et al. 1998). Transgenic epithelial cells show a downregulation of Shc phosphorylation and less activated extracellular signal-regulated kinase (ERK) and c-Jun N-terminal kinase (JNK) mitogen-activated protein kinases (MAPKs). Focal adhesion kinase (FAK) is not activated, suggesting an additional mechanism of activation to the ECM signal (Farraldo et al. 1998, 2000, 2001). Similar results have been documented for the expression of β_1 integrin-CD8 chimera in primary keratinocytes, which also leads to reduced ERK activation upon adhesion, but does not affect FAK phosphorylation (Zhu et al. 1999).

Deletion of the β_4 integrin cytoplasmic domain, which in vitro is able to bind and activate Shc in a phosphorylation-dependent manner, reduces proliferation in the skin and intestine (Murgia et al. 1998; Dans et al. 2001).

Mice lacking both α_3 and α_6 integrins have a reduced cell proliferation in the apical ectodermal ridge (AER) of the developing limb (De Arcangelis et al.

1999). Deletion of the α_1 integrin gene results in decreased proliferation of dermal fibroblasts (Pozzi et al. 1998). In vitro culture of these fibroblasts demonstrated a failure to recruit and activate the adaptor protein Shc, which triggers the MAPK activation cascade leading to cell proliferation (Pozzi et al. 1998).

Deletion of the alternatively spliced C-terminal sequence of β_1 integrin results in early lethality at E8.5 (Hirsch et al. 2002). The phenotype shows overlaps with the α_4- and α_5-deficient mouse. Decreased proliferation and cell survival were observed in vivo and in vitro on isolated fibroblasts. These cells showed normal adhesion to fibronectin, but showed impaired FAK-dependent PI3 K activation. This could be rescued by the expression of a constitutively active form of Rac, showing that β_1 integrin induced Rac activation is essential for anchorage-dependent control of cell growth (Hirsch et al. 2002).

While several integrin-deficient mutants display proliferation defects, only minor changes in cell differentiation were observed so far after the loss of specific integrins. Ablation of β_1 integrin does not interfere with differentiation of neurons and neural crest-derived cells (Fässler and Meyer 1995), of fetal hematopoietic cells (Potocnik et al. 2000), or of keratinocytes (Brakebusch et al. 2000; Raghavan et al. 2000). A disturbed differentiation could be observed in growth plate chondrocytes of mice with a specific deletion of the β_1 integrin gene in cartilage. It is possible, however, that the differentiation defect is a result of the disorganized growth plate structure, and thus a secondary effect of β_1 deletion (Aszódi et al. 2003). A delayed differentiation has been reported for β_1-null myoblasts (Hirsch et al. 1998) and for blood vessel formation in β_1-null embryoid bodies (Bloch et al. 1997). These results were obtained in vitro and the observed differentiation delay might be compensated in vivo. On the other hand, teratomas created from β_1-null cells are unable to form an endothelial cell population, suggesting that β_1 integrins could be involved in endothelial differentiation, proliferation, or more likely, in survival (Bloch et al. 1997). Double knockouts for α_3 and α_6 integrin show normal keratinocyte differentiation, despite the absence of the major integrin receptors, $\alpha_3\beta_1$ and $\alpha_6\beta_4$ (De Arcangelis et al. 1999). Most $\alpha_8\beta_1$-deficient mice die at birth due to kidney failure. Surviving mice have inner ear defects that might be caused by impaired hair cell differentiation (Littlewood-Evans and Müller 2000).

It has been conclusively shown in vitro that integrin-mediated adhesion is a survival factor for many cell types (Giancotti and Ruoslahti 1999). Cell survival defects in vivo have been reported for α_5 integrin, which was shown to be important for the survival of neural crest cells (Goh et al. 1997). Impaired cell-death regulation of interdigital cells leads to syndactyly in α_3/α_6-deficient mice (De Arcangelis et al. 1999). A slight increase of cell death can be observed after β_1 loss in chondrocytes (Aszódi et al. 2003). In contrast, loss of β_1 integrin-mediated adhesion of basal keratinocytes does not result in cell death, which was expected from cell culture experiments (Brakebusch et al. 2000).

However, integrin-mediated cell survival can depend on the expression and ligation of integrin receptors, which is difficult to investigate by deleting integrin subunits. It has been shown in vitro that $\alpha_v\beta_3$ induces apoptosis in endothelial cells, when it is not bound to an extracellular ligand. Apoptosis is induced by caspase 8 activation and is independent from the cell adhesion by other integrin receptors (Stupack et al. 2001).

3
Early Embryonic Development

At least 12 different β_1 integrin receptors are inactivated after the deletion of the β_1 integrin gene. Mouse oocytes express high levels of β_1 integrin, which appears on the cell surface in association with α_3, α_5, and α_6 subunits (Hierck et al. 1993; Tarone et al. 1993; Sutherland et al. 1993). Fertilization of β_1-null oocytes is unaffected and the development is normal until peri-implantation, possibly due to the presence of maternal β_1 integrin mRNA and protein (Brakebusch et al. 1997).

At the peri-implantation stage, inner cell mass cells (ICM) facing the cavity of the blastocyst differentiate into primitive endodermal cells and lay down a basement membrane (BM), which is crucial for the formation of ectoderm and the amniotic cavity. In β_1-deficient mouse blastocysts the endodermally derived BM fails to form, which results in peri-implantation lethality characterized by an ICM failure (Fässler and Meyer 1995; Stephens et al. 1995; Aumailley et al. 2000). The function of β_1 integrin during this process has been confirmed in embryoid bodies. Dispersed wild-type embryonic stem cells form embryoid bodies that develop an outer endodermal layer, form a subendodermal basement membrane, and differentiate to form epiblast and a central proamniotic-like cavity (Coucouvanis and Martin 1995; Murray and Edgar 2001). Embryoid bodies that are β_1 integrin-deficient do not express heterotrimeric laminin and do not make basement membranes, epiblast differentiation, and cavitation. Rescue of β_1 loss can be achieved by administration of exogenous laminin. This restores basement membranes along with epiblast differentiation and cavitation (Li et al. 2002).

Eight integrin heterodimers $\alpha_3\beta_1$, $\alpha_4\beta_1$, $\alpha_5\beta_1$, $\alpha_8\beta_1$, $\alpha_v\beta_1$, $\alpha_v\beta_3$, $\alpha_v\beta_6$, and $\alpha_{IIb}\beta_3$ can bind fibronectin. Deletion of any of the single integrin α subunits does not result in an embryonic phenotype as strong as in β_1-deficient mice. The deletion of α_4 integrin, which forms heterodimers with β_1 and β_7 and can bind to fibronectin and VCAM-1, leads to lethality at two different stages. Embryos deficient for α_4 integrin die either around E9.5–E11.5, due to a failure of allantois–chorion fusion during placentation, or between E11.5 and E14, due to developmental heart defects affecting epicardial and coronary vessels (Yang et al. 1995). Mice lacking VCAM-1 show similar defects (Gurtner et al. 1995; Kwee et al. 1995).

Mice deficient for α_5-integrin show, depending on the genetic background, embryonic lethality around E9.5-E10 with variable degrees of embryonic and extra-embryonic defects in the posterior trunk and yolk sac mesodermal structures (Yang et al. 1993, 1999). Interactions of $\alpha_5\beta_1$ integrin with fibronectin are not essential for the initial commitment of mesodermal cells, but are crucial for maintenance of mesodermal derivatives during postgastrulation stages and also for the survival of some neural crest cells (Goh et al. 1997). Cells derived from α_5-deficient mice migrate on fibronectin matrices, which suggests that other fibronectin-binding integrins compensate in the α_5-null mouse (Yang et al. 1995).

Mutants for α_7 and α_9 show no embryonic phenotype, but develop muscular dystrophy after birth or die due to bilateral chylothorax postnatally (Mayer et al. 1997; Huang et al. 2000). Mice lacking α_8-integrin have small or absent kidneys and most newborns die postnatally due to kidney failure. Animals with one functioning kidney survive but develop inner ear defects (Müller et al. 1997).

Of the four collagen-binding $\beta 1$ integrin receptors—α_1, α_2, α_{10}, and α_{11}—deletion of α_1 and α_2 does not result in any observed abnormalities during early embryonic development (Gardner et al. 1996; Holtkötter et al. 2002). Adult α_2-deficient mice have only mild hemostasis defects (Holtkötter 2002). Mice lacking α_{11} integrin have no obvious phenotype (D. Gullberg, personal communication). No reports have been published for the deletion of α_{10} integrin.

Integrins $\alpha_3\beta_1$ and $\alpha_6\beta_1$ are receptors for laminins, components of the basement membrane which underlies all epithelial cells. Mice deficient for α_3 integrin develop defects in kidney, lung, and skin (Kreidberg et al. 1996; diPersio et al. 1997). Mice which lack $\alpha_6\beta_1$ and $\alpha_6\beta_4$ integrins show defects in the laminar organization of the developing cerebral cortex and retina, and develop severe skin blistering (Georges-Labouesse et al. 1996, 1998).

The α_v integrin subunit associates with the β_1, β_3, β_5, β_6, and β_8 subunits. Integrins $\alpha_v\beta_1$, $\alpha_v\beta_3$, and $\alpha_v\beta_5$ can bind to fibronectin and vitronectin; integrin $\alpha_v\beta_6$ interacts with fibronectin, vitronectin, tenascin-C, and transforming growth factor (TGF)-β latency-associated peptide (LAP)1 and LAP3; and $\alpha_v\beta_8$ binds to fibronectin and LAP1 (Plow et al. 2000; Annes et al. 2002; Mu et al. 2002). Embryos deficient for α_v integrin develop normally until E9.5; however, around 80% of α_v-deficient mice die between E10 and E12, due to placental defects. These defects are characterized by a poorly developed labyrinthine zone and reduced interdigitation of fetal and maternal vessels. The remaining α_v-null mice die at birth and exhibit intracerebral and intestinal hemorrhages and cleft palates (Bader et al. 1998). The α_v-null phenotype might be due to a lack of fibronectin binding, since vitronectin, tenascin-C, and osteopontin-null mice show no obvious phenotype during early mouse development (Saga et al. 1992; Zheng et al. 1995; Liaw et al. 1998; Gustafsson and Fässler 2000).

Double mutants have been investigated for α_3/α_4, α_3/α_5, α_4/α_5, and α_5/α_v integrin subunits. No obvious differences from the additive phenotypes of the single mutants were observed in α_3/α_4, α_3/α_5, and α_4/α_5 double knockouts (Yang et al. 1999). Embryos deficient for both α_5 and α_v integrin die between E7.5 and E8 due to a severe gastrulation defect with a lack of anterior mesoderm (Yang et al. 1999). This phenotype is more severe than the single knockouts for α_v and α_5, suggesting redundant functions of these fibronectin receptors. Interestingly, α_v/α_5 double knockouts die even earlier than fibronectin-null mice, indicating that ligands other than fibronectin are also important for the in vivo function of these receptors.

4
Hematopoiesis and Inflammation

Hematopoietic stem cells (HSC) are generated in the yolk sac and in the para-aortic splanchnopleure/aorta-gonad mesonephros region. They can be found in the fetal blood of mice after the onset of circulation at around E8.5. At E10 they start to colonize the fetal liver and later thymus, spleen, other lymphoid organs, and the bone marrow. In adult mice, HSC reside in the bone marrow, but differentiated leukocytes circulate through the body. Site-specific adhesion and migration is achieved by integrins which are on circulating blood cells in a low-affinity state, ensuring that they do not make inappropriate interactions with ligands normally present on blood or endothelial cells. Chemokines released by the endothelium or the surrounding tissue during inflammation shift the leukocyte integrin into a high-affinity state. To leave the blood, leukocytes attach loosely to activated endothelium via selectins and begin to roll. The activated integrins bind to endothelial cell adhesion molecules such as ICAMs and VCAM-1, and firm adhesion of the blood cells to the vessel wall is established. Finally, the leukocytes cross the endothelial cell layer and underlying BM and migrate into the extravascular tissue.

Analysis of β_1-deficient chimeric mice revealed that β_1 integrin is essential for the homing of hematopoietic stem cells to liver, spleen, thymus, and bone marrow. Progenitor cells that lack β_1 integrins are unable to attach to the vessel walls and are thus sequestered in the blood circulation (Hirsch et al. 1996; Potocnik et al. 2000). In the presence of cytokines, β_1-null precursor cells differentiate normally in vitro, indicating that β_1 integrins are not essential for the differentiation of hematopoietic stem cells (Hirsch et al. 1996; Potocnik et al. 2000). In adult mice, β_1 integrin is dismissible for HSC retention in the BM, hematopoiesis, and trafficking of lymphocytes. However, β_1 integrins seem to be important for the primary IgM response. After immunization with T cell-dependent antigens, no IgM and an increased IgG response can be observed in mice with a deletion of the β_1 integrin gene restricted to the hematopoietic system. T cell-independent type 2 antigens induce only reduced IgG and IgM responses (Brakebusch et al. 2002).

The β_7 integrin subunit associates with to α_4 and α_E integrin subunits. An 80%–90% reduction of lymphocyte migration to the Peyer's patches and a reduced number of lamina propria and intraepithelial lymphocytes can be observed in β_7-deficient mice (Wagner et al. 1996). Integrin $\alpha_4\beta_7$ binds to mucosal addressin cell adhesion molecule (MadCAM)-1 which is expressed on high endothelial venules in the gut (Berlin et al. 1993; Briskin et al. 1997). The migration of lymphocytes to the Peyer's patches is mediated by $\alpha_4\beta_7$ binding to Mad-CAM-1. Mice lacking MadCAM-1 display very small Peyer's patches only visible by microscopic inspection (Pabst et al. 2000), and α_4-null T cell migration to Peyer's patches is impaired (Arroyo et al. 1996). E-cadherin is expressed on epithelial cells and recognized by $\alpha_E\beta_7$ integrin. Targeted disruption of the α_E gene leads to a reduction of T cells only in the lamina propria and gut epithelium

(Schön et al. 1999). Both β_7 and L-selectin act in a synergistic way to promote lymphocyte migration. Deletion of L-selectin in addition to β_7 integrin almost completely abolishes lymphocyte migration to Peyer's patches and in addition reduces migration into mesenteric lymph nodes (Steeber et al. 1998; Wagner et al. 1998).

The α_4 integrin subunit associates with β_1 and β_7 integrin. Early embryonic lethality of α_4-null mice made it necessary to study the function of α_4 integrin in the hematopoietic system in α_4-null chimeric mice or by cell transfer experiments. Chimeric mice have no α_4-null erythrocytes, almost no α_4-null B-lymphoid cells, and only few α_4-null myeloid cells, indicating an important role of α_4 integrins in postnatal hematopoietic development (Arroyo et al. 1999). Mice deficient for α_4-integrin have normal T cells until 1 month after birth, when T cells start to decrease in number. Cell transfer experiments have shown that α_4 deficient T cells develop in the bone marrow, at do not enter the circulation (Arroyo et al. 1996). However, α4-null T cells that have entered the circulation are able, although with reduced activity, to migrate into inflamed peritoneum (Arroyo et al. 2000) and α4-deficient pre-B cells can transmigrate in vitro (Arroyo et al. 1999). Proliferation of α4-null precursor cells might also be decreased since they showed poor mitotic activity in vitro (Arroyo et al. 1999). VCAM-1-deficient mice have normal hematopoiesis, suggesting that the α_4-null phenotype is caused by impaired interactions of $\alpha_4\beta_1$ and $\alpha_4\beta_7$ with fibronectin (Friedrich et al. 1996). However, VCAM-1-null mice show a defective migration of lymphocytes to the bone marrow (Koni et al. 2001; Leuker et al. 2001). Since this effect is not seen in β_1-null bone marrow chimera (Brakebusch et al. 2002) and in β_7-null mice, there might be additional receptors for VCAM-1 which mediate this effect.

Hematopoietic progenitors express $\alpha_5\beta_1$ and $\alpha_6\beta_1$ integrins in addition to $\alpha_4\beta_1$. Individual knockouts of the α_5 or α_6 integrin subunit do not interfere with HSC homing (Arroyo et al. 1996; Taverna et al. 1998; Arroyo et al. 2000).

Integrin β_2 is specifically expressed on leukocytes. It associates with α_L [lymphocyte function-associated antigen (LFA)-1], α_M (Mac-1), α_X and α_D subunits. Ligand binding includes members of the ICAM family (Plow et al. 2000). Integrin $\alpha_M\beta_2$ binds to inactivated complement factor (iC3b), fibrinogen, and factor X; $\alpha_X\beta_2$ to iC3b and type I collagen (Garnotel et al. 2000); and $\alpha_D\beta_2$ to VCAM-1 (Van der Vieren et al. 1999). Mice lacking β_2 integrin have increase 1 numbers of neutrophils and display a variable decrease of neutrophil extravasation, depending on the model of inflammation (Mizgerd et al. 1997; Scharfetter-Kochanek et al. 1998; Jung and Ley 1999; Grabbe et al. 2002). In the microcirculation, leukocytes show a gradual β_2 integrin-dependent decrease in rolling velocity that is correlated with an increase in intracellular free calcium concentration before arrest. When β_2 integrins are absent, the arrest of rolling leukocytes is severely reduced (Kunkel et al. 2000). Similarly, β_2-deficient dendritic precursor cells accumulate less efficiently in the lung (Schneeberger et al. 2000). T cell proliferation after stimulation by staphylococcal enterotoxin or major histocompatibility complex alloantigens is defective in β_2-deficient mice (Scharfetter-

Kochanek et al. 1998). Humans with a mutation in the β_2 gene develop leukocyte adhesion deficiency type I (LAD-1) with a massive leukocytosis, recurrent bacterial infections, impaired wound healing, and a severe gingivitis. As in mice, the neutrophil extravasation is severely disturbed.

Four α subunits are known to associate with β_2 integrin, of which only $\alpha_L\beta_2$ and $\alpha_M\beta_2$ integrins have been investigated in transgenic mouse models. No knockouts have been reported so far for α_X and α_D integrin. In the absence of $\alpha_L\beta_2$, immune responses against systemic viral infections are normal, but alloantigen-triggered T cell proliferation and cytotoxicity are severely impaired, leading to defective host-versus-graft reaction and abrogated tumor rejection (Schmits et al. 1996; Shier et al. 1996, 1999). The reduction of extravasation is similar to β_2-deficient mice and homing of lymphocytes to peripheral lymph nodes and, to a lesser degree, to mesenteric lymph nodes and Peyer's patches is impaired (Berlin-Rufenach et al. 1999). Mice lacking $\alpha_M\beta_2$, however, show an increase of neutrophil extravasation in response to tumor necrosis factor (TNF)-α (Ding et al. 1999). In contrast, extravasation was normal in an acute glomerulonephritis model, but $\alpha_M\beta_2$-null neutrophils did not remain in the tissue, apparently due to absent Fcγ binding of the neutrophils and failure to initiate sufficient adhesion (Tang et al. 1997; van Spriel et al. 2001). Neutrophils deficient for $\alpha_M\beta_2$ are also unable to bind to fibrinogen coated disks and display impaired phagocytosis and degranulation leading to a delayed neutrophil apoptosis (Coxon et al. 1996; Lu et al. 1997). Mast cells are reduced in some, but not all, locations of $\alpha_M\beta_2$-deficient mice (Lu et al. 1997; Rosenkranz et al. 1998). Unexpectedly, mice lacking $\alpha_M\beta_2$ or its ligand ICAM-1 are obese, suggesting a role of $\alpha_M\beta_2$ in the regulation of fat metabolism (Dong et al. 1997).

Apart from the regulation of adhesion and migration, $\alpha_L\beta_2$-ICAM-1 have additional function in the inflammatory response. In a murine autoimmune diabetes-1 model, $\alpha_L\beta_2$-deficient T cells showed a lower cytotoxicity and diminished expression of interleukin (IL)-4 during primary CD4 T cell responses (Camacho et al. 2001).

TGF-β1 and TGF-β3 are regulated by arginine-glycine-aspartic acid (RGD)-binding integrins. TGF-β1 can be activated by $\alpha_v\beta_6$ (Annes et al. 2002; Munger et al. 1999) and $\alpha_v\beta_8$ (Mu et al. 2002) binding to LAP1. In addition, $\alpha_v\beta_6$ binds to LAP3 and can activate latent TGF-β3 but not TGF-β2 (Annes et al. 2002). The $\alpha_v\beta_1$ and $\alpha_5\beta_1$ integrins also bind to LAP1, but are not able to activate TGF-β1 (Munger et al. 1998; Annes et al. 2002).

Loss of $\alpha_v\beta_6$ reduces the amount of active TGF-β1 in epithelia, which at least partially mimics a local TGF-β1 deficiency. Mutant mice exhibit juvenile baldness due to macrophage infiltration of the dermis and demonstrate hallmarks of asthma such as increased airway responsiveness and an infiltration of activated B and T cells into the lung (Munger 1999). Mice deficient for β_6 integrin show normal embryonic development and wound healing (Huang et al. 1996).

5
Platelet Function

When platelets contact injured or diseased blood vessel walls they attach to the subendothelial matrix, become activated, and are crosslinked to form thrombi which finally seal the defective blood vessel. The attachment of platelets to collagen is believed to be of great importance in vivo. It has been shown that glycoprotein VI (GPVI) is the main mediator of this interaction. GPVI also activates β_1 and β_3 integrins, which is a prerequisite for firm adhesion and thrombus growth (Nieswandt et al. 2001). The conditional deletion of β_1 integrin and the receptors $\alpha_2\beta_1$, $\alpha_5\beta_1$, and $\alpha_6\beta_1$ on megakaryocytes does not lead to significant changes in platelet counts or bleeding time, demonstrating that β_1 integrins are not essential for initial platelet adhesion (Nieswandt et al. 2001). Similarily, α_2-deficient mice have normal platelet counts and bleeding times. However, in the presence of an antibody against GPVI, adhesion of β_1-deficient or of α_2-deficient, but not wild-type, platelets is abrogated (Nieswandt et al. 2001; Holtkötter et al. 2002). Thus, $\alpha_2\beta_1$ plays only a supportive, rather than an essential, role in platelet–collagen interactions.

Integrin $\alpha_{IIb}\beta_3$ interacts directly with fibrinogen and indirectly with collagen via von Willebrand factor and is crucially important for the aggregation and adhesive spreading of platelets during hemostasis (Shattil et al. 1998). Various agonists such as thrombin, adenosine diphosphate (ADP), and collagen can induce the activation of the $\alpha_{IIb}\beta_3$ integrin receptor by "inside-out" signaling, allowing binding to fibrinogen. Ligand binding to $\alpha_{IIb}\beta_3$ results in "outside-in" signaling with subsequent calcium mobilization, tyrosine phosphorylation of numerous proteins including β_3 integrin itself, and cytoskeletal rearrangement (Shattil et al. 1998). Patients with a lack of functional $\alpha_{IIb}\beta_3$ on their platelets suffer from Glanzmann thrombasthenia. They display impaired platelet aggregation and prolonged bleeding times. The same phenotype was replicated in mice lacking the β_3 or the α_{IIb} integrin gene (Hodivala-Dilke et al. 1999; Tronik-Le Roux et al. 2000). Mice in which the ability for "outside-in" signaling has been disturbed by the replacement of two cytoplasmic tyrosines of the β_3 subunit are impaired in the late phase of platelet aggregation. They display defects in clot retraction in vitro and an increased tendency for rebleeding in once clotted tail wounds in vivo, indicating an instability in hemostatic plug formation (Law et al. 1999). A similar phenotype with an instability of arterial thrombi has been described for CD40L which binds to $\alpha_{IIb}\beta_3$ (Andre et al. 2002).

6
Vasculo- and Angiogenesis

Integrins $\alpha_1\beta_1$, $\alpha_2\beta_1$, $\alpha_3\beta_1$, $\alpha_5\beta_1$, $\alpha_6\beta_1$, $\alpha_v\beta_1$, $\alpha_v\beta_3$, $\alpha_v\beta_5$, $\alpha_6\beta_4$, and $\alpha_v\beta_8$ are expressed on endothelial cells and differentially regulated during angiogenesis (Kennel et al. 1992; el Gabalawy and Wilkins 1993; Creamer et al. 1995; Gingras et al. 1995; Jaspars et al. 1996; Zhu et al. 2002). Integrins $\alpha_4\beta_1$ and $\alpha_7\beta_1$ can be found on vascular smooth muscle cells (Duplaa et al. 1997; Yao et al. 1997).

Targeted null mutation of the β_1 integrin deletes all endothelial integrins except $\alpha_v\beta_3$, $\alpha_v\beta_5$, $\alpha_v\beta_8$, and $\alpha_6\beta_4$. There is strong evidence for an important role of β_1 integrin in blood vessel formation in vivo. First, chimeric mice derived from β_1-null embryonic stem (ES) cells lack β_1-null endothelial cells at least in the liver (Fässler and Meyer 1995). Secondly, β_1-null ES cells fail to contribute to the endothelial cells of the blood vessels of β_1-null teratomas (Bloch et al. 1997). In vitro differentiation of β_1-null ES cells into embryoid bodies shows that endothelial cells are formed, but that vasculogenesis is significantly delayed and responsiveness to vascular endothelial growth factor (VEGF) is impaired (Bloch et al. 1997).

Mice lacking the α_1 subunit show normal development of the blood vessel system (Gardner 1996), but have reduced tumor angiogenesis (Pozzi et al. 2000). The decrease in tumor angiogenesis has been explained by an over-expression of matrix metalloproteinases (MMP)7 and 9. MMP expression allows remodeling of the ECM and vessel invasion by degrading the ECM. Increased MMP expression, however, also leads to an elevation of angiostatin, a strong angiogenesis inhibitor that is thought to be responsible for the reduced tumor angiogenesis in α_1-deficient mice. In addition, isolated α_1-null endothelial cells from adult lung display reduced proliferation on both α_1-dependent and α_1-independent substrates (Pozzi et al. 2000). Thus, α_1 integrins seem to have different impact on embryonic, adult, and tumor angiogenesis.

Mice deficient for α_2 show no obvious vascular defects (Holtkötter et al. 2002), whereas α_3-deficient mice show reduced branching and a distended lumen of glomerular capillaries (Kreidberg et al. 1996). This could result from an abnormal formation of the capillary structure of the glomerulus or from a failure of podocytes to provide adequate scaffolding for the forming capillaries. In addition, these mutant mice have a lung defect with reduced branching of the conducting airway (Kreidberg et al. 1996) and show an alteration of the basal membrane organization of the submandibular gland (Menko et al. 2001). Most mice lacking integrin α_4 die during embryonic development due to defects in chorion allantois fusion at E10.5 (Yang et al. 1995). Animals that develop a functional placenta show defects in epicardial formation and coronary heart vessels (Yang et al. 1995). However, it is not clear if the coronary vessel defect is a direct consequence of the loss of α_4 or an indirect secondary defect due to the loss of the epicardium. Mice lacking the α_5 subunit have impaired development of the extraembryonic and embryonic vasculature (Yang et al. 1993). At E9.5, extraembryonic blood islands are not fused properly, vessel formation is impaired, and primitive blood cells leak into the exocoelomic space. The α_5-null embryos themselves form distended and leaky hearts and blood vessels that contain only a few primitive blood cells. Deletion of the major ligand of $\alpha_5\beta_1$, fibronectin, results in a similar, but more pronounced phenotype which is influenced by the genetic background (George et al. 1993, 1997). In C57BL/6 mutants, the yolk sac is completely devoid of vessels. Embryonic hearts, however, are formed, although myocardial and endocardial cells are disorganized resulting in a bulbous heart tube. Endothelial cells in the aorta lack contact with the surrounding mesenchyme. On a 129/Sv background the defects are more severe. Endothelial cells are able to differentiate, but fail to assemble into vessels. While fibronectin-deficient mice already show defects in initial vasculogenesis, α_5-deficient mice initiate vasculogenesis, but are unable to pursue proper formation and maintenance of blood vessels. This suggests that, in the absence of α_5, other fibronectin receptors realize early steps of vasculogenesis.

In addition to the β_1 integrins, endothelial cells express at least four members of the α_v-integrin subfamily; $\alpha_v\beta_1$, $\alpha_v\beta_3$, $\alpha_v\beta_5$, and $\alpha_v\beta_8$. The $a_v\beta_3$ and $a_v\beta_5$ integrins are involved in growth factor-induced angiogenesis (Brooks et al. 1994; Friedlander et al. 1995). Antagonist of α_v integrin disrupt vascular development in the embryo and block pathological angiogenesis in chorioallantoic membrane (CAM) assays (Brooks et al. 1994), in tumor models (Brooks et al. 1995), and in neovascularization studies of the mouse retina (Friedlander et al. 1995; Hammes et al. 1996), making this integrin subunit an attractive target for therapeutic intervention (Eliceiri and Cheresh 2001; Rupp and Little 2001). Blocking antibodies to inhibit tumor vascularization are currently evaluated in clinical trials for treatment of cancer, arthritis, and ischemic retinopathy (Gutheil et al. 2000). However α_v-null mice, develop normally until E9.5, when around 80% of the embryos die due to placental defects. The remaining 20% die at birth, showing intracerebral and intestinal hemorrhages and cleft palates but no defects in endothelial proliferation, migration, tube formation, branching, or basement membrane assembly (Bader et al. 1998). Normal vascular development has also been reported for null mutants of many α_v ligands including vitronectin (Zheng et al. 1995), tenascin-C (Forsberg et al. 1996; Saga et al. 1992), osteopontin (Liaw et al. 1998), fibrinogen (Suh et al. 1995), perlecan (Costell et al. 1999), and von Willebrand factor (Denis et al. 1998).

Two pathways of growth factor-induced angiogenesis have been identified in which basic fibroblast growth factor (bFGF) induces angiogenesis via integrin $\alpha_v\beta_3$ ligation, whereas VEGF induces angiogenesis via the ligation of integrin $\alpha_v\beta_5$ (Friedländer et al. 1995). Deletion of VEGF results in embryonic lethality in heterozygous mice between E8.5 and 9.5 (Carmeliet et al. 1996; Ferrara et al. 1996). VEGF injection into the blood or the brain of β_5-deficient mice results in a significantly reduced vascular permeability compared to β_3-deficient mice which display a normal response. VEGF induces Src-dependent phosphorylation of FAK which then interacts with $\alpha_v\beta_5$ integrin to trigger vascular responses in vivo (Eliceiri et al. 2001). VEGF-R1-deficient mice have normal hematopoietic progenitors, but stroke impaired blood vessel formation (Fong et al. 1995)

However, the loss of β_3 and/or β_5 integrins does not lead to obvious defects in vascular development (Hodivala-Dilke et al. 1999; Huang et al. 2000; Reynolds et al. 2002) and induced tumors in β_3- and/or β_5-deficient mice show enhanced, rather than reduced, angiogenesis (Reynolds et al. 2002). A possible explanation is that $\alpha_v\beta_3$ acts as a survival factor which allows cell survival if bound to the extracellular matrix, but induces apoptosis in its unbound state, as shown for

$\alpha_v\beta_3$ endothelial cells in vitro (Stupack et al. 2001). Blocking antibodies against α_v disrupt extracellular interactions of $\alpha_v\beta_3$ integrins and decrease angiogenesis by inducing apoptosis. In contrast, $\alpha_v\beta_3$-deficient cells are independent of adhesion-regulated apoptosis and thus show enhanced vessel formation (Cheresh and Stupack 2002).

Mice deficient for β_8 integrin share many similarities to the α_v mutants with early defects in placental development and later deficits in formation and stabilization of the vascularisation of the central nervous system (Zhu et al. 2002).

Mice lacking α_6 or β_4 integrin show no blood vessel defects (Georges-Labouesse et al. 1996; van der Neut et al. 1996).

7
Nervous System

The function of β_1 integrin in the nervous system has been investigated in chimeric mice and mice with a conditional deletion of β_1 in the brain. Chimeric mice showed normal neuronal migration and differentiation. However, mice that upon cre-mediated deletion lack the β_1 integrin subunit in neurons and glia die after birth with severe brain malformations. Cortical hemispheres and cerebellar folia fuse and cortical laminae are perturbed (Graus-Porta et al. 2001). These defects result from a disorganization of the cortical marginal zone, where β_1 integrins are supposed to regulate glial endfeet anchorage, meningeal basement membrane remodeling, and formation of the Cajal-Retzius cell layer. The phenotype of the β_1-deficient mice resembles pathological changes observed in human cortical dysplasias, suggesting that defective integrin function contributes to the development of some of these diseases (Graus-Porta et al. 2001). Abnormal laminar organization has also been observed in α_6 and α_3/α_6 double-null mice. Single deletion of the α_6 subunit results in a disorganization of the developing cerebral cortex and retina. In addition, ectopic neuroblastic outgrowth on the brain surface and in the eye was observed (Georges-Labouesse et al. 1998). In the α_3/α_6 double-knockout mice, the cortical disorganization appears earlier and is more severe. Compared to α_6-deficient mice, α_3/α_6 double mutants display additional abnormalities including exencephaly, syndactyly, and kidney defects (De Arcangelis et al. 1999). An abnormal laminin deposition has been observed in α_6 single- and α_3/α_6 double-mutant mice. Ablation of the ligand laminin α_5 gene leads to a brain phenotype similar to the α_3/α_6 double knockouts (Miner et al. 1998; Miner and Li 2000), indicating that the phenotype is caused by a disrupted interaction with laminin α_5. The importance of a normal BM composition is underlined by the phenotype of perlecan-deficient mice. Although a BM is initially assembled, mechanical stress leads to BM deterioration, which causes abnormal expansion of neuroepithelium, neuronal ectopias, and exencephaly in the expanding brain (Costell et al. 1999).

Involvement of integrins during nerve regeneration has been suggested by increased expression of $\alpha_7\beta_1$ integrin on axons and growth cones during peripheral nerve regeneration. An impaired axonal regeneration has been confirmed in

α_7-null mutants (Werner et al. 2000). The deletion of laminin-2, a major ligand for $\alpha_7\beta_1$ leads to muscular dystrophy and peripheral nerve dysmyelination due to an inability of Schwann cells to sort bundles of axons (Hodges et al. 1997). Schwann cell-specific disruption of β_1 integrin causes a severe neuropathy. Schwann cells deficient from β_1 do not extend or maintain normal processes around axons, but some Schwann cells form normal myelin, possibly due to the presence of other laminin receptors such as dystroglycan and $\alpha_6\beta_4$ integrin (Feltri et al. 2002). Similarly, β_1 compensation might be responsible for the normal myelinization of peripheral nerves in β_4-deficient mice (Frei et al. 1999). The consequences of deleting α_4 and α_5 integrin in the peripheral nerve system have been investigated by grafting experiments to overcome early lethality in α_4- and α_5-deficient embryos. In the absence of α_5, Schwann cell differentiation is unaffected, but the proliferation of early progenitor cells is reduced. In α_4-deficient explants, survival of progenitor cells is impaired in a cell density-dependent fashion (Haack and Hynes 2001).

Integrin $\alpha_8\beta_1$ is localized to the apical hair cell surface during formation of stereocilia in the inner ear. Most integrin α_8-null mice die soon after birth. However, a few survive until adulthood and display hearing and balance defects. In these mice, stereocilia start to develop, but deteriorate in a subpopulation of hair cells. FAK recruitment to the apical hair cell is impaired, suggesting that $\alpha_8\beta_1$ integrin and FAK are involved in the regulation of assembly or maintenance of the stereocilia cytoskeleton (Littlewood-Evans and Müller 2000). The early expression of α_3 and α_6 integrins during development of the mammalian inner ear suggests that they may be involved in the molecular processes that define epithelial boundaries and guide sensory innervation (Davies and Holley 2002). However, no data on inner ear phenotypes of α_3- or α_6-deficient mice are currently available.

8
Striated and Cardiac Muscle

During muscle development, two splice variants of β_1 integrin are expressed in muscle precursor cells and fetal muscle. The cytoplasmic β_{1A} splice variant is initially expressed and is substituted after birth by the β_{1D} variant (Belkin et al. 1996). Concomitant with the change to β_{1D} integrin, the expression of α_1, α_3, α_4, α_5, α_6, α_7, α_9, and α_v is downregulated and only the α_7 integrin is expressed by adult muscle cells (Bouvard et al. 2001).

Integrin-deficient Drosophila myoblasts fail to fuse into proper myocytes. However, in β_1-null chimeric mice, β_1-deficient myoblasts migrate to their normal destinations and fuse with wild-type myoblasts. The overall contribution of β_1-null cells to the muscle is 2%–28% (Hirsch et al. 1998). A delay of myotube formation can be observed in β_1-null embryoid bodies (Hirsch et al. 1998; Rohwedel et al. 1998), suggesting compensation by wild-type cells in vivo. Both chimeras and adult mice with a conditional deletion of β_1 integrin were used to investigate β_1 function in the heart. Chimeras showed a low contribution of β_1-

null cells in the heart and in areas with contribution of β_1-null cells, ultrastructural analysis revealed alterations in the sarcomeric architecture (Fässler et al. 1996). Using a conditional approach, β_1 integrin was deleted in most of the ventricular cardiac myocytes. The level of β_{1D} integrin in the heart was reduced to 18% of control levels. These mice were viable, but displayed myocardial fibrosis at age 5 weeks that by age 6 months had developed into a dilated cardiomyopathy (Shai et al. 2002). Transgenic mice expressing a dominant-negative form of β_1 integrin, in which the extracellular domain of CD4 is fused to the transmembrane and cytoplasmic domain of β_1 integrin, die around birth and display fibrotic changes in the heart. Lower levels of the transgene lead only to hypertrophic changes in the heart (Keller et al. 2001). Replacement of β_{1D} with β_{1A} in the heart results in mild cardiac defects, with increased levels of atrial natriuretic peptide (ANP), a vasorelaxant diminishing volume overload and hypertension. The increased expression of ANP suggests that the β_{1A} subunit, at least in the heart, is not fully compensating for β_{1D} (Baudoin et al. 1998). During embryonic development, $\alpha_5\beta_1$ integrin is expressed in adhesion plaque-like structures along the myotube (Lakonishok et al. 1992), but gets downregulated in adult muscle. Mice deficient for α_5 integrin die due to mesodermal defects even before muscle is formed. Chimeric mice with a high contribution of α_5-null myoblasts to the muscle develop muscular dystrophy, characterized by giant muscle fibers, vacuoles, centrally located nuclei, and reduced adhesion and survival of α_5-null myoblasts (Taverna et al. 1998). Overexpression of a constitutively active form of α_5 integrin in the heart results in electrocardiographic abnormalities, cardiomyopathy, and death within 1 month after birth (Valencik and McDonald 2001).

Integrin $\alpha_7\beta_1$ is the most abundant integrin in skeletal muscle and expressed during all stages of muscle development (Bao et al. 1993; George-Weinstein et al. 1993). In skeletal muscle, it binds to laminin 2 and laminin 4 (von der Mark et al. 1991; Yao et al. 1996; Schöber et al. 2000). Integrin α_7 mRNA undergoes tissue-specific and developmentally-regulated alternative splicing in its intra- and extracellular domain (Collo et al. 1993; Song et al. 1993; Ziober et al. 1993; Martin et al. 1996). Mice deficient for $\alpha_7\beta_1$ show a progressive muscular dystrophy with a disruption of the myotendinous junctions (Mayer et al. 1997). Ultrastructurally, interdigitations at the myotendinous junctions are lost and myofilaments retract from the sarcolemmal membrane, basement membranes are broadened and laminin α_2 is mislocalized. The lateral side of the myofibers remains morphologically normal. In contrast, mice that lack dystrophin have normal myotendinous junctions but lesions at the lateral side of the myotube, suggesting that $\alpha7\beta1$ is a major organizer of the myotendinous junction, whereas the dystrophin–glycoprotein complex is important for lateral adhesion of muscle cells (Miosge et al. 1999). Mutations in the α_7 gene have also been identified in patients suffering from congenital myopathies characterized by delayed motor milestones (Hayashi et al. 1998). A similar phenotype with congenital muscular dystrophy occurs also in man and mouse when laminin α_2 expression is lost (Hodges et al. 1997). Mice that lack both dystrophin and utrophin develop a severe muscular dystrophy similar to Duchenne muscular dystrophy. Twofold overexpression of α_7 integrin partially compensates for the absence of the dystrophin- and utrophin-mediated linkage systems and alleviates many of the symptoms (Burkin et al. 2001). Integrin $\alpha_4\beta_1$ had been implicated in the formation of secondary myotubes (Rosen et al. 1992). However, neither α_4-null chimeric mice nor α_4-null embryoid bodies show defects in myotube development (Yao et al. 1996). Similarly, no abnormalities in muscular developmental were observed upon deletion of VCAM-1, a ligand for $\alpha_4\beta_1$ integrin (Gurtner et al. 1995; Kwee et al. 1995). Single deletions of α_1, α_3, α_4, α_6, α_9, and α_v integrins also do not result in perturbation of muscular development.

9
Skeleton

Chondrocytes, bone-depositing osteoblasts, and bone resorbing osteoclasts are the major cell types of the skeleton and express a number of integrin receptors at their surfaces. Chondrocytes express $\alpha_1\beta_1$, $\alpha_2\beta_1$, $\alpha_3\beta_1$, $\alpha_5\beta_1$, $\alpha_6\beta_1$, $\alpha_{10}\beta_1$, $\alpha_v\beta_3$, and $\alpha_v\beta_5$ integrins (Dürr et al. 1993; Loeser et al. 1995; Salter et al. 1995; Camper et al. 2001). Integrins $\alpha_1\beta_1$, $\alpha_2\beta_1$ (Dürr et al. 1993), and $\alpha_{10}\beta_1$ (Camper et al. 1998) bind to type II collagen; $\alpha_1\beta_1$ interacts with matrilin-1 (Makihira et al. 1999) and collagen type VI (Loeser 1997), $\alpha_2\beta_1$ binds to chondroadherin (Camper et al. 1997); $\alpha_5\beta_1$ and $\alpha_6\beta_1$ have been shown to interact with fibronectin and laminin-1, respectively (Dürr et al. 1993; Dürr et al. 1996); and $\alpha_v\beta_3$ and $\alpha_v\beta_5$ are putative receptors for fibronectin, vitronectin, and osteopontin (Dürr et al. 1993).

The majority of mice with a deletion of the β_1 gene in chondrocytes die at birth and develop severe chondrodysplasia characterized by disproportionate dwarfism, disorganized growth plate, abnormal chondrocyte morphology, impaired differentiation, reduced proliferation, increased apoptosis, and perturbation of cytokinesis giving rise to an increased number of binucleated cells (Aszódi et al. 2003). Mice lacking fibronectin specifically in cartilage develop without apparent skeletal abnormalities (Aszódi et al. 2003). These data suggest an essential role for β_1 integrin binding to type II collagen for the process of endochondral ossification (Aszódi et al. 2003).

Integrin β_1 Integrin function in bone generation was tested using transgenic mice expressing a dominant-negative β_1 integrin subunit under the control of the osteoblast-specific osteocalcin promoter. The mice display a decreased rate of cortical bone formation and reduced bone mass of cortical and flat bones. Bone mass becomes normal in older male mice, but not in female mice (Zimmerman et al. 2000). Deletion of α_1 or α_2 results in no skeletal phenotype despite the severe phenotype with the absence of β_1 integrin. No reports have been published for the deletion of $\alpha10$ integrin. This suggests compensation between the different collagen II binding integrin receptors, or a major role for $\alpha_{10}\beta_1$.

Single deletion of α_3 or α_6 integrin subunits results in no obvious skeletal abnormalities. However, α_3/α_6 double-knockout mice display exencephaly due to incomplete neural tube closure, kinked tail, and limb anomalies (De Arcangelis et al. 1999). Detailed analyses of the limb anomalies revealed discontinuity of the surface ectoderm of the distal limb and defective formation of the AER, shortening and abnormal shape of the long bones, lack of digit separation, and fusion of phalanges between digits 2 and 3. Since single α_3 or α_6 mutants do not show such defects, the observations suggest redundancy of these integrins in the AER and the limb bud. Abnormalities of the distal limbs similar to the α_3/α_6 double knockout are present in laminin α_5 knockout mice (Miner et al. 1998), indicating that α_3 and α_6 integrins are the major cell surface receptors for α_5 laminin chains in the distal limb ectoderm.

Mice deficient in β_3 integrin suffer from osteosclerosis and hypocalcemia (McHugh et al. 2000) because osteoclasts fail to form the proper ruffled membrane important for their resorptive function. Osteoclasts deficient for β_3 integrin fail to spread in culture and lack the characteristic cortical actin rings, suggesting that $\alpha_v\beta_3$-mediated signals are important for the organization of cytoskeleton in these cells. No skeletal abnormalities during embryonic development have been reported after deletion of the α_v subunits (Bader et al. 1998).

10
Kidney

Integrin $\alpha_8\beta_1$ is essential for kidney development. Mice carrying a deletion of the α_8 integrin subunit show abnormal growth and branching of the ureteric bud and defective recruitment of mesenchymal cells into epithelial structures (Müller et al. 1997). The phenotype varies in different mouse strains, presumably due to modifier genes (Müller et al. 1997). Integrin $\alpha_8\beta_1$-deficient mice which survive to adulthood display an increased susceptibility to glomerular capillary destruction after experimentally induced desoxycorticosterone-salt hypertension, indicating that mesangial α_8 integrin contributes to maintaining the integrity of the glomerular capillary tuft during mechanical stress (Hartner et al. 2002). Integrin $\alpha_8\beta_1$ can bind fibronectin, tenascin-C, vitronectin, osteopontin, and nephronectin. Fibronectin, tenascin-C and vitronectin are, however, not expressed during this stage of kidney development. Osteopontin, which also binds $\alpha_8\beta_1$, had been proposed as the $\alpha_8\beta_1$ ligand in kidney, but osteopontin-null mice develop no apparent phenotype in the kidney (Denda et al. 1998; Rittling et al. 1998). Nephronectin was recently identified as a new ligand for $\alpha_8\beta_1$ in kidney and might be involved in the phenotype of the $\alpha_8\beta_1$-deficient mouse (Brandenberger et al. 2001). It will be interesting to see whether a loss of nephronectin mimics the α_8-null phenotype in kidney.

Apart from $\alpha_8\beta_1$ integrin, only $\alpha_3\beta_1$ mutants show a kidney-related phenotype. Integrin α_3-deficient mice display a disorganization of the glomerular basement membrane. Glomerular podocytes seem unable to form mature foot processes, suggesting that α_3 integrin might be important for basal membrane organization. The phenotype might, however, also result from an abnormal formation of the capillary structure of the glomerulus.

11
Skin

Human keratinocytes express several integrins, including $\alpha_2\beta_1$, $\alpha_3\beta_1$, $\alpha_5\beta_1$, $\alpha_9\beta_1$, $\alpha_6\beta_4$, and $\alpha_v\beta_5$ (Adams et al. 1991; Hertle et al. 1991). Basal keratinocytes adhere to the basement membrane via specialized adhesion junctions called hemidesmosomes. Keratinocytes that become committed to terminal differentiation detach from the basement membrane, migrate into the suprabasal layers, and terminally differentiate to form the stratum corneum. Binding to the basement membrane is mainly dependent on $\alpha_6\beta_4$, while $\alpha_3\beta_1$ seems to be more involved in migration of keratinocytes. In the absence of both α_3 and α_6 or β_4 integrin, basal keratinocytes can initially attach to the basal lamina and proliferate, indicating additional adhesion mechanisms (DiPersio et al. 2000). A candidate receptor for maintaining adhesion and proliferation could be α-dystroglycan.

Mutations in the α_6 or β_4 integrin genes in humans cause epidermolysis bullosa. Patients suffer from severe blister formation leading, in most cases, to early postnatal lethality (Vidal et al. 1995; Pulkkinen et al. 1997; Pulkkinen and Uitto 1999). A similar perinatal lethal phenotype with absence of hemidesmosomes and subsequent detachment of the epidermis is seen in α_6- and β_4-deficient mice. No disruption of the basal lamina has been observed in these mice (Dowling et al. 1996; Georges-Labouesse et al. 1996; van der Neut et al. 1996). Deletion of one of the subchains of laminin-5, the ligand for $\alpha_6\beta_4$ integrin, leads to lethal junctional epidermolysis bullosa in patients (Pulkkinen and Uitto 1999). Mice lacking laminin α_3 develop severe blistering of the skin and abnormal hemidesmosomes without involvement of the basal lamina (Ryan et al. 1999).

A disruption of the basement membrane occurs in mice deficient for α_3. The mice die perinatally due to defects in kidney and lung organogenesis (Kreidberg et al. 1996), but also show mild blisters caused by rupture of the basement membrane (DiPersio et al. 1997). Keratinocyte-restricted deletion of the β_1 integrin gene during early development results in perinatal lethality. These mice display severe blister formation of the skin with failure of basement membrane assembly and hemidesmosome instability (Raghavan et al. 2000). If keratinocyte-specific deletion of the β_1 integrin gene occurs around birth, keratinocytes with an aberrant morphology and reduced proliferation rate can be observed. They are, however, still able to terminally differentiate (Brakebusch et al. 2000). Migration and adhesion of β_1-null keratinocytes to collagen type I, laminin 1 and collagen type IV is impaired (Grose et al. 2002). Mice deficient for β_1 integrin in keratinocytes show severe defects in wound healing, with a delayed re-epithelization of the wound and an abnormal epithelial architecture after healing (Grose et al. 2002).

12
Tumorigenesis

Integrin functions are not only important for physiological processes, but also for tumor growth, invasion and metastasis, and for tumor-related processes such as angiogenesis and immune defense against tumors. Although there are numerous papers describing the functions of integrins for tumorigenesis in vitro, there is currently only limited data generated from the in vivo situation.

In epithelial cells, engagement of $\alpha_6\beta_4$ promotes cell cycle progression by recruitment of the adapter protein Shc to the α_4 cytoplasmic domain with subsequent activation of the Ras-MAPK cascade (Mainiero et al. 1995; Mainiero et al. 1997). It was also shown that expression of this integrin in $\alpha_6\beta_4$-deficient breast carcinoma cells markedly enhances their invasive potential through a preferential targeting of PI3 K activity (Shaw et al. 1997). In addition, $\alpha_6\beta_4$ can promote the PKB/Akt-dependent survival of carcinoma cells that lack functional p53 (Bachelder et al. 1999).

Following the hepatocyte growth factor (HGF) binding to Met or upon Met constitutive activation, neoplastic cells become invasive and start to form metastases (Jeffers et al. 1996; Meiners et al. 1998). Physical association between $\alpha_6\beta_4$ integrin and Met tyrosine kinase has been shown. Upon Met activation, β_4 is tyrosine phosphorylated and combines with Shc and PI3 K. This binding activity of $\alpha_6\beta_4$ is independent of the integrin adhesive role and resides in the β_4 cytoplasmic domain. In β_4-deficient cells or, if Shc recruitment is prohibited, Met is unable to activate the signaling pathways above the threshold level required for induction of invasive growth and metastasis (Trusolino et al. 2001).

While overexpression of $\alpha_6\beta_4$ increased the invasive potential of tumor cells in the skin, overexpression of $\alpha_3\beta_1$ has the opposite effect. Integrins $\alpha_3\beta_1$ and $\alpha_2\beta_1$ have been implicated in the invasive growth of squamous cell carcinomas because of their altered expression in tumor cells (Stamp and Pignatelli 1991). Ectopic expression of $\alpha_3\beta_1$ integrin in the suprabasal epidermal layers results in a lower frequency of conversion of experimentally induced papillomas to malignant squamous cell carcinomas compared to $\alpha_2\beta_1$ transgenic or wild-type mice. In addition, $\alpha_3\beta_1$ transgenic papillomas displayed a diminished proliferative capacity and higher grade of differentiation (Owens and Watt 2001).

The influence of β_1 integrin on metastasis and tissue invasion has been investigated by tail vein injection of Ras-Myc transformed fibroblast β_1-null and β_1-expressing cell lines. Fibroblasts expressing β_1 integrins formed bigger lung metastases and additional small metastases in the liver (Brakebusch et al. 1999). ESb murine T lymphoma cells invade muscle tissues and meninges after the loss of β_1 integrin (Stroeken et al. 1998), suggesting that β_1 integrin expression has an influence on the localization of forming metastases.

Epithelial cells that are not attached to matrix undergo apoptosis (Ruoslahti and Reed 1994). An additional cell survival signal, which is independent of cell adhesion by other integrins, has been described for β_1 and β_3 integrins. Tumor cells which express β_1 or β_3 integrins undergo apoptosis when the integrins are not bound to an extracellular ligand. Apoptosis is induced independent of cell adhesion and is achieved by activation of caspase 8 by the cytoplasmic tails of β_1 and β_3 integrin (Stupack et al. 2001).

Integrins are also involved in immune defense against tumor cells. Peripheral mononuclear cells (PMN), which attack tumor cells, require $\alpha_M\beta_2$ for the FcR-mediated cytotoxicity. PMNs deficient for $\alpha_L\beta_2$ integrins exhibit defective spreading on Ab-coated targets, impaired formation of immunologic synapses, and absent antibody-dependent cellular cytotoxicity, which is important for tumor cytolysis (van Spriel et al. 2001). Mice deficient for $\alpha_L\beta_2$ integrin normal cytotoxic T cell responses against systemic infections. However, they do not reject immunogenic tumors grafted into footpads and do not demonstrate priming response against tumor-specific antigen. Thus, $\alpha_L\beta_2$ deficiency causes a selective defect in induction of peripheral immune responses whereas responses to systemic infection are normal (Schmits et al. 1996).

13
Summary and Perspective

Gene targeting techniques have become a valuable tool to analyze protein function in vivo and to reevaluate data that have been produced in vitro. Almost all integrin subunits have been deleted up to date by conventional gene targeting techniques and analysis of these mice has confirmed many in vitro findings, and has also revealed new aspects of integrin function.

Conventional targeting techniques allow insights in integrin function in embryonic development and also help to establish cell lines which can be used to study in vivo observations at a molecular level in vitro. Redundancy between different integrin receptors can be investigated by the generation of double kockouts.

However, due to embryonic lethality, integrin function in specific embryonic and adult tissues or in aging, wound healing, tumor development, and degenerative processes cannot easily be addressed. Conditional gene targeting approaches have allowed researchers to investigate the function of embryonic-lethal integrins in adult tissues. Conditional targeted mice have thus far only been generated for β_1 integrin. However, the published data show the power of the approach by highlighting β_1 integrin function during skeletal development, brain and peripheral nerve development, hematopoiesis, heart function, and wound healing (Brakebusch et al. 2000, 2002; Potocnik et al. 2000; Raghavan et al. 2000; Graus-Porta et al. 2001; Feltri et al. 2002; Grose et al. 2002; Shai et al. 2002; Aszódi et al. 2003).

Drawbacks of conditional gene targeting lie in the availability of Cre expressing mouse strains. Onset of expression and specificity of Cre expression are dependent on the transgenic line and might not always correspond to the required and desired expression pattern. Cre expression in spermatids can result in chromosomal rearrangements, which are not restricted to the inserted loxP sites (Schmidt et al. 2000; Loonstra et al. 2001). Recombination frequencies depend on the achieved levels of Cre expression, and in addition, they differ from gene to gene. Cre mouse strains that result in a very high recombination frequency on one gene locus might prove less efficient on another one. Finally, cells that are still expressing the targeted protein might compensate for the protein loss in the targeted cells (Vooijs et al. 2001).

Gene targeting techniques are not only confined to the ablation of specific genes. The generation of knock-in mouse strains carrying distinct mutations enables the analysis of integrin signaling in vivo, which has so far been mainly restricted to cell culture experiments (Baudoin et al. 1998). Thus, the analysis of integrin function in specific processes will enhance our understanding of such central mechanisms as cell migration, proliferation, and differentiation but also of more complex processes such as tissue remodeling, thrombosis, tumor development, and inflammation.

Acknowledgements. We would like to thank Kathryn Rodgers for carefully reading the manuscript. RF is supported by the Max-Planck Society and the Fonds der Chemischen Industrie.

References

Adams JC, Watt FM (1991) Expression of β1, β3, β4, and β5 integrins by human epidermal keratinocytes and non-differentiating keratinocytes. J Cell Biol 115:829–841

Andre P, Prasad KS, Denis CV, He M, Papalia JM, Hynes RO, Phillips DR, Wagner DD (2002) CD40L stabilizes arterial thrombi by a β3 integrin-dependent mechanism. Nat Med 8:247–252

Annes JP, Rifkin DB, Munger JS (2002) The integrin $\alpha v \beta$6 binds and activates latent TGFβ3. FEBS Lett 511:65–68

Arnaout MA, Spits H, Terhorst C, Pitt J, Todd RF III (1984) Deficiency of a leukocyte surface glycoprotein (LFA-1) in two patients with Mo1 deficiency: effects of cell activation on Mo1/LFA-1 surface expression in normal and deficient leukocytes. J Clin Invest 74:1291–1300

Arroyo AG, Yang JT, Rayburn H, Hynes RO (1996) Differential requirements for α4 integrins during fetal and adult hematopoiesis. Cell 85:997–1008

Arroyo AG, Yang JT, Rayburn H, Hynes RO (1999) α4 integrins regulate the proliferation/differentiation balance of multilineage hematopoietic progenitors in vivo. Immunity 11:555–566

Arroyo AG, Taverna D, Whittaker CA, Strauch UG, Bader BL, Rayburn H, Crowley D, Parker CM, Hynes RO (2000) In vivo roles of integrins during leukocyte development and traffic: insights from the analysis of mice chimeric for α5, αv, and α4 integrins. J Immunol 165:4667–4675

Aszódi A, Hunzicker EB, Brackebusch C, Sakai T, Sakai K, Fässler R (2003) Crucial role of β1 integrins-type II collagen interactions in endochondral ossification. submitted

Aumailley M, Pesch M, Tunggal L, Gaill F, Fässler R (2000) Altered synthesis of laminin 1 and absence of basement membrane component deposition in β1 integrin-deficient embryoid bodies. J Cell Sci 113:259–268

Bachelder RE, Marchetti A, Falcioni R, Soddu S, Mercurio AM (1999) Activation of p53 function in carcinoma cells by the α6β4 integrin. J Biol Chem 274:20733–20737

Bader BL, Rayburn H, Crowley D, Hynes RO (1998) Extensive vasculogenesis, angiogenesis, and organogenesis precede lethality in mice lacking all αv integrins. Cell 95:507–519

Bao ZZ, Lakonishok M, Kaufman S, Horwitz AF (1993) $\alpha 7\beta 1$ integrin is a component of the myotendinous junction on skeletal muscle. J Cell Sci 106:579–589

Baudoin C, Goumans MJ, Mummery C, Sonnenberg A (1998) Knockout and knockin of the $\beta 1$ exon D define distinct roles for integrin splice variants in heart function and embryonic development. Genes Dev 12:1202–1216

Beatty PG, Ochs HD, Harlan JM, Price TH, Rosen H, Taylor RF, Hansen JA, Klebanoff SJ (1984) Absence of monoclonal-antibody-defined protein complex in a boy with abnormal leucocyte function. Lancet I:535–537

Belkin AM, Zhidkova NI, Balzac F, Altruda F, Tomatis D, Maier A, Tarone G, Koteliansky VE, Burridge K (1996) $\beta 1$D integrin displaces the $\beta 1$A isoform in striated muscles: localization at junctional structures and signaling potential in nonmuscle cells. J Cell Biol 132:211–226

Berlin C, Berg EL, Briskin MJ, Andrew DP, Kilshaw PJ, Holzmann B, Weissman IL, Hamann A, Butcher EC (1993) $\alpha 4\beta 7$ integrin mediates lymphocyte binding to the mucosal vascular addressin MAdCAM-1. Cell 74:185

Berlin-Rufenach C, Otto F, Mathies M, Westermann J, Owen MJ, Hamann A, Hogg N (1999) Lymphocyte migration in lymphocyte function-associated antigen (LFA)-1-deficient mice. J Exp Med 189:1467–1478

Bloch W, Forsberg E, Lentini S, Brakebusch C, Martin K, Krell HW, Weidle UH, Addicks K, Fässler R (1997) $\beta 1$ integrin is essential for teratoma growth and angiogenesis. J Cell Biol 139:265–278

Bouvard D, Brakebusch C, Gustafsson E, Aszódi A, Bengtsson T, Berna A, Fässler R (2001) Functional consequences of integrin gene mutations in mice. Circ Res 89:211–223

Bowden RA, Ding ZM, Donnachie EM, Petersen TK, Michael LH, Ballantyne CM, Burns AR (2000) Role of $\alpha 4$ integrin and VCAM-1 in CD18-independent neutrophil migration across mouse cardiac endothelium. Circ Res 90:562–569

Brakebusch C, Hirsch E, Potocnik A, Fässler R (1997) Genetic analysis of $\beta 1$ integrin function: confirmed, new and revised roles for a crucial family of cell adhesion molecules. J Cell Sci 110:2895–2904

Brakebusch C, Grose R, Quondamatteo F, Ramirez A, Jorcano JL, Pirro A, Svensson M, Herken R, Sasaki T, Timpl R, Werner S, Fässler R (2000) Skin and hair follicle integrity is crucially dependent on $\beta 1$ integrin expression on keratinocytes. Embo J 19:3990–4003

Brakebusch C, Fillatreau S, Potocnik A, Wilhelm P, Svensson M, Kearney P, Körner H, Gray D, Fässler R (2002) $\beta 1$ integrin is not essential for hematopoiesis, but for the T cell-dependent IgM antibody response. Immunity 16:465–477

Brandenberger R, Schmidt A, Linton J, Wang D, Backus C, Denda S, Müller U, Reichardt LF (2001) Identification and characterization of a novel extracellular matrix protein nephronectin that is associated with integrin $\alpha 8\beta 1$ in the embryonic kidney. J Cell Biol 154:447–458

Briskin M, Winsor-Hines D, Shyjan A, Cochran N, Bloom S, Wilson J, McEvoy LM, Butcher EC, Kassam N, Mackay CR, Newman W, Ringler DJ (1997) Human mucosal addressin cell adhesion molecule-1 is preferentially expressed in intestinal tract and associated lymphoid tissue. Am J Pathol 151:97

Brooks PC, Montgomery AM, Rosenfeld M, Reisfeld RA, Hu T, Klier G, Cheresh DA (1994) Integrin $\alpha v\beta 3$ antagonists promote tumor regression by inducing apoptosis of angiogenic blood vessels. Cell 79:1157–1164

Brooks PC, Stromblad S, Klemke R, Visscher D, Sarkar FH, Cheresh DA (1995) Antiintegrin $\alpha v\beta 3$ blocks human breast cancer growth and angiogenesis in human skin. J Clin Invest 96:1815–1822

Burkin DJ, Wallace GQ, Nicol KJ, Kaufman DJ, Kaufman SJ (2001) Enhanced expression of the $\alpha7\beta1$ integrin reduces muscular dystrophy and restores viability in dystrophic mice. J Cell Biol 152:1207–1218

Camacho SA, Heath WR, Carbone FR, Sarvetnick N, LeBon A, Karlsson L, Peterson PA, Webb SR (2001) A key role for ICAM-1 in generating effector cells mediating inflammatory responses. Nat Immunol 2:523–529

Camper L, Heinegard D, Lundgren-Akerlund E (1997) Integrin $\alpha2\beta1$ is a receptor for the cartilage matrix protein chondroadherin. J Cell Biol 138:1159–1167

Camper L, Hellman U, Lundgren-Akerlund E (1998) Isolation, cloning, and sequence analysis of the integrin subunit $\alpha10$, a $\beta1$-associated collagen binding integrin expressed on chondrocytes. J Biol Chem 273:20383–20389

Camper L, Holmvall K, Wangnerud C, Aszódi A, Lundgren-Akerlund E (2001) Distribution of the collagen-binding integrin $\alpha10\beta1$ during mouse development. Cell Tissue Res 306:107–116

Carmeliet P, Ferreira V, Breier G, Pollefeyt S, Kieckens L, Gertsenstein M, Fahrig M, Vandenhoeck A, Harpal K, Eberhardt C, Declercq C, Pawling J, Moons L, Collen D, Risau W, Nagy A (1996) Abnormal blood vessel development and lethality in embryos lacking a single VEGF allele. Nature 380:435–439

Cheresh DA, Stupack DG (2002) Integrin-mediated death: an explanation of the integrin-knockout phenotype? Nat Med 8:193–194

Collo G, Starr L, Quaranta V (1993) A new isoform of the laminin receptor integrin $\alpha7\beta1$ is developmentally regulated in skeletal muscle. J Biol Chem 268:19019–19024

Costell M, Gustafsson E, Aszódi A, Morgelin M, Bloch W, Hunziker E, Addicks K, Timpl R, Fässler R (1999) Perlecan maintains the integrity of cartilage and some basement membranes. J Cell Biol 147:1109–1122

Coucouvanis E, Martin GR (1995) Signals for death and survival: a two-step mechanism for cavitation in the vertebrate embryo. Cell 83:279–287

Coxon A, Rieu P, Barkalow FJ, Askari S, Sharpe AH, von Andrian UH, Arnaout MA, Mayadas TN (1996) A novel role for the $\beta2$ integrin CD11b/CD18 in neutrophil apoptosis: a homeostatic mechanism in inflammation. Immunity 5:653–666

Creamer D, Allen M, Sousa A, Poston R, Barker J (1995) Altered vascular endothelium integrin expression in psoriasis. Am J Pathol 147:1661–1667

Dans M, Gagnoux-Palacios L, Blaikie P, Klein S, Mariotti A, Giancotti FG (2001) Tyrosine phosphorylation of the $\beta4$ integrin cytoplasmic domain mediates Shc signaling to extracellular signal-regulated kinase and antagonizes formation of hemidesmosomes. J Biol Chem 276:1494–502

Dana N, Todd RF III, Pitt J, Springer TA, Arnaout MA (1984) Deficiency of a surface membrane glycoprotein (Mo1) in man. J Clin Invest 73:153–159

Davies D, Holley MC (2002) Differential expression of $\alpha3$ and $\alpha6$ integrins in the developing mouse inner ear. J Comp Neurol 445:122–132

De Arcangelis A, Mark M, Kreidberg J, Sorokin L, Georges-Labouesse E (1999) Synergistic activities of $\alpha3$ and $\alpha6$ integrins are required during apical ectodermal ridge formation and organogenesis in the mouse. Development 126:3957–3968

Dedhar S, Hannigan GE (1996) Integrin cytoplasmic interactions and bidirectional transmembrane signalling. Curr Opin Cell Biol 8:657–669

Denda S, Reichardt LF, Müller U (1998) Identification of osteopontin as a novel ligand for the integrin $\alpha8\beta1$ and potential roles for this integrin-ligand interaction in kidney morphogenesis. Mol Biol Cell 9:1425–1435

Denis C, Methia N, Frenette PS, Rayburn H, Ullman-Cullere M, Hynes RO, Wagner DD (1998) A mouse model of severe von Willebrand disease: defects in hemostasis and thrombosis. Proc Natl Acad Sci U S A 95:9524–9529

Ding ZM, Babensee JE, Simon SI, Lu H, Perrard JL, Bullard DC, Dai XY, Bromley SK, Dustin ML, Entman ML, Smith CW, Ballantyne CM (1999) Relative contribution of LFA-1 and Mac-1 to neutrophil adhesion and migration. J Immunol 163:5029–5038

DiPersio CM, Hodivala-Dilke KM, Jaenisch R, Kreidberg JA, Hynes RO (1997) $\alpha3\beta1$ Integrin is required for normal development of the epidermal basement membrane. J Cell Biol 137:729–742

DiPersio CM, van Der Neut R, Georges-Labouesse E, Kreidberg JA, Sonnenberg A, Hynes RO (2000) $\alpha3\beta1$and $\alpha6\beta4$ integrin receptors for laminin-5 are not essential for epidermal morphogenesis and homeostasis during skin development. J Cell Sci 113:3051–3062

Dong ZM, Gutierrez-Ramos JC, Coxon A, Mayadas TN, Wagner DD (1997) A new class of obesity genes encodes leukocyte adhesion receptors. Proc Natl Acad Sci U S A 94:7526–7530

Dowling J, Yu QC, Fuchs E (1996) $\beta4$ integrin is required for hemidesmosome formation, cell adhesion and cell survival. J Cell Biol 134:559–572

Dürr J, Goodman S, Potocnik A, von der Mark H, von der Mark K (1993) Localization of $\beta1$-integrins in human cartilage and their role in chondrocyte adhesion to collagen and fibronectin. Exp Cell Res 207:235–244

Dürr J, Lammi P, Goodman SL, Aigner T, von der Mark K (1996) Identification and immunolocalization of laminin in cartilage. Exp Cell Res 222:225–233

Duplaa C, Couffinhal T, Dufourcq P, Llanas B, Moreau C, Bonnet J (1997) The integrin very late antigen-4 is expressed in human smooth muscle cell. Involvement of $\alpha4$ and vascular cell adhesion molecule-1 during smooth muscle cell differentiation. Circ Res 80:159–169

el Gabalawy H, Wilkins J (1993) $\beta1$ (CD29) integrin expression in rheumatoid synovial membranes: an immunohistologic study of distribution patterns. J Rheumatol 20:231–237

Eliceiri BP, Cheresh DA (2001) Adhesion events in angiogenesis. Curr Opin Cell Biol 13:563–568

Eliceiri BP, Puente XS, Hood JD, Stupack DG, Schlaepfer DD, Huang XZ, Sheppard D, Cheresh DA (2002) Src-mediated coupling of focal adhesion kinase to integrin $\alpha(v)\beta5$ in vascular endothelial growth factor signaling. J Cell Biol 157:149–160

Elliott BE, Ekblom P, Pross H, Niemann A, Rubin K (1994) Anti-$\beta1$ integrin IgG inhibits pulmonary macrometastasis and the size of micrometastases from a murine mammary carcinoma. Cell Adhes Commun 1:319–332

Faraldo MM, Deugnier MA, Lukashev M, Thiery JP, Glukhova MA (1998) Perturbation of $\beta1$-integrin function alters the development of murine mammary gland. Embo J 17:2139–2147

Faraldo MM, Deugnier MA, Thiery JP, Glukhova MA (2000) Development of mammary gland requires normal $\beta1$-integrin function. Adv Exp Med Biol 480:169–174

Faraldo MM, Deugnier MA, Thiery JP, Glukhova MA (2001) Growth defects induced by perturbation of $\beta1$-integrin function in the mammary gland epithelium result from a lack of MAPK activation via the Shc and Akt pathways. EMBO Rep 2:431–437

Fässler R, Meyer M (1995) Consequences of lack of $\beta1$ integrin gene expression in mice. Genes Dev 9:1896–1908

Fässler R, Rohwedel J, Maltsev V, Addicks K, Hescheler J, Wobus AM (1996) Loss of $\beta1$ integrin function results in abnormal specification of cardiac cells during mouse ES cell-derived cardiogenesis. J Cell Sci 109:2989–2999

Feltri ML, Graus Porta D, Previtali SC, Nodari A, Migliavacca B, Cassetti A, Littlewood-Evans A, Reichardt LF, Messing A, Quattrini A, Müller U, Wrabetz L (2002) Conditional disruption of $\beta1$ integrin in Schwann cells impedes interactions with axons. J Cell Biol 156:199–209

Ferrara N, Carver-Moore K, Chen H, Dowd M, Lu L, O'Shea KS, Powell-Braxton L, Hillan KJ, Moore MW (1996) Heterozygous embryonic lethality induced by targeted inactivation of the VEGF gene. Nature 380:439–442

Fong GH, Rossant J, Gertsenstein M, Breitman ML (1995) Role of the Flt-1 receptor tyrosine kinase in regulating the assembly of vascular endothelium. Nature 376:66–70

Forsberg E, Hirsch E, Frohlich L, Meyer M, Ekblom P, Aszódi A, Werner S, Fässler R (1996) Skin wounds and severed nerves heal normally in mice lacking tenascin-C. Proc Natl Acad Sci U S A 93:6594–6599

Frei R, Dowling J, Carenini S, Fuchs E, Martini R (1999) Myelin formation by Schwann cells in the absence of $\beta4$ integrin. Glia 27:269–274

Friedlander M, Brooks PC, Shaffer RW, Kincaid CM, Varner JA, Cheresh DA (1995) Definition of two angiogenic pathways by distinct αv integrins. Science 270:1500–1502

Friedrich C, Cybulsky MI, Gutierrez-Ramos JC (1996) Vascular cell adhesion molecule-1 expression by hematopoiesis- supporting stromal cells is not essential for lymphoid or myeloid differentiation in vivo or in vitro. Eur J Immunol 26:2773–2780

Gardner H, Kreidberg J, Koteliansky V, Jaenisch R (1996) Deletion of integrin $\alpha1$ by homologous recombination permits normal murine development but gives rise to a specific deficit in cell adhesion. Dev Biol 175:301–313

Garnotel R, Rittie L, Poitevin S, Monboisse JC, Nguyen P, Potron G, Maquart FX, Randoux A, Gillery P (2000) Human blood monocytes interact with type I collagen through $\alpha x\beta2$ integrin (CD11c-CD18, gp150–95). J Immunol 164:5928–5934

George EL, Georges-Labouesse EN, Patel-King RS, Rayburn H, Hynes RO (1993) Defects in mesoderm, neural tube and vascular development in mouse embryos lacking fibronectin. Development 119:1079–1091

George EL, Baldwin HS, Hynes RO (1997) Fibronectins are essential for heart and blood vessel morphogenesis but are dispensable for initial specification of precursor cells. Blood 90:3073–3081

Georges-Labouesse E, Mark M, Messaddeq N, Gansmüller A (1998) Essential role of $\alpha6$ integrins in cortical and retinal lamination. Curr Biol 8:983–986

Georges-Labouesse E, Messaddeq N, Yehia G, Cadalbert L, Dierich A, Le Meur M (1996) Absence of integrin $\alpha6$ leads to epidermolysis bullosa and neonatal death in mice. Nat Genet 13:370–373

George-Weinstein M, Foster RF, Gerhart JV, Kaufman SJ (1993) In vitro and in vivo expression of $\alpha7$ integrin and desmin define the primary and secondary myogenic lineages. Dev Biol 156:209–229

Giancotti FG (2000) Complexity and specificity of integrin signalling. Nat Cell Biol 2:E13–14

Giancotti FG, Ruoslahti E (1999) Integrin signaling. Science 285:1028–1032

Gingras MC, Roussel E, Bruner JM, Branch CD, Moser RP (1995) Comparison of cell adhesion molecule expression between glioblastoma multiforme and autologous normal brain tissue. J Neuroimmunol 57:143–153

Goh KL, Yang JT, Hynes RO (1997) Mesodermal defects and cranial neural crest apoptosis in $\alpha5$ integrin-null embryos. Development 124:4309–4319

Grabbe S, Varga G, Beissert S, Steinert M, Pendl G, Seeliger S, Bloch W, Peters T, Schwarz T, Sunderkötter C, Scharffetter-Kochanek K (2002) $\beta2$ integrins are required for skin homing of primed T cells but not for priming naive T cells. J Clin Invest 109:183–192

Graus-Porta D, Blaess S, Senften M, Littlewood-Evans A, Damsky C, Huang Z, Orban P, Klein R, Schittny JC, Müller U (2001) $\beta1$-class integrins regulate the development of laminae and folia in the cerebral and cerebellar cortex. Neuron 31:367–379

Grose R, Hutter C, Bloch W, Watt FM, Fässler R, Brakebusch C, Werner S (2002) A crucial role of $\beta1$ integrin for keratinocyte migration in vitro and during cutaneous wound repair. Development 129:2303–2315

Gurtner GC, Davis V, Li H, McCoy MJ, Sharpe A, Cybulsky MI (1995) Targeted disruption of the murine VCAM1 gene: essential role of VCAM-1 in chorioallantoic fusion and placentation. Genes Dev 9:1–14

Gustafsson E, Fässler R (2000) Insights into extracellular matrix functions from mutant mouse models. Exp Cell Res 261:52–68

Gutheil JC, Campbell TN, Pierce PR, Watkins JD, Huse WD, Bodkin DJ, Cheresh DA (2000) Targeted antiangiogenic therapy for cancer using Vitaxin: a humanized monoclonal antibody to the integrin $\alpha v \beta 3$. Clin Cancer Res 6:3056–3061

Haack H, Hynes RO (2001) Integrin receptors are required for cell survival and proliferation during development of the peripheral glial lineage. Dev Biol 233:38–55

Hammes HP, Brownlee M, Jonczyk A, Sutter A, Preissner KT (1996) Subcutaneous injection of a cyclic peptide antagonist of vitronectin receptor-type integrins inhibits retinal neovascularization. Nat Med 2:529–533

Hartner A, Cordasic N, Klanke B, Müller U, Sterzel RB, Hilgers KF (2002) The $\alpha 8$ integrin chain affords mechanical stability to the glomerular capillary tuft in hypertensive glomerular disease. Am J Pathol 160:861–867

Hayashi YK, Chou FL, Engvall E, Ogawa M, Matsuda C, Hirabayashi S, Yokochi K, Ziober BL, Kramer RH, Kaufman SJ, Ozawa E, Goto Y, Nonaka I, Tsukahara T, Wang JZ, Hoffman EP, Arahata K (1998) Mutations in the integrin $\alpha 7$ gene cause congenital myopathy. Nat Genet 19:94–97

Hertle MD, Adams JC, Watt FM (1991) Integrin expression during human epidermal development in vivo and in vitro. Development 112:193–206

Hierck BP, Thorsteinsdottir S, Niessen CM, Freund E, Iperen LV, Feyen A, Hogervorst F, Poelmann RE, Mummery CL, Sonnenberg A (1993) Variants of the $\alpha 6 \beta 1$ laminin receptor in early murine development: distribution, molecular cloning and chromosomal localization of the mouse integrin $\alpha 6$ subunit. Cell Adhes Commun 1:33–53

Hirsch E, Iglesias A, Potocnik AJ, Hartmann U, Fässler R (1996) Impaired migration but not differentiation of haematopoietic stem cells in the absence of $\beta 1$ integrins. Nature 380:171–175

Hirsch E, Lohikangas L, Gullberg D, Johansson S, Fässler R (1998) Mouse myoblasts can fuse and form a normal sarcomere in the absence of $\beta 1$ integrin expression. J Cell Sci 111:2397–2409

Hirsch E, Barberis L, Brancaccio M, Azzolino O, Xu D, Kyriakis JM, Silengo L, Giancotti FG, Tarone G, Fassler R, Altruda F (2002) Defective Rac-mediated proliferation and survival after targeted mutation of the $\beta 1$ integrin cytodomain. J Cell Biol 157:481–492

Hodges BL, Hayashi YK, Nonaka I, Wang W, Arahata K, Kaufman SJ (1997) Altered expression of the $\alpha 7 \beta 1$ integrin in human and murine muscular dystrophies. J Cell Sci 110:2873–2881

Hodivala-Dilke KM, McHugh KP, Tsakiris DA, Rayburn H, Crowley D, Ullman-Cullere M, Ross FP, Coller BS, Teitelbaum S, Hynes RO (1999) $\beta 3$-integrin-deficient mice are a model for Glanzmann thrombasthenia showing placental defects and reduced survival. J Clin Invest 103:229–238

Holtkötter O, Nieswandt B, Smyth N, Müller W, Hafner M, Schulte V, Krieg T, Eckes B (2002) Integrin $\alpha 2$-deficient mice develop normally, are fertile, but display partially defective platelet interaction with collagen. J Biol Chem 277:10789–10794

Huang XZ, Wu JF, Cass D, Erle DJ, Corry D, Young SG, Farese RV Jr, Sheppard D (1996) Inactivation of the integrin $\beta 6$ subunit gene reveals a role of epithelial integrins in regulating inflammation in the lung and skin. J Cell Biol 133:921–928

Huang X, Griffiths M, Wu J, Farese RV Jr, Sheppard D (2000) Normal development, wound healing, and adenovirus susceptibility in $\beta 5$-deficient mice. Mol Cell Biol 20:755–759

Hynes RO (1992) Integrins: versatility, modulation, and signaling in cell adhesion. Cell 69:11–25

Jaspars LH, De Melker AA, Bonnet P, Sonnenberg A, Meijer CJ (1996) Distribution of laminin variants and their integrin receptors in human secondary lymphoid tissue. Colocalization suggests that the $\alpha 6 \beta 4$-integrin is a receptor for laminin-5 in lymphoid follicles. Cell Adhes Commun 4:269–279

Jeffers M, Rong S, Woude GF (1996) Hepatocyte growth factor/scatter factor-Met signaling in tumorigenicity and invasion/metastasis. J Mol Med 74:505–513

Jung U, Ley K (1999) Mice lacking two or all three selectins demonstrate overlapping and distinct functions for each selectin. J Immunol 162:6755–6762

Keller RS, Shai SY, Babbitt CJ, Pham CG, Solaro RJ, Valencik ML, Loftus JC, Ross RS (2001) Disruption of integrin function in the murine myocardium leads to perinatal lethality, fibrosis, and abnormal cardiac performance. Am J Pathol 158:1079–1090

Kennel SJ, Godfrey V, Ch'ang LY, Lankford TK, Foote LJ, Makkinje A (1992) The β4 subunit of the integrin family is displayed on a restricted subset of endothelium in mice. J Cell Sci 101:145–150

Koni PA, Joshi SK, Temann UA, Olson D, Burkly L, Flavell RA (2001) Conditional Vascular Cell Adhesion Molecule 1 Deletion in Mice. Impaired lymphocyte migration to bone marrow. J Exp Med 193:741–754

Kreidberg JA, Donovan MJ, Goldstein SL, Rennke H, Shepherd K, Jones RC, Jaenisch R (1996) α3β1 integrin has a crucial role in kidney and lung organogenesis. Development 122:3537–3547

Kunkel EJ, Dunne JL, Ley K (2000) Leukocyte arrest during cytokine-dependent inflammation in vivo. J Immunol 164:3301–3308

Kwee L, Baldwin HS, Shen HM, Stewart CL, Buck C, Buck CA, Labow MA (1995) Defective development of the embryonic and extraembryonic circulatory systems in vascular cell adhesion molecule (VCAM-1) deficient mice. Development 121:489–503

Lakonishok M, Muschler J, Horwitz AF (1992) The α5β1 integrin associates with a dystrophin-containing lattice during muscle development. Dev Biol 152:209–220

Law DA, DeGuzman FR, Heiser P, Ministri-Madrid K, Killeen N, Phillips DR (1999) Integrin cytoplasmic tyrosine motif is required for outside-in αIIbβ3 signalling and platelet function. Nature 401:808–811

Leuker CE, Labow M, Müller W, Wagner N (2001) Neonatally induced inactivation of the vascular cell adhesion molecule 1 gene impairs b cell localization and t cell-dependent humoral immune response. J Exp Med 193:755–768

Li S, Carbonetto S, Fässler R, Smyth N, Edgar D, Yurchenco PD (2002) Matrix assembly, regulation and survival functions of laminin and its receptors in embryonic stem cell differentiation. J Cell Biol 157:1279–1290

Liaw L, Birk DE, Ballas CB, Whitsitt JS, Davidson JM, Hogan BL (1998) Altered wound healing in mice lacking a functional osteopontin gene (spp1). J Clin Invest 101:1468–1478

Littlewood-Evans A, Müller U (2000) Stereocilia defects in the sensory hair cells of the inner ear in mice deficient in integrin α8β1. Nat Genet 24:424–428

Loeser RF (1997) Growth factor regulation of chondrocyte integrins. Differential effects of insulin-like growth factor 1 and transforming growth factor β on α1β1 integrin expression and chondrocyte adhesion to type VI collagen. Arthritis Rheum 40:270–276

Loeser RF, Carlson CS, McGee MP (1995) Expression of β1 integrins by cultured articular chondrocytes and in osteoarthritic cartilage. Exp Cell Res 217:248–257

Loonstra A, Vooijs M, Berna Beverloo H, Al Allak B, van Drunen E, Kanaar R, Berns A, Jonkers J (2001) Growth inhibition and DNA damage induced by Cre recombinase in mammalian cells PNAS 98:9209–9214

Lu H, Smith CW, Perrard J, Bullard D, Tang L, Shappell SB, Entman ML, Beaudet AL, Ballantyne CM (1997) LFA-1 is sufficient in mediating neutrophil emigration in Mac-1- deficient mice. J Clin Invest 99:1340–1350

Mainiero F, Pepe A, Wary KK, Spinardi L, Mohammadi M, Schlessinger J, Giancotti FG (1995) Signal transduction by the α6β4 integrin: distinct β4 subunit sites mediate recruitment of Shc/Grb2 and association with the cytoskeleton of hemidesmosomes. EMBO J 14:4470–4481

Mainiero F, Murgia C, Wary KK, Curatola AM, Pepe A, Blumemberg M, Westwick JK, Der CJ, Giancotti FG (1997) The coupling of $\alpha 6\beta 4$ integrin to Ras-MAP kinase pathways mediated by Shc controls keratinocyte proliferation. EMBO J 16:2365–2375

Makihira S, Yan W, Ohno S, Kawamoto T, Fujimoto K, Okimura A, Yoshida E, Noshiro M, Hamada T, Kato Y (1999) Enhancement of cell adhesion and spreading by a cartilage-specific noncollagenous protein, cartilage matrix protein (CMP/Matrilin-1), via integrin $\alpha 1\beta 1$. J Biol Chem 274:11417–11423

Martin PT, Kaufman SJ, Kramer RH, Sanes JR (1996) Synaptic integrins in developing, adult, and mutant muscle: selective association of $\alpha 1$, $\alpha 7A$, and $\alpha 7B$ integrins with the neuromuscular junction. Dev Biol 174:125–139

Mayer U, Saher G, Fässler R, Bornemann A, Echtermeyer F, von der Mark H, Miosge N, Pöschl E, von der Mark K (1997) Absence of integrin $\alpha 7$ causes a novel form of muscular dystrophy. Nat Genet 17:318–323

McEver RP, Baenziger NL, Majerus PW (1980) Isolation and quantitation of the platelet membrane glycoprotein deficient in thrombasthenia using a monoclonal hybridoma antibody. J Clin Invest 66:1311–1318

McHugh KP, Hodivala-Dilke K, Zheng MH, Namba N, Lam J, Novack D, Feng X, Ross FP, Hynes RO, Teitelbaum SL (2000) Mice lacking $\beta 3$ integrins are osteosclerotic because of dysfunctional osteoclasts. J Clin Invest 105:433–440

Meiners S, Brinkmann V, Naundorf H, Birchmeier W (1998) Role of morphogenetic factors in metastasis of mammary carcinoma cells. Oncogene 16:9–20

Menko AS, Kreidberg JA, Ryan TT, Van Bockstaele E, Kukuruzinska MA (2001) Loss of $\alpha 3\beta 1$ integrin function results in an altered differentiation program in the mouse submandibular gland. Dev Dyn 220:337–349

Miner JH, Li C (2000) Defective glomerulogenesis in the absence of laminin $\alpha 5$ demonstrates a developmental role for the kidney glomerular basement membrane. Dev Biol 217:278–289

Miner JH, Cunningham J, Sanes JR (1998) Roles for laminin in embryogenesis: exencephaly, syndactyly, and placentopathy in mice lacking the laminin $\alpha 5$ chain. J Cell Biol 143:1713–1723

Miosge N, Klenczar C, Herken R, Willem M, Mayer U (1999) Organization of the myotendinous junction is dependent on the presence of $\alpha 7\beta 1$ integrin. Lab Invest 79:1591–1599

Mizgerd JP, Kubo H, Kutkoski GJ, Bhagwan SD, Scharffetter-Kochanek K, Beaudet AL, Doerschuk CM (1997) Neutrophil emigration in the skin, lungs, and peritoneum: different requirements for CD11/CD18 revealed by CD18-deficient mice. J Exp Med 186:1357–1364

Mu D, Cambier S, Fjellbirkeland L, Baron JL, Munger JS, Kawakatsu H, Sheppard D, Broaddus VC, Nishimura SL (2002) The integrin $\alpha v\beta 8$ mediates epithelial homeostasis through MT1-MMP-dependent activation of TGF-$\beta 1$. J Cell Biol 157:493–507

Müller U, Wang D, Denda S, Meneses JJ, Pedersen RA, Reichardt LF (1997) Integrin $\alpha 8\beta 1$ is critically important for epithelial-mesenchymal interactions during kidney morphogenesis. Cell 88:603–613

Munger JS, Harpel JG, Giancotti FG, Rifkin DB (1998) Interactions between growth factors and integrins: latent forms of transforming growth factor-β are ligands for the integrin $\alpha v\beta 1$. Mol Biol Cell 9:2627–2638

Munger JS, Huang X, Kawakatsu H, Griffiths MJ, Dalton SL, Wu J, Pittet JF, Kaminski N, Garat C, Matthay MA, Rifkin DB, Sheppard D (1999) The integrin $\alpha v\beta 6$ binds and activates latent TGF$\beta 1$: a mechanism for regulating pulmonary inflammation and fibrosis. Cell 96:319–328

Murgia C, Blaikie P, Kim N, Dans M, Petrie HT, Giancotti FG (1998) Cell cycle and adhesion defects in mice carrying a targeted deletion of the integrin $\beta 4$ cytoplasmic domain. Embo J 17:3940–3951

Murray P, Edgar D (2001) Regulation of the differentiation and behaviour of extra-embryonic endodermal cells by basement membranes. J Cell Sci 114:931–939

Nieswandt B, Brakebusch C, Bergmeier W, Schulte V, Bouvard D, Mokhtari-Nejad R, Lindhout T, Heemskerk JW, Zirngibl H, Fässler R (2001) Glycoprotein VI but not $\alpha2\beta1$ integrin is essential for platelet interaction with collagen. EMBO J 20:2120–2130

Owens DM, Watt FM (2001) Influence of $\beta1$ integrins on epidermal squamous cell carcinoma formation in a transgenic mouse model: $\alpha3\beta1$, but not $\alpha2\beta1$, suppresses malignant conversion. Cancer Res 61:5248–5254

Pabst O, Förster R, Lipp M, Engel H, Arnold HH (2000) NKX2.3 is required for MAd-CAM-1 expression and homing of lymphocytes in spleen and mucosa-associated lymphoid tissue. Embo J 19:2015–2023

Plow EF, Haas TA, Zhang L, Loftus J, Smith JW (2000) Ligand binding to integrins. J Biol Chem 275:21785–21788

Potocnik AJ, Brakebusch C, Fässler R (2000) Fetal and adult hematopoietic stem cells require $\beta1$ integrin function for colonizing fetal liver, spleen, and bone marrow. Immunity 12:653–663

Pozzi A, Wary KK, Giancotti FG, Gardner HA (1998) Integrin $\alpha1\beta1$ mediates a unique collagen-dependent proliferation pathway in vivo. J Cell Biol 142:587–594

Pozzi A, Moberg PE, Miles LA, Wagner S, Soloway P, Gardner HA (2000) Elevated matrix metalloprotease and angiostatin levels in integrin $\alpha1$ knockout mice cause reduced tumor vascularization. Proc Natl Acad Sci U S A 97:2202–2207

Pulkkinen L, Uitto J (1999) Mutation analysis and molecular genetics of epidermolysis bullosa. Matrix Biol 18:29–42

Pulkkinen L, Kimonis VE, Xu Y, Spanou EN, McLean WH, Uitto J (1997) Homozygous $\alpha6$ integrin mutation in junctional epidermolysis bullosa with congenital duodenal atresia. Hum Mol Genet 6:669–674

Raghavan S, Bauer C, Mundschau G, Li Q, Fuchs E (2000) Conditional ablation of $\beta1$ integrin in skin. Severe defects in epidermal proliferation, basement membrane formation, and hair follicle invagination. J Cell Biol 150:1149–1160

Reynolds LE, Wyder L, Lively JC, Taverna D, Robinson SD, Huang X, Sheppard D, Hynes RO, Hodivala-Dilke KM (2002) Enhanced pathological angiogenesis in mice lacking $\beta3$ integrin or $\beta3$ and $\beta5$ integrins. Nat Med 8:27–34

Rittling SR, Matsumoto HN, McKee MD, Nanci A, An XR, Novick KE, Kowalski AJ, Noda M, Denhardt DT (1998) Mice lacking osteopontin show normal development and bone structure but display altered osteoclast formation in vitro. J Bone Miner Res 13:1101–1111

Rohwedel J, Guan K, Zuschratter W, Jin S, Ahnert-Hilger G, Fürst D, Fässler R, Wobus AM (1998) Loss of $\beta1$ integrin function results in a retardation of myogenic, but an acceleration of neuronal, differentiation of embryonic stem cells in vitro. Dev Biol 201:167–184

Rosen GD, Sanes JR, LaChance R, Cunningham JM, Roman J, Dean DC (1992) Roles for the integrin VLA-4 and its counter receptor VCAM-1 in myogenesis. Cell 69:1107–1119

Rosenkranz AR, Coxon A, Maurer M, Gurish MF, Austen KF, Friend DS, Galli SJ, Mayadas TN (1998) Impaired mast cell development and innate immunity in Mac-1 (CD11b/CD18, CR3)-deficient mice. J Immunol 161:6463–6467

Ruoslahti E, Reed JC (1994) Anchorage dependence, integrins, and apoptosis. Cell 77:477–478

Rupp PA, Little CD (2001) Integrins in vascular development. Circ Res 89:566–572

Ryan MC, Lee K, Miyashita Y, Carter WG (1999) Targeted disruption of the LAMA3 gene in mice reveals abnormalities in survival and late stage differentiation of epithelial cells. J Cell Biol 145:1309–1323

Saga Y, Yagi T, Ikawa Y, Sakakura T, Aizawa S (1992) Mice develop normally without te-
    nascin. Genes Dev 6:1821–1831
Salter DM, Godolphin JL, Gourlay MS (1995) Chondrocyte heterogeneity: immunohisto-
    logically defined variation of integrin expression at different sites in human fetal
    knees. J Histochem Cytochem 43:447–457
Scharffetter-Kochanek K, Lu H, Norman K, van Nood N, Munoz F, Grabbe S, McArthur
    M, Lorenzo I, Kaplan S, Ley K, Smith CW, Montgomery CA, Rich S, Beaudet AL
    (1998) Spontaneous skin ulceration and defective T cell function in CD18 null mice. J
    Exp Med 188:119–131
Schmidt EE, Taylor DS, Prigge JR, Barnett S, Capecchi MR (2000) Illegitimate Cre-depen-
    dent chromosome rearrangements in transgenic mouse spermatids. Proc Natl Acad
    Sci USA 97:13702–13707
Schmits R, Kundig TM, Baker DM, Shumaker G, Simard JJ, Duncan G, Wakeham A,
    Shahinian A, van der Heiden A, Bachmann MF, Ohashi PS, Mak TW, Hickstein DD
    (1996) LFA-1-deficient mice show normal CTL responses to virus but fail to reject
    immunogenic tumor. J Exp Med 183:1415–1426
Schneeberger EE, Vu Q, LeBlanc BW, Doerschuk CM (2000) The accumulation of dendrit-
    ic cells in the lung is impaired in CD18-/- but not in ICAM-1-/- mutant mice. J Im-
    munol 164:2472–2478
Schöber S, Mielenz D, Echtermeyer F, Hapke S, Pöschl E, von der Mark H, Moch H, von
    der Mark K (2000) The role of extracellular and cytoplasmic splice domains of α7-
    integrin in cell adhesion and migration on laminins. Exp Cell Res 255:303–313
Schön MP, Arya A, Murphy EA, Adams CM, Strauch UG, Agace WW, Marsal J, Donohue
    JP, Her H, Beier DR, Olson S, Lefrancois L, Brenner MB, Grusby MJ, Parker CM
    (1999) Mucosal T lymphocyte numbers are selectively reduced in integrin αE
    (CD103)-deficient mice. J Immunol 162:6641–6649
Schwartz MA, Schaller MD, Ginsberg MH (1995) Integrins: emerging paradigms of signal
    transduction. Annu Rev Cell Dev Biol 11:549–599
Shai SY, Harpf AE, Babbitt CJ, Jordan MC, Fishbein MC, Chen J, Omura M, Leil TA,
    Becker KD, Jiang M, Smith DJ, Cherry SR, Loftus JC, Ross RS (2002) Cardiac myo-
    cyte-specific excision of the β1 integrin gene results in myocardial fibrosis and cardi-
    ac failure. Circ Res 90:458–464
Shattil SJ, Kashiwagi H, Pampori N (1998) Integrin signaling: the platelet paradigm.
    Blood 91:2645–2657
Shaw LM, Rabinovitz I, Wang HH, Toker A, Mercurio AM (1997) Activation of phospho-
    inositide 3-OH kinase by the α6β4 integrin promotes carcinoma invasion. Cell
    91:949–960
Shier P, Otulakowski G, Ngo K, Panakos J, Chourmouzis E, Christjansen L, Lau CY, Fung-
    Leung WP (1996) Impaired immune responses toward alloantigens and tumor cells
    but normal thymic selection in mice deficient in the β2 integrin leukocyte function-
    associated antigen-1. J Immunol 157:5375–5386
Shier P, Ngo K, Fung-Leung WP (1999) Defective CD8+ T cell activation and cytolytic
    function in the absence of LFA-1 cannot be restored by increased TCR signaling. J
    Immunol 163:4826–4832
Song WK, Wang W, Sato H, Bielser DA, Kaufman SJ (1993) Expression of α7 integrin cy-
    toplasmic domains during skeletal muscle development: alternate forms, conforma-
    tional change, and homologies with serine/threonine kinases and tyrosine phospha-
    tases. J Cell Sci 106:1139–1152
Stamp GWH and Pignatelli M (1991) Distribution of β1, α1, α2, and α3 integrin chains in
    basal cell carcinomas. J Pathol 163:307–313
Steeber DA, Tang ML, Zhang XQ, Müller W, Wagner N, Tedder TF (1998) Efficient lym-
    phocyte migration across high endothelial venules of mouse Peyer's patches requires
    overlapping expression of L-selectin and β7 integrin. J Immunol 161:6638–6647

Stephens LE, Sutherland AE, Klimanskaya IV, Andrieux A, Meneses J, Pedersen RA, Damsky CH (1995) Deletion of β1 integrins in mice results in inner cell mass failure and peri-implantation lethality. Genes Dev 9:1883–1895

Stroeken PJ, van Rijthoven EA, van der Valk MA, Roos E (1998) Targeted disruption of the β1 integrin gene in a lymphoma cell line greatly reduces metastatic capacity. Cancer Res 58:1569–1577

Stupack DG, Puente XS, Boutsaboualoy S, Storgard CM, Cheresh DA (2001) Apoptosis of adherent cells by recruitment of caspase-8 to unligated integrins. J Cell Biol 155:459–70

Suh TT, Holmback K, Jensen NJ, Daugherty CC, Small K, Simon DI, Potter S, Degen JL (1995) Resolution of spontaneous bleeding events but failure of pregnancy in fibrinogen-deficient mice. Genes Dev 9:2020–2033

Sutherland AE, Calarco PG, Damsky CH (1993) Developmental regulation of integrin expression at the time of implantation in the mouse embryo. Development 119:1175–1186

Tang T, Rosenkranz A, Assmann KJ, Goodman MJ, Gutierrez-Ramos JC, Carroll MC, Cotran RS, Mayadas TN (1997) A role for Mac-1 (CDIIb/CD18) in immune complex-stimulated neutrophil function in vivo: Mac-1 deficiency abrogates sustained Fcg receptor- dependent neutrophil adhesion and complement-dependent proteinuria in acute glomerulonephritis. J Exp Med 186:1853–1863

Tarone G, Russo MA, Hirsch E, Odorisio T, Altruda F, Silengo L, Siracusa G (1993) Expression of β1 integrin complexes on the surface of unfertilized mouse oocyte. Development 117:1369–1375

Taverna D, Disatnik MH, Rayburn H, Bronson RT, Yang J, Rando TA, Hynes RO (1998) Dystrophic muscle in mice chimeric for expression of α5 integrin. J Cell Biol 143:849–859

Tronik-Le Roux D, Roullot V, Poujol C, Kortulewski T, Nurden P, Marguerie G (2000) Thrombasthenic mice generated by replacement of the integrin α(IIb) gene: demonstration that transcriptional activation of this megakaryocytic locus precedes lineage commitment. Blood 96:1399–1408

Trusolino L, Bertotti A, Comoglio PM (2001) A signaling adapter function for $\alpha6\beta4$ integrin in the control of HGF-dependent invasive growth. Cell 30;107:643–654

Valencik ML, McDonald JA (2001) Cardiac expression of a gain-of-function α(5)-integrin results in perinatal lethality. Am J Physiol Heart Circ Physiol 280:H361–367

van der Neut R, Krimpenfort P, Calafat J, Niessen CM, Sonnenberg A (1996) Epithelial detachment due to absence of hemidesmosomes in integrin β4 null mice. Nat Genet 13:366–369

van der Vieren M, Crowe DT, Hoekstra D, Vazeux R, Hoffman PA, Grayson MH, Bochner BS, Gallatin WM, Staunton DE (1999) The leukocyte integrin αDβ2 binds VCAM-1: evidence for a binding interface between I domain and VCAM-1. J Immunol 163:1984–1990

van Spriel AB, Leusen JH, van Egmond M, Dijkman HB, Assmann KJ, Mayadas TN, van de Winkel JG (2001) Mac-1 (CD11b/CD18) is essential for Fc receptor-mediated neutrophil cytotoxicity and immunologic synapse formation. Blood 97:2478–2486

Vidal F, Aberdam D, Miquel C, Christiano AM, Pulkkinen L, Uitto J, Ortonne JP, Meneguzzi G (1995) Integrin β4 mutations associated with junctional epidermolysis bullosa with pyloric atresia. Nat Genet 10:229–234

von der Mark H, Durr J, Sonnenberg A, von der Mark K, Deutzmann R, Goodman SL (1991) Skeletal myoblasts utilize a novel β1-series integrin and not $\alpha6\beta1$ for binding to the E8 and T8 fragments of laminin. J Biol Chem 266:23593–23601

Vooijs M, Jonkers J, Berns A (2001) A highly efficient ligand-regulated Cre recombinase mouse line shows that LoxP recombination is position dependent. EMBO Reports 2:292–297

Wagner N, Löhler J, Kunkel EJ, Ley K, Leung E, Krissansen G, Rajewsky K, Müller W (1996) Critical role for β7 integrins in formation of the gut-associated lymphoid tissue. Nature 382:366–370

Wagner N, Löhler J, Tedder TF, Rajewsky K, Müller W, Steeber DA (1998) L-selectin and β7 integrin synergistically mediate lymphocyte migration to mesenteric lymph nodes. Eur J Immunol 28:3832–3839

Werner A, Willem M, Jones LL, Kreutzberg GW, Mayer U, Raivich G (2000) Impaired axonal regeneration in α7 integrin-deficient mice. J Neurosci 20:1822–1830

Yang JT, Rayburn H, Hynes RO (1993) Embryonic mesodermal defects in α5 integrin-deficient mice. Development 119:1093–1105

Yang JT, Rayburn H, Hynes RO (1995) Cell adhesion events mediated by α4 integrins are essential in placental and cardiac development. Development 121:549–560

Yang JT, Bader BL, Kreidberg JA, Ullman-Cullere M, Trevithick JE, Hynes RO (1999) Overlapping and independent functions of fibronectin receptor integrins in early mesodermal development. Dev Biol 215:264–277

Yao CC, Ziober BL, Sutherland AE, Mendrick DL, Kramer RH (1996) Laminins promote the locomotion of skeletal myoblasts via the α7 integrin receptor. J Cell Sci 109:3139–3150

Yao CC, Breuss J, Pytela R, Kramer RH (1997) Functional expression of the α7 integrin receptor in differentiated smooth muscle cells. J Cell Sci 110:1477–1487

Zheng X, Saunders TL, Camper SA, Samuelson LC, Ginsburg D (1995) Vitronectin is not essential for normal mammalian development and fertility. Proc Natl Acad Sci U S A 92:12426–12430

Zhu AJ, Haase I, Watt FM (1999) Signaling via β1 integrins and mitogen-activated protein kinase determines human epidermal stem cell fate in vitro. Proc Natl Acad Sci USA 96:6728–6733

Zhu J, Motejlek K, Wang D, Zang K, Schmidt A, Reichardt LF (2002) beta8 integrins are required for vascular morphogenesis in mouse embryos. Development 12:2891–2903

Zimmerman D, Jin F, Leboy P, Hardy S, Damsky C (2000) Impaired bone formation in transgenic mice resulting from altered integrin function in osteoblasts. Dev Biol 220:2–15

Ziober BL, Vu MP, Waleh N, Crawford J, Lin CS, Kramer RH (1993) Alternative extracellular and cytoplasmic domains of the integrin α7 subunit are differentially expressed during development. J Biol Chem 268:26773–26783

Part 3
Nervous System

Transgenic Mouse Models in the Analysis of Neurotransmitter Release Mechanisms

N. Brose[1] · J. Rettig[2]

[1] Abteilung Molekulare Neurobiologie, Max-Planck-Institut für Experimentelle Medizin, Herrmann-Rein-Straße 3, 37075 Göttingen, Germany
e-mail: brose@em.mpg.de
[2] Physiologisches Institut, Universität des Saarlandes, Gebäude 59, 66424 Homburg, Germany
e-mail: jrettig@uniklinik-saarland.de

Abstract The release of neurotransmitter molecules from synaptic vesicles is of outmost importance for the communication between cells in the nervous system. Before their fusion with the plasma membrane, vesicles undergo a multistep process which is tightly regulated by a large number of proteins. After fusion, a similarly complex protein machinery is involved in the recycling of the vesicle membrane. In addition, many proteins modulate the amount of neurotransmitter being released, accounting at least in part for the tremendous plasticity of human brain function. Here we review the current knowledge that has been gained by the targeted disruption of genes encoding presynaptic proteins in mice. In the first chapters, we discuss those proteins which have been assigned to a specific step in the synaptic vesicle cycle. In particular, we cover proteins involved in transmitter and ion transport into synaptic vesicles, in synaptic vesicle docking and priming, in Ca^{2+} signaling and sensing, and in the fusion process itself. Next, we discuss proteins which are not required for neurotransmitter release, but which modulate its extent and thus most likely play a role in synaptic plasticity. Finally, we review what is known about pharmacological tools which interfere with neurotransmitter release. It can be expected that the use of transgenic mouse models will continue to increase over the coming years and that this strategy will help to finally unravel the secrets of neurotransmitter release.

Keywords Neurotransmitter release · Secretion · Synaptic transmission · Exocytosis · Endocytosis · Docking · Priming · Fusion · Synaptic plasticity

1
Introduction

The complexity of our central nervous system is what distinguishes humans from other animals on our planet. In this context, the distinguishing factor is not simply the sheer size of the brain (dolphins, for example, have a larger brain than humans) or the number of nerve cells present. Rather, differences in the wiring patterns between nerve cells that form functional networks as well as subtle differences in the function and regulation of genes and/or proteins involved in central nervous system processes appear to account for the striking computing power of the human brain in comparison to other nervous systems.

The connecting part between two nerve cells is called a synapse, and each of the 100 billion nerve cells in our brain forms on average about 1,000 synapses with other nerve cells. The interplay of neurons within this gigantic network, i.e., the temporal and spatial organization of the signals they communicate, leads ultimately to behavior and higher brain functions like self-awareness or language. It is evident that such a complex system is prone to various levels of dysfunction, expressed in severe disorders like epilepsy, depression, schizophrenia, Parkinson's disease, or Alzheimer's disease. Thus, in order to understand human brain function and the accompanying disorders, one first has to understand the basic mechanisms underlying communication between nerve cells. This communication process occurs at the synapse and is called synaptic transmission. The sending (presynaptic) nerve cell releases neurotransmitter into the synaptic cleft through Ca^{2+}-dependent fusion of synaptic vesicles with the presynaptic membrane, and the receiving cell transduces this chemical signal back into an electrical one through opening of neurotransmitter-gated ion channels on the postsynaptic membrane. It is widely accepted that modulation of synaptic strength in either positive or negative direction forms the molecular basis of the plasticity of the human brain, which underlies learning and memory processes as well as multiple pathophysiological alterations of brain function.

Plastic modulation of synaptic transmission is achieved in vivo through a multitude of pre- and postsynaptic processes. With a special focus on mutant mouse models used as research tools, we summarize here the remarkable progress that has been made over the past few years in understanding the composition of the molecular machinery that mediates and modifies neurotransmitter release from the presynaptic cell. Some of the proteins discussed in this context are possible targets for pharmacological interventions aiming at the therapeutic interference with the transmitter release process in neurological and psychiatric diseases.

2
The Synaptic Vesicle Cycle

As mentioned above, synaptic transmission starts with the fusion of a synaptic vesicle with the presynaptic plasma membrane. The release of the neurotransmitter from the interior of the synaptic vesicle is initiated by the opening of presynaptic Ca^{2+} channels which are gated by the action potential-induced depolarization. These channels are not distributed evenly over the entire presynapse, but are highly localized to a small membrane area called active zone (Heuser and Reese 1973; Heuser et al. 1974). The active zone can be visualized by electron microscopy as a dense thickening of the presynaptic membrane that is caused by the enrichment of electron-dense, proteinaceous material. Just like the opposing postsynaptic density, the active zone represents a specialized area, since it is the only area of the presynaptic membrane where fusion of synaptic vesicles occurs. Consequently, the active zone has to contain a large variety of proteins which mediate and maintain the exocytotic process. Indeed, research over the last decade has identified many proteins which are localized to the active zone. Some of these are expressed exclusively in that area, and those molecules are thought to fulfill specific functions related to Ca^{2+} dependent fusion of synaptic vesicles (Garner et al. 2002; see below).

The presynaptic terminal represents the endpoint of a nerve cell axon, and as such can be centimeters away from the cell soma where new proteins are synthesized. Therefore, the availability of presynaptic proteins mediating fusion would soon become a rate-limiting problem if the proteins involved would be used only for a single round of fusion. The cell circumvents this potential problem by recycling the synaptic vesicle membrane with its protein components through Clathrin-mediated endocytosis (Brodin et al. 2000; see Fig. 1). The retrieval of fused vesicle membrane occurs about a micrometer away from the edge of an active zone. It starts with the binding of the tetrameric adaptor protein (AP)-2 to this membrane area (Schmid 1997), probably aided by the interaction of AP-2 with the synaptic vesicle membrane protein synaptotagmin (Haucke and De Camilli 1999), phosphoinositides and phospholipase D. AP-2 attaches the clathrin coat consisting of hexagons and pentagons of clathrin and the monomeric adaptor protein AP-180 to the plasma membrane. Accessory proteins like endophilin are then required to generate invaginated coated pits (Ringstad et al. 1999; Schmidt et al. 1999), before the neck region narrows and the vesicle pinches off—a process called fission—with the help of other accessory proteins like dynamin and amphiphysin (Schmid et al. 1998; Takei et al. 1999). After the endocytic vesicle has left the plasma membrane, it is rapidly

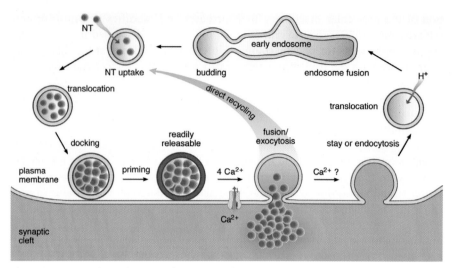

Fig. 1 Synaptic vesicles undergo a cyclic process in the presynaptic terminal. After refilling with neurotransmitter and acidification, they translocate to the active zone of the plasma membrane where they are anchored through a process called docking. Docked vesicles are then rendered fusion-competent by a process called priming. Elevation of intraterminal $[Ca^{2+}]$ through opening of voltage-gated calcium channels leads to fusion of synaptic vesicles with the plasma membrane and the release of neurotransmitter into the synaptic cleft. The vesicle membrane is then retrieved through clathrin-mediated endocytosis, and the majority fuses with endosomal compartments in the presynapse. Alternatively, empty vesicles can be directly refilled with neurotransmitter without passing through endosomes. Note that the third endocytotic pathway mentioned in the text, the "kiss-and-stay-mechanism," has been omitted in this figure for clarity

uncoated by the uncoating ATPase Hsc70 and auxilin (Ungewickell 1999). Most likely, synaptojanin, a polyphosphoinositide phosphatase, is also involved in this process (Cremona et al. 1999).

The majority of uncoated vesicles then passes through a second process of fusion and budding with the endosomal membrane, aided by the synaptic vesicle proteins Rab5 and Vti1 (Fischer von Mollard et al. 1994; Antonin et al. 2000). An alternative endocytic pathway is the direct return to the release site as a fully functional synaptic vesicle (Cremona and De Camilli 1997; Gad et al. 1998; Murthy and Stevens 1998; see Fig. 1). Recently, a third alternative has been postulated in which a small population of synaptic vesicles do not fuse entirely with the plasma membrane and thus do not undergo clathrin-mediated endocytosis, but remain after their partial emptying at the release site and can immediately repeat their partial fusion (Pyle et al. 2000; Stevens and Williams 2000). This attractive hypothesis has been termed "reuse mechanism" (Pyle et al. 2000) or, reminiscent of the hotly debated kiss-and-run mechanism, the "kiss-and-stay mechanism" (Südhof 2000). The overall physiological picture emerging from these different vesicle cycles is that the largest pool of vesicles recycles through endosomes but contributes very little to release while the small resident pool is the most active in release.

Before reuse, synaptic vesicles have to be re-filled with neurotransmitter molecules. This uptake mechanism is mediated by the corresponding neurotransmitter transporters (Liu and Edwards 1997; Eiden 2000; Iversen 2000) and is driven by an electrochemical gradient that is generated by a vacuolar proton pump consisting of at least 13 subunits (Stevens and Forgac 1997). The neurotransmitter-filled vesicle then translocates to the active zone, a process in which the synaptic vesicle protein synapsin plays an instrumental role (Hilfiker et al. 1999; Ferreira and Rapoport 2002). At the active zone, the vesicle is anchored to its future release site at the plasma membrane through a process called docking (see Fig. 1). Although the docking process can be nicely visualized with evanescent-field fluorescence microscopy, where it is characterized by a large reduction in lateral mobility of the vesicle (Steyer and Almers 1999; Oheim and Stühmer 2000), little is known about the molecules involved in this step. Docked vesicles, however, are not ready to fuse upon Ca^{2+} influx, but have to be rendered fusion-competent by a process called priming. Considerable progress has been made over the last few years in identifying priming factors, and members of the presynaptic Munc13 protein family appear to be essential for this reaction (Brose et al. 2000; see below). Once vesicles have been primed, they enter the release-ready pool from which they can fuse in a Ca^{2+}- and SNARE protein-dependent manner.

3
Mouse Genetic Analysis of the Presynaptic Transmitter Release Process: The Pros and Cons

The presynaptic transmitter release machinery is one of the most extensively studied functional protein networks in nerve cell biology. Indeed, due to their ideal biochemical accessibility, synaptic vesicles, the key cellular organelles in the transmitter release process, are among the best characterized subcellular compartments, with most of their protein components biochemically identified and cloned (Fernandez-Chacon and Südhof 1999). Complementing this information, numerous plasma membrane or active zone resident and cytosolic proteins have been identified as mediators or important regulators of neurotransmitter release (Garner et al. 2002).

With the advent of the gene knockout technology, the phase of identification and cloning of presynaptic proteins involved in neurotransmitter release, which started in the early 1980s, has been followed by a wave of mouse genetic studies on proteins involved in presynaptic function. Since publication of the synapsin 1 knockout in 1993 (Rosahl et al. 1993), over 30 genes coding for protein components of the neurotransmitter release machinery have been deleted or mutated in mice (Table 1). The information yielded by these studies has been of extraordinary importance for our current understanding of the mechanisms of neurotransmitter secretion.

Table 1 Mouse genetic analysis of presynaptic proteins involved in transmitter release

Protein	Protein type and function	Mutation and phenotype	Reference(s)
Presynaptic Ca^{2+} channels			
Cacna1a	Subunit α_{1A} of P/Q-type Ca^{2+} channel	KO: Lethal at P28; elimination of P/Q-type Ca^{2+} currents; synaptic transmission and secretion from chromaffin cells maintained at reduced levels and more reliant on other Ca^{2+} channel subtypes; ataxia and dystonia	Jun et al. 1999; Aldea et al. 2002
		Cacna1a^{tg} (tottering); P^{601}L point mutation between TMD S5 and S6 of repeat II: Altered P/Q-type Ca^{2+} channel expression/ characteristics; reduced transmitter release; reduced synaptic transmission at parallel fiber→Purkinje cell synapses; cerebellar cell death; ataxia, dyskinesia, absence seizures	Fletcher et al. 1996; Ayata et al. 2000; Matsushita et al. 2002
		Cacna1a^{tg-la} (leaner); exon skipping (frame shift and novel sequence after L^{1921}) and/or intron read through (frame shift and novel sequence after Q^{1967}) due to a point mutation in the splice donor site of the unspliced intron: Altered P/Q-type Ca^{2+} channel characteristics; reduced transmitter release; cerebellar cell death; reduced viability; ataxia; absence seizures	Fletcher et al. 1996; Ayata et al. 2000
		Cacna1a^{tg-rol} (rolling Nagoya); R^{1262}G point mutation in TMD S4 of repeat III: Reduced voltage sensitivity of P/Q-type Ca^{2+}channels; cerebellar cell death; ataxia	Mori et al. 2000
		Cacna1a^{rkr} (rocker); T^{1310}K point mutation between TMD S5 and S6 in repeat III: Altered P/Q-type Ca^{2+} channel expression/ characteristics; aberrant morphology of cerebellar neurons; ataxia; absence seizures	Zwingman et al. 2001
Cacna1b	Subunit α_{1B} of N-type Ca^{2+} channel	KO: Elimination of N-type Ca^{2+}currents; disorders of the sympathetic nervous system (e.g., baroreflex reduced); suppression of inflammatory and neuropathic pain	Hatakeyama et al. 2001; Ino et al. 2001; Saegusa et al. 2001; Kim et al. 2001
Cacna1e	Subunit α_{1E} of R-type Ca^{2+} channel	KO: Altered pain responses	Saegusa et al. 2000

Table 1 (continued)

Protein	Protein type and function	Mutation and phenotype	Reference(s)
Synaptic vesicle components			
ClC-3 (vesicular Cl⁻ channel)	Integral membrane protein of SVs; translocates Cl^- (charge balance)	KO: Impaired acidification of SVs; severe postnatal degeneration of retina and hippocampus	Stobrawa et al. 2001
CSP	Peripheral membrane protein of SVs (fatty acylation); putative synaptic cochaperone	KO: Reduced growth rate and viability	Preliminary characterization in: Tobaben et al. 2001
DOC2α	C_2 domain protein associated with SVs; Munc18 interactor	KO: Impaired short- and long-term synaptic plasticity and learning	Sakaguchi et al. 1999
Rab3A	Small G protein; postulated ole in SV targeting and late steps of SV fusion	KO: Impaired short- and long-term synaptic plasticity (mossy fiber LTP); increased glutamate release; perturbed SV trafficking and docking	Geppert et al. 1994a; Geppert et al. 1997; Castillo et al. 1997; Leenders et al. 2001
Rabphilin 3A	Rab3A binding C_2 domain protein associated with SVs	KO: No phenotypic changes detected	Schluter et al. 1999
SCAMP 1	Integral membrane protein of SVs	KO: Fusion pore function suggested (required for full execution of stable exocytosis in mast cells)	Fernandez-Chacon et al. 1999
SV2A	Integral membrane proteins of SVs (homology to bacterial transporters); multiple suggested functions	KO: Decreased readily releasable SV pool size; decreased evoked transmission	Janz et al. 1999b; Crowder et al. 1999; Xu and Bajjalieh 2001
SV2B	Integral membrane proteins of SVs (homology to bacterial transporters); multiple suggested functions	KO: Mild	Janz et al. 1999b
SV2A/SV2B		DKO: Severe; altered short-term synaptic plasticity (facilitation) suggested to be due to changed Ca^{2+} sensitivity of release machinery or altered Ca^{2+} homeostasis	Janz et al. 1999b

Table 1 (continued)

Protein	Protein type and function	Mutation and phenotype	Reference(s)
Synapsin 1	Peripheral membrane phosphoprotein of SVs; postulated role in SV tethering to cytoskeletal components, vesicle mobilization, synaptogenesis	KO: Altered short-term synaptic plasticity (increased PPF); increased seizure propensity; impaired axon outgrowth and synaptogenesis; reduced SV number and SV protein levels	Rosahl et al. 1993 and 1995; Chin et al. 1995; Li et al. 1995; Terada et al. 1999
Synapsin 2	Peripheral membrane phosphoprotein of SVs; postulated role in SV tethering to cytoskeletal components, vesicle mobilization, synaptogenesis	KO: Altered short-term synaptic plasticity (synaptic depression and reduced PTP); increased seizure propensity; reduced SV number and SV protein levels; learning deficits	Rosahl et al. 1995; Silva et al. 1996; Ferreira et al. 1995
Synapsin 3	Peripheral membrane protein of SVs	KO: Increased recycling SV pool ize; reduced IPSCs but not EPSCs; impaired axon outgrowth	Feng et al. 2002
Synapsin 1/synapsin 2		DKO: Aggravated phenotype; altered short-term synaptic plasticity (synaptic depression and reduced PTP); increased seizure propensity; reduced SV number and SV protein levels; learning deficits	Rosahl et al. 1995; Silva et al.1996
Synaptobrevin 2	Integral membrane protein of SVs; v-SNARE protein; substrate of clostridial neurotoxins; function in vesicle fusion	KO: Lethal (P0); completely paralyzed; normal brain development; readily releasable SV pool size and spontaneous fusion reduced by 90%; evoked Ca^{2+} dependent fusion reduced by 99%	Schoch et al. 2001
Synaptogyrin 1	Integral membrane protein of SVs	KO: Altered post-tetanic potentiation; partly redundant with Synaptophysin 1	Janz et al. 1999a
Synaptophysin 1	Integral membrane protein of SVs; multiple suggested functions	KO: Mild SV alterations in rod photoreceptors; mild deficit in activity dependent synaptogenesis; partly redundant with synaptogyrin 1	Eshkind and Leube 1995; McMahon et al. 1996; Spiwoks-Becker et al. 2001; Tarsa and Goda 2002
Synaptogyrin 1/synaptophysin 1		DKO: Impaired short and long-term synaptic plasticity	Janz et al. 1999a

Table 1 (continued)

Protein	Protein type and function	Mutation and phenotype	Reference(s)
Synaptotagmin 1	Integral membrane protein of SVs; Ca^{2+} binding protein; function as Ca^{2+} sensor	KO: Lethal (P0); fast, synchronous component of Ca^{2+}-triggered release dramatically reduced; readily releasable SV pool size and fusion normal	Geppert et al. 1994b
		$R^{233}Q$ KI: Reduced Ca^{2+} sensitivity of release machinery	Fernandez-Chacon et al. 2001
		$D^{232}N$ KI: Increased synaptic depression during repetitive stimulation	Fernandez-Chacon et al. 2002
		$D^{238}N$ KI: No phenotypic changes detected	Fernandez-Chacon et al. 2002
Synaptotagmin 4	Integral membrane protein of SVs	KO: Deficits in motor coordination and hippocampus dependent learning	Ferguson et al. 2000
VMAT 2 (vesicular monoamine transporter)	Integral membrane protein of SVs; transports monoamines	KO: Lethal (P0); heterozygotes are hypersensitive to amphetamine, cocaine, MPTP; susceptible to lethal cardiac arrhythmias	Wang et al. 1997; Fon et al. 1997; Takahashi et al. 1997; Fumagalli et al. 1999; Itokawa et al. 1999; Travis et al. 2000; Uhl et al. 2000
ZnT-3 (vesicular Zn^{2+} transporter)	Integral membrane protein of SVs; translocates Zn^{2+}	KO: Increased susceptibility to seizures	Cole et al. 1999
Cytosolic regulators of transmitter release			
Complexin 1	SNARE complex binding protein	KO: Motor coordination deficits	Reim et al. 2001
Complexin 2	SNARE complex binding protein	KO: Impaired long-term synaptic plasticity	Takahashi et al. 1999; Reim et al. 2001
Complexin 1/complexin 2		DKO: Lethal (P0); reduced evoked transmitter release and Ca^{2+} sensitivity of release machinery (altered Ca^{2+} sensing or SNARE complex function)	Reim et al. 2001
Rab3 GEP	Rab3 GDP/GTP exchange protein	KO: Lethal (P0); strongly impaired transmitter release and reduced number of total/docked SVs	Tanaka et al. 2001
RabGDIα	Rab GDP dissociation inhibitor	KO: Altered short-term synaptic plasticity (facilitation); hyperexcitability; hypersensitivity to bicuculline	Ishizaki et al. 2000

Table 1 (continued)

Protein	Protein type and function	Mutation and phenotype	Reference(s)
Presynaptic plasma membrane and active zone components			
CL1	Heptahelical transmembrane receptor for α latrotoxin	KO: Reduced α latrotoxin sensitivity	Tobaben et al 2002
Munc13–1	Presynaptic active zone component; Syntaxin regulator; essential for SV priming	KO: Lethal (P0); readily releasable SV pool size and spontaneous and evoked Ca^{2+} dependent fusion reduced by 90%; pecific for glutamatergic neurons; remaining activity (Munc13–2 dependent) has dramatically changed short-term synaptic plasticity characteristics	Augustin et al. 1999; Rosenmund et al. 2002
		$H^{567}K$ KI: Lethal (P0); normal evoked and spontaneous release; increased synaptic depression upon high frequency stimulation; no diacylglycerol/phorbol ester sensitivity of transmitter release	Rhee et al. 2002
Munc13–2	Presynaptic active zone component; role in SV priming	KO: Slightly altered short-term synaptic plasticity	Rosenmund et al. 2002; Varoqueaux et al. 2002
Munc13–3	Presynaptic active zone component; role in SV priming; cerebellum specific	KO: Reduced release probability (increased PPF) at parallel fiber →Purkinje cell synapses; impaired motor learning	Augustin et al. 2001
Munc13–1/Munc13–2		DKO: Lethal (P0); completely paralyzed; largely normal brain development and synaptogenesis; complete lack of primed SVs, and spontaneous and evoked release	Rosenmund et al. 2002; Varoqueaux et al. 2002
Munc18–1	Syntaxin regulator	KO: Lethal (P0); completely paralyzed; complete loss of spontaneous or evoked release in central neurons; reduced vesicle docking in chromaffin cells; secondary degeneration in brain stem and spinal cord	Verhage et al. 2000; Voets et al. 2001
Neurexin 1α	Presynaptic cell adhesion molecule; receptor for α-latrotoxin	KO: Reduced α latrotoxin sensitivity	Geppert et al. 1998

Table 1 (continued)

Protein	Protein type and function	Mutation and phenotype	Reference(s)
CL1/neurexin 1α		DKO: Reduced α latrotoxin sensitivity; cooperative role of the two receptors in mediating the toxin effects on transmitter release	Tobaben et al. 2002
RIM-1	Presynaptic active zone component; Rab3 effector; Munc13 regulator	KO: Reduced release probability and impaired short-term plasticity; impaired mossy fiber LTP (like Rab3A KO)	Castillo et al. 2002; Schoch et al. 2002
SNAP-25	Peripheral membrane protein of plasma membrane (fatty acylation); t-SNARE protein; substrate of clostridial neurotoxins; function in SV fusion	KO: Lethal (P0); completely paralyzed; normal brain development; dramatic reduction in spontaneous and evoked transmitter release in central synapses; reduced evoked release but ncreased frequency of spontaneous events at neuromuscular junction	Washbourne et al. 2002
Presynaptic endocytosis machinery			
Amphiphysin 1	Dynamin binding protein; regulator of endocytosis	KO: Co-reduction of Amphiphysin 2; defective cell free assembly of endocytic protein scaffolds; defects in synaptic vesicle recycling; propensity to seizures; learning deficits	Di Paolo et al. 2002
Synaptojanin	Polyphosphoinositide phosphatase; egulator of endocytosis	KO: Increased PIP_2 levels; clathrin coated vesicles accumulate in the presynaptic cytomatrix; increased synaptic depression during and reduced recovery from high frequency stimulation; multiple neurological and cognitive deficits	Cremona et al. 1999; Luthi et al. 2001

CL1, CIRL/Latrophilin 1; CSP, cystein string protein; DOC2α, double C_2 domain protein α; DKO, double knockout; GEP, GDP/GTP exchange protein; GDI, GDP dissociation inhibitor; KI, knock in; KO, knockout; LTP, long-term potentiation; PIP_2, phosphatidylinositol-4,5-bisphosphate; PPF, paired pulse facilitation; PTP, posttetanic potentiation; PX, postnatal day x; RIM, Rab3 interacting molecule; SNAP-25, synaptosomal associated protein of 25 kDa; SV, synaptic vesicle; SCAMP, secretory carrier membrane protein; SV2, synaptic vesicle associated membrane protein 2; TMD, transmembrane domain.

In the past, the gene knockout approach to the study of presynaptic function has received repeated criticism which focused on three principal pitfalls: (1) redundancy of protein function, because other isoforms or pathways may compromise the result of a single knockout; (2) for proteins with multiple functional domains participating in distinct processes, the deletion mutant phenotype may have a mixed character and may be difficult to interpret; and (3) for a protein with multiple essential functions, developmentally later roles may not be uncovered by a standard knockout. However, all these limitations can be—and in many cases have been—overcome by using alternative approaches and more sophisticated technology.

Ten years of gene knockout studies on presynaptic function have shown that the problem of redundancy is eminent because almost all proteins involved in the control of neurotransmitter release belong to complex families of multiple isoforms. As a consequence, elimination of even some of the most abundant presynaptic proteins is of surprisingly little functional consequence as is evident from the phenotypes of synaptophysin 1 (Eshkind and Leube 1995; Mcmahon et al. 1996), synaptogyrin 1 (Janz et al. 1999a), synapsin 1 or synapsin 2 (Rosahl et al. 1993, 1995; Chin et al. 1995; Li et al. 1995; Terada et al. 1999), SV2A or SV2B (Janz et al. 1999b; Crowder et al. 1999), complexin 1 or complexin 2 (Reim et al. 2001), and Munc13-2 or Munc13-3 knockouts (Augustin et al. 2001; Varoqueaux et al. 2002). However, subsequent studies showed that in all these cases the problem of redundancy can be circumvented by introducing multiple knockouts in a gene family, thus revealing interesting insights into the complex functional interplay between members of the respective families (Rosahl et al. 1995; Janz et al. 1999a,b; Reim et al. 2001; Varoqueaux et al. 2002). With respect to the functional analysis of individual protein domains, introduction of point mutations into proteins by homologous recombination has proved to be a powerful research tool. In the case of synaptotagmin 1, this approach has identified the C_2A domain as a key regulatory module involved in the Ca^{2+} sensing function of synaptotagmin 1 (Fernandez-Chacon et al. 2001 and 2002; see below). Likewise, the introduction of a point mutation into the C_1 domain of Munc13-1 has led to the identification of this protein as the only relevant presynaptic target of the diacylglycerol second messenger pathway (Rhee et al. 2002; see below). Although it has not been applied in the context of deletion mutations in genes coding for components of the presynaptic release machinery, the technology of inducible and tissue-specific knockouts allows a spatially and temporally more restricted and detailed analysis of knockout phenotypes.

An additional, frequently mentioned point of criticism with respect to the use of knockouts in the analysis of presynaptic function (as well as in other research areas) concerns the chronic nature of knockouts, together with the possibility of compensation mechanisms coming into play (Augustine et al. 1996). In this context, experimental approaches such as interference with protein expression and function using antisense oligonucleotides, RNAi, or peptide, protein and antibody injections are propagated as alternatives that may surpass the usefulness of gene knockouts in mice. However, in the case of antisense experiments and RNAi, the time between the respective manipulation and the assay of effects is in the range of days, and therefore not dramatically different from the time scale of brain development in utero. Moreover, attempts to perturb presynaptic function in various preparations by protein or antibody injection are characterized by a number of caveats, including the problem of in vivo specificity of the corresponding peptides, proteins, and antibodies in use. With respect to "compensatory" changes in protein levels after gene knockout, such compensatory upregulation of homologous isoforms after elimination of a particular protein family member is rare. In the case of the deletion of the α_{1A} subunit of the P/Q-type Ca^{2+} channel, functional compensation via upregulation of N-type and R-type channels has been described (Jun et al. 1999; Aldea et al. 2002). However, it is currently unknown whether this compensation is based on changes at the transcriptional or translational level or caused by altered channel protein stability or modulation (Jun et al. 1999; Aldea et al. 2002). What is frequently observed after deletion of genes encoding presynaptic proteins is the parallel destabilization/downregulation of proteins that are not structurally related to the deleted protein but function in the same molecular pathway (e.g., in the case of synapsin 1/2, synaptophysin 1, Munc18-1, Munc13-1, or RIM1 knockouts; Rosahl et al. 1993, 1995; McMahon et al. 1996; Verhage et al. 2000; Augustin et al. 2001; Betz et al. 2001; Schoch et al. 2002). It is questionable whether in any of the documented cases the altered protein levels serve to ameliorate an otherwise more deleterious phenotype or whether these changes likely contribute to the mutant phenotype and thus compromise the interpretation of the phenotype observed (see, e.g., Schoch et al. 2002). Rather, concomitant changes in the levels of proteins that are functionally but not structurally related to the deleted protein have provided interesting insights into functional protein networks that had previously been unknown (e.g., in the case of Munc13-1, RIM1, and complexin 1; Augustin et al. 1999; Reim et al. 2001; Betz et al. 2001; Schoch et al. 2002).

A major advantage of mouse gene knockout studies in the analysis of transmitter release mechanisms is the fact that phenotypic changes can readily be studied in cultured nerve cells. As a consequence, even (or particularly) perinatally lethal phenotypes are very informative, since neurons can be cultured from late embryonic stages and analyzed electrophysiologically, morphologically, and biochemically in culture. Moreover, novel viral transfection technologies can be applied in cultured nerve cells from knockout mice, thus allowing rescue experiments and structure–function analyses of relevant protein domains on the deletion mutant background. Indeed, the combination of gene knockout and viral rescue experiments using the Semliki Forest Virus system has allowed a speed, detail, and complexity of genetic analysis of transmitter release mechanisms in cultured mouse neurons which approaches a level that is otherwise only achieved in genetically more amenable model organisms such as *Caenorhabditis elegans* and *Drosophila* (Betz et al. 2001; Rhee et al. 2002; Rosenmund et al. 2002).

4
Insights from Mouse Genetic Analyses
of the Presynaptic Transmitter Release Process

Table 1 summarizes the current literature on gene knockout studies involving proteins that are relevant for the transmitter release process. In several cases, the observed phenotypic changes are surprisingly mild and do not allow us to define a molecular function for the proteins studied. Interestingly, in some cases the apparent lack of phenotypic changes contradicts theories on the essential function of the deleted proteins that had been based on numerous biochemical and cell biological studies. Examples include synaptophysin 1 (Eshkind and Leube 1995; McMahon et al. 1996) or rabphilin 3A (Schlüter et al. 1999), but have to be interpreted with caution because of the possible presence of functionally redundant homologues (Janz et al. 1999a). Indeed, it is likely that the role of proteins whose deletion in mice has so far not provided the expected functional insights will be determined once systematic mouse genetic studies involving other members of the corresponding gene family reach completion (as has been the case with complexins or Munc13s; Augustin et al. 1999, 2001; Reim et al. 2001; Rosenmund et al. 2002; Varoqueaux et al. 2002).

While the "curse" of redundancy may have compromised the interpretation of certain deletion mutant phenotypes, it is not a general problem. Rather, many knockout analyses have initially led to a cell biological and physiological characterization of the functional role of the proteins under investigation, thus allowing researchers to relate the particular protein to a defined trafficking step in the transmitter release process. Subsequent studies based on the initial characterization of these mutant phenotypes, some involving the knockout/viral rescue approach discussed above, have then resulted in a detailed molecular model of protein function. In the following section, we are discussing some of the most informative gene knockout studies of presynaptically relevant proteins with a focus on recent developments (for related reviews on earlier knockout studies in mice see Brose 1998; Fernandez-Chacon and Südhof 1999).

4.1
Transmitter and Ion Transport into Synaptic Vesicles

The energy needed for the uptake of neurotransmitters into synaptic vesicles is provided by a vacuolar-type proton pump which generates an electrochemical gradient across the vesicle membrane. Depending on the type of transmitter carrier present on the vesicle, the ΔpH or the $\Delta\Psi$ component of this electrochemical gradient is utilized for transmitter uptake (Reimer et al. 1998). The primary structures of several mammalian vesicular glutamate (VGLUT1–3; Ni et al. 1994; Aihara et al. 2000; Takamori et al. 2001; Gras et al. 2002), γ-aminobutyric acid (GABA) (VGAT; Mcintire et al. 1997; Sagne et al. 1997), and monoamine transporters (VMAT1 and 2; Erickson et al. 1992; Liu et al. 1992) are known. Vesicle acidification and uptake of certain transmitters require flux of counterions, in particular Cl⁻ (Maycox and Jahn 1990). Accordingly, synaptic vesicles contain at least one type of Cl⁻ channel, ClC-3 (Stobrawa al. 2001). In addition, transporters for Zn^{2+} (Palmiter et al. 1996) and other proteins with structural homology to transporter proteins but unknown function (e.g., SV2) are present on synaptic vesicles (Lowe et al. 1988).

Among the neurotransmitter transporter genes, only the VMAT2 gene has been deleted in mice (Fon et al. 1997; Takahashi et al. 1997; Wang et al. 1997; Fumagalli et al. 1999; Itokawa et al. 1999; Travis et al. 2000; Uhl et al. 2000). While homozygous mutants show a perinatally lethal phenotype, heterozygous animals survive into adulthood, are viable and fertile, but show increased mortality. Interestingly, heterozygous VMAT2 deletion mutant mice are characterized by reduced catecholamine release, which is indicative of reduced transmitter uptake and shows that the activity of vesicular neurotransmitter transporters may be rate-limiting (Takahashi et al. 1997). Heterozygous VMAT2 mutants show increased heart rates and blood pressure under anesthesia, as well as increased QT intervals in telemetrically measured EKGs, which could be the basis of the increased mortality observed (Takahashi et al. 1997; Itokawa et al. 1999). In addition, heterozygous VMAT2 mutants exhibit strikingly altered responses to various pharmacological agents that target monoaminergic transmission: increased amphetamine- and cocaine-induced locomotion, increased methamphetamine and 1-methyl-4-phenyl-1,2,3,6-tetrahydropyridine (MPTP) toxicity, and reduced amphetamine reward and sensitization to amphetamine. Moreover, heterozygous VMAT2 mutants display enhanced age-related changes. In view of these data, one focus of current research on VMAT2 function is on polymorphisms in the human VMAT2 gene and their possible role in variant drug responses and diseases such as Parkinson's disease or substance abuse (Uhl et al. 2000).

As mentioned above, synaptic vesicles contain channels/carriers for several different ions, some of which are necessary for normal transmitter uptake activity. The broadly expressed ClC-3 Cl⁻ channel, for example, is specifically localized to synaptic vesicles and endosomal compartments of neurons (Stobrawa et al. 2001). ClC-3-deficient mutant mice are viable, presumably because of the presence of other Cl⁻ channels on synaptic vesicles, but characterized by massive degeneration of the retina and hippocampus. Synaptic vesicles from homozygous ClC-3 mutants acidify at lower rates compared to controls, but glutamate uptake into vesicles is not reduced when assayed in vitro. In fact, miniature excitatory postsynaptic current (mEPSCs), and evoked EPSCs are slightly increased in the mutants, possibly due to increased glutamate loading of vesicles as would be expected by the increase in $\Delta\Psi$ after reduction of vesicular Cl⁻ conductance. This increase in glutamate loading of vesicles in vivo could cause excitotoxic levels of glutamate in the brain, which in turn would lead to the observed specific degeneration of retina and hippocampus (Stobrawa et al. 2001). Taken together, the data obtained on ClC-3-deficient mice demonstrate the importance of vesicular Cl⁻ channels for the control of glutamate release. It is likely that more dramatic consequences of the ClC-3 deletion are occluded by the presence of additional vesicular Cl⁻ channels.

In addition to neurotransmitters and Cl⁻, a subset of synaptic vesicles (e.g., in mossy fiber terminals of the hippocampal CA3 region) accumulates high levels of Zn^{2+}, which may serve as a regulator of glutamatergic transmission at *N*-methyl-D-aspartate (NMDA) receptors. Zn^{2+} is transported into synaptic vesicles by the ZnT-3 transporter. Elimination of ZnT-3 in deletion mutant mice has very minor consequences. Mutant mice have slightly increased seizure propensity but are otherwise normal. While these data indicate that vesicular Zn^{2+} has a protective neuromodulatory role, the presence of the alternative Zn^{2+} transporter ZnT4 may compensate for the loss of ZnT-3 and occlude additional, more severe consequences of the ZnT-3 deletion (Palmiter et al. 1996; Huang and Gitschier 1997).

4.2
Synaptic Vesicle Tethering/Docking

Synaptic vesicle tethering/docking is a morphologically defined step in the synaptic vesicle cycle that describes the state of close physical contact between the vesicular and plasma membranes. Functionally, the pool of docked vesicles is thought to define the pool of vesicles that is immediately available for release (Schikorski and Stevens 2001). While electron microscopical data indicate that tethered/docked vesicles at the presynaptic active zone are linked to the plasma membrane by proteinaceous material (Harlow et al. 2001), the molecular identity of tethering/docking proteins is unclear.

Irrespective of the actual step in the synaptic vesicle cycle involved, many deletion mutations that lead to dramatic changes of transmitter release in mice have very little effect on synaptic ultrastructure in general and the distribution of synaptic vesicles within the synapse in particular. For example, almost complete arrest of vesicle priming and transmitter release in Munc13-1 deletion mutants (Augustin et al. 1999) or almost complete block of Ca^{2+}-dependent exocytosis in synaptotagmin 1 deletion mutants (Geppert et al. 1994b) leaves the muber of docked vesicles as well as other vesicle pools unaffected (which is in striking contrast to the respective deletion mutations in *C. elegans*; see, e.g., Jorgensen et al. 1995; Richmond et al. 1999).

Only very few deletion mutations in mice lead to ultrastructural changes at the level of vesicle distribution in the synaptic terminal. The overall number of synaptic vesicles in nerve terminals is reduced in synapsin 1/2 and Rab3 GDP/GTP exchange protein (GEP) deletion mutant neurons, but the reasons for these phenotypic changes are not known (Rosahl et al. 1993, 1995; Tanaka et al. 2001). In the case of Rab3 GEP, the deletion mutation is likely to interfere with Rab-dependent vesicle trafficking and cause mistargeting and destabilization of transport vesicles. Rab3-deficient nerve terminals are characterized by a deficit in activity-dependent recruitment and tethering/docking of synaptic vesicles to the plasma membrane, indicating one role of Rab3 proteins in vesicle targeting and tethering/docking to the presynaptic active zone as postulated on the basis of their homology to yeast Ypt proteins (Leenders et al. 2001).

The only deletion mutation of a presynaptically relevant gene that seems to interfere directly and specifically with vesicle tethering/docking is the Munc18-1 deletion (Voets et al. 2001). Munc18-1 belongs to an evolutionarily conserved family of syntaxin interactors that are essential for fusion in yeast, invertebrates, and vertebrates. Deletion of Munc18-1 in mice leads to a complete loss of regulated secretory activity in neurons (Verhage et al. 2000). Mutant mice are completely paralyzed at birth and characterized by widespread neurodegeneration, due to a specific role of Munc18-1 in neuronal survival rather than to the lack of synaptic activity (Varoqueaux et al. 2002). However, surviving synapses in the central nervous system of Munc18-1 mutant mice are ultrastructurally normal. In contrast, the number of tethered/docked secretory granules in Munc18-1-deficient chromaffin cells is reduced to 10% of control values, causing a comparable reduction of secretory activity in these cells (Voets et al. 2001). It is unclear why loss of Munc18-1 leads to reduced vesicle tethering/docking in chromaffin cells and why this effect is not seen in synapses of the central nervous system. Vertebrate Munc18-1 and many related proteins in other organisms are thought to act via Syntaxin and its homologues with which they form a stable complex (Misura et al. 2000). This Munc18-1/syntaxin complex may act as a vesicle tethering/docking receptor in the chromaffin cell plasma membrane that interacts with a vesicular proteinaceous component (e.g., a Rab/Rab effector complex or DOC2α). In synapses of the central nervous system, this Munc18-1-dependent vesicle tethering/docking can be bypassed by an unknown mechanism.

4.3
Synaptic Vesicle Priming

Before docked vesicles can fuse with the plasma membrane in response to an increase in the intracellular Ca^{2+} concentration, they have to be primed to fusion competence. The size of the pool of primed, readily releasable synaptic vesicles can be determined by a neuron's response to hypertonic sucrose solutions. This priming process, which had originally been postulated on the basis of combined electrophysiological and morphological analyses of synaptic fatigue, is now known to be mediated by the presynaptic active zone components Munc13-1, -2, and -3 (Augustin et al. 1999; Brose et al. 2000; Augustin et al. 2001; Varoqueaux et al. 2002).

Munc13 proteins are among the very few known proteins that are specifically localized to presynaptic active zones (Betz et al. 1998; Augustin et al. 2001). Depending on the isoform involved, deletion of Munc13 proteins leads to phenotypic alterations that range from mild changes in synaptic plasticity (Munc13-2 and Munc13-3; Augustin et al. 2001; Varoqueaux et al. 2002) to an almost complete lack of fusion competent vesicles and synaptic transmitter release (Munc13-1; Augustin et al. 1999). This variability of phenotypic consequences is due to a complex redundancy among Munc13 isoforms. Once all Munc13 variants expressed in a nerve cell are deleted, the readily releasable vesicle pool and spontaneous and evoked release of glutamate and GABA (the only transmitters tested in these mutant mice so far) are completely abolished, demonstrating that Munc13-mediated vesicle priming is essential for transmitter release (Varoqueaux et al. 2002).

At the molecular level, Munc13 proteins are thought to mediate their priming function by regulating the activity of syntaxins. Many syntaxins can adopt two alternative conformations (Dulubova et al. 1999), one "closed," unable to enter SNARE complexes, and stabilized by Munc18, and one "open," competent to form SNARE complexes, and stabilized by Munc13 proteins. Munc13 proteins are thought to mediate vesicle priming by "opening" syntaxins, thereby promoting SNARE complex formation (Brose et al. 2000), a model that recently received direct support by data obtained in elegant genetic studies on Munc13 homologues in *C. elegans* (Richmond et al. 2001). This model, according to which the activity of the t-SNARE syntaxin is controlled by the active zone-specific Munc13 proteins, would also explain why transmitter release from synapses in the central nervous system is spatially restricted to presynaptic active zones although the t-SNAREs syntaxin and SNAP-25 are not restricted to this area but rather spread out over the entire axonal plasma membrane.

Interestingly, the different Munc13 isoforms appear to have different priming characteristics and subcellular distributions. In studies on individual hippocampal glutamatergic neurons (which only express Munc13-1 and Munc13-2) in autaptic culture, deletion of Munc13-1 was shown to cause a 90% loss of priming activity due to the shut down of 90% of all synapses. The remaining 10% of active synapses are exclusively dependent on Munc13-2 and release transmitter with normal release probability. In contrast to the majority of synapses in these neurons—which are dependent on Munc13-1, silenced in the Munc13-1 mutant, and show profound synaptic depression during high-frequency stimulation—the Munc13-2-dependent synapses that are uncovered in the Munc13-1 deletion mutant phenotype show pronounced and transient augmentation of synaptic transmitter release. These data indicate that presynaptic boutons formed by a single axon of a hippocampal glutamatergic neuron are differentially equipped with Munc13 priming factors which in turn differ with respect to their short-term plasticity characteristics (Augustin et al. 1999; Rosenmund et al. 2002). This mechanism of differential expression of Munc13 isoforms at individual synapses may represent a general mechanism that controls short-term synaptic plasticity and contributes to the heterogeneity of synaptic information coding (Rosenmund et al. 2002).

As the only protein class of the presynaptic release machinery, Munc13 isoforms contain a C_1 domain and are regulated by the intracellular second messenger diacylglycerol and its phorbol ester analogues. This feature resembles characteristics of classical and novel protein kinase C isoforms and identifies Munc13 proteins as potential targets of the diacylglycerol second messenger pathway that may act in parallel with protein kinase C variants (Betz et al. 1998). Indeed, recent evidence suggests that Munc13 proteins, rather than protein kinase C isoforms, are the only relevant targets of diacylglycerol and phorbol esters in the control of presynaptic neurotransmitter release. When mice are mutated by homologous recombination such that their hippocampal neurons express only one diacylglycerol-/phorbol ester-insensitive Munc13 variant—a genotype that can be generated by crossing the Munc13-1^{H567K} knock-in mutation (expressing a diacylglycerol/phorbol ester insensitive Munc13-1) into the Munc13-2 deletion mutant background—transmitter release from hippocampal neurons is no longer sensitive to the stimulating effects of phorbol esters and otherwise characterized by a reduction in activity-dependent vesicle priming that leads to a perinatally lethal phenotype (Rhee et al. 2002).

Apart from Munc13 proteins, RIM1 and its invertebrate homologues are active zone proteins that may be involved in the control of synaptic vesicle priming. RIM1 binds to Munc13-1 and the ubiquitously expressed Munc13 isoform ubMunc13-2 and controls their priming activity (Betz et al. 2001), and neurons in RIM1 deletion mutant mice exhibit phenotypic changes that are compatible with a reduction in vesicle priming and synaptic release probability. Moreover, Munc13-1 levels are reduced by 60% in RIM1-deficient brains, indicating that the two proteins function in the same protein interaction cascade (Schoch et al. 2002). Indeed, deletion of the RIM1 homologue Unc-10 in *C. elegans* (Koushika et al. 2001) leads to phenotypic changes that are very similar to, but more moderate than those observed after elimination of the Munc13 homologue Unc-13 (Richmond et al. 1999), demonstrating that Munc13 and RIM isoforms function in the same vesicle priming pathway that regulates syntaxin activity.

4.4
Presynaptic Ca^{2+} Signaling and Sensing

Stimulus-secretion coupling, i.e., the transduction of an arriving action potential into transmitter release at the synapse, is initiated by the opening of voltage-activated Ca^{2+} channels in response to the action potential-induced depolarization. The Ca^{2+} channels involved in triggering fast neurotransmitter release at synapses are of the high voltage activated P/Q and N type. In some synapses, R-type Ca^{2+} channels also contribute to the presynaptic Ca^{2+} signal that triggers transmitter release. The increase in intracellular [Ca^{2+}] that follows opening of voltage-activated Ca^{2+} channels—10–20 μM may suffice to trigger physiological release patterns (Bollmann et al. 2000; Schneggenburger and Neher 2000)—directly triggers synaptic vesicle fusion with a very short delay of some 100–200 μs. For this fast effect of Ca^{2+} on vesicle fusion, a Ca^{2+} sensor is required at the site of exocytosis. Given the kinetic characteristics of the Ca^{2+} triggering effect on synaptic exocytosis, the corresponding exocytotic Ca^{2+} sensor must exhibit highly cooperative Ca^{2+} binding and a Ca^{2+} affinity of some 10–20 μM. In view of these requirements, the best candidates for exocytotic Ca^{2+} sensors belong to the synaptotagmin family (see Südhof 2002; Chapman 2002 for recent reviews of the extensive literature). However, alternative Ca^{2+} sensors are also discussed. For example, components of the SNARE complex may act as Ca^{2+} sensors that trigger secretory vesicle exocytosis (Sorensen et al. 2002).

So far, all Ca^{2+} channels that are most relevant for synaptic transmitter release have been deleted in mice: Cacna1a (P/Q-type α_{1A} subunit; Jun et al. 1999; Aldea et al. 2002); Cacna1b (N-type α_{1B} subunit; Hatekayama et al. 2001; Ino et al. 2001; Saegusa et al. 2001; Kim et al. 2001); and Cacna1e (R-type α_{1E} subunit; Saegusa et al. 2000). In all cases, the respective pharmacologically characterized Ca^{2+} current is eliminated. Interestingly, the phenotypic consequences of these mutations are very mild and synaptic transmitter release is maintained, albeit often at reduced levels. Transmitter release is slightly reduced in the Cacna1a deletion mutant but maintained at robust levels, because other Ca^{2+} channel types are upregulated and functionally compensate the loss of P/Q-type channels. However, it is currently unknown whether this compensation is based on changes at the transcriptional or translational level or caused by altered channel protein stability or modulation (Jun et al. 1999; Aldea et al. 2002). At the behavioral level, Cacna1a deletion mutants are characterized by ataxia and dystonia which are paralleled by morphological changes in the cerebellum (Jun et al. 1999). Similar phenotypic alterations in mice are found in carriers of a number of spontaneous or chemically induced mutations in the Cacna1a gene that lead to partial loss of P/Q-type Ca^{2+} channel function (Cacna1a^{tg}; Cacna1a^{tg-la}; Cacna1a^{tg-rol}; Cacna1a^{rkr}; Fletcher et al. 1996; Ayata et al. 2000; Mori et al. 2000; Zwingman et al. 2001; Matsushita et al. 2002). Elimination of N- or R-type Ca^{2+} channels after Cacna1b or Cacna1e deletion mainly causes changes in pain responses, making the respective mouse lines interesting model systems in the analysis and treatment of pain (Saegusa et al. 2000, 2001; Hatakeyama et al. 2001; Ino et al. 2001; Kim et al. 2001). With respect to the role of different voltage-gated Ca^{2+} channels in neurotransmitter release, the data obtained on deletion mutant mice demonstrate a striking functional redundancy among presynaptic Ca^{2+} channels that can be modulated in a dynamic manner. Even minor changes in Ca^{2+} signaling due to channel deletion lead to developmental and functional deficits that are characterized by aberrant cerebellar development and cerebellar dysfunction in the case of P/Q-type Ca^{2+} channels or by altered pain responses in the case of N- and R-type Ca^{2+} channels.

As mentioned above, synaptotagmins may act as the exocytotic Ca^{2+} sensors that convert the presynaptic Ca^{2+} signal into vesicle fusion. In the central nervous system, synaptotagmin 1 is the most abundant synaptotagmin isoform. Like several other members of the synaptotagmin family, synaptotagmin 1 binds Ca^{2+} ions via two C_2 domains. Depending on the C_2 domain involved, Ca^{2+} binding leads to secondary acidic phospholipid or target protein binding. Among the protein interactors of synaptotagmin 1, syntaxin and SNAP-25 are thought to be most relevant for the postulated Ca^{2+} sensor role (Chapman 2002; Südhof 2002). Deletion of synaptotagmin 1 in mice leads to an almost complete block of Ca^{2+}-dependent transmitter release, while the size of the readily releasable vesicle pool remains largely unaffected (Geppert et al. 1994b), a phenotype that is compatible with a Ca^{2+} sensor function of synaptotagmin 1. The functional relevance of Ca^{2+} binding to synaptotagmin 1 is most clearly demonstrated by subtle point mutations in the synaptotagmin 1 gene. Introduction of an $R^{233}Q$ point mutation in the C_2A domain of synaptotagmin 1 reduces the apparent Ca^{2+} affinity of this domain (Fernandez-Chacon et al. 2001). When the same point mutation is introduced into the murine synaptotagmin 1 gene by homologous recombination, mutant nerve cells exhibit a reduced Ca^{2+} sensitivity of transmitter release, indicating that synaptotagmin 1 indeed functions as the exocytotic Ca^{2+} sensor (Fernandez-Chacon et al. 2001). Surprisingly, analogous genomic mutations in the Ca^{2+} binding site of the synaptotagmin 1 C_2A domain, which cause loss of Ca^{2+} binding in vitro, have hardly any phenotypic consequences (Fernandez-Chacon et al. 2002). Recent data obtained in *Drosophila* support the findings obtained in mice and show that Ca^{2+} binding to the C_2B domain of synaptotagmin is essential for Ca^{2+}-induced transmitter release (Mackler et al. 2002; Robinson et al. 2002). Taken together, genetic data from mice and *Drosophila* indicate that synaptotagmins are indeed the presynaptic exocytotic Ca^{2+} sensors. Their C_2 domains appear to act in concert to sense increases in Ca^{2+} concentrations and trigger Ca^{2+}-dependent vesicle fusion. Whether this effect is due to Ca^{2+}-dependent phospholipid binding or a Ca^{2+}-dependent interaction of synaptotagmins with SNARE proteins or other components of the presynaptic release machinery is still unknown.

Apart from mutations in the murine Ca^{2+} channel and synaptotagmin 1 genes, only two other mouse deletion mutants that lack presynaptic proteins show changes in the Ca^{2+} sensitivity of neurotransmitter release: SV2A/B double mutants and complexin 1/2 double mutants (Janz et al. 1999b; Reim et al. 2001). In both cases, it is unknown how exactly this changed Ca^{2+} sensitivity of release is brought about. SV2A and B may function in Ca^{2+} sequestration into synaptic vesicles such that their elimination changes presynaptic Ca^{2+} homeostasis (Janz et al. 1999b). Complexins 1 and 2, on the other hand, are stoichiometric components of a subpopulation of SNARE complexes and likely to affect the apparent Ca^{2+} sensitivity of transmitter release by altering SNARE complex function or SNARE complex interaction with the exocytotic Ca^{2+} sensor (e.g., synaptotagmin 1; Reim et al. 2001).

4.5
Synaptic Vesicle Fusion

Despite the identification of proteins that are essential for the actual fusion reaction of synaptic vesicles, the molecular mechanism of fusion remains a matter of controversy. The fact that the synaptic vesicle v-SNARE synaptobrevin/VAMP 2 and the plasma membrane t-SNAREs syntaxin 1 and SNAP-25 are essential for vesicle fusion is evident from the fact that their specific proteolytic cleavage by several clostridial neurotoxins completely abolishes vesicle fusion without affecting other properties of synaptic terminals (see, e.g., Südhof et al. 1993 for a review of the pioneering work on clostridial toxins). The three synaptic SNARE proteins (as well as several homologous SNARE proteins from different intracellular compartments) form a thermodynamically highly stable complex, the SNARE complex, whose association is thought to pull vesicle and plasma membrane into close proximity and drive the actual fusion reaction (Weber et al. 1998; Sutton et al. 1998; Jahn and Südhof 1999). Alternative molecular models that mainly originate from data obtained in analyses of yeast vacuolar fusion and sea urchin egg cortical granule fusion view the actual vesicle fusion step to be independent of SNAREs. However, support for these models in the context of synaptic neurotransmitter release is currently lacking.

Among the known synaptic SNAREs, synaptobrevin/VAMP 2 and SNAP-25 have been genetically eliminated in mice (Schoch et al. 2001; Washbourne et al. 2002). In both cases, mutants are completely paralyzed and die at birth because evoked and spontaneous transmitter release are almost completely blocked. However, nerve cells from both mutants still exhibit detectable vesicular exocytosis. In particular, spontaneous vesicle fusion rates are surprisingly high despite the postulated essential role of synaptobrevin/VAMP 2 and SNAP-25 in vesicle fusion. At present, it is not clear whether the fact that synaptobrevin/VAMP 2 and SNAP-25 deletion mutants still show spontaneous vesicle fusion is indicative of SNARE-independent fusion mechanisms. In fact, it is likely that alternative homologous SNAREs compensate partially for the loss of synaptobrevin/VAMP 2 and SNAP-25. Thus, all currently available data on SNARE deletion mutants are compatible with the idea that SNAREs mediate the actual vesicle fusion reaction. Additional support for the SNARE model of membrane fusion is provided by the fact that complete elimination of Munc13-mediated synaptic vesicle priming, which is thought to involve activation of the t-SNARE syntaxin as a key mechanistic step, leads to a complete arrest of spontaneous and evoked transmitter release (Varoqueaux et al. 2002).

4.6
Synaptic Plasticity

Dynamic changes in the efficacy of synaptic transmission in the central nervous system are essential for proper brain function. Long-lasting changes of synaptic transmission efficacy, as observed in long-term potentiation and long-term depression, are thought to be the basis of learning and memory processes in the brain.

Changes in short-term synaptic plasticity processes such as paired pulse facilitation and other forms of synaptic facilitation, post-tetanic potentiation, or synaptic augmentation are observed in a large number of mouse deletion mutants lacking presynaptic proteins (see Table 1). In many cases, these changes reflect subtle deficits in overall presynaptic function that appear to be most readily detectable in short-term synaptic plasticity paradigms. In the case of Munc13 priming proteins, the changes in short-term synaptic plasticity that are observable in the respective deletion mutant neurons are due to protein intrinsic features/differences (Rosenmund et al. 2002). In fact, Munc13 priming activity appears to be regulated directly and indirectly by changes in intracellular Ca^{2+}

concentrations that cause short-term plastic changes of presynaptic activity (Rhee et al. 2002; Rosenmund et al. 2002).

As seen with respect to short-term plasticity, changes in long-term synaptic plasticity are often observed after genetic interference with presynaptic function (see Table 1). In fact, changes in long-term potentiation are among the most frequently observed phenotypic alterations in deletion-mutant mice with a central nervous system dysfunction. It is unlikely that this is because all of the respective deleted proteins are directly involved in the molecular mechanism of long-term potentiation. Rather, induction and maintenance of long-term potentiation appear to be very sensitive even to subtle changes in synaptic transmission and other nerve cell functions such that mild deficits have indirect consequences for long-term changes of synaptic efficacy.

Among the mouse deletion mutants that lack presynaptically relevant proteins, only two yielded direct insights into possible mechanisms of long-term potentiation: in mice lacking the small GTPase Rab3A (Castillo et al. 1997) and in mice lacking the Rab3 effector RIM1 (Castillo et al. 2002), mossy fiber long-term potentiation in the hippocampal CA3 region is abolished. In contrast to NMDA receptor-dependent long-term potentiation, mossy fiber long-term potentiation has a principal presynaptic component and requires activation of protein kinase A, indicating that presynaptic substrates of protein kinase A are involved. In view of the fact that RIM1 is a Rab3A effector and a substrate for protein kinase A, it is possible that the increases in transmitter release during mossy fiber long-term potentiation are caused by a mechanism that involves a GTP- and phosphorylation-dependent interaction of Rab3A and RIM1 at the contact site between synaptic vesicle and active zone (Castillo et al. 2002). Munc13 proteins, which are regulated by direct interaction with RIM1 (Betz et al. 2001), may represent an additional protein component involved in mossy fiber long-term potentiation. In fact, the essential role of Munc13 proteins in determining presynaptic transmitter release efficacy in mice (Augustin et al. 1999, 2001; Rosenmund et al. 2002; Varoqueaux et al. 2002) indicates that Munc13 proteins may be a main target of regulation in mossy fiber long-term potentiation.

5
Pharmacological Interference with Transmitter Release

Evidently, control of the synaptic vesicle cycle is mediated by a complex cascade of protein–protein interactions. In most of the published cases, these interactions involve poorly defined protein regions. Examples of interactions of clearly defined domains and/or crystal structures thereof are rare and include the SNARE complex without and with complexin (Sutton et al. 1998; Chen et al. 2002) the Rab3A/Rabphilin3A complex (Ostermeier and Brunger 1999), or the Munc18-1/syntaxin 1A complex (Misura et al. 2000). So far, none of the documented protein–protein interactions involved in neurotransmitter release are known to be perturbed by defined small molecules that might be developed into pharmacologically relevant drugs. Given the central role of neurotransmitter release in brain function, a systematic pharmacological analysis of the presynaptic transmitter release process and the underlying protein–protein interactions using combinatorial chemical libraries represents a promising aim of future research efforts.

While such pharmacological interference with presynaptic protein–protein interactions is a realistic vision at best, several individual components of the presynaptic release machinery are established or potential drug targets for whose analysis the mutant mouse models described above may serve as important experimental test systems. Voltage-gated Ca^{2+} channels, for example, are known to be blocked by a number of toxins that are also useful therapeutically in the treatment of pain. In this context, the Cacna1a, Cacna1b, and Cacna1e deletion mutant mice will serve as important model organisms for the development of new drugs (Jun et al. 1999; Saegusa et al. 2000, 2001; Hatakeyama et al. 2001; Ino et al. 2001; Kim et al. 2001; Aldea et al. 2002). At the level of neurotransmitter uptake, the example of the VMAT blocker reserpine, which was one of the first antihypertensive and antipsychotic agents used clinically, is proof of the principle that synaptic vesicle neurotransmitter transporters are useful drug targets. In particular, the known vesicular glutamate transporters VGLUT1–3 (Ni et al. 1994; Aihara et al. 2000; Takamori et al. 2001; Gras et al. 2002) are interesting targets in this context because they are differentially expressed in different brain regions such that isoform-specific inhibitors would allow quite specific interference with glutamatergic transmission. Unfortunately, corresponding mouse mutants that might serve as model systems for the development of VGLUT-specific drugs are not available yet. Finally, a number of presynaptically relevant proteins contain defined protein domains for which small molecule activators and inhibitors are known. One of the most interesting examples is the Munc13family of vesicle priming proteins which contain a central C_1 domain that is activated by diacylglycerol or phorbol esters and inhibited by calphostin C (Betz et al. 1998; Rhee et al. 2002). Given the essential role of Munc13-mediated vesicle priming and the differences between the various known Munc13 isoforms with respect to their expression pattern and priming function, Munc13 proteins may serve as interesting targets for pharmacological interference with transmitter release in different transmitter systems once isoform-specific inhibitors or activators have been developed. Corresponding mutant mice that would be helpful to characterize such Munc13 isoform-specific pharmacological agents are already available (Augustin et al. 1999, 2001; Varoqueaux et al. 2002).

References

Aihara Y, Mashima H, Onda H, Hisano S, Kasuya H, Hori T, Yamada S, Tomura H, Yamada Y, Inoue I, Kojima I, Takeda J (2000) Molecular cloning of a novel brain-type Na(+)-dependent inorganic phosphate cotransporter. J Neurochem 74:2622–2625
Aldea M, Jun K, Shin HS, Andres-Mateos E, Solis-Garrido LM, Montiel C, Garcia AG, Albillos A (2002) A perforated patch-clamp study of calcium currents and exocytosis in

chromaffin cells of wild-type and alpha(1A) knockout mice. J Neurochem 81:911–921

Antonin W, Riedel D, Fischer von Mollard G (2000) The SNARE Vti1a-beta is localized to small synaptic vesicles and participates in a novel SNARE complex. J Neurosci 20:5724–5732

Augustin I, Korte S, Rickmann M, Kretzschmar HA, Südhof TC, Herms JW, Brose N (2001) The cerebellum-specific Munc13 isoform Munc13-3 regulates cerebellar synaptic transmission and motor learning in mice. J Neurosci 21:10–17

Augustin I, Rosenmund C, Südhof TC, Brose N (1999) Munc 13-1 is essential for fusion competence of glutamatergic synaptic vesicles. Nature 400:457–461

Augustine GJ, Burns ME, DeBello WM, Pettit DL, Schweizer FE (1996) Exocytosis:proteins and perturbations. Annu Rev Pharmacol Toxicol 36:659–701

Ayata C, Shimizu-Sasamata M, Lo EH, Noebels JL, Moskowitz MA (2000) Impaired neurotransmitter release and elevated threshold for cortical spreading depression in mice with mutations in the alpha1A subunit of P/Q type calcium channels. Neuroscience 95:639–645

Betz A, Ashery U, Rickmann M, Augustin I, Neher E, Südhof TC, Rettig J, Brose N (1998) Munc13-1 is a presynaptic phorbol ester receptor that enhances neurotransmitter release. Neuron 21:123–136

Betz A, Thakur P, Junge HJ, Ashery U, Rhee JS, Scheuss V, Rosenmund C, Rettig J, Brose N (2001) Functional interaction of the active zone proteins Munc13-1 and RIM1 in synaptic vesicle priming. Neuron 30:183–196

Bollmann JH, Sakmann B, Borst JG (2000) Calcium sensitivity of glutamate release in a calyx-type terminal. Science 289:953–957

Brodin L, Löw P, Shupliakov O (2000) Sequential steps in clathrin-mediated synaptic vesicle endocytosis. Curr Opin Neurobiol 10:312–320

Brose N (1998) Synaptic vesicle proteins—a genetic approach. In: Linial M, Grasso A, Lazarovici M (eds) Cellular and molecular mechanisms of toxin action—secretory systems. Harwood, Amsterdam, p 45

Brose N, Rosenmund C, Rettig J (2000) Regulation of transmitter release by Unc-13 and its homologues. Curr Opin Neurobiol 10:303–311

Castillo PE, Janz R, Südhof TC, Tzounopoulos T, Malenka RC, Nicoll RA (1997) Rab3A is essential for mossy fibre long-term potentiation in the hippocampus. Nature 388:590–593

Castillo PE, Schoch S, Schmitz F, Südhof TC, Malenka RC (2002) RIM1alpha is required for presynaptic long-term potentiation. Nature 415:327–330

Chapman ER (2002) Synaptotagmin: A Ca^{2+} sensor that triggers exocytosis? Nat Rev Mol Cell Biol 3:498–508

Chen X, Tomchick DR, Kovrigin E, Arac D, Machius M, Südhof TC, Rizo J (2002) Three-dimensional structure of the complexin/SNARE complex. Neuron 33:397–409

Chin LS, Li L, Ferreira A, Kosik KS, Greengard P (1995) Impairment of axonal development and of synaptogenesis in hippocampal neurons of synapsin I-deficient mice. Proc Natl Acad Sci USA 92:9230–9234

Cole TB, Wenzel HJ, Kafer KE, Schwartzkroin PA, Palmiter RD (1999) Elimination of zinc from synaptic vesicles in the intact mouse brain by disruption of the ZnT3 gene. Proc Natl Acad Sci USA 96:1716–1721

Cremona O, De Camilli P (1997) Synaptic vesicle endocytosis. Curr Opin Neurobiol 7:323–330

Cremona O, Di Paolo G, Wenk MR, Luthi A, Kim WT, Takei K, Daniell L, Nemoto Y, Shears SB, Flavell RA, McCormick DA, De Camilli P (1999) Essential role of phosphoinositide metabolism in synaptic vesicle recycling. Cell 99:179–188

Crowder KM, Gunther JM, Jones TA, Hale BD, Zhang HZ, Peterson MR, Scheller RH, Chavkin C, Bajjalieh SM (1999) Abnormal neurotransmission in mice lacking synaptic vesicle protein 2A (SV2A). Proc Natl Acad Sci USA 96:15268–15273

Di Paolo G, Sankaranarayanan S, Wenk MR, Daniell L, Perucco E, Caldarone BJ, Flavell R, Picciotto MR, Ryan TA, Cremona O, De Camilli P (2002) Decreased synaptic vesicle recycling efficiency and cognitive deficits in amphiphysin 1 knockout mice. Neuron 33:789–804

Dulubova I, Sugita S, Hill S, Hosaka M, Fernandez I, Südhof TC, Rizo J (1999) A conformational switch in syntaxin during exocytosis: role of munc18. EMBO J 18:4372–4382

Eiden LE (2000) The vesicular neurotransmitter transporters: current perspectives and future prospects. FASEB J 14:2396–2400

Erickson JD, Eiden LE, Hoffman BJ (1992) Expression cloning of a reserpine-sensitive vesicular monoamine transporter. Proc Natl Acad Sci USA 89:10993–10997

Eshkind LG, and Leube RE (1995) Mice lacking synaptophysin reproduce and form typical synaptic vesicles. Cell Tissue Res 282:423–433

Feng J, Chi P, Blanpied TA, Xu Y, Magarinos AM, Ferreira A, Takahashi RH, Kao HT, McEwen BS, Ryan TA, Augustine GJ, Greengard P (2002) Regulation of neurotransmitter release by synapsin III. J Neurosci 22:4372–4380

Ferguson GD, Anagnostaras SG, Silva AJ, Herschman HR (2000) Deficits in memory and motor performance in synaptotagmin IV mutant mice. Proc Natl Acad Sci USA 97:5598–5603

Fernandez-Chacon R, Alvarez de Toledo G, Hammer RE, Südhof TC (1999) Analysis of SCAMP1 function in secretory vesicle exocytosis by means of gene targeting in mice. J Biol Chem 274:32551–32554

Fernandez-Chacon R, Konigstorfer A, Gerber SH, Garcia J, Matos MF, Stevens CF, Brose N, Rizo J, Rosenmund C, Südhof TC (2001) Synaptotagmin I functions as a calcium regulator of release probability. Nature 410:41–49

Fernandez-Chacon R, Shin O-H, Konigstorfer A, Matos M, Meyer A, Garcia J, Gerber SH, Rizo J, Südhof TC, Rosenmund C (2002) Structure/function analysis of Ca^{2+} binding to the C_2A-domain of Synaptotagmin 1. J Neurosci, in press

Fernandez-Chacon R, Südhof TC (1999) Genetics of synaptic vesicle function: toward the complete functional anatomy of an organelle. Annu Rev Physiol 61:753–776

Ferreira A, Han H, Greengard P, Kosik KS (1995) Suppression of Synapsin II inhibits the formation and maintenance of synapses in hippocampal culture. Proc Natl Acad Sci USA 92:9225–9229

Ferreira A, Rapoport M (2002) The synapsins: beyond the regulation of neurotransmitter release. Cell Mol Life Sci 59:589–595

Fischer von Mollard G, Stahl B, Walch-Solimena C, Takei K, Daniels L, Khoklatchev A, De Camilli P, Südhof TC, Jahn R (1994) Localization of Rab5 to synaptic vesicles identifies endosomal intermediate in synaptic vesicle recycling pathway. Eur J Cell Biol 65:319–326

Fletcher CF, Lutz CM, O'Sullivan TN, Shaughnessy JD Jr, Hawkes R, Frankel WN, Copeland NG, Jenkins NA (1996) Absence epilepsy in tottering mutant mice is associated with calcium channel defects. Cell 87:607–617

Fon EA, Pothos EN, Sun BC, Killeen N, Sulzer D, Edwards RH (1997) Vesicular transport regulates monoamine storage and release but is not essential for amphetamine action. Neuron 19:1271–1283

Fumagalli F, Gainetdinov RR, Wang YM, Valenzano KJ, Miller GW, Caron MG (1999) Increased methamphetamine neurotoxicity in heterozygous vesicular monoamine transporter 2 knockout mice. J Neurosci 19:2424–2431

Gad H, Löw P, Zotova E, Brodin L, Shupliakov O (1998) Dissociation between Ca^{2+}-evoked synaptic vesicle exocytosis and clathrin-mediated endocytosis at a central vertebrate synapse. Neuron 21:607–616

Garner CC, Zhai RG, Gundelfinger ED, Ziv NE (2002) Molecular mechanisms of CNS synaptogenesis. Trends Neurosci 25:251–258

Geppert M, Bolshakov VY, Siegelbaum SA, Takei K, De Camilli P, Hammer RE, Südhof TC (1994a) The role of Rab3A in neurotransmitter release. Nature 369:493–497

Geppert M, Goda Y, Hammer RE, Li C, Rosahl TW, Stevens CF, Südhof TC (1994b) Synaptotagmin I: a major Ca^{2+} sensor for transmitter release at a central synapse. Cell 79:717–727

Geppert M, Goda Y, Stevens CF, Südhof TC (1997) The small GTP-binding protein Rab3A regulates a late step in synaptic vesicle fusion. Nature 387:810–814

Geppert M, Khvotchev M, Krasnoperov V, Goda Y, Missler M, Hammer RE, Ichtchenko K, Petrenko AG, Südhof TC (1998) Neurexin I alpha is a major alpha-latrotoxin receptor that cooperates in alpha-latrotoxin action. J Biol Chem 273:1705–1710

Gras C, Herzog E, Bellenchi GC, Bernard V, Ravassard P, Pohl M, Gasnier B, Giros B, El Mestikawy S (2002) A third vesicular glutamate transporter expressed by cholinergic and serotoninergic neurons. J Neurosci 22:5442–5451

Harlow ML, Ress D, Stoschek A, Marshall RM, McMahan UJ (2001) The architecture of active zone material at the frog's neuromuscular junction. Nature 409:479–484

Hatakeyama S, Wakamori M, Ino M, Miyamoto N, Takahashi E, Yoshinaga T, Sawada K, Imoto K, Tanaka I, Yoshizawa T, Nishizawa Y, Mori Y, Niidome T, Shoji S (2001) Differential nociceptive responses in mice lacking the alpha(1B) subunit of N-type Ca^{2+} channels. Neuroreport 12:2423–2427

Haucke V, De Camilli P (1999) AP-2 recruitment to synaptotagmin stimulated by tyrosine-based endocytic motifs. Science 285:1268–1271

Heuser JE, Reese TS (1973) Evidence for recycling of synaptic vesicle membrane during transmitter release at the frog neuromuscular junction. J Cell Biol 57:315–344

Heuser JE, Reese TS, Landis DM (1974) Functional changes in frog neuromuscular junctions studied with freeze-fracture. J Neurocytol 3:109–131

Hilfiker S, Pieribone VA, Czernik AJ, Kao HT, Augustine GJ, Greengard P (1999) Synapsins as regulators of neurotransmitter release. Philos Trans R Soc Lond B Biol Sci 354:269–279

Huang L, Gitschier J (1997) A novel gene involved in zinc transport is deficient in the lethal milk mouse. Nat Genet 17:292–297

Ino M, Yoshinaga T, Wakamori M, Miyamoto N, Takahashi E, Sonoda J, Kagaya T, Oki T, Nagasu T, Nishizawa Y, Tanaka I, Imoto K, Aizawa S, Koch S, Schwartz A, Niidome T, Sawada K, Mori Y (2001) Functional disorders of the sympathetic nervous system in mice lacking the alpha 1B subunit (Cav 2.2) of N-type calcium channels. Proc Natl Acad Sci USA 98:5323–5328

Ishizaki H, Miyoshi J, Kamiya H, Togawa A, Tanaka M, Sasaki T, Endo K, Mizoguchi A, Ozawa S, and Takai Y (2000) Role of rab GDP dissociation inhibitor alpha in regulating plasticity of hippocampal neurotransmission. Proc Natl Acad Sci USA 97:11587–11592

Itokawa K, Sora I, Schindler CW, Itokawa M, Takahashi N, Uhl GR (1999) Heterozygous VMAT2 knockout mice display prolonged QT intervals: possible contributions to sudden death. Brain Res Mol Brain Res 71:354–357

Iversen L (2000) Neurotransmitter transporters: fruitful targets for CNS drug discovery. Mol Psychiatry 5:357–362

Jahn R, Südhof TC (1999) Membrane fusion and exocytosis. Annu Rev Biochem 68:863–911

Janz R, Südhof TC, Hammer RE, Unni V, Siegelbaum SA, Bolshakov VY (1999a) Essential roles in synaptic plasticity for synaptogyrin I and synaptophysin I. Neuron 24:687–700

Janz R, Goda Y, Geppert M, Missler M, Südhof TC (1999b) SV2A and SV2B function as redundant Ca^{2+} regulators in neurotransmitter release. Neuron 24:1003–1016

Jorgensen EM, Hartwieg E, Schuske K, Nonet ML, Jin Y, Horvitz HR (1995) Defective recycling of synaptic vesicles in synaptotagmin mutants of Caenorhabditis elegans. Nature 378:196–199

Jun K, Piedras-Renteria ES, Smith SM, Wheeler DB, Lee SB, Lee TG, Chin H, Adams ME, Scheller RH, Tsien RW, Shin HS (1999) Ablation of P/Q-type Ca^{2+} channel currents, altered synaptic transmission, and progressive ataxia in mice lacking the alpha(1A)-subunit. Proc Natl Acad Sci USA 96:15245–15250

Kim C, Jun K, Lee T, Kim SS, McEnery MW, Chin H, Kim HL, Park JM, Kim DK, Jung SJ, Kim J, Shin HS (2001) Altered nociceptive response in mice deficient in the alpha(1B) subunit of the voltage-dependent calcium channel. Mol Cell Neurosci 18:235–245

Koushika SP, Richmond JE, Hadwiger G, Weimer RM, Jorgensen EM, Nonet ML (2001) A post-docking role for active zone protein Rim. Nat Neurosci 4:997–1005

Leenders AG, Lopes da Silva FH, Ghijsen WE, Verhage M (2001) Rab3a is involved in transport of synaptic vesicles to the active zone in mouse brain nerve terminals. Mol Biol Cell 12:3095–3102

Li L, Chin LS, Shupliakov O, Brodin L, Sihra TS, Hvalby O, Jensen V, Zheng D, McNamara JO, Greengard P, Andersen P (1995) Impairment of synaptic vesicle clustering and of synaptic transmission, and increased seizure propensity, in synapsin I-deficient mice. Proc Natl Acad Sci USA 92:9235–9239

Liu Y, Edwards RH (1997) The role of vesicular transport proteins in synaptic transmission and neural degeneration. Annu Rev Neurosci 20:125–156

Liu Y, Peter D, Roghani A, Schuldiner S, Prive GG, Eisenberg D, Brecha N, Edwards RH (1992) A cDNA that suppresses MPP+ toxicity encodes a vesicular amine transporter. Cell 70:539–551

Lowe AW, Madeddu L, Kelly RB (1988) Endocrine secretory granules and neuronal synaptic vesicles have three integral membrane proteins in common. J Cell Biol 106:51–59

Lüthi A, Di Paolo G, Cremona O, Daniell L, De Camilli P, McCormick DA (2001) Synaptojanin 1 contributes to maintaining the stability of GABAergic transmission in primary cultures of cortical neurons. J Neurosci 21:9101–9111

Mackler JM, Drummond JA, Loewen CA, Robinson IM, Reist NE (2002) The C_2B Ca^{2+}-binding motif of synaptotagmin is required for synaptic transmission in vivo. Nature 418:340–344

Matsushita K, Wakamori M, Rhyu IJ, Arii T, Oda S, Mori Y, Imoto K (2002) Bidirectional alterations in cerebellar synaptic transmission of tottering and rolling Ca^{2+} channel mutant mice. J Neurosci 22:4388–4398

Maycox PR, Hell JW, Jahn R (1990) Amino acid neurotransmission: spotlight on synaptic vesicles. Trends Neurosci 13:83–87

McIntire SL, Reimer RJ, Schuske K, Edwards RH, Jorgensen EM (1997) Identification and characterization of the vesicular GABA transporter. Nature 389:870–876

McMahon HT, Bolshakov VY, Janz R, Hammer RE, Siegelbaum SA, Südhof TC (1996) Synaptophysin, a major synaptic vesicle protein, is not essential for neurotransmitter release. Proc Natl Acad Sci USA 93:4760–4764

Misura KM, Scheller RH, Weis WI (2000) Three-dimensional structure of the neuronal-Sec1-syntaxin 1a complex. Nature 404:355–362

Mori Y, Wakamori M, Oda S, Fletcher CF, Sekiguchi N, Mori E, Copeland NG, Jenkins NA, Matsushita K, Matsuyama Z, Imoto K (2000) Reduced voltage sensitivity of activation of P/Q-type Ca^{2+} channels is associated with the ataxic mouse mutation rolling Nagoya (tg(rol)). J Neurosci 20:5654–5662

Murthy VN, Stevens CF (1998) Synaptic vesicles retain their identity through the endocytic cycle. Nature 392:497–501

Ni B, Rosteck PR Jr, Nadi NS, Paul SM (1994) Cloning and expression of a cDNA encoding a brain-specific Na^{+}-dependent inorganic phosphate cotransporter. Proc Natl Acad Sci USA 91:5607–5611

Oheim M, Stühmer W (2000) Tracking chromaffin granules on their way through the actin cortex. Eur Biophys J 29:67–89

Ostermeier C, Brunger AT (1999) Structural basis of Rab effector specificity: crystal structure of the small G protein Rab3A complexed with the effector domain of rab-philin-3A. Cell 96:363–374

Palmiter RD, Cole TB, Quaife CJ, Findley SD (1996) ZnT-3, a putative transporter of zinc into synaptic vesicles. Proc Natl Acad Sci USA 93:14934–14939

Pyle JL, Kavalali ET, Piedras-Renteria ES, Tsien RW (2000) Rapid reuse of readily releasable pool vesicles at hippocampal synapses. Neuron 28:221–231

Reim K, Mansour M, Varoqueaux F, McMahon HT, Südhof TC, Brose N, Rosenmund C (2001) Complexins regulate a late step in Ca^{2+}-dependent neurotransmitter release. Cell 104:71–81

Reimer RJ, Fon EA, Edwards RH (1998) Vesicular neurotransmitter transport and the presynaptic regulation of quantal size. Curr Opin Neurobiol 8:405–412

Rhee JS, Betz A, Pyott S, Reim K, Varoqueaux F, Augustin I, Hesse D, Südhof TC, Takahashi M, Rosenmund C, Brose N (2002) Beta phorbol ester- and diacylglycerol-induced augmentation of transmitter release is mediated by Munc13 s and not by PKCs. Cell 108:121–133

Richmond JE, Davis WS, Jorgensen EM (1999) UNC-13 is required for synaptic vesicle fusion in C. elegans. Nat Neurosci 2:959–964

Richmond JE, Weimer RM, Jorgensen EM (2001) An open form of syntaxin bypasses the requirement for UNC-13 in vesicle priming. Nature 412:338–341

Ringstad N, Gad H, Löw P, DiPaolo G, Brodin L, Shupliakov O, De Camilli P (1999) Endophilin/SH3P4 is required for the transition from early to late stages in clathrin-mediated synaptic vesicles endocytosis. Neuron 24:143–154

Robinson IM, Ranjan R, Schwarz TL (2002) Synaptotagmins I and IV promote transmitter release independently of Ca^{2+} binding in the C_2A domain. Nature 418:336–340

Rosahl TW, Geppert M, Spillane D, Herz J, Hammer RE, Malenka RC, Südhof TC (1993) Short-term synaptic plasticity is altered in mice lacking synapsin I. Cell 75:661–670.

Rosahl TW, Spillane D, Missler M, Herz J, Selig DK, Wolff JR, Hammer RE, Malenka RC, Südhof TC (1995) Essential functions of synapsins I and II in synaptic vesicle regulation. Nature 375:488–493

Rosenmund C, Sigler A, Augustin I, Reim K, Brose N, Rhee JS (2002) Differential control of vesicle priming and short-term plasticity by Munc13 isoforms. Neuron 33:411–424

Saegusa H, Kurihara T, Zong S, Kazuno A, Matsuda Y, Nonaka T, Han W, Toriyama H, Tanabe T (2001) Suppression of inflammatory and neuropathic pain symptoms in mice lacking the N-type Ca^{2+} channel. EMBO J 20:2349–2356

Saegusa H, Kurihara T, Zong S, Minowa O, Kazuno A, Han W, Matsuda Y, Yamanaka H, Osanai M, Noda T, Tanabe T (2000) Altered pain responses in mice lacking alpha 1E subunit of the voltage-dependent Ca^{2+} channel. Proc Natl Acad Sci USA 97:6132–6137

Sagne C, El Mestikawy S, Isambert MF, Hamon M, Henry JP, Giros B, Gasnier B (1997) Cloning of a functional vesicular GABA and glycine transporter by screening of genome databases. FEBS Lett 417:177–183

Sakaguchi G, Manabe T, Kobayashi K, Orita S, Sasaki T, Naito A, Maeda M, Igarashi H, Katsuura G, Nishioka H, Mizoguchi A, Itohara S, Takahashi T, Takai Y (1999) Doc2alpha is an activity-dependent modulator of excitatory synaptic transmission. Eur J Neurosci 11:4262–4268

Schikorski T, Stevens CF (2001) Morphological correlates of functionally defined synaptic vesicle populations. Nat Neurosci 4:391–395

Schlüter OM, Schnell E, Verhage M, Tzonopoulos T, Nicoll RA, Janz R, Malenka RC, Geppert M, Südhof TC (1999) Rabphilin knockout mice reveal that rabphilin is not required for rab3 function in regulating neurotransmitter release. J Neurosci 19:5834–5846

Schmid SL (1997) Clathrin-coated vesicle formation and protein sorting: an integrated process. Annu Rev Biochem 66:511–548

Schmid SL, McNiven MA, De Camilli P (1998) Dynamin and its partners: a progress report. Curr Opin Cell Biol 10:504–512

Schmidt A, Wolde M, Thiele C, Fest W, Kratzin H, Podtelejnikov AV, Witke W, Huttner WB, Söling HD (1999) Endophilin I mediates synaptic vesicle formation by transfer of arachidonate to lysophosphatidic acid. Nature 401:133–141

Schneggenburger R, Neher E (2000) Intracellular calcium dependence of transmitter release rates at a fast central synapse. Nature 406:889–893

Schoch S, Castillo PE, Jo T, Mukherjee K, Geppert M, Wang Y, Schmitz F, Malenka RC, Südhof TC (2002) RIM1alpha forms a protein scaffold for regulating neurotransmitter release at the active zone. Nature 415:321–326

Schoch S, Deak F, Konigstorfer A, Mozhayeva M, Sara Y, Südhof TC, Kavalali ET (2001) SNARE function analyzed in synaptobrevin/VAMP knockout mice. Science 294:1117–1122

Silva AJ, Rosahl TW, Chapman PF, Marowitz Z, Friedman E, Frankland PW, Cestari V, Cioffi D, Südhof TC, Bourtchuladze R (1996) Impaired learning in mice with abnormal short-lived plasticity. Curr Biol 6:1509–1518

Sorensen JB, Matti U, Wei SH, Nehring RB, Voets T, Ashery U, Binz T, Neher E, Rettig J (2002) The SNARE protein SNAP-25 is linked to fast calcium triggering of exocytosis. Proc Natl Acad Sci USA 99:1627–1632

Spiwoks-Becker I, Vollrath L, Seeliger MW, Jaissle G, Eshkind LG, Leube RE (2001) Synaptic vesicle alterations in rod photoreceptors of synaptophysin-deficient mice. Neuroscience 107:127–142

Stevens CF, Williams JH (2000) "Kiss and run" exocytosis at hippocampal synapses. Proc Natl Acad Sci USA 97:12828–12832

Stevens TH, Forgac M (1997) Structure, function and regulation of the vacuolar (H^+)-ATPase. Annu Rev Cell Dev Biol 13:779–808

Steyer JA, Almers W (1999) Tracking single secretory granules in live chromaffin cells by evanescent-field fluorescence microscopy. Biophys J 76:2262–2271

Stobrawa SM, Breiderhoff T, Takamori S, Engel D, Schweizer M, Zdebik AA, Bosl MR, Ruether K, Jahn H, Draguhn A, Jahn R, Jentsch TJ (2001) Disruption of ClC-3, a chloride channel expressed on synaptic vesicles, leads to a loss of the hippocampus. Neuron 29:185–196

Südhof TC (2000) The synaptic vesicle cycle revisited. Neuron 28:317–320

Südhof TC (2002) Synaptotagmins: why so many? J Biol Chem 277:7629–7632

Südhof TC, De Camilli P, Niemann H, Jahn R (1993) Membrane fusion machinery: insights from synaptic proteins. Cell 75:1–4

Sutton RB, Fasshauer D, Jahn R, Brunger AT (1998) Crystal structure of a SNARE complex involved in synaptic exocytosis at 2.4 A resolution. Nature 395:347–353

Takahashi N, Miner LL, Sora I, Ujike H, Revay RS, Kostic V, Jackson-Lewis V, Przedborski S, Uhl GR (1997) VMAT2 knockout mice: heterozygotes display reduced amphetamine-conditioned reward, enhanced amphetamine locomotion, and enhanced MPTP toxicity. Proc Natl Acad Sci USA 94:9938–9943

Takahashi S, Ujihara H, Huang GZ, Yagyu KI, Sanbo M, Kaba H, Yagi T (1999) Reduced hippocampal LTP in mice lacking a presynaptic protein: complexin II. Eur J Neurosci 11:2359–2366

Takamori S, Rhee JS, Rosenmund C, Jahn R (2001) Identification of differentiation-associated brain-specific phosphate transporter as a second vesicular glutamate transporter (VGLUT2). J Neurosci 21:RC182

Takei K, Slepnev VI, Haucke V, De Camilli P (1999) Functional partnership between amphiphysin and dynamin in clathrin-mediated endocytosis. Nat Cell Biol 1:33–39

Tanaka M, Miyoshi J, Ishizaki H, Togawa A, Ohnishi K, Endo K, Matsubara K, Mizoguchi A, Nagano T, Sato M, Sasaki T, Takai (2001) Role of Rab3 GDP/GTP exchange protein in synaptic vesicle trafficking at the mouse neuromuscular junction. Mol Biol Cell 12:1421–1430

Tarsa L, Goda Y (2002) Synaptophysin regulates activity-dependent synapse formation in cultured hippocampal neurons. Proc Natl Acad Sci 99:1012–1016

Terada S, Tsujimoto T, Takei Y, Takahashi T, Hirokawa N (1999) Impairment of inhibitory synaptic transmission in mice lacking synapsin I. J Cell Biol 145:1039–1048

Tobaben S, Südhof TC, Stahl B (2002) Genetic analysis of alpha-latrotoxin receptors reveals functional interdependence of CIRL/latrophilin 1 and neurexin 1 alpha. J Biol Chem 277:6359–6365.

Tobaben S, Thakur P, Fernandez-Chacon R, Südhof TC, Rettig J, Stahl B (2001) A trimeric protein complex functions as a synaptic chaperone machine. Neuron 31:987–999

Travis ER, Wang YM, Michael DJ, Caron MG, Wightman RM (2000) Differential quantal release of histamine and 5-hydroxytryptamine from mast cells of vesicular monoamine transporter 2 knockout mice. Proc Natl Acad Sci USA 97:162–167

Uhl GR, Li S, Takahashi N, Itokawa K, Lin Z, Hazama M, Sora I (2000) The VMAT2 gene in mice and humans: amphetamine responses, locomotion, cardiac arrhythmias, aging, and vulnerability to dopaminergic toxins. FASEB J 14:2459–2465

Ungewickell E (1999) Wrapping the package. Proc Natl Acad Sci USA 96:8809–8810

Varoqueaux F, Sigler A, Rhee JS, Brose N, Enk C, Reim K, Rosenmund C (2002) Total arrest of spontaneous and evoked synaptic transmission but normal synaptogenesis in the absence of Munc13-mediated vesicle priming. Proc Natl Acad Sci USA 99:9037–9042

Verhage M, Maia AS, Plomp JJ, Brussaard AB, Heeroma JH, Vermeer H, Toonen RF, Hammer RE, van den Berg TK, Missler M, Geuze HJ, Südhof TC (2000) Synaptic assembly of the brain in the absence of neurotransmitter secretion. Science 287:864–869

Voets T, Toonen RF, Brian EC, de Wit H, Moser T, Rettig J, Südhof TC, Neher E, Verhage M (2001) Munc18-1 promotes large dense-core vesicle docking. Neuron 31:581–591

Wang YM, Gainetdinov RR, Fumagalli F, Xu F, Jones SR, Bock CB, Miller GW, Wightman RM, Caron MG (1997) Knockout of the vesicular monoamine transporter 2 gene results in neonatal death and supersensitivity to cocaine and amphetamine. Neuron 19:1285–1296

Washbourne P, Thompson PM, Carta M, Costa ET, Mathews JR, Lopez-Bendito G, Molnar Z, Becher MW, Valenzuela CF, Partridge LD, Wilson MC (2002) Genetic ablation of the t-SNARE SNAP-25 distinguishes mechanisms of neuroexocytosis. Nat Neurosci 5:19–26

Weber T, Zemelman BV, McNew JA, Westermann B, Gmachl M, Parlati F, Sollner TH, Rothman JE (1998) SNAREpins: minimal machinery for membrane fusion. Cell 92:759–772

Xu T, Bajjalieh SM (2001) SV2 modulates the size of the readily releasable pool of secretory vesicles. Nat Cell Biol 3:691–698

Zwingman TA, Neumann PE, Noebels JL, Herrup K (2001) Rocker is a new variant of the voltage-dependent calcium channel gene Cacna1a. J Neurosci 21:1169–1178

Analysis of GABA Receptor Assembly and Function in Targeted Mutant Mice

U. Rudolph

Institute of Pharmacology and Toxicology,
Winterthurerstrasse 190, 8057 Zürich, Switzerland
e-mail: rudolph@pharma.unizh.ch

Abstract GABA is the major inhibitory neurotransmitter in the central nervous system, acting via ionotropic GABA$_A$ receptors and metabotropic GABA$_B$ receptors. GABA$_A$ receptors are molecular substrates for the regulation of vigilance, anxiety, muscle tension, epileptogenic activity and memory functions and the enhancement of GABA$_A$ receptor-mediated fast synaptic inhibition is the basis of the pharmacotherapy of various neurological and psychiatric disorders. The GABA$_B$ receptor is a target for the treatment of spasticity, migraine headache and musculoskeletal pain. GABA$_A$ receptors are pentameric complexes assembled from a repertoire of at least 18 subunits (α_1–α_6, β_1–β_3, γ_1–γ_3, δ, ε, θ, ρ_1–ρ_3), whereas GABA$_B$ receptors are heterodimers composed of the GABA$_{B1}$ and GABA$_{B2}$ subunits. Two kinds of GABA$_A$ receptor-targeted mutant mice have been generated: (1) knock-out mice which lack individual GABA$_A$ receptor subunits (α_1, α_5, α_6, β_2, β_3, γ_2, δ, ρ_1) and (2) knock-in mice which carry point mutations affecting the action of modulatory drugs [α_1(H101R), α_2(H101R), α_3(H126R) and α_5(H105R)]. With regard to the GABA$_B$ receptor, the GABA$_{B1}$ receptor subunit has been knocked out. Whereas the knockout mice have provided information primarily with respect to regulation of subunit gene transcription, receptor assembly and some physiological functions of individual receptor subtypes, the point-mutated knock-in mice, in which specific GABA$_A$ receptor subtypes are insensitive to diazepam, have revealed the contribution of individual receptor subtypes to the broad pharmacological spectrum of diazepam. The insights obtained studying targeting mutant mice are expected to aid in the development of novel subtype-specific drugs with fewer side effects than the drugs currently in clinical use.

Keywords GABA receptor · Neurotransmitter · Central nervous system · Benzodiazepines · Diazepam · Anxiolysis · Hypnosis · Fear conditioning

1
Introduction

γ-Aminobutyric acid (GABA) is the major inhibitory neurotransmitter in the central nervous system. It is synthesized in presynaptic terminals from glutamate by the enzyme glutamic acid decarboxylase (GAD), stored in vesicles and released into the synaptic cleft by an action potential. GABA binds to postsynaptic ionotropic GABA$_A$ receptors, which mediate fast responses, and pre- and postsynaptic metabotropic, G protein-coupled GABA$_B$ receptors, which mediate slow responses. Binding of GABA to the GABA$_A$ receptor is followed in a matter of milliseconds—in most cases—by an influx of chloride ions, leading to hyperpolarization and thus functional inhibition of the postsynaptic neuron. GABA$_B$ receptors are found both pre- and postsynaptically. Their activation inhibits basal and forskolin-stimulated adenylyl cyclase activity, decreases Ca^{2+} conductance and increases K$^+$ conductance (for review see Bowery et al. 2002). GABA is removed from the synaptic cleft by GABA transporters and metabolized in a transamination reaction (Fig. 1). This review is mainly focussed on the analysis of assembly and function of GABA$_A$ receptors.

GABA$_A$ receptors belong to the superfamily of ligand-gated ion channels and are pentameric membrane protein complexes that operate as GABA-gated chloride channels. They have an extracellular N-terminal domain, four putative transmembrane domains, and an extracellular C-terminal domain. The second transmembrane domain presumably lines the channel. The third intracellular

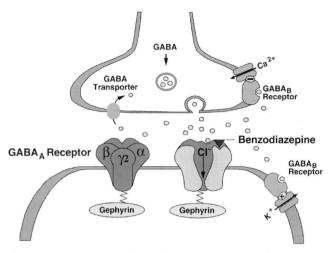

Fig. 1 GABAergic synapse. Scheme of a GABAergic synapse, depicting major elements of signal transduction. Postsynaptic GABA$_A$ receptors are pentameric ligand-gated ion channels assembled from various types of subunits. On the cytoplasmatic site they are indirectly linked to gephyrin. Metabotropic GABA$_B$ receptors are found pre- and postsynaptically and regulate Ca^{2+} and K^+ conductances. (Adapted from Möhler et al. 2002)

loop contains consensus sequences for phosphorylation by protein kinases. On the cytoplasmic side, most GABA$_A$ receptors appear to be linked indirectly to the cytoskeletal protein gephyrin via the γ_2 subunit (Essrich et al. 1998). There are seven classes of subunits with mostly multiple variants (α_1–α_6, β_1–β_3, γ_1–γ_3, δ, ε, θ, ρ_1–ρ_3). Among themselves, α subunits share greater than ca. 70% amino acid sequence identity, whereas from one subunit class to another, the identity is in the range of ca. 30%–40%. Most GABA$_A$ receptors are composed of α, β and γ subunits with $\alpha 1\beta 2,3\gamma 2$ being the most abundant receptor subtype (Fritschy et al. 1992), representing more than half of all GABA$_A$ receptors (Möhler et al. 1995; McKernan and Whiting 1996).

GABA$_A$ receptors play an essential role in regulating the excitability of the brain. Their activity is modulated by a variety of therapeutic agents, including benzodiazepines, barbiturates, neurosteroids and general anaesthetics (Fig. 2). The $\alpha 1$ subunit is by far the most abundant α subunit and expressed for instance in cerebral cortex, cerebellar cortex, hippocampus and thalamus. The other α subunits have more restricted distribution patterns. For instance, the $\alpha 2$ subunit is largely expressed is hippocampus, striatum and amygdala, the $\alpha 3$ subunit in monoaminergic and serotonergic neurons of the brain stem, in basal forebrain cholinergic neurons and in the reticular nucleus of the thalamus, the $\alpha 4$ subunit in the thalamus, the $\alpha 5$ subunit in the hippocampus and the $\alpha 6$ subunit in cerebellar granule cells (Fritschy and Möhler 1995). Among the β subunits, the β_2 subunit is the most abundant (55%–60% of GABA$_A$ receptors), followed by the β_3 and the β_1 subunits (19%–26% and 16%–18% of GABA$_A$ receptors, respectively) (Benke et al. 1994). The by far most abundant γ subunit is γ_2

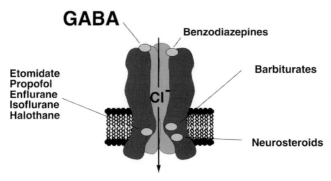

Fig. 2 Model of a GABA$_A$ receptor and its binding sites. In addition to the binding site for the neurotransmitter GABA, GABA$_A$ receptors have modulatory sites for a variety of ligands including benzodiazepines, barbiturates, neurosteroids and general anaesthetics such as isoflurane, enflurane, halothane, etomidate and propofol. The positioning and size of these sites is arbitrary. One subunit has been removed to visualize the pore. (Adapted from Möhler et al. 1996)

(ca. 90% of all γ subunit-containing receptors), whereas γ_1 and γ_3 are rare. In some instances, receptors contain a δ subunit presumably instead of a γ subunit. The GABA binding site is most likely located at the interface between α and β subunits. The binding site for modulatory benzodiazepines is, however, most likely located at the interface between α and γ subunits (Stephenson et al. 1990; Smith and Olsen 1995). Recombinant receptors consisting of α and β subunits only are activated by GABA, but a γ subunit is necessary to convey modulation by benzodiazepines (Pritchett et al. 1989). The GABA$_A$ receptors containing the α_1, α_2, α_3 and α_5 subunits (in addition to β and γ subunits) are sensitive to modulation by classical benzodiazepines such as diazepam, whereas receptors containing the α_4 and α_6 subunits are not.

2
GABA$_A$ Receptor Subunit Expression and Assembly

2.1
Regulation of Subunit Gene Transcription Following Gene Inactivation

When individual components of multimeric receptor complexes are lacking due to a gene knockout, the question arises whether the missing subunit is replaced by another subunit of the same class, whether there are compensatory up- or downregulations of other GABA$_A$ receptor subunits, whether the expression of GABA$_A$ receptor subunits and composition of GABA$_A$ receptor complexes are altered in a particular brain region or neuron or whether there is no change detectable at the transcriptional and/or translational level apart from the subunit in question following the knockout of a receptor subunit.

In γ_2 subunit knockout mice, which die shortly after birth, the protein levels of the subunits α_1, α_2, α_3, $\beta_{2,3}$, γ_1 and γ_3 were unaltered as shown by immunoblotting, indicating that in this case there are no major up- or downregulations of other receptor subunits (Günther et al. 1995). In β_2 and β_3 subunit knockout mice, other β subunits were unable to substitute for the lacking β subunit (Homanics et al. 1997b; Sur et al. 2001).

Inactivation of the α_6 subunit gene, which is expressed in cerebellar granule cells, did not change the levels of α_1, $\beta_{2,3}$, and γ_2 subunit in the cerebellum, as shown by radioligand binding and α_1 subunit immunohistochemistry. However, in Western blotting there was a trend towards lower levels of the α_1 subunit protein (Jones et al. 1997). In an α_6 knockout generated independently, the mRNA levels for α_1, α_3, β_2, γ_2 and δ were unaltered, while diazepam-insensitive [^{3}H]Ro15-4513 binding to cerebellar granule cells was reduced, consistent with the loss of receptors containing the α_6 subunit (Homanics et al. 1997a). However, when the α_6 knockout mice generated by Wisden and collaborators (Jones et al. 1997) were examined in more detail, the composition of receptors found in the cerebellum was shown to be altered. Immunoprecipitation and ligand binding revealed that the total number of GABA$_A$ receptors was reduced by ca. 50% in the cerebellum of α_6 knockout mice. The amounts of β_2, β_3 and γ_2 subunits were reduced by ca. 50%, 20% and 40%, respectively, as detected by immunoblotting. The proportion of receptors containing β_3 subunits was increased in the cerebellum of α_6 knockout mice, indicating that the remaining GABA$_A$ receptors display an overall altered subunit distribution (Nusser et al. 1999). In the same α_6 knockout mice, it was also found that the expression of the α_1 and β_2 genes in the forebrain was reduced by ca. 43% and 25%, respectively, as assessed by immunoblotting. The expression of the γ_2 and β_3 subunits was not changed. These changes are most likely due to elements in the neomycin-resistance gene that was used for generating the α_6 knockout, which affect the transcription of neighbouring genes. In the genome, the genes for GABA$_A$ receptor subunits are clustered. A cluster containing the α_1, α_6, β_2, and γ_2 subunit genes is located on mouse chromosome 11. Thus, elements in the neomycin-resistance gene appear to reduce the expression of the neighbouring genes (Uusi-Oukari et al. 2000). This artefact may limit the usefulness of this animal model, since it may be difficult to decide whether e.g. a behavioural phenotypic abnormality is due to the lack of the α_6 subunit or due to the downregulation of α_1 and β_2 in the forebrain.

In α_1 knockout mice, more than 50% of total GABA$_A$ receptors are lost. However, the expression of α_2 and α_3 subunits is increased by 42% as seen in quantitative immunoprecipitation experiments, which can be viewed as a compensatory upregulation. In addition, the abundance of α_6 subunits in the cerebellum was reduced by ca. 38%, as assessed by radioligand binding (Sur et al. 2001). Thus, the lack of the α_1 subunit causes compensatory changes in the expression of several other subunits, indicating that phenotypes seen in these animals should be interpreted with these changes in mind.

In the β_2 knockout mice, the expression of the α subunits α_1–α_6 was reduced by ca. 39%–62%, indicating that the β_2 subunits also associate with α subunits other than α_1 (Sur et al. 2001).

2.2
Subunits Required for Receptor Assembly

Most GABA$_A$ receptors contain α, β and γ subunits. Mutant animals lacking individual subunits have provided information on whether all three subunit types are required to form receptors in the brain. As already mentioned, in α_1 knockout mice, more than 50% of total GABA$_A$ receptors are lost, indicating that in the absence of the α_1 subunit, the respective receptors normally containing the α_1 subunit are not formed (Sur et al. 2001). In α_5 knockout mice, the α_5 GABA$_A$ receptors, which are located primarily in the hippocampus, appear to be lost, without detectable upregulation of other α subunits. However, since even in the hippocampus, α_5 GABA$_A$ receptors only represent ca. 20% of all GABA$_A$ receptors, it might be difficult to detect potential minor changes in subunit expression (Collinson et al. 2002). Interestingly, in hippocampal pyramidal cells of mice lacking the α_5 subunit (and the γ_3 subunit) due to chromosomal deletions on both alleles which have been generated by random mutagenesis (Culiat et al. 1994), the α_2 subunits remained targeted to the axon initial segments and did not replace the α_5 subunit at their somatic and dendritic sites, indicating that each receptor subtype is programmed for a specific subcellular localization (Fritschy et al. 1998).

In the β_2 knockout mice, where the expression of all α subunits was reduced dramatically (39%–69%) (Sur et al. 2001) and in the β_3 knockout mice, where also about half of the GABA$_A$ receptors were lost (Homanics et al. 1997b), the receptors normally incorporating the knocked-out subunit were apparently largely not formed. In contrast, the number of GABA$_A$ receptors was apparently unchanged in γ_2 knockout mice as shown by immunoblotting. However, the number of benzodiazepine binding sites was reduced by 90% (Günther et al. 1995). The apparent $\alpha\beta$ receptors had a normal dose–response curve for GABA, but the single channel conductance was reduced (Günther et al. 1995; Lorez et al. 2000) and while the benzodiazepine response was missing, the response to barbiturates was retained (Günther et al. 1995). These results show that receptors containing of α and β subunits can be assembled in the brain (though not properly clustered, see Essrich et al. 1998). Extrapolated from a previous study on recombinant receptors (Baumann et al. 2001), these $\alpha\beta$ receptors most likely contain two α and three β subunits. The lack of the γ_2 subunit affects responses to both GABA and benzodiazepines. Thus, whereas receptors are not assembled when the respective α or β subunits are missing, receptors most likely consisting of only α and β subunits can be assembled and inserted into the plasma membrane in the absence of a γ subunit.

The δ subunit preferentially assembles with the α_4 subunit in the forebrain. In δ subunit knockout mice (Mihalek et al. 1999), the level of γ_2 was increased and the level of α_4 decreased in immunoblots of forebrain membranes, while the level of α_1 was unaltered. As shown by immunoprecipitation with an antiserum recognizing γ_2, the remaining α_4 subunits were more often associated with γ_2 subunits. This was paralleled by an increase in diazepam-insensitive benzodiazepine binding sites in receptor autoradiography (Korpi et al. 2002). These data support the idea of selective subunit assembly based on subunit availability and their competition in assembly mechanisms. Similarly, in a separate study, it was shown that γ_2 subunit expression was increased and α_4 subunit expression was decreased in areas of the forebrain normally expressing the δ subunit (Peng et al. 2002).

In the α_6 knockout mice, the δ subunit mRNA was present in cerebellar granule cells at the same level as in wild type, however, a δ subunit-specific antibody failed to detect the δ subunit in immunoprecipitation, immunocytochemistry and immunoblot analysis. These findings indicate a post-translational loss of the δ subunit in the absence of the α_6 subunit and thus indicate a specific partnership between the α_6 and δ subunits (Jones et al. 1997).

3
GABA$_A$ Receptor Function

In the following paragraph we will review the lessons learned from gene knockouts and knock-ins with a particular emphasis on behavioural phenotypes.

3.1
Gene Knockout Studies

The following GABA$_A$ receptors subunits have been knocked out: α_1, α_5, α_6, β_2, β_3, γ_2, δ, and ρ_1. Selected phenotypes of these mice are summarized in Table 1.

3.1.1
α_1 Subunit

Since the majority of diazepam-sensitive GABA$_A$ receptors contain the α_1 subunit, it is somewhat surprising that α_1 knockout mice are viable, although underrepresented in offspring from heterozygote crosses, indicating that there is some lethality. Apart from the changes in subunit expression described above ("Regulation of Subunit Gene Transcription Following Gene Inactivation"), α_1 knockout mice had lower body weights (ca. 30%) until the age of at least 3 months and exhibited a tremor when handled. They did not display any major deficits in beam balancing and swimming ability tests. The level of spontaneous locomotor activity and exploration and the performance on the rotating rod were similar to wild type (Sur et al. 2001). Further behavioural analysis was not reported. In an independently generated line of α_1 knockout mice, the developmental changes of inhibitory synaptic currents in cerebellar neurons seen in wild type mice were absent (Vicini et al. 2001).

Table 1 Overview of selected phenotypes of GABA$_A$ receptor subunit knockout mice

α_1	No spontaneous seizures Normal locomotor activity and motor performance	Sur et al. 2001; Vicini et al. 2001
α_5	Improved performance in a hippocampus-dependent task (spatial learning)	Collinson et al. 2002
α_6	Posttranslational loss of δ subunit in cerebellum Increased expression of TASK-1 K$^+$ channels	Jones et al. 1997; Homanics et al. 1997a; Brickley et al. 2001
β_2	Increased locomotor activity in novel environment No spontaneous seizures	Sur et al. 2001
β_3	Cleft palate Neonatally lethal (ca. 90%) Hyperactive Spontaneous seizures Hyperresponsive Motor impairment	Homanics et al. 1997b; DeLorey et al. 1998
$\gamma 2$	Homozygotes: Neonatally lethal Defects in postsynaptic clustering of GABA$_A$ receptors Heterozygotes: Reduction of synaptic clustering e.g. in hippocampus, chronic anxiety Heightened responsiveness in trace fear conditioning and ambiguous cue discrimination	Gunther et al. 1995; Essrich et al. 1998; Crestani et al. 1999
δ	Attenuation of responses to neuroactive steroids Reduced ethanol consumption Attenuated withdrawal from chronic ethanol exposure Reduced anticonvulsant effect of ethanol	Mihalek et al. 1999, 2001
ρ_1	Alteration of the& excitation/inhibition balance between second and third retinal neurons	McCall et al. 2002

3.1.2
α_5 Subunit

α_5 Knockout mice display no overt phenotypic abnormalities. Motor performance and coordination were also normal. The benzodiazepine chlordiazepoxide retained its anxiolytic-like action in these mice. Strikingly, in the Morris water maze test of spatial learning, α_5 knockout mice find the platform earlier than wild type mice, indicating that in a hippocampus-dependent task these mice show a significantly improved performance. In the two-way active avoidance paradigm, which is thought to be hippocampus-independent, the performance of α_5 knockout mice and wild type mice was indistinguishable. Evidence for the specific alteration of hippocampal functions were also obtained in point-mutated α_5(H105R) mice (Crestani et al. 2002; see also Sect. 3.2.5). Thus, the α_5-containing GABA$_A$ receptors play a central role in cognitive processes. This is in line with the localization of α_5 subunits predominantly in dendritic regions of the CA1–CA3 fields of the hippocampus. In fact, the amplitude of the IPSCs was decreased in the CA1 region of hippocampal slices from α_5 knockout mice, and the paired-pulse facilitation of field EPSP (fEPSP) amplitudes was enhanced. Taken together, these results suggest that an inverse agonist selective for α_5-containing GABA$_A$ receptors may be useful as a drug enhancing cognitive functions (Collinson et al. 2002)

3.1.3
α_6 Subunit

Two lines of α_6 knockout mice have been generated independently. For one of these lines, its was reported that the mice showed the same level of exploratory activity in the open field as wild type mice, and the same behaviour on the rotating rod and the horizontal wire (Jones et al. 1997). However, in the rotating rod test, α_6 knockout mice were significantly more impaired by diazepam than wild type mice (Korpi et al 1999). This is surprising since the α_6-containing GABA$_A$ receptors are diazepam-insensitive. Thus, these changes may be due to compensatory alterations in the cerebellum or due to the fact that the expression of the diazepam-sensitive GABA$_A$ receptors containing the α_1 and β_2 subunits in the forebrain is decreased due to the presence of the neomycin resistance cassette in the α_6 gene (see Sect. 2.1). Ethanol produced similar impairments of the rotating rod performance in α_6 knockout and wild type mice (Korpi et al. 1999). In the other α_6 knockout mouse line, the duration of the loss of the righting reflex in response to ethanol, enflurane and halothane was the same as in wild type mice. In addition, the tail-clamp/withdrawal response to enflurane was also identical in both genotypes (Homanics et al. 1997a). Thus, the α_6-containing GABA$_A$ receptors do not appear to be relevant for mediating the behavioural responses to these agents. Perhaps most importantly, the α_6 knockout mice have provided an insight into mechanisms involved in the regulation of tonic inhibition. In cerebellar granule cells from these mice, a tonic conductance, which is dependent on the presence of the GABA$_A$ receptor α_6 subunit, is absent. However, the response of these cells to excitatory synaptic input is unaltered. This appears to be due to an increased voltage-independent K$^+$ conductance maintaining normal neuronal behaviour, with properties characteristic of the two-pore-domain K$^+$ channel TASK-1 (Brickley et al. 2001).

3.1.4
β_2 Subunit

The β_2 subunit is the most abundant of the three β subunits. Nevertheless, the β_2 knockout mice had no obvious phenotypic abnormalities, normal body weights and did not display major deficits in the rotating rod, beam balancing and swimming ability tests. When β_2 knockout mice were placed in a novel environment, they exhibited a higher level of locomotor activity than wild type mice, although they habituated to a similar degree as wild type mice. The basis for this observation is not known (Sur et al. 2001). Further behavioural studies on these mice have not been reported.

3.1.5
β_3 Subunit

Mice lacking the β_3 subunit have been generated by random radiation-induced mutagenesis before GABA$_A$ receptor subunit knockout mice became available. Deletion mutants have been identified which encompass the pink-eyed dilution (p) locus on mouse chromosome 7, which is located close to a cluster of the genes encoding the α_5, β_3 and γ_3 subunits. Various deletion mutants were identified, which had also lost the genes encoding the γ_3 subunit, the γ_3 and the α_5 subunits or the γ_3, α_5 and the β_3 subunits (Culiat et al. 1993; Nakatsu et al. 1993; Culiat et al. 1994). It was observed that while mice lacking the γ_3 and α_5 subunits are viable without apparent major deficits, mice lacking the γ_3, α_5 and the β_3 subunits mostly die within a short period of time, presumably due to a cleft palate which interferes with sucking milk. When the β_3 subunit was expressed as a transgene in mice lacking these three subunits on their chromosomes, the cleft palate phenotype was rescued, strongly suggesting that the lack of the β_3 subunit gene was indeed responsible for the cleft palate (Culiat et al. 1995).

When the β_3 subunit was knocked out by gene targeting, ca. 90% of the mice died within 24 h of birth, which is similar to the frequencies observed in the radiation-induced mutants mentioned above. The penetrance of the cleft palate phenotype was only ca. 57% in the knockouts, which may reflect differences in genetic background or the contribution of other genes deleted in the radiation-induced mutants. It is noteworthy that the β_3 knockout mice were analysed on a hybrid (129 Sv/SvJ x C57BL/6 J) background and not on an inbred background. Frequently, phenotypes are less severe on a hybrid background. Nevertheless, in the β_3 knockout mice not all lethality was due to cleft palate to which feeding problems can be attributed. The precise cause of the mortality not dependent on cleft palate is not known. Surviving β_3 knockout mice are runted until weaning but achieve a normal body weight in adulthood (Homanics et al. 1997b). They show features which are strikingly similar to Angelman syndrome in humans. These include hyperactivity, poor learning and memory, poor motor coordination, repetitive stereotypical behaviour (running continuously in tight circles), seizures and EEG abnormalities (DeLorey et al. 1998). These findings suggest that the impaired expression of the β_3 subunit may contribute to at least some clinical features of Angelman syndrome in humans. Further phenotypic abnormalities of β_3 knockout mice that have been described are an enhanced responsiveness to low-intensity thermal stimuli and that the GABA$_A$ receptor agonist tetrahydroisoxazolopyridinol (THIP) does not produce antinociception (Ugarte et al. 2000). However, the fact that the antinociceptive effect of the GABA$_B$ receptor agonist baclofen was also reduced in β_3 knockout mice indicates that the function of other neurotransmitter receptor systems is also affected by the knockout (Ugarte et al. 2000). With respect to the response to anaesthetic agents, the duration of the loss of the righting reflex in response to midazolam and etomidate, but not to pentobarbital, ethanol, enflurane and halothane were reduced in β_3 knockout mice. The immobilizing action of enflurane and halothane as determined in a tail clamp/withdrawal assay, was decreased in β_3 knockout mice (Quinlan et al. 1998). This indicates that β_3-containing GABA$_A$ receptors may play a role in the mediation of some responses to selected general anaesthetics. However, the altered sensory threshold and the demonstration that other neurotransmitter receptors are also functionally impaired by the β_3 knockout warrant some caution in interpreting these studies. Since the loss of the righting reflex and the tail-clamp/withdrawal reflex are thought to be largely mediated at the spinal level and the β_3 subunit is abundant in the spinal cord, it can be speculated that the spinal β_3 GABA$_A$ receptors are involved in mediating actions of general anaesthetics. Interestingly, in electrophysiological studies on the spinal cord, the sensitivity of evoked responses did not differ between β_3 knockout and wild type mice, which was, however, coupled with a decreased role for GABA$_A$ receptors in mediating the actions of enflurane in the β_3 knockout. It was concluded that the mutation led to a quantitative change in the molecular basis for anaesthetic depression of spinal neurotransmission in a fashion not predicted by the mutation itself (Wong et al. 2001). These changes might be due to developmental and/or adaptive changes in response to the β_3 knockout. In another set of experiments, it was found that locomotor stimulation induced by cocaine was greater in β_3 knockout compared to wild type mice (Resnick et al. 1999). The mechanisms underlying this effect are not known.

An endogenous unsaturated fatty acid amide, oleamide, has sleep-enhancing actions in mice. It decreases sleep latency and wake time, while it increases non-rapid eye movement and total sleep in wild type mice. All of these effects are missing in the β_3 knockout mice, indicating that oleamide mediates its sleep effects via β_3-containing GABA$_A$ receptors (Laposky et al. 2001).

In electrophysiological studies in slices, GABA-mediated inhibition was abolished in reticular nucleus, but unaffected in relay cells, consistent with the observation that the β_3 subunit is largely restricted to the reticular nucleus in rodent thalamus. Oscillatory synchrony was dramatically intensified, suggesting that recurrent inhibitory connections within the reticular nucleus act as "desynchronizers" (Huntsman et al. 1999).

3.1.6
γ_2 Subunit

Historically, the γ_2 subunit was the first GABA$_A$ receptor subunit to be knocked out by gene targeting. Homozygous γ_2 knockout mice die typically in the first few days after birth. The oldest animal survived for 18 days (Günther et al. 1995). The animals displayed a defect in postsynaptic clustering of GABA$_A$ receptors, indicating that the γ_2 subunit is essential for postsynaptic clustering in vivo (Essrich et al. 1998). The survivors exhibited increased body and limb movements following birth, and later impaired grasping and righting reflexes and an abnormal gait (Günther et al. 1995). More than 90% of the benzodiazepine binding sites were absent in the brain of neonatal mice and the single channel conductance level and the Hill coefficient were reduced, as they are in recombinant $\alpha\beta$ receptors (Günther et al. 1995). It is conceivable that the lack of postsynaptic clustering and/or the decreased conductance level are directly related to the lethality of the phenotype. When the γ_3 subunit was expressed ectopically in the γ_2 knockout background, synaptic clustering was restored. However, this did not rescue the lethal γ_2 knockout phenotype (Baer et al. 1999). In mice that are heterozygous for the γ_2-null mutation, $\gamma_2^{+/-}$ mice, the synaptic clustering was reduced, mainly in hippocampus and cerebral cortex. These mice displayed an enhanced behavioural inhibition towards natural aversive stimuli and heightened responsiveness in trace fear conditioning and ambiguous cue discrimination learning. Thus, these mice represent a model of chronic anxiety, suggesting that GABA$_A$ receptor dysfunction may underlie a predisposition of patients to anxiety disorders. The anxiety-related behavioural inhibition of γ_2 heterozygous mice was reversed by diazepam, which is in line with the observation in humans that subjects with high anxiety scores are more sensitive to the anxiolytic actions of benzodiazepines than controls (Crestani et al. 1999).

The γ_2 subunit consists of a short and a long form, γ_{2S} and γ_{2L}, respectively, which arise by alternative splicing. γ_{2S} Differs from γ_{2L} by the inclusion of an exon coding for eight additional amino acids. These amino acids are located in the third intracellular loop and include a consensus sequence for protein kinase C phosphorylation. It has been proposed that these eight amino acids which are unique to γ_{2L} are required for the potentiating action of ethanol at the GABA$_A$ receptor (Wafford et al. 1991). Mice lacking the exon encoding these eight amino acids displayed electrophysiological responses to ethanol indistinguishable from wild type. Likewise, the behavioural effects of ethanol such as loss of the righting reflex, anxiolytic-like effect, acute functional tolerance, chronic withdrawal hyperexcitability and hyperlocomotor activity were not affected by the lack of these eight amino acids. Thus, the γ_{2L}-specific exon is not required for the modulatory action of ethanol at GABA$_A$ receptors and its behavioural effects (Homanics et al. 1999). In a separate set of experiments, transgenic overexpression of γ_{2S} or γ_{2L} rescued the lethal γ_2 knockout phenotype, indicating that the both forms are functionally equivalent in this respect (Baer et al. 2000).

3.1.7
δ Subunit

The role of the δ subunit has been enigmatic, perhaps in part because GABA$_A$ receptors containing α, β and δ subunits are not modulated by diazepam. At the electrophysiological level, a significantly faster miniature inhibitory postsynaptic current decay time was found in hippocampal slices from δ knockout mice, with no change in miniature inhibitory postsynaptic current amplitude or frequency. In δ subunit knockout mice, the duration of the loss of the righting reflex was significantly shorter in response to the neurosteroids alphaxalone and pregnanolone, but not in response to pentobarbital, propofol, midazolam, etomidate and ketamine. Thus, the attenuation of the responses to neuroactive steroids is strikingly selective. In the elevated plus maze, the neurosteroid ganaxolone has no anxiolytic-like effect in δ knockout mice, in contrast to wild type mice. Likewise, ganaxolone failed to prolong pentylenetetrazole-induced absence-like immobilization in δ knockout mice, indicating that GABA$_A$ receptors containing the δ subunit are involved in mediating the anxiolytic-like and pro-absence effects of neurosteroids. The duration of the loss of the righting reflex in response to halothane and the tail clamp/withdrawal response to halothane and enflurane were unaltered in the δ knockout mice. Contextual and tone fear conditioning were indistinguishable from wild type in the δ knockout, indicating that learning and memory associated with fear conditioning are normal (Mihalek et al. 1999). Furthermore, δ knockout mice display reduced consumption of ethanol, attenuated withdrawal from chronic ethanol exposure and a reduced anticonvulsant effect of ethanol. The anxiolytic-like and hypothermic responses to ethanol were indistinguishable from wild type, as were the development of acute and chronic tolerance (Mihalek et al. 2001).

3.1.8
ρ_1 Subunit

The ionotropic GABA receptors consisting of ρ subunits display different properties than the receptor subtypes described above. In particular, they are not sensitive to bicuculline and are now frequently termed GABA$_C$ receptors (Bormann 2000), whereas in the official IUPHAR nomenclature these receptors are subsumed under GABA$_A$ receptors (Barnard et al. 1998). In the retina the expression of these receptors is largely restricted to the terminals of retinal bipolar cells. These terminals transmit the visual signal to amacrine and ganglion cells. When the ρ_1 subunit was knocked out, the overall retinal and rod bipolar cell morphology was normal. However, immunohistochemical and electrophysiological measurements revealed that the expression of "GABA$_C$" receptors was eliminated. Electroretinogram (ERG) analysis revealed that only inner retinal function was altered, indicating an alteration of the excitation/inhibition balance between second and third order retinal neurons (McCall et al. 2002).

3.2
Point Mutation Studies

Although studies with knockout mice have provided important insights into the function of GABA$_A$ receptor subtypes, their limitations, including adaptive changes during development and a high complexity or even lethality of the phenotype, can make interpretation of findings difficult. However, gene-targeting technology also allows for the introduction of more subtle mutations into the mouse genome, e.g. point mutations. α Subunits that, when incorporated into recombinant receptor complexes with β and γ subunits, can bind diazepam (α_1,

α_2, α_3, and α_5) contain a histidine residue at a conserved homologous position (101, 101, 126, and 105, respectively), whereas the α subunits α_4 and α_6 contain an arginine residue at this position. When the histidine residue in the α_1 subunit was replaced by an arginine subunit, recombinant $\alpha_1\beta_2\gamma_2$ receptors became diazepam-insensitive (Wieland et al. 1992). This observation was later extended to the α_2, α_3 and α_5 subunits (Benson et al. 1998). Thus, for all diazepam-sensitive α subunits, the exchange of a histidine to an arginine residue represents a genetic switch, with which a specific GABA$_A$ receptor subtype can be rendered diazepam-insensitive.

Diazepam is a prototypic classical benzodiazepine, which is used clinically for its anxiolytic, sedative, hypnotic, anticonvulsant and myorelaxant actions. Until recently, it was not known whether specific drug effects would be mediated by defined GABA$_A$ receptor subtypes. It would in particular be desirable to develop drugs which have a more selective profile than the benzodiazepines currently in clinical use, e.g. an anxiolytic without sedative side effects. To explore the pharmacological role of defined GABA$_A$ receptor subtypes, α_1(H101R), α_2(H101R), α_3(H126R) and α_5(H105R) mice were generated (Rudolph et al. 1999; McKernan et al. 2000; Löw et al. 2000; Crestani et al. 2002). The diazepam effects that are normally mediated by the now mutated GABA$_A$ receptor subtype are expected to be absent in the respective mouse lines. Conversely, any diazepam effect that is present in a particular mouse line must be mediated by one or more of the available wild type receptor subtypes. This point-mutation strategy was designed to leave the physiological function of the mutated GABA$_A$ receptors intact and thus avoid the problems associated with typical knockouts, e.g. compensatory regulations. Analysis by immunoblotting, immunohistochemistry and immunofluorescence revealed that the mutant receptor subunits were expressed at normal levels with unaltered regional and subcellular distributions. The notable exception are the α_5(H105R) mice, where the abundance of the (extrasynaptic) α_5 subunit is reduced in the hippocampus only (not in other brain regions). The regional and subcellular localization were, however, unchanged. The significance of this finding will be discussed later.

3.2.1
Sedation, Anterograde Amnesia, and Anticonvulsant Activity of Diazepam Are Mediated by α_1-Containing GABA$_A$ Receptors

In α_1(H101R) mice, diazepam failed to reduce horizontal motor activity and the latency to enter the dark compartment in the passive avoidance paradigm. The specificity of the latter effect was confirmed with scopolamine, which retained its amnesic action in α_1(H101R) mice (Rudolph et al. 1999). In α_2(H101R), α_3(H126R) and α_5(H105R) mice, diazepam still elicited its sedative action (Löw et al. 2000; Crestani et al. 2002). Thus, the sedative and the anterograde amnesic effects of diazepam are mediated by GABA$_A$ receptors containing the α_1 subunit. The sedative action of the imidazopyridine zolpidem, a widely used hypnotic, which has a high affinity for α_1-containing GABA$_A$ receptors, an intermediate affinity for α_2- and α_3-containing GABA$_A$ receptors and no affinity for α_5-containing GABA$_A$ receptors, was also absent in α_1(H101R) mice, indicating that α_1-containing GABA$_A$ receptors are also mediating the sedative action of zolpidem (Crestani et al. 2000a).

It has been observed that when the mice are tested in a novel and thus exciting and stressful environment, diazepam may increase the locomotor activity in α_1(H101R) mice. This locomotor stimulant effect is thus likely to be mediated by α_2-, α_3-, or α_5-containing GABA$_A$ receptors (McKernan et al. 2000; Crestani et al. 2000b). In contrast, in a familiar environment, diazepam decreases motor activity in wild type but not in α_1(H101R) mice (Rudolph et al. 1999). Thus, the novelty or familiarity of the test environment is a parameter that critically affects the motor behaviour.

The anticonvulsant activity of diazepam was assessed using the pentylenetetrazole convulsion test. Diazepam, given 30 min before the pentylenetetrazole, can protect wild type mice from tonic seizures. This protective effect was reduced in α_1(H101R) mice (Rudolph et al. 1999), but not in α_2(H101R), α_3(H126R) and α_5(H105R) mice (Löw et al. 2000; Crestani et al. 2002). Thus, the anticonvulsant activity of diazepam is mediated in part by α_1-containing GABA$_A$ receptors. It is possible that the remainder of the anticonvulsant action of diazepam will require at least two different GABA$_A$ receptor subtypes to act in concert. Whereas diazepam displays activity against myoclonic jerks in wild type mice and to a significantly reduced degree in α_1(H101R) mice, zolpidem did not display this kind of activity even in wild type mice. However, zolpidem was active against tonic convulsions in wild type mice but not in α_1(H101R) mice, indicating that this activity of zolpidem is entirely mediated by α_1-containing GABA$_A$ receptors (Crestani et al. 2000a).

3.2.2
Anxiolytic-Like Activity of Diazepam Is Mediated via α_2-Containing GABA$_A$ Receptors

Since the anxiolytic-like activity of diazepam, as assessed in two ethological tests of anxiety, the light-dark choice test and the elevated plus maze test, was still present in the α_1(H101R) mice, it is likely to be mediated by GABA$_A$ receptors not containing the α_1 subunit. In the light-dark choice test and the elevated plus maze test, diazepam increased the time the mice spent in the lit compartment or the open arms, respectively, in wild type mice, α_3(H126R) mice and α_5(H105R) mice, but not in α_2(H101R) mice (Löw et al. 2000; Crestani et al. 2002). This indicates that α_2-containing GABA$_A$ receptors, which constitute only ca. 15% of the diazepam-sensitive GABA$_A$ receptors (Marksitzer et al. 1993) but not α_3- or α_5-containing GABA$_A$ receptors, mediate the anxiolytic-like action of diazepam. The finding that GABA$_A$ receptors containing the α_2 subunit mediate the anxiolytic-like action of diazepam is consistent with the expression of this subunit in brain regions that are involved in emotional stimulus processing, e.g. amygdala and hippocampus (Fritschy and Möhler 1995).

Table 2 Proposed roles of GABA$_A$ receptor subtypes in benzodiazepine action based on analysis of point-mutated α subunit knock-in mice. The functional roles of GABA$_A$ receptor subtypes defined by the presence of the α_1, α_2, α_3 or α_5 subunits mediating particular actions of diazepam are indicated

	α_1	α_2	α_3	α_5
Sedation	+	−	−	−
Anterograde amnesia	+	ND	ND	ND
Anticonvulsant activity	+	−	−	−
Anxiolysis-	+	−	−	−
Myorelaxation	−	+	+	+

ND, not determined; +, response is absent in the mouse line carrying a point mutation in the subunit in question and thus mediated by the respective receptor subtype; −, response is present in the mutant mouse line and apparently not mediated by the respective receptor subtype.
Original data are from Rudolph et al. (1999), McKernan et al. (2000), Low et al. (2000) and Crestani et al.& (2002).

3.2.3
Myorelaxant Activity of Diazepam Is Mediated via α_2-, α_3- and α_5-Containing GABA$_A$ Receptors

The myorelaxant activity was assessed in the horizontal wire test. In wild type mice, diazepam impairs the grasping reflex and the animals are not able to grasp the wire firmly. This activity of diazepam was completely preserved in α_1(H101R) mice (Rudolph et al. 1999; McKernan et al. 2000). In α_2(H101R) mice, however, it was absent at a dose of 10 mg/kg diazepam, which is myorelaxant in wild type mice. At a higher dose (30 mg/kg), diazepam had some residual myorelaxant effect in α_2(H101R) mice. These findings were specific, since the myorelaxant action of the GABA$_B$ receptor agonist baclofen is not different in α_2(H101R) and wild type mice. In α_3(H126R) mice, diazepam has a myorelaxant effect at 10 and 30 mg/kg, but at 30 mg/kg this effect is reduced compared to wild type mice (Crestani et al. 2001). In α_5(H105R) mice, diazepam is not myorelaxant at 10 mg/kg, and at 30 mg/kg its effect was smaller compared to wild type (Crestani et al. 2002). Thus, the myorelaxant action of diazepam appears to be mediated by GABA$_A$ receptors containing the α_2, α_3 or α_5 subunits. These findings are consistent with the presence of these subunits in the spinal cord. The results of the studies on the function of individual receptor subtypes described so far are summarized in Table 2.

3.2.4
Diazepam-Induced Changes in the EEG

As pointed out previously, the sedative action of diazepam is mediated by GABA$_A$ receptors containing the α_1 subunit. It was therefore expected that the hypnotic activity of diazepam would also be mediated by this receptor subtype. However, in α_1(H101R) mice, 3 mg/kg diazepam reduced the amount of initial

REM sleep similar as in wild type mice. Furthermore, the increase in power density above 21 Hz in non-REM sleep and waking and the suppression of slow-wave activity (0.75 Hz–4 Hz) in non-REM sleep were seen in both α_1(H101R) and wild type mice, being even more pronounced in the α_1(H101R) mice. Also, the number of brief awakenings per hour of sleep was decreased and thus sleep continuity enhanced by diazepam only in α_1(H101R) mice. These findings suggest that the diazepam-induced changes in the EEG and possibly its hypnotic action may not be mediated by GABA$_A$ receptors containing the α_1 subunit and that the sedative and hypnotic actions of diazepam may be considered qualitatively different phenomena mediated by different neuronal circuits (Tobler et al. 2001).

3.2.5
Physiological Functions of α_5-Containing GABA$_A$ Receptors

Whereas in α_1(H101R), α_2(H101R) and α_3(H126R) mice the mutant subunits have been found to be expressed at normal levels, the expression of the mutant α_5 subunits in α_5(H105R) mice was reduced in hippocampal pyramidal cells by ca. 30%, but not in other brain regions. However, the laminar distribution of the α_5 subunit in the hippocampus was unchanged. The reasons for this selective reduction are not known. In contrast to the α_1, α_2 and α_3 subunits, the α_5 subunits are largely located extrasynaptically (except in the spinal cord). Perhaps, assembly and/or targeting of these extrasynaptic receptors are affected by the point mutation, whereas these processes are not significantly affected by the mutation with respect to synaptic receptors. In α_5(H105R) mice, the sedative, anticonvulsant and anxiolytic-like actions of diazepam were indistinguishable from wild type. Only the muscle relaxant action of diazepam was reduced in these mutant mice (Crestani et al. 2002).

The hippocampus plays an essential role in certain types of associative learning and memory. When a tone (conditioned stimulus) and a foot shock (unconditioned stimulus) are paired, associative learning involves the hippocampus when tone and foot shock are separated by a time interval (trace fear conditioning) but not when they co-terminate or overlap (delay fear conditioning). When the α_5(H105R) mice were tested in a delay fear conditioning paradigm, the amount of freezing was indistinguishable to wild type mice. However, in trace fear conditioning, the α_5(H105R) mice showed an enhanced percentage of freezing compared to wild type mice. Thus, the α_5(H105R) mice show a response different from wild type mice only in the hippocampus-dependent task, which is compatible with the reduced expression of α_5 subunits in the hippocampus of α_5(H105R) mice (Crestani et al. 2002). Interestingly, in the γ_2 knockout heterozygous mice described above (Section 3.1.6)—which display a loss of benzodiazepine-binding sites in the CA1 and CA3 regions of 35% and 28%, respectively—in trace fear conditioning, the time spent freezing to the tone was also significantly increased (Crestani et al. 1999). These studies demonstrate that, most likely, GABA$_A$ receptors containing the α_5 subunit and the γ_2 subunit are crucial for this response. There is also evidence for the involvement of excitatory neurotransmitter receptors in trace fear conditioning. Mice lacking the N-methyl-D-aspartate (NMDA) receptor subunit NR1 in CA1 pyramidal cells only (NR1.AC1-KO mutant) failed to memorize the tone-shock association in fear conditioning when tone and shock are temporally separated by a trace but not in delay fear conditioning, when the trace was removed (Huerta et al. 2000). Thus, hippocampal NMDA receptors and GABA$_A$ receptors containing the α_5 subunit and/or γ_2 subunit apparently have opposite roles in trace fear conditioning.

4
GABA$_B$ Receptor Function

The GABA$_B$ receptor agonist baclofen is used clinically for the treatment of spasticity, where it is a drug of choice, and also for migraine headache, musculoskeletal pain, pain associated with trigeminal neuralgia, stroke and spinal cord injury. Nevertheless, its effectiveness as an analgesic is only moderate. Preliminary evidence suggests that baclofen also reduces the craving for cocaine in humans (Ling et al. 1998). Its utility is limited by side-effects such as sedation. Thus, it would be desirable to develop drugs with more specific clinical profiles. There is, however, so far no unequivocal evidence for the existence for multiple GABA$_B$ receptor subtypes. Functional GABA$_B$ receptors are heterodimers composed of GABA$_{B1}$ and GABA$_{B2}$ receptor subunits. These two receptor subunits have 54% similarity and 35% homology and seven putative transmembrane domains. The agonist appears to bind to the GABA$_{B1}$ subunit, whereas the GABA$_{B2}$ subunit couples to G proteins (for review see Bowery et al. 2002). The GABA$_{B1}$ subunit alone is not transported to the plasma membranes and remains trapped in the endoplasmic reticulum (Couve et al. 1998). In GABA$_{B1}$ knockout mice, of which two lines have been generated independently (Prosser et al. 2001; Schuler et al. 2001), the expression of GABA$_{B2}$ is strongly downregulated, indicating that GABA$_{B1}$ is required for stable GABA$_{B2}$ expression. Tissues from these mice do not respond to GABA$_B$ receptor agonists and have lost detectable pre- and postsynaptic responses, indicating that the GABA$_{B1}$ subunit is an essential component of the GABA$_B$ receptor and that all GABA$_{B2}$ protein is associated with GABA$_{B1}$. Whereas one of the knockout lines, which was studied on a 129/Ola x C57BL/6J hybrid background, has a relatively short life span (up to 27 days) due to generalized epilepsy resulting in premature death (Prosser et al. 2001), the other line, which was kept on a Balb/c background, had a life expectancy of at least 140 days despite the occurrence of tonic-clonic and, less frequently, absence seizures (Schuler et al. 2001; Bowery et al. 2002). The GABA$_{B1}$ knockout mice displayed increased locomotor activity, and the GABA$_B$ receptor agonist baclofen did not impair motor coordination in the rotating rod test and did not induce hypothermia. In the hot plate, tail flick and paw pressure tests the knockout mice displayed hyperalgesia. Passive avoidance learning was impaired, indicating a marked negative effect of the knockout on memory performance (Schuler et al. 2001). Heterozygous animals showed enhanced prepulse inhibition responses, indicating increased sensorimotor gating mechanisms (Prosser et al. 2001). The studies on the $GABA_{B1}$ knockout mice did not reveal any evidence for pharmacologically distinct $GABA_B$ receptor subtypes. Generation and analysis of animals with elimination of either the $GABA_{B1(a)}$ or $GABA_{B1(b)}$ splice variants, which have different transcriptional start sites, may reveal whether they have different functional properties.

5
Outlook

Studies on $GABA_A$ receptor subunit knockout and knock-in mice have provided significant insights into the physiological and pharmacological role of $GABA_A$ receptors in general and specific receptor subtypes in particular that would have been difficult or impossible to obtain without gene targeting. The next "wave" in the study of in vivo functions of $GABA_A$ receptors are expected to be conditional subunit knockouts. The ability to delete genes in a temporally and spatially controlled fashion should open up new avenues for research and help to achieve an unprecedented level of precision in the analysis.

Acknowledgements. The work on the α subunit point-mutated mice described in this review was mostly performed in Hanns Möhler's laboratory at the Institute of Pharmacology and Toxicology, University of Zürich in close collaboration with Florence Crestani, Karin Löw, Ruth Keist, Jean-Marc Fritschy and Dietmar Benke and was supported by a grant from the Swiss National Science Foundation. The author thanks Hanns Möhler, Florence Crestani and Jean-Marc Fritschy for critically reading the manuscript.

References

Baer K, Essrich C, Benson JA, Benke D, Bluethmann H, Fritschy JM, Lüscher B (1999) Postsynaptic clustering of γ-aminobutyric acid type A receptors by the γ3 subunit in vivo. Proc Natl Acad Sci USA 96:12860–12865

Baer K, Essrich C, Balsiger S, Wick MJ, Harris RA, Fritschy JM, Lüscher B (2000) Rescue of γ2 subunit-deficient mice by transgenic overexpression of the $GABA_A$ receptor γ2S or γ2L subunit isoforms. Eur J Neurosci 12:2639–2643

Barnard EA, Skolnick P, Olsen RW, Mohler H, Sieghart W, Biggio G, Braestrup C, Bateson AN, Langer SZ (1998) International Union of Pharmacology. XV. Subtypes of γ-aminobutyric acid$_A$ receptors: classification on the basis of subunit structure and receptor function. Pharmacol Rev50:291–313

Baumann SW, Baur R, Sigel E (2001) Subunit arrangement of γ-aminobutyric acid type A receptors. J Biol Chem. 276:36275–36280

Benke D, Fritschy JM, Trzeciak A, Bannwarth W, Möhler H (1994) Distribution, prevalence, and drug binding profile of gamma-aminobutyric acid type A receptor subtypes differing in the beta-subunit variant. J Biol Chem 269:27100–27107

Benson JA, Low K, Keist R, Mohler H, Rudolph U. (1998) Pharmacology of recombinant γ-aminobutyric acid$_A$ receptors rendered diazepam-insensitive by point-mutated α-subunits. FEBS Lett 431:400–404

Bormann J (2000) The 'ABC' of GABA receptors, Trends Pharmacol Sci 21:16–19

Bowery NG, Bettler B, Froestl W, Gallagher JP, Marshall F, Raiteri M, Bonner TI, Enna SJ (2002) International Union of Pharmacology. XXXIII. Mammalian γ-Aminobutyric Acid$_B$ Receptors: Structure and Function. Pharmacol Rev 54:247–264

Brickley SG, Revilla V, Cull-Candy SG, Wisden W, Farrant M (2001) Adaptive regulation of neuronal excitability by a voltage-independent potassium conductance. Nature 409:88–92

Collinson N, Kuenzi FM, Jarolimek W, Maubach KA, Cothliff R, Sur C, Smith A, Otu FM, Howell O, Atack JR, McKernan RM, Seabrook GR, Dawson GR, Whiting PJ, Rosahl TW (2002) Enhanced Learning and Memory and Altered GABAergic Synaptic Transmission in Mice Lacking the α5 Subunit of the GABA$_A$ Receptor. J Neurosci 22:5572–5580

Couve A, Filippov AK, Connolly CN, Bettler B, Brown DA, Moss SJ (1998) Intracellular retention of recombinant GABA$_B$ receptors. J Biol Chem 273:26361–26367

Crestani F, Lorez M, Baer K, Essrich C, Benke D, Laurent JP, Belzung C, Fritschy JM, Lüscher B, Möhler H. (1999) Decreased GABA$_A$ receptor clustering results in enhanced anxiety and a bias for threat cues. Nat Neurosci 2:833–839

Crestani F, Martin JR, Mohler H, Rudolph U (2000a) Mechanism of action of the hypnotic zolpidem in vivo. Br J Pharmacol 131:1251–1254

Crestani F, Martin JR, Mohler H, Rudolph U. (2000b) Resolving differences in GABA$_A$ receptor mutant mouse studies. Nat Neurosci 3:1059

Crestani F, Löw K, Keist R, Mandelli M, Möhler H, Rudolph U. (2001) Molecular targets for the myorelaxant action of diazepam. Mol Pharmacol 59:442–445

Crestani F, Keist R, Fritschy JM, Benke D, Vogt K, Prut L, Bluthmann H, Mohler H, Rudolph U. (2002) Trace fear conditioning involves hippocampal α5 GABA$_A$ receptors. Proc Natl Acad Sci USA 99:8980–8985

Culiat CT, Stubbs L, Nicholls RD, Montgomery CS, Russell LB, Johnson DK, Rinchik EM. (1993) Concordance between isolated cleft palate in mice and alterations within a region including the gene encoding the β3 subunit of the type A γ-aminobutyric acid receptor. Proc Natl Acad Sci USA 90:5105–5109

Culiat CT, Stubbs LJ, Montgomery CS, Russell LB, Rinchik EM (1994) Phenotypic consequences of deletion of the γ3, α5, or β3 subunit of the type A γ-aminobutyric acid receptor in mice. Proc Natl Acad Sci USA 91:2815–2818

Culiat CT, Stubbs LJ, Woychik RP, Russell LB, Johnson DK, Rinchik EM. (1995) Deficiency of the β3 subunit of the type A γ-aminobutyric acid receptor causes cleft palate in mice. Nat Genet 11:344–346

DeLorey TM, Handforth A, Anagnostaras SG, Homanics GE, Minassian BA, Asatourian A, Fanselow MS, Delgado-Escueta A, Ellison GD, Olsen RW (1998) Mice lacking the β3 subunit of the GABA$_A$ receptor have the epilepsy phenotype and many of the behavioral characteristics of Angelman syndrome. J Neurosci 18:8505–8514

Essrich C, Lorez M, Benson JA, Fritschy JM, Luscher B (1998) Postsynaptic clustering of major GABA$_A$ receptor subtypes requires the γ2 subunit and gephyrin. Nat Neurosci 1:563–571

Fritschy JM, Benke D, Mertens S, Oertel WH, Bachi T, Möhler H (1992). Five subtypes of type A γ-aminobutyric acid receptors identified in neurons by double and triple immunofluorescence staining with subunit-specific antibodies. Proc Natl Acad Sci USA 89:6726–6730

Fritschy JM, Möhler H (1995) GABA$_A$-receptor heterogeneity in the adult rat brain: differential regional and cellular distribution of seven major subunits. J Comp Neurol 359:154–194

Fritschy JM, Johnson DK, Mohler H, Rudolph U. (1998) Independent assembly and subcellular targeting of GABA(A)-receptor subtypes demonstrated in mouse hippocampal and olfactory neurons in vivo. Neurosci Lett 249:99–102

Günther U, Benson J, Benke D, Fritschy JM, Reyes G, Knoflach F, Crestani F, Aguzzi A, Arigoni M, Lang Y, Bluethmann H, Möhler H, Lüscher B (1995) Benzodiazepine-insensitive mice generated by targeted disruption of the γ2 subunit gene of γ-aminobutyric acid type A receptors. Proc Natl Acad Sci USA 92:7749–7753

Homanics GE, Ferguson C, Quinlan JJ, Daggett J, Snyder K, Lagenaur C, Mi ZP, Wang XH, Grayson DR, Firestone LL (1997a) Gene knockout of the α6 subunit of the γ-aminobutyric acid type A receptor: lack of effect on responses to ethanol, pentobarbital, and general anesthetics. Mol Pharmacol 51:588–596

Homanics GE, DeLorey TM, Firestone LL, Quinlan JJ, Handforth A, Harrison NL, Krasowski MD, Rick CE, Korpi ER, Makela R, Brilliant MH, Hagiwara N, Ferguson C, Snyder K, Olsen RW (1997b). Mice devoid of γ-aminobutyrate type A receptor β3 subunit have epilepsy, cleft palate, and hypersensitive behavior. Proc Natl Acad Sci USA 94:4143–4148.

Homanics GE, Harrison NL, Quinlan JJ, Krasowski MD, Rick CE, de Blas AL, Mehta AK, Kist F, Mihalek RM, Aul JJ, Firestone LL (1999) Normal electrophysiological and behavioral responses to ethanol in mice lacking the long splice variant of the γ2 subunit of the γ-aminobutyrate type A receptor. Neuropharmacology 38:253–265

Huerta PT, Sun LD, Wilson MA, Tonegawa S (2000) Formation of temporal memory requires NMDA receptors within CA1 pyramidal neurons. Neuron 25:473–480

Huntsman MM, Porcello DM, Homanics GE, DeLorey TM, Huguenard JR. (1999) Reciprocal inhibitory connections and network synchrony in the mammalian thalamus. Science 283:541–543.

Jones A, Korpi ER, McKernan RM, Pelz R, Nusser Z, Makela R, Mellor JR, Pollard S, Bahn S, Stephenson FA, Randall AD, Sieghart W, Somogyi P, Smith AJ, Wisden W (1997) Ligand-gated ion channel subunit partnerships: GABA_A receptor α6 subunit gene inactivation inhibits δ subunit expression. J Neurosci 17:1350–1362.

Korpi ER, Koikkalainen P, Vekovischeva OY, Makela R, Kleinz R, Uusi-Oukari M, Wisden W (1999) Cerebellar granule-cell-specific GABA_A receptors attenuate benzodiazepine-induced ataxia: evidence from α6-subunit-deficient mice. Eur J Neurosci 11:233–240

Korpi ER, Mihalek RM, Sinkkonen ST, Hauer B, Hevers W, Homanics GE, Sieghart W, Luddens H (2002) Altered receptor subtypes in the forebrain of GABA_A receptor δ subunit-deficient mice: recruitment of γ2 subunits. Neuroscience 109:733–743

Laposky AD, Homanics GE, Basile A, Mendelson WB (2001) Deletion of the GABA_A receptor β3 subunit eliminates the hypnotic actions of oleamide in mice. Neuroreport 12:4143–4147

Ling W, Shoptaw S, Majewska D (1998) Baclofen as a cocaine anti-craving medication: a preliminary clinical study. Neuropsychopharmacology 18:403–404

Lorez M, Benke D, Luscher B, Mohler H, Benson JA (2000) Single-channel properties of neuronal GABA_A receptors from mice lacking the γ2 subunit. J Physiol 527.1:11–31

Löw K, Crestani F, Keist R, Benke D, Brunig I, Benson JA, Fritschy JM, Rulicke T, Bluethmann H, Möhler H, Rudolph U (2000) Molecular and neuronal substrate for the selective attenuation of anxiety. Science 290:131–134

Marksitzer R, Benke D, Fritschy JM, Trzeciak A, Bannwarth W, Mohler H (1993) GABA_A-receptors: drug binding profile and distribution of receptors containing the α2-subunit in situ. J Recept Res 13:467–477

McCall MA, Lukasiewicz PD, Gregg RG, Peachey NS (2002) Elimination of the ρ1 subunit abolishes GABA_C receptor expression and alters visual processing in the mouse retina. J Neurosci 22:4163–4174

McKernan RM, Whiting PJ (1996) Which GABA_A-receptor subtypes really occur in the brain? Trends Neurosci 19:139–143

McKernan RM, Rosahl TW, Reynolds DS, Sur C, Wafford KA, Atack JR, Farrar S, Myers J, Cook G, Ferris P, Garrett L, Bristow L, Marshall G, Macaulay A, Brown N, Howell O, Moore KW, Carling RW, Street LJ, Castro JL, Ragan CI, Dawson GR, Whiting PJ (2000) Sedative but not anxiolytic properties of benzodiazepines are mediated by the GABA_A receptor α1 subtype. Nat Neurosci 3:587–592

Mihalek RM, Banerjee PK, Korpi ER, Quinlan JJ, Firestone LL, Mi ZP, Lagenaur C, Tretter V, Sieghart W, Anagnostaras SG, Sage JR, Fanselow MS, Guidotti A, Spigelman I, Li Z, DeLorey TM, Olsen RW, Homanics GE (1999) Attenuated sensitivity to neuroactive steroids in γ-aminobutyrate type A receptor δ subunit knockout mice. Proc Natl Acad Sci USA 96:12905–12910

Mihalek RM, Bowers BJ, Wehner JM, Kralic JE, VanDoren MJ, Morrow AL, Homanics GE (2001) GABA$_A$-receptor δ subunit knockout mice have multiple defects in behavioral responses to ethanol. Alcohol Clin Exp Res 25:1708–1718

Möhler H, Benke D, Benson J, Lüscher B, Fritschy JM (1995) GABA$_A$-receptor subtypes in vivo: cellular localization, pharmacology and regulation. Adv Biochem Psychopharmacol 48:41–56

Möhler H, Fritschy JM, Lüscher B, Rudolph U, Benson J, Benke D (1996) The GABA$_A$ receptors. From subunits to diverse functions. In: Narahashi T (ed.), Ion Channels, Volume 4, Plenum Press, New York, pp 89–113

Möhler H, Fritschy JM, Rudolph U (2002) A new benzodiazepine pharmacology. J Pharmacol Exp Ther 300:2–8

Nakatsu Y, Tyndale RF, DeLorey TM, Durham-Pierre D, Gardner JM, McDanel HJ, Nguyen Q, Wagstaff J, Lalande M, Sikela JM, Olsen RW, Tobin AJ, Brilliant MH (1993) A cluster of three GABA$_A$ receptor subunit genes is deleted in a neurological mutant of the mouse p locus. Nature 364:448–450

Nusser Z, Ahmad Z, Tretter V, Fuchs K, Wisden W, Sieghart W, Somogyi P (1999) Alterations in the expression of GABAA receptor subunits in cerebellar granule cells after the disruption of the α6 subunit gene. Eur J Neurosci111:1685–1697

Peng Z, Hauer B, Mihalek RM, Homanics GE, Sieghart W, Olsen RW, Houser CR. GABA$_A$ receptor changes in d subunit-deficient mice: altered expression of α4 and γ2 subunits in the forebrain. J Comp Neurol 446:179–197

Pritchett DB, Sontheimer H, Shivers BD, Ymer S, Kettenmann H, Schofield PR, Seeburg PH (1989) Importance of a novel GABA$_A$ receptor subunit for benzodiazepine pharmacology. Nature 338:582–585

Quinlan JJ, Homanics GE, Firestone LL (1998) Anesthesia sensitivity in mice that lack the β3 subunit of the γ-aminobutyric acid type A receptor. Anesthesiology 88:775–780

Prosser HM, Gill CH, Hirst WD, Grau E, Robbins M, Calver A, Soffin EM, Farmer CE, Lanneau C, Gray J, Schenck E, Warmerdam BS, Clapham C, Reavill C, Rogers DC, Stean T, Upton N, Humphreys K, Randall A, Geppert M, Davies CH, Pangalos MN (2001) Epileptogenesis and enhanced prepulse inhibition in GABA$_{B1}$-deficient mice. Mol Cell Neurosci 17:1059–1070

Resnick A, Homanics GE, Jung BJ, Peris J. (1999) Increased acute cocaine sensitivity and decreased cocaine sensitization in GABA$_A$ receptor β3 subunit knockout mice. J Neurochem 73:1539–1548

Rudolph U, Crestani F, Benke D, Brunig I, Benson JA, Fritschy JM, Martin JR, Bluethmann H, Mohler H (1999) Benzodiazepine actions mediated by specific γ-aminobutyric acid$_A$ receptor subtypes. Nature 401:796–800

Schuler V, Lüscher C, Blanchet C, Klix N, Sansig G, Klebs K, Schmutz M, Heid J, Gentry C, Urban L, Fox A, Spooren W, Jaton AL, Vigouret J, Pozza M, Kelly PH, Mosbacher J, Froestl W, Kaslin E, Korn R, Bischoff S, Kaupmann K, van der Putten H, Bettler B (2001) Epilepsy, hyperalgesia, impaired memory, and loss of pre- and postsynaptic GABA$_B$ responses in mice lacking GABA$_{B1}$. Neuron 31:47–58

Smith GB, Olsen RW (1995) Functional domains of GABA$_A$ receptors. Trends Pharmacol Sci 16:162–168

Stephenson FA, Duggan MJ, Pollard S (1990) The γ2 subunit is an integral component of the γ-aminobutyric acid$_A$ receptor but the α1 polypeptide is the principal site of the agonist benzodiazepine photoaffinity labeling reaction. J Biol Chem 265:21160–21165.

Sur C, Wafford KA, Reynolds DS, Hadingham KL, Bromidge F, Macaulay A, Collinson N, O'Meara G, Howell O, Newman R, Myers J, Atack JR, Dawson GR, McKernan RM, Whiting PJ, Rosahl TW (2001) Loss of the major GABA$_A$ receptor subtype in the brain is not lethal in mice. J Neurosci 21:3409–3418

Tobler I, Kopp C, Deboer T, Rudolph U (2001) Diazepam-induced changes in sleep: role of the α1 GABA$_A$ receptor subtype. Proc Natl Acad Sci USA 98:6464–6469

Ugarte SD, Homanics GE, Firestone LL, Hammond DL (2000) Sensory thresholds and the antinociceptive effects of GABA receptor agonists in mice lacking the β3 subunit of the GABA$_A$ receptor. Neuroscience 95:795–806

Uusi-Oukari M, Heikkila J, Sinkkonen ST, Makela R, Hauer B, Homanics GE, Sieghart W, Wisden W, Korpi ER (2000) Long-range interactions in neuronal gene expression: evidence from gene targeting in the GABA$_A$ receptor β2-α6-α1-γ2 subunit gene cluster. Mol Cell Neurosci 16:34–41

Vicini S, Ferguson C, Prybylowski K, Kralic J, Morrow AL, Homanics GE (2001) GABA$_A$ receptor α1 subunit deletion prevents developmental changes of inhibitory synaptic currents in cerebellar neurons. J Neurosci 21:3009–3016

Wafford KA, Burnett DM, Leidenheimer NJ, Burt DR, Wang JB, Kofuji P, Dunwiddie TV, Harris RA, Sikela JM (1991) Ethanol sensitivity of the GABA$_A$ receptor expressed in Xenopus oocytes requires 8 amino acids contained in the γ2L subunit. Neuron 7:27–33

Wieland HA, Luddens H, Seeburg PH (1992) A single histidine in GABA$_A$ receptors is essential for benzodiazepine agonist binding. J Biol Chem 267:1426–1429.

Wong SM, Cheng G, Homanics GE, Kendig JJ (2001) Enflurane actions on spinal cords from mice that lack the β3 subunit of the GABA$_A$ receptor. Anesthesiology 95:154–164

Neurotrophic Factors

M. Sendtner

Institut für Klin. Neurobiologie, University of Würzburg,
Josef-Schneider-Str.11, 97080 Würzburg, Germany
e-mail: sendtner@mail.uni-wuerzburg.de

Abstract Since the discovery of nerve growth factor (NGF) and original observations that limiting quantities of this protein regulate survival of distinct populations of neurons during development, a broad variety of neurotrophic factors has been identified. These factors are members of several gene families and promote their effects though specific membrane receptors which either include transmembrane receptor tyrosine kinases or classical cytokine receptor subunits such as gp130. Neurotrophic factors do not only regulate neuronal survival but also neural differentiation, neurite outgrowth, synapse formation, transmitter synthesis and release. Additional functions in other organs than the nervous systems have also been identified. Mouse models in which the genes for these factors are specifically deleted have played an important role in our present understanding of the physiological function of these molecules. These findings are summarized and discussed in this review.

Key words Neuronal cell death · Neurotrophins · Neurogenesis · Glial-derived neurotrophin factor · Ciliary neurotrophic factor

1
Neurotrophic Factors and Developmental Neuronal Death:
Nerve Growth Factor

In higher vertebrates, many types of neurons are generated in excess. A significant proportion of the newly generated cells are eliminated during development. Studies by Victor Hamburger and Rita Levi-Montalcini (Levi-Montalcini 1987) have shown that target tissues play a central role in this process by providing limiting quantities of survival factors to neurons, in particular those projecting to peripheral targets such as muscle, skin, or blood vessels. In 6-day-old chick embryos, the lumbar part of the spinal cord contains about 20,000 motoneurons of which about 8,000 are lost until embryonic day 12 (see Oppenheim 1991 for review). Experiments by Victor Hamburger (Hamburger 1934, 1958) showed that limb or wing bud removal in early chick embryos leads to virtually complete loss of corresponding motoneurons. Conversely, the implantation of an additional limb anlage results in an increased number of motoneurons projecting to the enlarged target area (Holliday and Hamburger 1975). These experiments were the first steps in the discovery of nerve growth factor (NGF). Experiments with sarcoma tissue as a replacement of target tissue (Levi-Montalcini et al. 1954) demonstrated enhanced survival of sympathetic neurons in the paravertebral ganglia and subpopulations of sensory neurons, but not of spinal motoneurons. These data indicated that distinct survival factors are responsible for various populations of neurons. After the identification of NGF as a specific survival factor for sympathetic and subpopulations of sensory neurons, subsequent experiments showed that this protein is produced in the target of these neurons and transported in the axons to the cell bodies after binding to specific receptors (Thoenen and Barde 1980; Ginty and Segal 2002). These findings with NGF have guided research in the field of neurotrophic factors. During the past few decades, researchers have concentrated on discovering factors with analogous function for motoneurons and other types of neurons.

Experiments performed to understand the mechanisms of developmental cell death of motoneurons have played an essential role in establishing the hypothesis that target tissues influence development and maintenance of innervating neurons. Since 1989, a broad variety of factors with survival-promoting activity for motoneurons and many other types of neurons were identified, and evidence has accumulated that various neurotrophic factors exist in target tissues, such as skeletal muscle, and regulate survival of innervating cells during development (reviewed by Thoenen et al. 1993). Animal models in which the genes for these factors were eliminated have played a crucial role in determining the physiological significance of these molecules in this context. For example, mice lacking endogenous NGF (Crowley et al. 1994) show enhanced loss of sympathetic and sensory neurons in spinal dorsal root ganglia, but do not show increased cell death in the population of central cholinergic neurons in the basal forebrain or basal nucleus of Meynert, a specific population of neurons which is highly responsive to NGF treatment under physiological and pathophysiological conditions (Li et al. 1995b; Hartikka and Hefti 1988). Similarly, although motoneurons are highly responsive to BDNF (Oppenheim et al. 1992; Sendtner et al. 1992a), the second member of the neurotrophin family which was identified (Leibrock et al. 1989), mice lacking brain-derived neurotrophic factor (BDNF) do not show any reduction in motoneuron numbers (Conover et al. 1995; Liu et al. 1995), despite major abnormalities in other populations of neurons. Thus, compensatory effects by other neurotrophic factors could be unravelled. In addition, these mouse mutants proved very helpful to discover and investigate the role of these neurotrophic factors for neuronal function, in particular in neurite outgrowth, synaptogenesis and synaptic activity. This chapter will summarize some of these findings, with specific emphasis on the role of these mouse mutants for understanding the function of neurotrophic factors in the motor system.

2
Neurotrophins

2.1
Receptors for Neurotrophins: Dual Role of p75^{NTR} in Neuronal Survival

NGF is the prototypic target-derived trophic factor (reviewed by Barde 1990). Its biological activities are limited to specific populations of peripheral and central neurons. The biological effects of nerve growth factor on responsive neurons are mediated by a low-affinity receptor which is common to all neurotrophins (p75^{NTR}) and through a specific high-affinity receptor (trk-A; see Eide et al. 1993). The p75^{NTR} receptor is highly expressed in motoneurons during embryonic development. Expression drops to undetectable levels after birth, and only after nerve lesion or in degenerative diseases, in particular in neurodegenerative disorders such as amyotrophic lateral sclerosis, it is re-expressed (Kerkhoff et al. 1993; Seeburger et al. 1993). For some time, it was thought that the biological functions of NGF on survival and neurite outgrowth were exclusively mediated though the trk-A transmembrane tyrosine kinase receptor. Only in recent years have we seen clear evidence for an involvement of the p75^{NTR} receptor in signal transduction (Dechant and Barde 1997; Kaplan and Miller 2000). The p75^{NTR} receptor also mediates pro-apoptotic signalling responses (Rabizadeh et al. 1993; Bothwell 1996), but reports on this function in transgenic mouse models were confusing. Initial reports on enhanced survival of cholinergic neurons in the basal forebrain in p75^{NTR} knockout mice had to be revisited (Van der Zee et al. 1996) and other data which are based on experiments with p75^{NTR} gene knockout mice and neuronal cultures derived from these mice showed that p75^{NTR} co-operates with trk receptors in mediating pro-survival effects (Wiese et al. 1999). The observation that p75^{NTR} preferentially binds pro-forms of neurotrophins (Lee et al. 2001) that have not yet been cleaved to the shorter mature neurotrophins has led to the hypotheses that (1) cleavage of neurotrophin precursor protein decides on pro- versus anti-apoptotic effects of these molecules, (2) neurotrophin precursor proteins mediate cell death via p75^{NTR}, and (3) mature neurotrophins mediate survival through trk receptors or complexes of trk and p75^{NTR} subunits.

These results correspond to pro-apoptotic effects of NGF on various types of neurons. For example, in newborn rats, the application of NGF increases the number of degenerating motoneurons after sciatic nerve lesion (Miyata et al. 1986) and after facial nerve lesion (Sendtner et al. 1992a). During embryonic development, endogenous NGF promotes cell death of retinal ganglion cells through p75^{NTR} (Frade et al. 1996). This scenario could also be relevant when p75^{NTR} is re-expressed in motoneurons, such as neurodegenerative disorders like amyotrophic lateral sclerosis (ALS).

The p75^{NTR} receptor is also involved in functions other than mediating cell death and survival signals. These functions have been observed long before neurotrophin receptors were identified on a molecular level. For example, trk-A is not expressed in motoneurons, whereas relatively high levels of p75^{NTR} are observed during development or after nerve lesion. The high expression of p75 explains why NGF can be taken up and retrogradely transported in embryonic motoneurons of newborn, but not adult rats (Stoeckel et al. 1975; Yan et al. 1988). Some effects of NGF have been observed in motoneurons, among them hypertrophy of a subpopulation of NGF-receptor-positive lumbar motoneurons (Koliatsos et al. 1991) or a short-term effect on neurite outgrowth in cultured embryonic motoneurons (Wayne and Heaton 1988; Wayne and Heaton 1990a,b). These effects are caused by activation of rhoA by direct interaction with p75^{NTR} (Yamashita et al. 1999).

2.2
Other Members of the Neurotrophin Family: BDNF, NT-3 and NT-4/5

In 1989, the gene for BDNF was cloned (Leibrock et al. 1989). BDNF is the second members of the neurotrophin family. Its discovery paved the way to identification of neurotrophin (NT)-3 (Hohn et al. 1990; Maisonpierre et al. 1990) and NT-4/5 (Berkemeier et al. 1991; Hallböök et al. 1991). BDNF and NT-4/5 specifically interact with trk-B, and NT-3 preferentially binds to trk-C receptors. All neurotrophins bind to the p75^{NTR} with similar affinity. The expression of the trk receptors defines the specificity for actions on various populations of neurons.

For example, motoneurons express full-length trk-B but not trk-A and therefore do not respond for their survival to NGF. A subpopulation of motoneurons also expresses trk-C, which is a specific cellular receptor for NT-3 (Henderson et al. 1993; Griesbeck et al. 1995). The positive effects of BDNF and NT-3 were discovered when these proteins were applied to lesioned motoneurons in newborn rats (Sendtner et al. 1992a; Yan et al. 1992) or to the allantoic membrane of developing chick embryos (Oppenheim et al. 1992). Although virtually all of the

Table 1 Neuronal losses in of mice with gene knockout for neurotrophins and trks

	Sensory neurons		Sympathetic	Motoneurons		Reference(s)
	Dorsal root ganglion	Trigeminal ganglion	Superior cervical ganglion	Facial nucleus	Spinal cord	
NGF	70%	75%	>95%	ND	ND	Crowley et al. 1994
BDNF	35%	30%	ND	NS	NS	Brady et al. 1999
NT-3	60%	60%	50%	ND	ND	Ernfors et al. 1994, 1995
NT-4/5	NS	NS	NS	NS	NS	Stucky et al. 1998
BDNF NT-4	NS	9%	ND	NS	NS	Conover et al. 1995; Liu et al. 1995
NT-3/BDNF	83%	74%	ND	ND	ND	Liebl et al. 1997
NT-3/BDNF/NT-4/5	92%	88%	47%	22%	20%	Pinon et al. 1996; Liu and Jaenisch 2000
TrkA	70–90%	70%	>95%	ND	ND	Silos-Santiago et al. 1995
TrkB	30%	60%	ND	ND	NS	Klein et al. 1993; DeChiara et al. 1995
TrkC	20%	21%	NS	ND	ND	Klein et al. 1994; Minichiello and Klein 996
TrkB/C	41%	ND	ND	ND	ND	Minichiello and Klein 1996

ND, not determined; NS, not shown.

motoneurons express trk-B, only a subpopulation of about 50%–60% of the motoneurons survive after BDNF administration in vivo (Sendtner et al. 1992a; Yan
et al. 1992) or in vitro (Henderson et al. 1993; Hughes et al. 1993). The reason
for this apparent discrepancy is still not clear. As this effect is both observed in
cultured motoneurons from different embryonic stages as well as in vivo in
postnatal motoneurons, it has to be assumed that the responsiveness of motoneurons to BDNF through trk-B does not simply increase during embryonic
development, but is regulated by other cellular or extracellular signals.

The genes for BDNF, NT-3 as well as the genes for the corresponding receptors trk-B and trk-C have been knocked out in mice (Table 1). Mice without
BDNF survive after birth, but feed poorly and usually die within 4 weeks. Histological examination has shown loss of sensory neurons in the dorsal root ganglia and in particular the vestibular and nodose ganglia (reviewed in Snider
1994). Interestingly, motoneurons are not reduced in BDNF-deficient mice. It
was speculated that this could be due to the presence of NT-4 in muscle and a
compensatory effect of this neurotrophin through trk-B which is shared as a receptor. However, mice in which both BDNF and NT-4 were deleted also did not
show enhanced motoneurons loss (Conover et al. 1995; Liu et al. 1995). Similarly, and in contrast to original reports (Klein et al. 1993), mice with inactivated
trk-B also do not show enhanced motoneuron (DeChiara et al. 1995) cell death.
The loss of sensory neurons was slightly higher in the trigeminal ganglia in
trk-B knockout mice (Klein et al. 1993) than in BDNF-deficient mice (Conover
et al. 1995). Highest loss of neurons in BDNF-deficient mice was observed in the
vestibular ganglion (90%–96% reduction) and in the nodose–petrosal ganglion
complex (60% loss). This result indicates that NT-4 does not compensate for
lack of BDNF in this neuronal population. Altogether, these analyses revealed
that the physiological requirement of these different population of neurons for
individual factors of the neurotrophin family vary, and that compensatory effects between various members of the neurotrophin family exist, but they are
not of major relevance for survival during development.

Many types of neurons also express trk-C, the specific receptor for NT-3, often in combination with trk-B. In particular, spinal motoneurons express relatively high levels of this receptor. This appears relevant, since NT-3 is the most
abundantly expressed neurotrophin in skeletal muscle, both during development and in the adult. For comparison, levels of BDNF expression in muscle are
very low (Griesbeck et al. 1995). From trk-C and NT-3 knockout mice, there is
good evidence that the γ-motoneurons innervating the muscle spindles are dependent on NT-3 for their physiological development (Ernfors et al. 1995; Kucera et al. 1995). However, NT-3 also supports survival of facial motoneurons after nerve lesion, a population of motoneurons which does not contain γ-mo-
toneurons (Sendtner et al. 1992a). Therefore, subpopulations of α-motoneurons
should also be responsive to NT-3. This is also suggested by the observation that
trk-C mRNA is highly expressed in spinal and brain stem motoneurons. During
embryonic development, the spinal motoneurons express NT-3 at relatively high
levels (Ernfors and Persson 1991). This suggested that NT-3 could function as

an autocrine factor during this period. However, gene ablation of NT-3 did not lead to reduced numbers of α-motoneurons. It appears that the NT-3 produced in motoneurons serves as a neurotrophic and axon-attractant for proprioceptive neurons which invade the spinal cord through the dorsal horn and make contacts with the ventral motoneurons. In addition, NT-3 from motoneurons could function on upper motoneurons, which have been shown to respond to this factor (Schnell et al. 1994).

NT-4/5 can also bind to trk-B and support motoneurons, most probably through this receptor. Therefore, redundancy of these two ligands in their function on motoneurons has been suggested (Hughes et al. 1993; Conover et al. 1995; Liu et al. 1995). However, this is not necessarily the case. Splice variants of trk-B have been identified with increased specificity for BDNF (Strohmaier et al. 1996), and it is not clear so far whether such splice variants with increased specificity for each of these ligands are expressed on motoneurons. This could be relevant for consideration of the therapeutic potential of these two ligands for treatment of neurodegenerative diseases.

NT-3 expression is detectable in skeletal muscle both during development and in the adult. After muscle denervation either by nerve transection or by transient blockade of neuronal transmission by injection of tetrodotoxin into the sciatic nerve, NT-4 expression is rapidly downregulated in adult rats (Griesbeck et al. 1995). Electrical stimulation of motor nerves leads to the opposite effect, a significant upregulation of NT-4 expression (Funakoshi et al. 1995). These data suggest that neuronal activity at the neuromuscular endplate has a significant influence on NT-4 expression in skeletal muscle, and NT-4 could be involved in regulating efficacy of neuromuscular transmission, as has been shown in co-cultures of Xenopus motoneurons and skeletal muscle after addition of NT-3 or BDNF (Lohof et al. 1993).

2.3
Pharmacological Potential of Neurotrophins: Lessons from Animal Models and Mouse Mutants

In contrast to ciliary neurotrophic factor (CNTF) (Shapiro et al. 1993; Fantuzzi et al. 1995) and leukaemia inhibitory factor (LIF) (Metcalf and Gearing 1989; Ryffel 1993), the systemic application of BDNF or NT-3 is well tolerated in animal models. However, animal studies in which these factors were applied for maintaining survival of motoneurons under various experimental conditions pointed to potential problems. The pharmacological application of BDNF, NT-4 or NT-3 to cell cultures or lesioned motoneurons in vivo supports less motoneurons than one would expect from the expression of trk-B or trk-C (Yan et al. 1992; Henderson et al. 1993). Moreover, the local administration of high amounts of BDNF to lesioned motor nerves in newborn rodents has only a transient effect in rescuing the corresponding motoneurons (Vejsada et al. 1994; Vejsada et al. 1995; Vejsada et al. 1998).

Levels of endogenous BDNF mRNA are extremely low in skeletal muscle, but upregulated after lesion of peripheral nerves (Griesbeck et al. 1995). This procedure leads to upregulation of BDNF mRNA production in Schwann cells, which starts at the end of the first week after lesion and increases continuously during the following 4 weeks (Meyer et al. 1992). At that time, levels of BDNF production are about tenfold higher than maximal levels of NGF, which can be observed a few days after nerve lesion. This scenario would make BDNF available to lesioned motoneurons only at later periods when the motor axons regenerate to their original muscle fibres. Therefore, a decreased responsiveness of lesioned motoneurons to BDNF within a few days after lesion would not be compatible with a functional role of this factor during the long period of axonal regrowth after nerve lesion. In order to test the hypothesis that BDNF has to be available continuously at physiological concentrations for lesioned motoneurons, recombinant adenoviruses were used for local overexpression of BDNF after motor nerve lesion in newborn rats (Gravel et al. 1997). Indeed, this procedure could lead to prolonged survival of motoneuron cell bodies. The molecular counterpart for the influence of concentration (Vejsada et al. 1994) and application mode (bolus vs. continuous application) might reside in the regulation of high-affinity BDNF receptor expression on the cell surface of motoneurons. Cell culture experiments with cerebellar granular cells have shown that high levels of BDNF can lead to a dramatic decrease of trk-B receptor expression on the cell surface, most probably due to a block in transfer of full-length trk-B binding sites from intracellular compartments to the cell surface (Carter et al. 1995). Such mechanisms could play a role in motoneurons when BDNF is pharmacologically administered. Currently, various efforts are being made to generate mouse mutants in which specific deletions and point mutations are made into the receptors in order to define specific elements which are responsible for transfer of receptors to the cell surface, for activation of specific signalling pathways in correlation with effects on neurite outgrowth, synaptic activity and neuronal survival. For example, mutation of the shc binding domain in trk-B revealed a specific need of this site for NT-4-mediated effects on survival of sensory neurons, but not for BDNF (Minichiello et al. 1998). Other mutants have been made and are currently being investigated, and these mouse models could help us define signalling pathways which are necessary for pharmacological effects of neurotrophic factors, and possible downstream targets which might be worth considering as target molecules for pharmacological treatment of neurodegenerative diseases.

3
CNTF and Functionally Related Molecules

CNTF was originally identified as a survival-promoting factor for cultured embryonic chick ciliary neurons present in high quantities in chick eye extracts (Adler et al. 1979; Barbin et al. 1984). This protein is also present in relatively high amounts in peripheral myelinating Schwann cells, so that this protein could be finally purified from this source and its gene cloned (Lin et al. 1989; Stöckli et al. 1989). CNTF differs from neurotrophins by its lack of a hydrophobic signal peptide, and thus it is not released via the conventional secretory pathway. Moreover, it is not expressed during embryonic development at a time when physiological cell death of motoneurons and other responsive neuronal populations occurs.

3.1
The CNTF Receptor Complex: Actions of Leukaemia Inhibitory Factor, Oncostatin M, Cardiotrophin-1 Are Mediated Through Shared Receptor Subunits

CNTF acts on responsive neurons via a receptor complex involving at least three subunits (Stahl and Yancopoulos 1994). The low-affinity receptor CNTFRα exists both in membrane-bound form and as a soluble binding protein in body fluids (Davis et al. 1993). The cell membrane-bound CNTFRα is linked via a glycosyl-phosphatidyl-inositol (GPI) anchor to the outer layer of the cell membrane and lacks a transmembrane domain. The expression of this receptor component is relatively high in the nervous system and in skeletal muscle.

The high-affinity receptor for CNTF involves two additional components, gp130, which has originally been identified as the signal-transducing component of the interleukin (IL)-6 receptor, and LIFRβ. This latter component can bind LIF with low affinity (Gearing et al. 1991). Involvement of gp130 and LIFRβ in the receptor complexes for CNTF, LIF, oncostatin-M (OSM) and cardiotrophin-1 (CT-1) (Gearing et al. 1992; Pennica et al. 1995) explains the overlapping activities of these factors in supporting motoneuron survival and function.

Mice have been generated in which the receptor components LIFRβ CNTFRα and gp130 have been eliminated (DeChiara et al. 1995; Li et al. 1995a; Yoshida et al. 1996). In all cases, the introduced gene defects are lethal, and enhanced cell death in motoneuron and sensory neuronal populations was observed in CNTFRα- and LIFRβ-deficient mice. Thus, it appears that ligands for the LIFRβ/CNTFRα constitute physiological endogenous survival factors for developing motoneurons and probably also other populations of neurons.

Mice in which the genes for CNTF (Masu et al. 1993), LIF (Escary et al. 1993; Sendtner et al. 1996) or CT-1 (Oppenheim et al. 2001) are eliminated, are much less affected than CNTFRα or LIFRβ mice. All these mutants are viable and do not show severe neurological deficits. CNTF$^{-/-}$ mice do not show any deficits at birth, but postnatally show enhanced motoneuron cell death which reaches a level of -20% at an age of 6 months. When LIF is deficient, there is no loss of neurons at any stage of development. However, in CNTF and LIF double-deficient mice, neuronal loss—in particular postnatal loss of motoneurons—is enhanced, leading to measurable neurological defects such as reduction of muscle strength by about 30% (Fig. 1). These data point to a significant degree of overlap and redundancy of CNTF and LIF on neuronal survival. CNTF does not only affect motoneuron survival, but also mitosis, differentiation and survival of

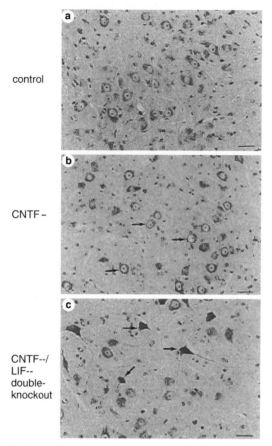

control

CNTF –

CNTF--/
LIF--
double-
knockout

Fig. 1a–c Morphology of motoneuron in the facial nucleus of control (**a**), CNTF (**b**) and CNTF/LIF (**c**) double-deficient mice. In CNTF$^{-/-}$ mice, loss of about 20% of the motoneurons is observed in 3-month-old mice (**b**), whereas LIF-deficient mice do not show enhanced cell death in this neuronal population. However, when these gene defects are combined, significantly enhanced neuronal loss is observed (**c**)

oligodendrocytes and corresponding precursor cells (Barres et al. 1993). Thus, the rate of mitosis of oligodendrocyte precursor cells in the optic nerve of CNTF$^{-/-}$ mice is reduced, and when an inflammatory disease is induced in the nervous system in these mice by myelin/oligodendrocyte glycoprotein (MOG)-peptide induced experimental autoimmune encephalomyelitis, the number of proliferation oligodendrocyte precursor cells was massively reduced, apoptosis of oligodendrocytes was enhanced, and degeneration of axons was observed, corresponding to more severe disease (Maurer et al. 2002).

Similarly, a role of CNTF was identified as a modifier gene by crossbreeding mice with transgenic mutant superoxide dismutase (SOD)1, a classical model of human motoneuron disease, with CNTF-deficient mice (Giess et al. 2002a). These mice show significantly earlier disease onset and higher loss of spinal motoneurons. These observation might be relevant insofar as a point mutation in the splice acceptor site for exon 2 of the human CNTF gene is quite abundant so that 2% of the human population are CNTF deficient (Takahashi et al. 1994). Although this mutation per se is not associated with any neurological defect, it modulates severity of disease when it occurs in combination with other genetic and epigenetic conditions which lead to familial or sporadic motoneuron disease (Giess et al. 2000b; Giess et al. 2002a) or multiple sclerosis (Giess et al. 2002b). Similarly, mutations in the LIF gene have been reported to be more abundant in patients with motoneuron disease than in controls (Giess et al. 2000a).

Mice with gene inactivation for CT-1 show enhanced loss of motoneurons during embryonic development (Oppenheim et al. 2001). Thus, this factor seems to be the only protein which so far has been clearly proven to act as a target derived neurotrophic factor for spinal motoneurons. However, there is no significant further loss of motoneurons during postnatal development. Thus CT-1 acts primarily during embryonic development, whereas CNTF and LIF seem to play a role in maintenance of motoneurons and other populations of neurons during postnatal development.

Nevertheless, the extent of motoneuron loss and the severity of the neurological deficit in CT-1-deficient mice is much less severe than in CNTFRα or LIFRβ mice. The discovery of cardiotrophin-like cytokine (CLC) as another ligand for CNTFRα (Elson et al. 2000) when bound to cytokine-like factor (CLF) has given a potential explanation for this observation, and efforts are currently made to investigate CLF-deficient mice (Alexander et al. 1999) in order to find out how the phenotype compares with CNTFRα gene knockout mice on a histopathological level.

3.2
Effects of CNTF and Other Neurotrophic Factors in Murine Animal Models for Motoneuron Disease

CNTF has been successfully used for experimental therapy in murine animal models for motoneuron disease. Systemic administration of CNTF to progressive motor neuropathy (pmn) (Sendtner et al. 1992b), wobbler (Mitsumoto et al. 1992) and motor neurodegenerative (mnd) (Helgren et al. 1992) mice showed significant effects on the course of the disease, although the mechanisms how CNTF achieves this effect might be different. The underlying gene defects in these mouse mutants have not been identified so far. However, chromosomal linkage data and experiments searching for mutations in candidate genes indicate that they are unrelated and that these mice are not defective of genes coding for these neurotrophic factors or their receptors. In the case of the mnd and wobbler mice, large inclusion bodies were observed in motoneurons which appeared during the course of the disease. Whereas the content of these inclusion bodies has not been identified in wobbler mice (Blondet et al. 1995), the mnd mouse has been described as an animal model of neural ceroid lipofuscinosis (corresponding to Batten's disease in humans) (Bronson et al. 1993). In the meantime, the underlying mutation in the mnd mouse has been identified as a single bp insertion at codon 90 of the CLN8 gene which defines a specific subgroup of neural ceroid lipofuscinosis in mouse and human. Surprisingly, significant effects of CNTF have been observed in this mouse mutant (Helgren et al. 1992; Winter et al. 1996). Recently, also the gene defect responsible for motoneuron disease in pmn mice was discovered (Bommel et al. 2002; Martin et al. 2002) as a point mutation leading to a single amino acid exchange in the tubulin specific chaperone E gene. This indicates that CNTF signalling interferes with a variety of cellular defects, also such defects which are not primarily caused by mutation in signalling molecules for neuronal survival pathways.

4
Glial-Derived Neurotrophic Factor

Glial-derived neurotrophic factor (GDNF) was identified in 1993 as a potent survival factor for midbrain dopaminergic neurons (Lin et al. 1993). It quickly became apparent that this protein, which shares distant structural homologies with members of the TGF-β gene family, is also an effective survival factor for other populations of neurons, in particular motoneurons. Half-maximal survival of cultured embryonic motoneurons is supported by 0.2 pg/ml GDNF, corresponding to 7 fM (Henderson et al. 1994). Thus GDNF is several orders of magnitude more potent than BDNF, CNTF or LIF. The same study showed no effect of GDNF on sensory, trigeminal or sympathetic neurons derived from embryonic or perinatal rats. Relatively high expression of GDNF was found in skeletal muscle, E15 hind-limb and Schwann cell cultures, and nerve lesions increase GDNF mRNA expression within 2 days to maximal levels. Therefore, a function of GDNF as an endogenous lesion factor for axotomized motoneurons (and probably other types of neurons) was proposed, resembling very much the function of LIF and CNTF.

An effect of GDNF on peripheral sympathetic and sensory neurons was observed in studies with chick embryos (Oppenheim et al. 1995). The application of GDNF to the chorioallantoic membrane led to increased motoneuron survival during the critical period of physiological cell death, but also increased the number of surviving sympathetic and sensory neurons.

Mice in which the GDNF gene was inactivated show renal agenesis and a complete lack of neurons in the autonomic ganglia of the gut which form the myenteric plexus (Moore et al. 1996; Pichel et al. 1996; Sanchez et al. 1996). Analysis of the nervous system identified deficits in several populations of sensory neurons, in particular from dorsal root, sympathetic and nodose ganglia. A small reduction in trigeminal and spinal lumbar motoneuronsin the range of 20% was found, but not in facial motoneurons. Thus, GDNF does not play a key role in regulating survival of motoneurons during embryonic development.

The GDNF receptor complex involves a low-affinity binding component (GFRα1) (Jing et al. 1996), which is linked to the membrane via a GPI-anchor, comparable to the CNTFRα. In contrast to the CNTF/LIF-receptor complex, signal transduction of GDNF and related molecules is mediated by a tyrosine kinase (c-ret) which associates with the GFRα receptors after ligand binding and transmits the ligand-induced signal to the cell (Durbec et al. 1996; Treanor et al. 1996; Trupp et al. 1996). Thus, Ret-deficient mice show similar severe defect in kidney development and in the enteric nervous system (Taraviras et al. 1999; Baloh et al. 2000).

The GDNF gene family now comprises three additional factors which also activate the RET tyrosine kinase receptor which is shared by all these ligands. These molecules have been named neurturin, persephin and artemin. They seem to bind with some preference to one of four α-receptors, named GFRα1, GFRα2, GFRα3 and GFRα4. GDNF preferentially binds to GFRα1, neurturin to GFRα2, artemin to GFRα3 and persephin to GFRα4. However, neurturin and artemin also bind to GFRα1, so there is a structural basis for functional overlap between these ligands. The genes for the RET tyrosine kinase, the GFRα receptors, GDNF and other ligands have been inactivated in mice by standard techniques. Mice with deficiency in RET (Schuchardt et al. 1994), GFRα1 (Enomoto et al. 1998), and GDNF (Moore et al. 1996; Pichel et al. 1996; Sanchez et al. 1996) die during development. GDNF- and GFRα1-deficient mice fail to develop kidneys and enteric neurons and die around birth. RET and GFRα1 are expressed in the embryonic ureteric bud and GDNF is found in the metanephrogenic mesenchyme to which the ureteric buds grow during development. In *RET*-deficient mice, in addition to the lack of kidneys, many apoptotic cells are found in the foregut, and these mice show a massive loss of sympathetic neurons in the superior cervical ganglia. In this respect, they differ from GDNF-deficient mice. Significant loss of neurons in the $GDNF^{-/-}$ mice is also observed in nodose and sensory dorsal root ganglia, whereas loss of motoneurons is in a range of 20%–30%, thus resembling $CT-1^{-/-}$ mice.

Neurturin binds preferentially to GFRα2, and gene knockout for this ligand or its corresponding α-receptor does not lead to severe developmental defects. The mice are born, and they develop and breed normally, without any major organ defects (Heuckeroth et al. 1999; Rossi et al. 1999). A decrease in density of the myenteric plexus was observed which correlates with the relatively high expression of the GFRα2 receptor in autonomic neurons within gut and bowel after birth. Also some reduction of GFRα2-expressing sensory neurons in the dorsal root ganglia of neurturin-deficient mice have been observed, in particular in a population of neurons conferring heat sensitivity. However, it is not yet clear whether this reflects a loss of this subpopulation or simply the fact that expression of GFRα2 is reduced and function is disturbed when the ligand is lacking.

Mice with gene knockout of GFRα3 have been generated (Nishino et al. 1999), and the phenotype of these mice indicates that artemin/GFRα3-signalling plays a major role for migration and differentiation of sympathetic neurons in the superior cervical ganglion. GFRα3-deficient mice show ptosis which is due to lack of innervation for lacrimal gland secretion. Interestingly, no major defect was observed in paravertebral sympathetic and sensory ganglia.

Mice with deficiency of GFRα4 have been generated (J.O. Hiltunen et al., personal communication), they seem to be viable and fertile, and no gross abnormalities have been observed so far (Airaksinen and Saarma 2002).

Altogether, a significant overlap of defects between the GDNF and the neurotrophin families was observed, indicating that these two families of neurotrophic factors act together in promoting migration, differentiation, survival and function of specific populations of neurons. Currently, many efforts are being made to investigate these functional co-operations in more detail, and mouse models, in particular mice in which individual gene defects are combined in double- and triple-mutant mice, play a major role in these studies.

5
Signalling Pathways for Neurotrophic Factor-Mediated Neuronal

Recent years have seen significant progress in the understanding of signalling pathways which mediate the various functions of neurotrophic factors in neuronal cells. The neurotrophins have served as a prototypic gene family for investigation of the signalling pathways which regulate survival and other effects in primary neurons (Segal and Greenberg 1996). A significant contribution to this research was provided by investigations employing the rat pheochromocytoma cell line PC12. Signalling through high-affinity neurotrophin receptors which include members of the trk gene family involves several pathways. Initiation of this signalling depends on the cytosolic tyrosine phosphatase Shc, the activation of PLC-γ and the activation of the PI-3-kinase/AKT-pathways directly at the level of the trk transmembrane tyrosine kinases.

The Shc adapter proteins have been focus of research, as they can couple trk-signalling to the Ras/mitogen-activated protein (MAP) kinase pathway, which has been shown to be involved in promoting neuronal survival and neurite outgrowth. Experiments with PC-12 cells (Bar-Sagi and Feramisco 1985) and with primary sympathetic neurons have shown that activated ras can support differentiation and survival of primary neurons (Borasio et al. 1993), respectively. At least in PC-12 cells, sustained activation of the MAPK pathway (Traverse et al. 1992; Aletta 1994; Wixler et al. 1996) seems to be responsible for the differentiation versus mitogenic effects, and it has been suggested that sustained activation of the MAPK pathway is also responsible for the neurotrophin-mediated survival effect in neuronal cell lines and primary neurons. Recently, a second ras-independent pathway for activation of the MAPK pathway was shown to be involved in mediating the differentiation effects of NGF (York et al. 1998). This redirects focus of interest on activation mechanisms upstream from ras and other small GTP-binding proteins which transduce the signal from receptor molecules to the MAPK and other intracellular signalling pathways.

In neurons, several forms of Shc exist, which are named ShcA, ShcB, and ShcC/N-shc (Cattaneo and Pelicci 1998). The expression of these Shc isoforms stands under strict control during development, and only little is known so far about whether differences in the expression of these Shc isoforms influence signal transduction downstream of trk receptors, for example by determining downstream targets involved in mediating cellular effects of neurotrophic factors including survival of specific neuronal cell types at a specific stage of development. Particular attention deserves the ratio of ShcA and ShcC expression. ShcC/N has been detected as a neuron-specific Shc isoform (Nakamura et al. 1996) which mediates the coupling of trk signalling to Ras activation. Whereas ShcA is expressed in a widespread manner in virtually all types of cells, ShcC expression is only found in the brain at late stages of development. Interestingly, the upregulation of ShcC corresponds to a downregulation of ShcA expression in the brain at a developmental stage when neuronal cells become postmitotic (Conti et al. 1997) and at least some populations of neurons including the motoneurons become dependent on neurotrophic factors for their survival. It is tempting to speculate that this switch from ShcA to ShC expression might be responsible for a switch in response to neurotrophic factors from a differentiation signal to a survival signal (Segal and Greenberg 1996). This could be of importance for understanding how motoneurons become responsible to neurotrophic factors for their survival during development.

Recent evidence from mice in which the Shc binding site in trk-B was mutated (Minichiello et al. 1998) suggest that differences between various neurotrophic factors exist in the utilization of this pathway for mediating survival and neurite outgrowtheffects. Mice in which the Shc binding site of trk-B is mutated show that NT-4-mediated survival effects were more dramatically reduced than BDNF-dependent differentiation or survival. These mice display a complete loss of the NT-4 dependent D-hair cells but no change in BDNF-dependent slowly adapting mechanotransducing sensory neurons. However, survival of motoneurons has not been investigated in such mice so far, and it remains to be demonstrated whether survival or functional properties in motoneurons are altered when the Shc binding site is mutated in the trk-B receptor.

Nevertheless, this report showed that significant differences exist between various ligands in the activation of downstream pathways, even if shared receptor components such as trkB in the case of BDNF and NT-4 are involved.

Besides the ras/MAPK pathway, a second pathway involving activation of PI-3 K seems to be highly important for neuronal survival (Dudek et al. 1997). Although direct association of PI-3 K with trk receptors has been found under specific experimental conditions (Obermeier et al. 1993), it is now widely accepted that Shc signalling plays a major role for activation of PI-3 K downstream of trks in neuronal cells (Baxter et al. 1995; Greene and Kaplan 1995; Datta et al. 1997). The PI-3 kinase in turn leads to activation of Akt, a serine/threonine kinase with broad spectrum of substrates including the pro-apoptotic Bad (Datta et al. 1997), caspase-9 (Cardone et al. 1998), the forkhead transcription factor FKHRL1 (Brunet et al. 1999) and IκB kinase (IKK)α kinase, leading to activation of the nuclear factor (NF)-κB pathway (Ozes et al. 1999; Romashkova and Makarov 1999). It remains to be seen which of these downstream pathways is responsible for neuronal survival during various stages of development and in the adult.

A third important pathway which could be of importance for neuronal survival is the activation of phospholipase C (PLC)γ1 (Obermeier et al. 1994; Segal and Greenberg 1996; Tinhofer et al. 1996). Activation of this pathway leads to increased release of free Ca^{2+} from intracellular stores, which in turn can activate cyclic AMP-response element binding protein (CREB) (Finkbeiner et al. 1997; Lonze and Ginty 2002). In addition, elevated intracellular Ca^{2+} levels have also been described to activate the small GTP-binding protein Rap1 but not Ras (Grewal et al. 2000). This leads to activation of B-raf but not to activation of Raf-1. In developing motoneurons, B-raf is expressed at relatively high levels during the period of physiological cell death (Wiese et al. 2001). Thus, a link between various pathways could exist, and increased levels of Ca^{2+} could contribute to activation of Rafs, which seem to play a central role both in activation of the MAPK pathway, and also as effector kinases for bcl-2. Rafs could phosphorylate BAD and thus inhibit its pro-apoptotic activity (Wang et al. 1994).

5.1
Characterization of Downstream Signalling Pathways Which Mediate the Neuronal Survival Response to Neurotrophins and CNTF: The Role of Members of the IAP Family

Not very much is known about the downstream signals involved in execution of neuronal cell death and neurotrophic factor-mediated survival. Research on the role bcl-2 has guided the way to our present knowledge. Overexpression of bcl-2 can significantly reduce the extent of physiological neuronal cell death during development (Dubois-Dauphin et al. 1994; Martinou et al. 1994). However, mice in which bcl-2 expression is abolished by homologous recombination show only a small reduction of motoneuron numbers at birth (Michaelidis et al. 1996), indicating either that bcl-2-related molecules can substitute or that bcl-2 is not physiologically necessary for motoneuron survival during development. Interestingly, motoneuron cell death is enhanced in the postnatal period, leading to loss of around 40% of facial motoneurons of 6-week-old bcl-2$^{-/-}$ mice. This suggests that bcl-2 becomes important for postnatal survival at least of subpopulations of motoneurons. However, this does not mean that bcl-2-deficient motoneurons lose their responsiveness to neurotrophic factors. Both BDNF and CNTF are still capable of rescuing motoneurons from lesion-induced cell death after facial nerve transection in newborn animals. Nevertheless, survival in response to these neurotrophic factors was lower in bcl-2-deficient mice, indicating that subpopulations depend on bcl-2 for survival after nerve lesion and/or that compensation by other anti-apoptotic members of the bcl-2 family is only incomplete in these cells.

Observations that neurons from BAX-deficient mice (Knudson et al. 1995; Deckwerth et al. 1998) are resistant against cell death after neurotrophic factor deprivation provide a second indication that mechanisms involving members of the bcl-2 family are involved, and that mitochondria play a role in motoneuron cell death. Recently, it has been shown that BAX-dependent release of cytochrome c from mitochondria plays an essential role in the initiation of cell death in NGF-deprived sympathetic neurons (Deshmukh and Johnson 1998). However, microinjection of cytochrome c into the cytoplasm could not initiate cell death when the primary sympathetic neurons were grown in the presence of NGF. Based on these observations, it was speculated that NGF leads to a rapid production of an intracellular protein, which protects cells from pro-apoptotic actions of cytochrome c (Newmeyer and Green 1998). Furthermore, it was concluded that such protective molecules are expressed at low basal levels and up-regulated within a short time after NGF exposure.

Members of the inhibitor of apoptosis/inhibitor of T cell apoptosis (IAP/ITA) family are candidates for such protective proteins. They inhibit the activation of procaspase-9 (Deveraux et al. 1998), which is initiated by cytochrome c and Apaf-1 (Slee et al. 1999; Stennicke et al. 1999). Furthermore, they inhibit the function of activated caspase-3, -6 and -7, and thus at least at two levels interfere with cellular programs for apoptosis (Deveraux et al. 1997, 1998). The identification and cloning of the chick *ita* gene (Digby et al. 1996), which encodes a protein of 611 amino acids with highest homology to the human cIAP-2 gene (also called HIAP-1 or MIHC), allowed us to investigate the involvement of this protein in NGF-mediated survival of developing chick sympathetic and sensory neurons. We could show that NGF rapidly induced ITA expression in cultured sympathetic and sensory neurons. This upregulation of ITA mRNA and protein levels involves the PI-3 K pathway. Overexpression of ITA in primary sensory and sympathetic neurons can promote neuronal survival in the absence of NGF, and antisense expression of ITA can abolish the NGF survival effect in sensory and sympathetic neurons. These actions are apparently mediated through the baculovirus IAP repeat (BIR domains) of the ITA protein, as expression of a BIR-deleted form of ITA, was without any effect on neuronal survival.

These data suggest that members of the IAP family which include the mammalian IAP-2 and XIAP are important molecules which are involved in the signalling machinery for neurotrophic factor-mediated survival of sympathetic and sensory neurons. The expression of inhibitors for caspases could be an essential mechanism which contributes to motoneurons survival once these caspases are activated, and they probably could be of high importance in protecting motoneurons to any kind of pro-apoptotic signalling which might occur during postnatal life and which has to be neutralized for further maintenance of these cells.

References

Adler, R., Landa, K.B., Manthorpe, M., and Varon, S. (1979) Cholinergic neurotrophic factors: intraocular distribution of trophic activity for ciliary neurons. Science *204*, 1434–1436

Airaksinen, M.S. and Saarma, M. (2002) The GDNF family: signalling, biological functions and therapeutic value. Nat.Rev.Neurosci. *3*, 383–394

Aletta, J.M. (1994) Differential effect of NGF and EGF on ERK in neuronally differentiated PC12 cells. Neuroreport 5, 2090–2092

Alexander, W.S., Rakar, S., Robb, L., Farley, A., Willson, T.A., Zhang, J.G., Hartley, L., Kikuchi, Y., Kojima, T., Nomura, H., Hasegawa, M., Maeda, M., Fabri, L., Jachno, K., Nash, A., Metcalf, D., Nicola, N.A., and Hilton, D.J. (1999) Suckling defect in mice lacking the soluble haemopoietin receptor NR6. Curr.Biol. 9, 605–608

Baloh, R.H., Enomoto, H., Johnson, E.M., Jr., and Milbrandt, J. (2000) The GDNF family ligands and recept. Curr.Opin.Neurobiol. 10, 103–110

Bar-Sagi, D. and Feramisco, J.R. (1985) Microinjection of the ras oncogene protein into PC12 cells induces morphological differentiation. Cell 42, 841–848

Barbin, G., Manthorpe, M., and Varon, S. (1984) Purification of the chick eye ciliary neuronotrophic factor. J.Neurochem. 43, 1468–1478

Barde, Y.-A. (1990) The nerve growth factor family. Progress in Growth Factor Research 2, 237–248

Barres, B.A., Jacobson, M.D., Schmid, R., Sendtner, M., and Raff, M.C. (1993) Does oligodendrocyte survival depend on axons? Current Biology 3, 489–497

Baxter, R.M., Cohen, P., Obermeier, A., Ullrich, A., Downes, C.P., and Doza, Y.N. (1995) Phosphotyrosine residues in the nerve-growth-factor receptor (Trk-A) Their role in the activation of inositolphospholipid metabolism and protein kinase cascades in phaeochromocytoma (PC12) cells. Eur.J.Biochem. 234, 84–91

Berkemeier, L.R., Winslow, J.W., Kaplan, D.R., Nikolics, K., Goeddel, D.V., and Rosenthal,A. (1991) Neurotrophin-5: A novel neurotrophic factor that activates trk and trkB. Neuron 7, 857–866

Blondet, B., Hantaz Ambroise, D., Ait Ikhlef, A., Cambier, D., Murawsky, M., and Rieger, F. (1995) Astrocytosis in wobbler mouse spinal cord involves a population of astrocytes which is glutamine synthetase-negative. Neurosci Lett 183, 179–182

Boemel, H., Xie, G., Rossoll, W., Wiese, S., Jablonka, S., Boehm, T., and Sendtner, M. (2002) Missense mutation in the tubulin-specific chaperone E (Tbce) gene in the mouse mutant progressive motor neuronopathy, a model of human motoneuron disease. Journal of Cell Biology 159, 563–569

Borasio,G.D., Markus,A., Wittinghofer,A., Barde,Y.A., and Heumann,R. (1993) Involvement of ras p21 in neurotrophin-induced response of sensory, but not sympathetic neurons. Journal of Cell Biology 121, 665–672

Bothwell, M. (1996) p75NTR: a receptor after all. Science 272, 506–507

Brady, R., Zaidi, S.I., Mayer, C., and Katz, D.M. (1999) BDNF is a target-derived survival factor for arterial baroreceptor and chemoafferent primary sensory neurons. J.Neurosci. 19, 2131–2142

Bronson, R.T., Lake, B.D., Cook, S., Taylor, S., and Davisson, M.T. (1993) Motor neuron degeneration of mice is a model of neuronal ceroid lipofuscinosis (Batten's disease) Ann.Neurol. 33, 381–385

Brunet, A., Bonni, A., Zigmond, M.J., Lin, M.Z., Juo, P., Hu, L.S., Anderson, M.J., Arden, K.C., Blenis, J., and Greenberg, M.E. (1999) Akt promotes cell survival by phosphorylating and inhibiting a Forkhead transcription factor. Cell 96, 857–868

Cardone, M.H., Roy, N., Stennicke, H.R., Salvesen, G.S., Franke, T.F., Stanbridge, E., Frisch,S., and Reed,J.C. (1998) Regulation of cell death protease caspase-9 by phosphorylation. SCIENCE 282, 1318–1321

Carter, B.D., Zirrgiebel, U., and Barde, Y.A. (1995) Differential regulation of p21ras activation in neurons by nerve growth factor and brain-derived neurotrophic factor. J Biol Chem 270, 21751–21757

Cattaneo, E. and Pelicci, P.G. (1998) Emerging roles for SH2/PTB-containing Shc adaptor proteins in the developing mammalian brain. Trends Neurosci. 21, 476–481

Conover, J.C., Erickson, J.T., Katz, D.M., Bianchi, L.M., Poueymirou, W.T., McClain, J., Pan, L., Helgren, M., Ip, N.Y., Boland, P., Friedman, B., Wiegand, S., Vejsada, R., Kato, A.C., DeChiara, T.M., and Yancopoulos, G.D. (1995) Neuronal deficits, not involving motor neurons, in mice lacking BDNF and/or NT4. Nature 375, 235–238

Conti, L., De Fraja, C., Gulisano, M., Migliaccio, E., Govoni, S., and Cattaneo, E. (1997) Expression and activation of SH2/PTB-containing ShcA adaptor protein reflects the pattern of neurogenesis in the mammalian brain. Proc.Natl.Acad.Sci.U.S.A 94, 8185–8190

Crowley, C., Spencer, S.D., Nishimura, M.C., Chen, K.S., Pitts-Meek, S., Armanini, M.P., Ling, L.H., McMahon, S.B., Shelton, D.L., Levinson, A.D., and Phillips, H.S. (1994) Mice lacking nerve growth factor display perinatal loss of sensory and sympathetic neurons yet develop basal forebrain cholinergic neurons. Cell 76, 1001–1011

Datta, S.R., Dudek, H., Tao, X., Masters, S., Fu, H., Gotoh, Y., and Greenberg, M.E. (1997) Akt phosphorylation of BAD couples survival signals to the cell- intrinsic death machinery. Cell 91, 231–241

Davis, S., Aldrich, T.H., Ip, N.Y., Stahl, N., Scherer, S., Farruggella, T., Distefano, P.S., Curtis, R., Panayotatos, N., Gascan, H., Chevalier, S., and Yancopoulos, G.D. (1993) Released form of cntf receptor-alpha component as a soluble mediator of cntf responses. SCIENCE 259, 1736–1739

Dechant, G. and Barde, Y.A. (1997) Signalling through the neurotrophin receptor p75NTR. Current Opinion in Neurobiology 7, 413–418

DeChiara, T.M., Vejsada, R., Poueymirou, W.T., Acheson, A., Suri, C., Conover, J.C., Friedman, B., McClain, J., Pan, L., Stahl, N., Ip, N.Y., Kato, A., and Yancopoulos, G.D. (1995) Mice lacking the CNTF receptor, unlike mice lacking CNTF, exhibit profound motor neuron deficits at birth. Cell 83, 313–322

Deckwerth, T.L., Easton, R.M., Knudson, C.M., Korsmeyer, S.J., and Johnson, E.M., Jr. (1998) Placement of the BCL2 family member BAX in the death pathway of sympathetic neurons activated by trophic factor deprivation. Exp.Neurol. 152, 150–162

Deshmukh, M. and Johnson, E.M., Jr. (1998) Evidence of a novel event during neuronal death: development of competence-to-die in response to cytoplasmic cytochrome c]. Neuron 21, 695–705

Deveraux, Q.L., Roy, N., Stennicke, H.R., Van Arsdale, T., Zhou, Q., Srinivasula, S.M., Alnemri, E.S., Salvesen, G.S., and Reed, J.C. (1998) IAPs block apoptotic events induced by caspase-8 and cytochrome c by direct inhibition of distinct caspases. EMBO J. 17, 2215–2223

Deveraux, Q.L., Takahashi, R., Salvesen, G.S., and Reed, J.C. (1997) X-linked IAP is a direct inhibitor of cell-death proteases. 1995Nature 388, 300–304

Digby,M.R., Kimpton,W.G., York,J.J., Connick,T.E., and Lowenthal,J.W. (1996) ITA, a vertebrate homologue of IAP that is expressed in T lymphocytes. DNA Cell Biol. 15, 981–988

Dubois-Dauphin, M., Frankowski, H., Tsujimoto, Y., Huarte, J., and Martinou, J.-C. (1994) Neonatal motoneurons overexpressing the bcl-2 protooncogene in transgenic mice are protected from axotomy-induced cell death. Proceedings of the national academy of science USA 91, 3309–3313

Dudek, H., Datta, S.R., Franke, T.F., Birnbaum, M.J., Yao, R., Cooper, G.M., Segal, R.A., Kaplan, D.R., and Greenberg, M.E. (1997) Regulation of neuronal survival by the serine-threonine protein kinase Akt. SCIENCE 275, 661–665

Durbec, P., Marcos Gutierrez, C.V., Kilkenny, C., Grigoriou, M., Wartiowaara, K., Suvanto, P., Smith, D., Ponder, B., Costantini, F., Saarma, M., Sariola, H., and Pachnis, V. (1996) GDNF signalling through the Ret receptor tyrosine kinase. Nature 381, 789–793

Eide, F.F., Lowenstein, D.H., and Reichardt, L.F. (1993) Neurotrophins and their receptors–Current concepts and implications for neurologic disease. Exp.Neurol. 121, 200–214

Elson, G.C., Lelievre, E., Guillet, C., Chevalier, S., Plun-Favreau, H., Froger, J., Suard, I., de Coignac, A.B., Delneste, Y., Bonnefoy, J.Y., Gauchat, J.F., and Gascan, H. (2000) CLF associates with CLC to form a functional heteromeric ligand for the CNTF receptor complex. Nat.Neurosci. 3, 867–872

Enomoto, H., Araki, T., Jackman, A., Heuckeroth, R.O., Snider, W.D., Johnson, E.M., Jr., and Milbrandt, J. (1998) GFR alpha1-deficient mice have deficits in the enteric nervous system and kidneys. Neuron 21, 317–324

Ernfors, P., Kucera, J., Lee, K.F., Loring, J., and Jaenisch, R. (1995) Studies on the physiological role of brain-derived neurotrophic factor and neurotrophin-3 in knockout mice. Int.J.Dev.Biol. 39, 799–807

Ernfors, P., Lee, K.-F., Kucera, J., and Jaenisch, R. (1994) Lack of neurotrophin-3 leads to deficiencies in the peripheral nervous system and loss of limb proprioceptive afferents. Cell 77, 503–512

Ernfors, P. and Persson, H. (1991) Developmentally regulated expression of NDNF/NT-3 mRNA in rat spinal cord motoneurons and expression of BDNF mRNA in embryonic dorsal root ganglion. European Journal of Neuroscience 3, 953–961

Escary, J.-L., Perreau, J., Duménil, D., Ezine, S., and Brûlet, P. (1993) Leukaemia inhibitory factor is necessary for maintenance of haematopoietic stem cells and thymocyte stimulation. Nature 363, 361–364

Fantuzzi, G., Benigni, F., Sironi, M., Conni, M., Carelli, M., Cantoni, L., Shapiro, L., Dinarello, C.A., Sipe, J.D., and Ghezzi, P. (1995) Ciliary neurotrophic factor (CNTF) induces serum amyloid A, hypoglycaemia and anorexia, and potentiates IL-1 induced corticosterone and IL-6 production in mice. Cytokine. 7, 150–156

Finkbeiner, S., Tavazoie, S.F., Maloratsky, A., Jacobs, K.M., Harris, K.M., and Greenberg, M.E. (1997) CREB: a major mediator of neuronal neurotrophin responses. Neuron 19, 1031–1047

Frade, J.M., Rodriguez Tebar, A., and Barde, Y.A. (1996) Induction of cell death by endogenous nerve growth factor through its p75 receptor. Development 383, 166–168

Funakoshi, H., Belluasdo, N., Arenas, E., Yamamoto, Y., Casabona, A., Persson, H., and Ibanez, C.F. (1995) Muscle-derived Neurotrophin-4 as an activity-dependent trophic signal for adult motor neurons. SCIENCE 268, 1495–1499

Gearing, D.P., Comeau, M.R., Friend, D.J., Gimpel, S.D., Thut, C.J., McGourty, J., Brasher, K.K., King, J.A., Gillis, S., Mosley, B., and et al (1992) The IL-6 signal transducer, gp130: an oncostatin M receptor and affinity converter for the LIF receptor. SCIENCE 255, 1434–1437

Gearing, D.P., Thut, C.J., VandeBos, T., Gimpel, S.D., Delaney, P.B., King, J., Price, V., Cosman, D., and Beckmann, M.P. (1991) Leukemia inhibitory factor receptor is structurally related to the IL-6 signal transducer, gp130. EMBO J. 10, 2839–2848

Giess, R., Beck, M., Goetz, R., Nitsch, R.M., Toyka, K.V., and Sendtner, M. (2000a) Potential role of LIF as a modifier gene in the pathogenesis of amyotrophic lateral sclerosis. Neurology 54, 1003–1005

Giess, R., Beck, M., Goetz, R., Nitsch, R.M., Toyka, K.V., and Sendtner, M. (2000b) Potential role of LIF as a modifier gene in the pathogenesis of amyotrophic lateral sclerosis Neurology 54, 1003–1005

Giess, R., Holtmann, B., Braga, M., Grimm, T., Muller-Myhsok, B., Toyka, K.V., and Sendtner, M. (2002a) Early onset of severe familial amyotrophic lateral sclerosis with a SOD-1 mutation: potential impact of CNTF as a candidate modifier gene. Am.J.-Hum.Genet. 70, 1277–1286

Giess, R., Maurer, M., Linker, R., Gold, R., Warmuth-Metz, M., Toyka, K.V., Sendtner, M., and Rieckmann, P. (2002b) Association of a null mutation in the CNTF gene with early onset of multiple sclerosis. Arch.Neurol. 59, 407–409

Ginty, D.D. and Segal, R.A. (2002) Retrograde neurotrophin signaling: Trk-ing along the axon. Curr.Opin.Neurobiol. 12, 268–274

Gravel, C., Götz, R., Lorrain, A., and Sendtner, M. (1997) Adenoviral gene transfer of ciliary neurotrophic factor and brain-derived neurotrophic factor leads to longterm survival of axotomized motoneurons. Nature Medicine 3, 765–770

Greene, L.A. and Kaplan, D.R. (1995) Early events in neurotrophin signalling via Trk and p75 receptors. Curr.Opin.Neurobiol. 5, 579–587

Grewal, S.S., Horgan, A.M., York, R.D., Withers, G.S., Banker, G.A., and Stork, P.J. (2000) Neuronal Calcium Activates a Rap1 and B-Raf Signaling Pathway via the Cyclic Adenosine Monophosphate-dependent Protein Kinase. Journal of Biological Chemistry 275, 3722–3728

Griesbeck, O., Parsadanian, A.Sh., Sendtner, M., and Thoenen, H. (1995) Expression of neurotrophins in skeletal muscle: Quantitative comparison and significance for motoneuron survival and maintenance of function. J.Neurosci.Res. 42, 21–33

Hallböök, F., Ibáñez, C.F., and Persson, H. (1991) Evolutionary studies of the nerve growth factor family reveal a novel member abundantly expressed in Xenopus ovary. Neuron 6, 845–858

Hamburger, V. (1934) The effects of wing bud extirpation on the development of the central nervous system in chick embryos. J.Exp.Zool. 68, 449–494

Hamburger, V. (1958) Regression versus peripheral control of differentiation in motor hyperplasia. Am.J.Anat. 102, 365–410

Hartikka, J. and Hefti, F. (1988) Comparison of nerve growth factor's effects on development of septum, striatum, and nucleus basalis cholinergic neurons in vitro. J.Neurosci.Res. 21, 352–364

Helgren, M.E., Friedman, B., Kennedy, M., Mullholland, K., Messer, A., Wong, V., and Lindsay, R.M. Ciliary neurotrophic factor (CNTF) delays motor impairments in the mnd mouse, a genetic model of motor neuron disease. Neurosci.Abstr. 267.11, 618. 1992

Henderson, C.E., Camu, W., Mettling, C., Gouin, A., Poulsen, K., Karihaloo, M., Rullamas, J., Evans, T., McMahon, S.B., Armanini, M.P., Berkemeier, L., Phillips, H.S., and Rosenthal,A. (1993) Neurotrophins promote motor neuron survival and are present in embryonic limb bud. Nature 363, 266–270

Henderson, C.E., Phillips, H.S., Pollock, R.A., Davies, A.M., Lemeulle, C., Armanini, M., Simpson, L.C., Moffet, B., Vandlen, R.A., Koliatsos, V.E., and et al (1994) GDNF: a potent survival factor for motoneurons present in peripheral nerve and muscle. SCIENCE 266, 1062–1064

Heuckeroth, R.O., Enomoto, H., Grider, J.R., Golden, J.P., Hanke, J.A., Jackman, A., Molliver, D.C., Bardgett, M.E., Snider, W.D., Johnson, E.M., Jr., and Milbrandt, J. (1999) Gene targeting reveals a critical role for neurturin in the development and maintenance of enteric, sensory, and parasympathetic neurons. Neuron 22, 253–263

Hohn, A., Leibrock, J., Bailey, K., and Barde, Y.-A. (1990) Identification and characterzation of a novel member of the nerve growth factor/brain-derived neurotrophic factor family. Nature 344, 339–341

Holliday,M. and Hamburger,V. (1975) Reduction of the naturally occuring motor neuron loss by enlargement of the periphery. J.Comp.Neurol. 170, 311–320

Hughes, R.A., Sendtner, M., and Thoenen, H. (1993) Members of several gene families influence survival of rat motoneurons in vitro and in vivo. J.Neurosci.Res. 36(6), 663–671

Jing, S., Wen, D., Yu, Y., Holst, P.L., Luo, Y., Fang, M., Tamir, R., Antonio, L., Hu, Z., Cupples, R., Louis, J.C., Hu, S., Altrock, B.W., and Fox, G.M. (1996) GDNF-induced activation of the ret protein tyrosine kinase is mediated by GDNFR-alpha, a novel receptor for GDNF. Cell 85, 1113–1124

Kaplan, D.R. and Miller, F.D. (2000) Neurotrophin signal transduction in the nervous system. Curr.Opin.Neurobiol. 10, 381–391

Kerkhoff, H., Troost, D., Louwerse, E.S., Van Dijk, M., Veldman, H., and Jennekens, F.G.I. (1993) Inflammatory cells in the peripheral nervous system in motor neuron disease. Acta Neuropathol.(Berl.) 85, 560–565

Klein, R., Silos-Santiago,I ., Smeyne, R.J., Lira, S.A., Brambilla, R., Bryant, S., Zhang, L., Snider, W.D., and Barbacid, M. (1994) Disruption of the neurotrophin-3 receptor gene trkC eliminates Ia muscle afferents and results in abnormal movements.Nature 368, 249–251

Klein, R., Smeyne, R.J., Wurst, W., Long, L.K., Auerbach, B.A., Joyner, A.L., and Barbacid, M. (1993) Targeted disruption of the trkB neurotrophin receptor results in nervous system lesions and neonatal death. Cell *75*, 113–122

Knudson, C.M., Tung, K.S., Tourtellotte, W.G., Brown, G.A., and Korsmeyer,S.J. (1995) Bax-deficient mice with lymphoid hyperplasia and male germ cell death. SCIENCE *270*, 96–99

Koliatsos, V.E., Shelton, D.L., Mobley, W.C., and Price, D.L. (1991) A novel group of nerve growth factor receptor-immunoreactive neurons in the ventral horn of the lumbar spinal cord. Brain Res. *541*, 121–128

Kucera, J., Ernfors, P., and Jaenisch, R. (1995) Reduction in the number of spinal motor neurons in neurotrophin-3-deficient mice. Neurosci. *69*, 312–330

Lee, R., Kermani, P., Teng, K.K., and Hempstead, B.L. (2001) Regulation of cell survival by secreted proneurotrophins. SCIENCE *294*, 1945–1948

Leibrock, J., Lottspeich, F., Hohn, A., Hofer, M., Hengerer, B., Masiakowski, P., Thoenen, H., and Barde, Y.-A. (1989) Molecular cloning and expression of brain-derived neurotrophic factor. Nature *341*, 149–152

Levi-Montalcini, R. (1987) The nerve growth factor: thirty-five years later. EMBO J. *6*, 1145–1154

Levi-Montalcini, R., Meyer, H., and Hamburger, V. (1954) In vitro experiments on the effects of mouse sarcomas 180 and 37 on the spinal and sympathetic ganglia of the chick embryo. Cancer Res. *14*, 49–57

Li, M., Sendtner, M., and Smith, A. (1995a) Essential function of LIF receptor in motor neurons. Nature *378*, 724–727

Li, Y., Holtzman, D.M., Kromer, L.F., Kaplan, D.R., Chua-Couzens, J., Clary, D.O., Knusel, B., and Mobley, W.C. (1995b) Regulation of TrkA and ChAT expression in developing rat basal forebrain: evidence that both exogenous and endogenous NGF regulate differentiation of cholinergic neurons. J.Neurosci. *15*, 2888–2905

Liebl, D.J., Tessarollo, L., Palko, M.E., and Parada, L.F. (1997) Absence of sensory neurons before target innervation in brain-derived neurotrophic factor-, neurotrophin 3-, and TrkC-deficient embryonic mice. J.Neurosci. *17*, 9113–9121

Lin, L.-F., Mismer, D., Lile, J.D., Armes, L.G., Butler III, E.T., Vannice, J.L., and Collins, F. (1989) Purification, cloning, and expression of ciliary neurotrophic factor (CNTF) SCIENCE *246*, 1023–1025

Lin, L.-F.H., Doherty, D.H., Lile, J.D., Bektesh, S., and Collins, F. (1993) GDNF: A glial cell line-derived neurotrophic factor for midbrain dopaminergic neurons. SCIENCE *260*, 1130–1132

Liu, X., Ernfors, P., Wu, H., and Jaenisch, R. (1995) Sensory but not motor neuron deficits in mice lacking NT4 and BDNF. Nature *375*, 238–240

Liu, X. and Jaenisch, R. (2000) Severe peripheral sensory neuron loss and modest motor neuron reduction in mice with combined deficiency of brain-derived neurotrophic factor, neurotrophin 3 and neurotrophin 4/5. Dev.Dyn. *218*, 94–101

Lohof, A.M., Ip, N.Y., and Poo, M. (1993) Potentiation of developing neuromuscular synapses by the neurotrophins NT-3 and BDNF. Nature *363*, 350–353

Lonze, B.E. and Ginty, D.D. (2002) Function and regulation of CREB family transcription factors in the nervous system. Neuron *35*, 605–623

Maisonpierre, P.C., Belluscio, L., Squinto, S.P., Ip, N.Y., Furth, M.E., Lindsay, R.M., and Yancopoulos, G.D. (1990) Neurotrophin-3: A neurotrophic factor related to NGF and BDNF. SCIENCE *247*, 1446–1451

Martin, N., Jaubert, J., Gounon, P., Salido, E., Haase, G., Szatanik, M., and Guenet, J.L. (2002) A missense mutation in Tbce causes progressive motor neuronopathy in mice. Nat.Genet. *32*, 443–447

Martinou, J.-C., Dubois-Dauphin, M., Staple, J.K., Rodriguez, I., Frankowski, H., Missotten, M., Albertini, P., Talabot, D., Catsicas, S., Pietra, C., and Huarte, J. (1994) Overexpression of BCL-2 in transgenic mice protects neurons from naturally occurring cell death and experimental ischemia. Neuron *13*, 1017–1030

Masu, Y., Wolf, E., Holtmann, B., Sendtner, M., Brem, G., and Thoenen, H. (1993) Disruption of the CNTF gene results in motor neuron degeneration. Nature365, 27–32

Maurer, M., Linker, R., Gold, R., Toyka, K.V., Sendtner, M., and Rieckmann, P. (2002) A Null Mutation in the CNTF Gene Is Not Associated With Early Onset of Multiple Sclerosis. Arch.Neurol. 59, 1974–1975

Metcalf, D. and Gearing, D.P. (1989) Fatal syndrome in mice engrafted with cells producing high levels of the leukemia inhibitory factor. Proc.Natl.Acad.Sci.U.S.A 86, 5948–5952

Meyer, M., Matsuoka, I., Wetmore, C., Olson, L., and Thoenen, H. (1992) Enhanced synthesis of brain-derived neurotrophic factor in the lesioned peripheral nerve: Different mechanisms are responsible for the regulation of BDNF and NGF mRNA. Journal of Cell Biology 119, 45–54

Michaelidis, T.M., Sendtner, M., Cooper, J.D., Airaksinen, M., Holtmann, B., Meyer, M., and Thoenen, H. (1996) Inactivation of the bcl-2 gene results in progressive degeneration of motoneurons, sensory and sympathetic neurons during early postnatal development. Neuron 17, 75–89

Minichiello, L., Casagranda, F., Tatche, R.S., Stucky, C.L., Postigo, A., Lewin, G.R., Davies, A.M., and Klein, R. (1998) Point mutation in trkB causes loss of NT4-dependent neurons without major effects on diverse BDNF responses. Neuron 21, 335–345

Minichiello, L. and Klein, R. (1996) TrkB and TrkC neurotrophin receptors cooperate in promoting survival of hippocampal and cerebellar granule neurons. Genes Dev. 10, 2849–2858

Mitsumoto, H., Ikeda, K., Wong, V., Lindsay, R.M., and Cedarbaum,J.M. Recombinant human ciliary neurotrophic factor (rHCNTF) improves muscle strength in wobbler mouse motor neuron disease. Genetics and cell biology of the motor neurone. Third international Symposium on ALS/MND. T6. 1992

Miyata, Y., Kashihara, Y., Homma, S., and Kuno, M. (1986) Effects of nerve growth factor on the survival and synaptic function of Ia sensory neurons axotomized in neonatal rats. J.Neurosci. 6, 2012–2018

Moore, M.W., Klein, R.D., Farinas, I., Sauer, H., Armanini, M., Phillips, H., Reichardt, L.F., Ryan, A.M., Carver Moore, K., and Rosenthal, A. (1996) Renal and neuronal abnormalities in mice lacking GDNF. Nature 382, 76–79

Nakamura, T., Sanokawa, R., Sasaki, Y., Ayusawa, D., Oishi, M., and Mori, N. (1996) N-Shc:a neural-specific adapter molecule that mediates signaling from neurotrophin/Trk to Ras/Mapk pathway. Oncogene 1111–1121

Newmeyer, D.D. and Green, D.R. (1998) Surviving the cytochrome seas. Neuron 21, 653–655

Nishino, J., Mochida, K., Ohfuji, Y., Shimazaki, T., Meno, C., Ohishi, S., Matsuda, Y., Fujii, H., Saijoh, Y., and Hamada, H. (1999) GFR alpha3, a component of the artemin receptor, is required for migration and survival of the superior cervical ganglion. Neuron 23, 725–736

Obermeier, A., Bradshaw, R.A., Seedorf, K., Choidas, A., Schlessinger, J., and Ullrich, A. (1994) Neuronal differentiation signals are controlled by nerve growth factor receptor/Trk binding sites for SHC and PLCgamma. EMBO J. 13, 1585–1590

Obermeier, A., Lammers, R., Wiesmuller, K.H., Jung, G., Schlessinger, J., and Ullrich, A. (1993) Identification of Trk binding sites for SHC and phosphatidylinositol 3'- kinase and formation of a multimeric signaling complex. Journal of Biological Chemistry 268, 22963–22966

Oppenheim, R.W. (1991) Cell death during development of the nervous system. Annu.Rev.Neurosci. 14, 453–501

Oppenheim, R.W., Houenou, L.J., Johnson, J.E., Lin, L.F., Li, L., Lo, A.C., Newsome, A.L., Prevette, D.M., and Wang, S. (1995) Developing motor neurons rescued from programmed and axotomy- induced cell death by GDNF. Nature 373, 344–346

Oppenheim, R.W., Qin-Wei, Y., Prevette, D., and Yan, Q. (1992) Brain-derived neurotrophic factor rescues developing avian motoneurons from cell death. Nature 360, 755–757

Oppenheim, R.W., Wiese, S., Prevette, D., Armanini, M., Wang, S., Houenou, L.J., Holt-mann, B., Gotz, R., Pennica, D., and Sendtner, M. (2001) Cardiotrophin-1, a Muscle-Derived Cytokine, Is Required for the Survival of Subpopulations of Developing Motoneurons. J.Neurosci. *21*, 1283–1291

Ozes, O.N., Mayo, L.D., Gustin, J.A., Pfeffer, S.R., Pfeffer, L.M., and Donner, D.B. (1999) NF-kappaB activation by tumour necrosis factor requires the Akt serine- threonine kinase. Nature *401*, 82–85

Pennica, D., Shaw, K.J., Swanson, T.A., Moore, M.W., Shelton, D.L., Zioncheck, K.A., Rosenthal, A., Taga, T., Paoni, N.F., and Wood, W.I. (1995) Cardiotrophin-1. Biological activities and binding to the leukemia inhibitory factor receptor/gp130 signaling complex. Journal of Biological Chemistry *270*, 10915–10922

Pichel, J.G., Shen, L., Sheng, H.Z., Granholm, A.C., Drago, J., Grinberg, A., Lee, E.J., Huang, S.P., Saarma, M., Hoffer, B.J., Sariola, H., and Westphal, H. (1996) Defects in enteric innervation and kidney development in mice lacking GDNF. Nature *382*, 73–76

Pinon, L.G., Minichiello, L., Klein, R., and Davies, A.M. (1996) Timing of neuronal death in trkA, trkB and trkC mutant embryos reveals developmental changes in sensory neuron dependence on Trk signalling. Development *122*, 3255–3261

Rabizadeh, S., Oh, J., Zhong, L., Yang, J., Bitler, C.M., Butcher, L.L., and Bredesen, D.E. (1993) Induction of apoptosis by the low-affinity NGF receptor. SCIENCE *261*, 345–348

Romashkova, J.A. and Makarov, S.S. (1999) NF-kappaB is a target of AKT in anti-apoptotic PDGF signalling Nature *401*, 86–90

Rossi,J., Luukko,K., Poteryaev,D., Laurikainen,A., Sun,Y.F., Laakso,T., Eerikainen,S., Tuominen,R., Lakso,M., Rauvala,H., Arumae,U., Pasternack,M., Saarma,M., and Airaksinen,M.S. (1999) Retarded growth and deficits in the enteric and parasympathetic nervous system in mice lacking GFR alpha2, a functional neurturin receptor. Neuron *22*, 243–252

Ryffel, B. (1993) Pathology induced by leukemia inhibitory factor. Int.Rev.Exp.Pathol. *34* Pt B, 69–72

Sanchez, M.P., Silos Santiago, I., Frisen, J., He, B., Lira, S.A., and Barbacid, M. (1996) Renal agenesis and the absence of enteric neurons in mice lacking GDNF. Nature *382*, 70–73

Schnell, L., Schneider, R., Kolbeck, R., Barde, Y.-A., and Schwab, M.E. (1994) Neurotrophin-3 enhances sprouting of corticospinal tract during development and after spinal cord lesion. Nature *367*, 170–173

Schuchardt, A., D'Agati, V., Larsson-Blomberg, L., Costantini, F., and Pachnis, V. (1994) Defects in the kidney and enteric nervous system of mice lacking the tyrosine kinase receptor Ret. Nature *367*, 380–383

Seeburger, J.L., Tarras, S., Natter, H., and Springer, J.E. (1993) Spinal cord motoneurons express p75[NGFR] and p145[trkB] mRNA in amyotrophic lateral sclerosis. Brain Res. *621*, 111–115

Segal, R.A. and Greenberg, M.E. (1996) Intracellular signaling pathways activated by neurotrophic factors. Annu.Rev.Neurosci. *19*, 463–489

Sendtner, M., Götz, R., Holtmann, B., Escary, J.-L., Masu, Y., Carroll, P., Wolf, E., Brehm, G., Brulet, P., and Thoenen, H. (1996) Cryptic physiological trophic support of motoneurons by LIF disclosed by double gene targeting of CNTF and LIF. Current Biology *6*, 686–694

Sendtner, M., Holtmann, B., Kolbeck, R., Thoenen, H., and Barde, Y.-A. (1992a) Brain-derived neurotrophic factor prevents the death of motoneurons in newborn rats after nerve section. Nature *360*, 757–758

Sendtner, M., Schmalbruch, H., Stöckli, K.A., Carroll, P., Kreutzberg, G.W., and Thoenen,H. (1992b) Ciliary neurotrophic factor prevents degeneration of motor neurons in mouse mutant progressive motor neuronopathy. Nature *358*, 502–504

Shapiro, L., Zhang, X.-X., Rupp, R.G., Wolff, S.M., and Dinarello, C.A. (1993) Ciliary neu-rotrophic factor is an endogenous pyrogen. Proceedings of the national academy of science USA *90*, 8614–8618

Silos-Santiago, I., Molliver, D.C., Ozaki, S., Smeyne, R.J., Fagan, A.M., Barbacid, M., and Snider, W.D. (1995) Non-TrkA-expressing small DRG neurons are lost in TrkA defi-cient mice. J.Neurosci. *15*, 5929–5942

Slee, E.A., Harte, M.T., Kluck, R.M., Wolf, B.B., Casiano, C.A., Newmeyer, D.D., Wang, H.G., Reed, J.C., Nicholson, D.W., Alnemri, E.S., Green, D.R., and Martin, S.J. (1999) Ordering the Cytochrome c-initiated Caspase Cascade: Hierarchical Activation of Caspases-2, -3, -6, -7, -8, and −10 in a Caspase-9- dependent Manner. Journal of Cell Biology *144*, 281–292

Snider, W.D. (1994) Functions of the neurotrophins during nervous system development: What the knockouts are teaching us. Cell *77*, 627–638

Stahl, N. and Yancopoulos, G.D. (1994) The tripartite CNTF receptor complex: Activation and signaling involves components shared with other cytokines. J.Neurobiol. *25*, 1454–1466

Stennicke, H.R., Deveraux, Q.L., Humke, E.W., Reed, J.C., Dixit, V.M., and Salvesen, G.S. (1999) Caspase-9 can Be activated without proteolytic processing. Journal of Biologi-cal Chemistry *274*, 8359–8362

Stöckli, K.A., Lottspeich, F., Sendtner, M., Masiakowski, P., Carroll, P., Götz, R., Lindholm, D., and Thoenen, H. (1989) Molecular cloning, expression and regional distribution of rat ciliary neurotrophic factor. Nature *342*, 920–923

Stoeckel, K., Schwab, M., and Thoenen, H. (1975) Specificity of retrograde transport of nerve growth factor (NGF) in sensory neurons: a biochemical and morphological study. Brain Res. *81*, 1–14

Strohmaier, C., Carter, B.D., Urfer, R., Barde, Y.A., and Dechant, G. (1996) A splice variant of the neurotrophin receptor trkB with increased specificity for brain-derived neuro-trophic factor. EMBO J. *15*, 3332–3337

Stucky, C.L., DeChiara, T., Lindsay, R.M., Yancopoulos, G.D., and Koltzenburg, M. (1998) Neurotrophin 4 is required for the survival of a subclass of hair follicle receptors. J.Neurosci. *18*, 7040–7046

Takahashi, R., Yokoji, H., Misawa, H., Hayashi, M., Hu, J., and Deguchi, T. (1994) A null mutation in the human *CNTF* gene is not causally related to neurological diseases. Nature Genet. *7*, 79–84

Taraviras, S., Marcos-Gutierrez, C.V., Durbec, P., Jani, H., Grigoriou, M., Sukumaran, M., Wang, L.C., Hynes, M., Raisman, G., and Pachnis, V. (1999) Signalling by the RET re-ceptor tyrosine kinase and its role in the development of the mammalian enteric ner-vous system. Development *126*, 2785–2797

Thoenen, H. and Barde, Y.-A. (1980) Physiology of nerve growth factor. Physiol.Rev. *60*, 1284–1335

Thoenen, H., Hughes, R.A., and Sendtner, M. (1993) Trophic support of motoneurons: Physiological, pathophysiological, and therapeutic implications. Exp.Neurol. *124*, 47–55

Tinhofer, I., Maly, K., Dietl, P., Hochholdinger, F., Mayr, S., Obermeier, A., and Grunicke, H.H. (1996) Differential Ca2+ signaling induced by activation of the epidermal growth factor and nerve growth factor receptors. Journal of Biological Chemistry *271*, 30505–30509

Traverse, S., Gomez, N., Paterson, H., Marshall, C., and Cohen, P. (1992) Sustained activa-tion of the mitogen-activated protein (MAP) kinase cascade may be required for dif-ferentiation of PC12 cells. Comparison of the effects of nerve growth factor and epi-dermal growth factor. Biochem.J. *288*, 351–355

Treanor, J.J., Goodman, L., de Sauvage, F., Stone, D.M., Poulsen, K.T., Beck, C.D., Gray, C., Armanini, M.P., Pollock, R.A., Hefti, F., Phillips, H.S., Goddard, A., Moore, M.W., Buj Bello, A., Davies, A.M., Asai, N., Takahashi, M., Vandlen, R., Henderson, C.E., and

Rosenthal, A. (1996) Characterization of a multicomponent receptor for GDNF. Nature *382*, 80–83

Trupp, M., Arenas, E., Fainzilber, M., Nilsson, A.S., Sieber, B.A., Grigoriou, M., Kilkenny, C., Salazar Grueso ,E., Pachnis, V., Arumae, U., Sariola, H., Saarma, M., and Ibanez, C.F. (1996) Functional receptor for GDNF encoded by the c-ret proto-oncogene. Nature *381*, 785–788

Van der Zee, C.E., Ross, G.M., Riopelle, R.J., and Hagg, T. (1996) Survival of cholinergic forebrain neurons in developing p75NGFR- deficient mice [retracted by Hagg T. In: Science 1999 Jul 16;285(5426):340]. SCIENCE *274*, 1729–1732

Vejsada, R., Sagot, Y., and Kato, A.C. (1994) BDNF-mediated rescue of axotomized motor neurones decreases with increasing dose. Neuroreport *5*, 1889–1892

Vejsada, R., Sagot, Y., and Kato, A.C. (1995) Quantitative comparison of the transient rescue effects of neurotrophic factors on axotomized motoneurons in vivo. Eur.J.Neurosci. *7*, 108–115

Vejsada, R., Tseng, J.L., Lindsay, R.M., Acheson, A., Aebischer, P., and Kato, A.C. (1998) Synergistic but transient rescue effects of BDNF and GDNF on axotomized neonatal motoneurons. Neuroscience *84*, 129–139

Wang, H.-G., Miyashita, T., Takayama, S., Sato, T., Torigoe, T., Krajewski, S., Tanaka, S., Hovey, L., III, Troppmair, J., Rapp, U.R., and Reed, J.C. (1994) Apoptosis regulation by interaction of Bcl-2 protein and Raf-1 kinase. Oncogene *9*, 2751–2756

Wayne, D.B. and Heaton, M.B. (1988) Retrograde transport of NGF by early chick embryo spinal cord motoneurons. Dev.Biol. *127*, 220–223

Wayne, D.B. and Heaton, M.B. (1990a) The ontogeny of specific retrograde transport of nerve growth factor by motoneurons of the brainstem and spinal cord. Dev.Biol. *138*, 484–498

Wayne, D.B. and Heaton, M.B. (1990b) The response of cultured trigeminal and spinal cord motoneurons to nerve growth factor. Dev.Biol. *138*, 473–483

Wiese, S., Metzger, F., Holtmann, B., and Sendtner, M. (1999) The role of p75NTR in modulating neurotrophin survival effects in developing motoneurons. Eur.J.Neurosci. *11*, 1668–1676

Wiese, S., Pei, G., Karch, C., Troppmair, J., Holtmann, B., Rapp, U.R., and Sendtner, M. (2001) Specific function of B-Raf in mediating survival of embryonic motoneurons and sensory neurons. Nat.Neurosci. *4*, 137–142

Winter, C.G., Saotome, Y., Saotome, I., and Hirsh, D. (1996) CNTF overproduction hastens onset of symptoms in motor neuron degeneration (mnd) mice. J.Neurobiol. *31*, 370–378

Wixler, V., Smola, U., Schuler, M., and Rapp, U. (1996) Differential regulation of Raf isozymes by growth versus differentiation inducing factors in PC12 pheochromocytoma cells. FEBS Letters *385*, 131–137

Yamashita, T., Tucker, K.L., and Barde, Y.A. (1999) Neurotrophin binding to the p75 receptor modulates Rho activity and axonal outgrowth. Neuron *24*, 585–593

Yan, Q., Elliott, J., and Snider, W.D. (1992) Brain-derived neurotrophic factor rescues spinal motor neurons from axotomy-induced cell death. Nature *360*, 753–755

Yan, Q., Snider, W.D., Pinzone, J.J., and Johnson, E.M., Jr. (1988) Retrograde transport of nerve growth factor (NGF) in motoneurons of developing rats: assessment of potential neurotrophic effects. Neuron *1*, 335–343

York, R.D., Yao, H., Dillon, T., Ellig, C.L., Eckert, S.P., McCleskey, E.W., and Stork, P.J. (1998) Rap1 mediates sustained MAP kinase activation induced by nerve growth factor. Nature *392*, 622–626

Yoshida, K., Taga, T., Saito, M., Suematsu, S., Kumanogoh, A., Tanaka, T., Fujiwara, H., Hirata, M., Yamagami, T., Nakahata, T., Hirabayashi, T., Yoneda, Y., Tanaka, K., Wang, W.Z., Mori, C., Shiota, K., Yoshida, N., and Kishimoto, T. (1996) Targeted disruption of gp130, a common signal transducer for the interleukin 6 family of cytokines, leads to myocardial and hematological disorders. Proc.Natl.Acad.Sci.U.S.A. *93*, 407–411

Genetic Analysis of the Endogenous Opioid System

J. E. Pintar[1] · B. L. Kieffer[2]

[1] Dept. Neuroscience and Cell Biology, UMDNJ-Robert Wood Johnson Medical School,
CABM Rm 326, 675 Hoes Lane, Piscataway, NJ 08854, USA
e-mail: pintar@cabm.rutgers.edu
[2] IGBMC, CNRS/INSERM/ULP, 1 rue Laurent Fries, 67404 Illkirch Cedex, France

Abstract The production and analysis of opioid system knockout (KO) mice deficient in one or more of the three opioid receptors (mu (MOR-1), delta (DOR-1), and kappa (KOR-1)) and the three precursor proteins encoding opioid system ligands (proenkephalin, prodynorphin, and proopiomelanocortin) have considerably enhanced our understanding of the roles of this complex system. All single and combinatorial KO mice with mutations in this system are viable with receptor mutations, in particular, generally accompanied by only minor compensations in other opioid system genes. These novel strains have been used to examine the contributions of the endogenous opioid system to both baseline behaviors and to actions of exogenous compounds. The effects of opioid system mutation on endogenous behavior are generally modest, but there are demonstrated effects of specific opioid system gene deletions on locomotion as well as emotional behaviors, and there is evidence for opposing actions of specific receptor systems on these processes. Exogenous administration of opioid system ligands has complemented and extended the findings of traditional pharmacology while unanticipated observations continue to emerge. For example, extensive analysis in multiple paradigms continues to demonstrate that essentially all actions of morphine are abolished following deletion of MOR-1, despite its significant binding to other receptor subtypes in vitro. In addition, requirements of DOR-1 and preproenkephalin for morphine tolerance but not dependence have been demonstrated, as have alternate systems that can mediate analgesic responses to delta ligands, and recent findings indicate that at least some traditional opioid receptor ligands retain activity even in mice lacking all classic opioid receptors. These recent results should help focus analysis of the genomic and proteomic alterations that accompany drug administration and opioid system mutation as well as characterization of conditional mutations of opioid system genes.

Keywords Opioid receptor · Delta opioid receptor · Mu opioid receptor · Kappa opioid receptor · Analgesia · Opioid pharmacology · Morphine tolerance · Morphine dependence · Anxiety · Locomotion

Abbreviations

ACTH	Corticotropin
βend	β-Endorphin
CFA	Complete Freund adjuvant
DAMGO	[D-Ala^2,MePhe^4,Gly-ol^5]Enkephalin
DOR	Delta-opioid receptor
DPDPE	Cyclic[D-penicillamine^2,D-penicillamine^5]enkephalin
GTPγS	Guanosine 5′-3-O-(thio)triphosphate
HPA	Hypothalamic-pituitary-adrenal axis
i.c.v.	Intracerebroventricular
it	Intrathecal
KOR	Kappa-opioid receptor
M6G	Morphine-6-glucuronide
MOR	Mu opioid receptor
MSH	Melanocyte stimulating hormone
Pdyn	Preprodynorphin
Penk	Preproenkephalin
POMC	Proopiomelanocortin
SIA	Stress-induced analgesia

1
Introduction

Since its isolation from the poppy seed, humans have used the prototypic opioid morphine not only because it relieves pain, but also because it produces feelings of euphoria and well-being. Morphine remains the most widely used treatment for several types of severe pain, while the synthetic diacetylation of morphine forms heroin, which remains one of the most addictive drugs of abuse. The endogenous receptors that are targets of these exogenous opiate drugs were first identified pharmacologically in the 1960s, when binding studies indicated that three major classes of opioid receptor sites exist, which continue to be designated as mu, delta, and kappa receptors. In the 1970s, Met- and Leu-enkephalin became the first endogenous ligands for opioid receptors to be identified, while isolation of β-endorphin and dynorphin peptides rapidly followed. The discovery of not only receptors for exogenous ligands but also prospective endogenous ligands for these receptors suggested that multiple new circuits could not only mediate effects of exogenous opiates but could be expected to modulate multiple endogenous physiologic processes as well.

Following discovery of this endogenous opioid system, its pharmacology has been extensively explored using an increasing number of morphine derivatives, additional natural products and multiple synthetic agonists and antagonists with demonstrated selectivity for the three major opioid receptor subclasses. These compounds have been used to characterize the effects on several physiologic processes, and have established that all three opioid receptor subclasses could participate in nociception, reward processes, and anxiety as well as other functions such as stress, respiration, food intake, gastrointestinal motility, and endocrine and immune activity. The information from this pharmacologic approach has recently been reviewed (see Vaccarino and Kastin 2000) and reinforces not only the complexity of the opioid system but also the critical role of this system in mediating the interaction and response of an organism to its environment.

Molecular approaches identified three opioid peptide precursor genes in the late 1970s, while genes encoding the receptors were not identified until over a decade later. Preproenkephalin (Penk), preprodynorphin (Pdyn) and proopiomelanocortin (POMC) genes encode several enkephalin peptides, several dynorphin-related peptides, and one copy of β-endorphin, respectively. These peptides, once liberated from their respective precursors by prohormone convertases, all express the canonical opioid receptor-binding sequence Tyr-Gly-Gly-Phe-Met/Leu sequence at their N-terminus. The opioid receptor proteins belong to the G protein-coupled receptor family, and form a four-member gene subfamily together with the orphanin FQ/nociceptin receptor discovered later by homology screening (Darland et al. 1998; Mogil and Pasternak 2001). Three genes encoding proteins with the pharmacology of the classic mu (MOR-1), delta (DOR-1) and kappa (KOR-1) receptors have been isolated and have alternatively designated Oprm, Oprd1 and Oprk1 using mouse genome nomenclature, or as MOP, DOP and KOP by the International Union of Pharmacology (IUPHAR). These three genes predict highly homologous receptor proteins (Kieffer 1995) and have similar genomic organization (Gaveriaux-Ruff and Kieffer 1999).

Homologous recombination technology has successfully produced mouse strains lacking all genes of the endogenous opioid system introduced above. These mice have already been extensively used to complement and extend classic pharmacologic approaches and several important applications of these mice have emerged. First, subtype-specific knockout (KO) mice have been used to assess genetically the molecular targets of prototypic opioid agonists or antagonists developed by pharmacology. In addition, behavioral phenotyping of each mutant strain has allowed for the contribution of each endogenous peptide and receptor to presumptive opioid-controlled behaviors to be re-assessed. Since several independently generated strains with mutations in the same gene have been produced and analyzed in similar paradigms, broad consensus on several aspects of opioid function have been reached. Nonetheless, several surprising results have emerged from this analysis, which provide a focus for current work. Here we will review much of the information from the study of opioid system KO mice and attempt to highlight the particularly significant advances provided by genetic analysis of this system. Analysis of the initial data from these strains has been summarized in prior reviews (Hayward and Low 1999; Kieffer 1999; Kieffer 2000). More recent data from an emerging area—the effect of opioid system KOs on responses to other substances of abuse— has recently been reviewed (Kieffer and Gaveriaux-Ruff 2002), where a more thorough discussion of immune and stress responses beyond the scope of this review can also be found.

2
Production of Opioid Receptor and Ligand Mutant Mice

2.1
Single and Combinatorial Opioid Receptor Knockout Mouse Lines

All opioid receptor genes have a similar organization (Gaveriaux-Ruff and Kieffer 1999) and their coding regions are included in three exons. The MOR-1 gene differs slightly in that the last twelve codons of the 3′ coding region, are found on a fourth coding exon. Several additional MOR-1 exons have also been identified in overlapping murine cosmid clones (Pan et al. 2001) and it will be of interest to determine whether these exons also exist in humans. Between two and five distinct targeting vectors for the MOR-1, DOR-1, and KOR-1 genes have been successfully used for homologous recombination. The mutant alleles produced by these targeting events are illustrated with references in Fig. 1a.

Five strains of mice have been produced that contain mutations in the MOR-1 locus (Matthes et al. 1996; Sora et al. 1997; Tian et al. 1997; Loh et al. 1998; Schuller et al. 1999). Three strains contain deletions of exon 1, though the extent of the deletion differs among the strains, a fourth contains an insertion

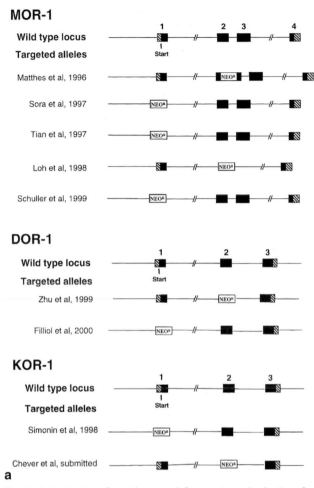

Fig. 1a, b Production of opioid system-deficient mice. **a** Production of opioid receptors-deficient. The wild-type locus and targeted alleles for independent MOR-1, DOR-1, and KOR-1 receptor KO mice. Introns are indicated by *solid lines*. Exons are represented by *boxes* and show coding (*black boxes*) and non-coding (*diagonal-containing boxes*) regions of the genes. The position of the neomycin-resistance cassette is indicated. Mice with the following genetic backgrounds were assayed in original reports: 129/SvxC57BL/6 (Matthes et al. 1996; Sora et al. 1997; Simonin et al. 1998; Filliol et al. 2000), 129/OlaxC57BL/6 (Loh et al. 1998), Swiss black hybrids (Tian et al. 1997), 129/SvEvxC57BL/6 (Schuller et al. 1999; Zhu et al. 1999; Chever et al. submitted). **b** Production of opioid peptide-deficient mice. The wild-type locus and targeted genomes are indicated for β-endorphin (POMC gene), preproenkephalin, and prodynorphin. Introns are represented by *solid lines*, while as in **a**, *black boxes* show the coding region of exons while *boxes with diagonal lines* indicate non-coding parts of the genes. The position of the neomycin-resistance cassette is indicated. A partial duplication of exon 3 occurred at the 3' end of Neo in the Penk mutant generated by König et al. Targeting of the POMC gene by Rubinstein et al. was designed as to delete βend only, while other POMC-derived peptides are intact. In original reports mutant mice harvest the following genetic backgrounds: 129/SvxC57BL/6 (Rubinstein et al. 1996; Zimmer et al. 2001), CD1 hybrids (König et al. 1996), 129SvEv-Tac for Sharifi et al. 2001), 129/SvEvxC57BL/6 (Nitsche et al. 2002)

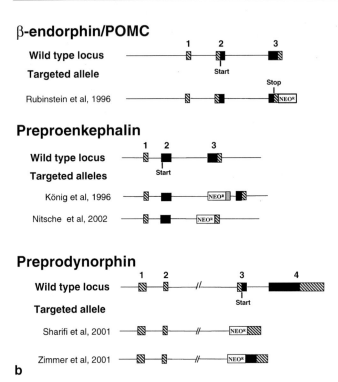

Fig. 1 b

of a Neo cassette into exon 2, while the fifth strain has a deletion of both exons 2 and 3. In homozygous mutant mice from all five strains, binding of [³H] DAM-GO, the prototypic mu-selective agonist was abolished, demonstrating that classic, pharmacologically defined mu receptor sites were deleted by all targeting strategies. Binding of one other highly selective mu ligand, [³H] endomorphin-2, is also absent from the one mutant strain tested (Monory et al. 2000). DAM-GO, morphine, and endomorphin 1 and 2 have also been examined for ability to activate G proteins; this ability is abolished in several MOR-1 mutants examined (Matthes et al. 1998; Mizoguchi et al. 1999; Monory et al. 2000; Narita et al. 1999; Park et al. 2000). These data indicate that all activation elicited by these compounds requires MOR-1 and, conversely, that these agonists are unable to initiate detectable G protein activation following possible binding to other receptors.

Two strains of mice have been produced that contain deletions of either exon 1 or exon 2 of murine DOR-1 (Zhu et al. 1999; Filliol et al. 2000). In both strains, binding of several radiolabeled delta-selective compounds with preferred specificity for either the pharmacologically defined delta-1 sites (DPDPE) or the delta-2 sites (deltorphin 1 and 2) were undetected in homozygous mutant mice after either homogenate or autoradiographic ligand binding. Binding of the general delta antagonist naltrindole was also significantly reduced in both strains. Taken together, these results demonstrate that the delta receptor subtypes postulated by classical pharmacology (see Zaki et al. 1996) arise from, or require, the DOR-1 gene.

Two lines of mice with deletions of either exon 1 or exon 2 of the murine KOR-1 gene have also been produced, binding the highly selective kappa agonist [^{3}H] CI-977 or [^{3}H]U-69,363, respectively (Simonin et al. 1998; V. Chever, submitted), could not be detected by homogenate binding and/or autoradiographic mapping, demonstrating that murine KOR-1 encodes the previously described kappa-1 receptor. The pharmacology of other kappa opioid receptor subtypes, a highly controversial area, has begun to be elucidated using combinatorial receptor KO mice as discussed below.

In summary, results from all nine KOs of individual opioid receptors have consistently shown that binding of prototypic radiolabelled opioid ligands selective for mu, delta, and kappa sites, respectively, is undetectable in all cognate MOR-1, DOR-1, and KOR-1 mutant strains. Interesting, binding in all heterozygous mutants examined have exhibited ~50% reductions in receptor number, which indicates that regulation of gene expression or receptor protein stability is not adjusted in the presence of a null allele. Thus, analysis of mice with half the number of functional receptors can have implications for identifying phenotypes where the full complement of receptors is required, as discussed below.

Homozygous mutant mice from all nine opioid receptor lines are viable, fertile, and have not shown any obvious morphologic deficits despite the widespread prenatal activation of each gene in both central and peripheral nervous systems as well as peripheral tissues of the mouse (Zhu et al. 1998; Zhu and Pintar 1998). While these normal phenotypes raised the possibility that receptor proteins might not be synthesized or activated during development, the ability of mu and delta agonists to stimulate G protein activation during prenatal stages has recently been demonstrated (Nitsche and Pintar 2003). In essentially all neural sites of fetal opioid receptor expression, the ability of both mu and delta ligands to stimulate G protein activation begins soon after cognate mRNA detection, though coupling is often slightly delayed from the time of specific mRNA appearance. One dramatic exception is the trigeminal ganglion, where mu ligand coupling is not present even at birth, though MOR-1 mRNA is robustly expressed soon after this ganglion forms. A significant conclusion from these studies is that the lack of major developmental effects of MOR-1 and DOR-1 receptors, at least, is not because these receptors are unable to activate G proteins before birth. Nonetheless, detailed morphological studies of neural and glial cell number, as well as detailed structural analysis of neural circuitry, have yet to be reported for the mature or developing brain for any mutant.

Mouse strains containing combinations of either two or all three individual opioid receptor subtype mutations have also recently been produced. Like each individual mutant, the double and triple opioid receptor mutant mice are viable and fertile. Two strains of mice lacking three distinct individual mutations include either the alleles reported by Matthes et al. (1996), Simonin et al. (1998), and Filliol et al. (2000) or those reported by Schuller et al. (1999), Zhu et al. (1999), and Chever (V. Chever, submitted). The first strain as expected lacks [³H] DAMGO, [³H] CI-977 and [³H] DPDPE binding sites in homogenate assays (Simonin et al. 2001), while the second strain shows a complete absence of [³H] naloxone binding, the prototype opioid antagonist, as assessed by both autora-diography and homogenate binding (Clarke et al. 2002). While these studies clearly support the opioid receptor specificity of ligands such as naloxone under the binding conditions used, low-affinity binding sites for these ligands might not be detected using standard binding conditions but could potentially have physiologic relevance that can be explored in these KO models.

2.2
Opioid Peptide Knockout Mouse Lines

Mice containing mutations in opioid peptide precursor genes have also been produced using the targeting strategies illustrated and referenced in Fig. 1b. The POMC precursor encodes several biologically active peptides including the opi-oid peptide β-endorphin. To specifically delete this peptide domain, which is the C-terminal peptide encoded by this precursor, a stop codon was introduced at the β-MSH-βend junction. In homozygous mutant mice containing this mu-tation, β-melanocyte-stimulating hormone (β-MSH) content and corticotropin (ACTH) immunoreactivity were unchanged while βend was absent, confirming that the mutation had successfully ablated production of the opioid peptide but had not altered processing of other POMC domains. A strain lacking the entire POMC coding region has also been reported (Yaswen et al. 1999); the absence of multiple peptides with distinct activities in addition to βend has thus far pre-vented changes arising specifically from the absence of βend to be identified.

Two strains of KO mice lacking the Penk gene have been reported. In the first (Konig et al. 1996), the targeting strategy truncated the enkephalin-coding re-gion (5′ part of exon 3) but also introduced an unexpected partial duplication of this exon. This mutation has nonetheless been useful since no met-enkephalin has been detected in the homozygous mutants. In the second mutant, the target-ing strategy deleted the entire region encoding the 5′ part of exon 3 (Ragnauth et al. 2001; Nitsche et al. 2002).

Two null mutations have also been introduced into the Pdyn gene by different laboratories and include either deletion of the whole coding region, spanning exons 3 and 4 in one KO, which eliminated Pdyn mRNA in homozygous mu-tants, or deletion of exon 3 and part of exon 4, which produced mice lacking all dynorphin peptides.

Thus mouse strains with mutations in each gene encoding opioid peptides have been produced. Mice heterozygous for the ligand mutations generally show half the peptide content, at least for βend and Penk, again making these mice useful for studies of ligand reserve. Like receptor-null mice, homozygous opioid ligand mutant mice do not show any obvious developmental defects or decreases in fecundity. Although there has been no report of triple-ligand KO mice yet, viable and fertile β-endorphin and Penk double mutant have been produced and used for experimental analysis (Hayward et al. 2002).

2.3
Compensatory Changes Accompanying Opioid System Mutation

Absence of one opioid system component throughout development might be expected to induce adaptive changes in either other molecules of the opioid system or functionally associated neurotransmitter systems as a compensation to maintain homeostasis. Such compensatory modifications could be subtle and would not necessarily require altered gene expression to be functionally relevant, especially since the known endogenous ligands such as βend and Penk have somewhat overlapping terminal fields and could be expected to bind both mu and delta receptors in vivo as they do in vitro.

Examinations of non-mutated opioid system components in several individual mutant strains have been undertaken to evaluate intra-opioid system compensation. In mice lacking an individual opioid receptor, levels of the two remaining receptors have been measured in both whole brain homogenates and with receptor autoradiography to provide anatomic resolution. In MOR-1-deficient mice, homogenate binding of several prototypic delta and kappa1 ligands were similar in wild-type and mutant mice (Matthes et al. 1996; Kitchen et al. 1997; Sora et al. 1997; Loh et al. 1998; Schuller et al. 1999; Chen et al. 2000). Mu and kappa agonist binding were also grossly similar in DOR-1-deficient mice (Zhu et al. 1999; Filliol et al. 2000) while DAMGO and deltorphin binding were unchanged in the KOR-1 homozygous mutant mice (V. Chever et al., submitted; Simonin et al. 1998). At the regional level, qualitative in situ hybridization did not reveal any major change in the level MOR-1 or DOR-1 expression in DOR-1 or MOR-1 receptor mutants respectively (Schuller et al. 1999; Zhu et al. 1999). More detailed quantitative autoradiographic receptor mapping has also been reported for each individual mutant, which has revealed at best subtle (10% on average) but regionally restricted downregulation of delta and kappa sites in MOR-1-deficient mice (Kitchen et al. 1997), upregulation of delta sites in the KOR-1 mutant mice (Slowe et al. 1999), and trend toward regional decreases of mu and kappa 1 sites in the DOR-1 mutant mice (Goody et al. 2002). Together, the data clearly indicate that the absence of one opioid receptor does not dramatically alter the expression of other opioid receptor genes. Mutation of the structurally related ORL-1 gene similarly does not significantly impact expression of any of the classical opioid receptors (Slowe et al. 2001)

Adaptations at the level of receptor coupling efficiency could occur in the absence of alterations in receptor binding. This possibility has not yet been fully explored but has been investigated most thoroughly in MOR-1 mutant mice. In these mice, SNC80- and deltorphin-stimulated $[^{35}S]GTP\gamma S$ binding was generally unchanged, suggesting integrity of delta receptor activation of G proteins (Matthes et al. 1998; Narita et al. 1999; Hosohata et al. 2000). DPDPE also stimulated [^{35}S]GTPγS binding with similar efficacy in wild-type and MOR-1 mutant mice (Matthes et al. 1998; Narita et al. 1999), although with slightly reduced efficacy in MOR-1 KO brain when a high dose was used (Park et al. 2000) as well as in the spinal cord (Hosohata et al. 2000). The later findings could reflect DPDPE occupancy of mu receptors in wild-type mice (Hosohata et al. 2000), which would produce an apparent overall lower efficacy in the MOR-1 mutants. DPDPE does show lower selectivity towards delta receptors compared to deltorphin (Corbett 1993; Matthes et al. 1998) and thus may bind both mu and delta receptors under specific experimental conditions. Detailed autoradiographic [^{35}S]GTPγS studies have not been reported in these mice to identify more restricted sites of regional coupling differences which could underlie the clear differences in delta agonist-mediated behavior that accompany MOR-1 mutation as discussed below.

The coupling of three different kappa agonists in MOR-1 mutant mice has also been explored and induced [^{35}S]GTPγS binding activities were comparable in wild-type and MOR-1-deficient mice (Matthes et al. 1998; Narita et al. 1999; Park et al. 2000). Thus, data so far strongly suggest that delta and kappa receptor coupling to G proteins is generally intact in the absence of mu receptors. Therefore the analysis of [^{35}S]GTPγS binding in MOR-1 KO mice thus far provides no evidence for mu/delta or mu/kappa interactions at the cellular level. The findings that ligand-stimulated downstream events, such as DPDPE-, deltorphin- and U50,488H-inhibition of cAMP production, are also unaffected in MOR-1 mutant mice (Matthes et al. 1998) is consistent with this notion. Analogous studies in DOR-1- and KOR-1-deficient mice have not yet been reported and, as mentioned above, a more restricted anatomic analysis or pharmacologic interventions successfully used in vitro (Jordan and Devi 1999; Rios et al. 2001) could conceivably uncover more discrete anatomically restricted changes that could be ascribed to receptor dimers.

Just as individual receptor deletion does not markedly modify expression of the other opioid receptors, opioid peptide deletion does not significantly alter levels of other opioid peptides. In βend-deficient mice, for example, dynorphin and enkephalin expression was unchanged (Rubinstein et al. 1996). Pdyn homozygous mutant showed normal Penk mRNA but slightly attenuated POMC transcript levels (Sharifi et al. 2001) while Penk KO mice displayed normal levels of dynorphin and βend immunoreactivity in striatal and hypothalamic extracts, respectively (Konig et al. 1996).

Since transmitter and peptide levels can often regulate the numbers of cognate receptors, experiments to determine whether absence of specific receptors modifies expression of endogenous ligands or, conversely, whether the absence of ligand alters receptor expression have been of interest. The absence of a receptor does not seem to regulate ligand expression since, at the RNA level, MOR-1, DOR-1, and KOR-1 mutants all show no obvious alteration in POMC, Penk, and Pdyn transcript levels, respectively, as demonstrated by in situ hybridization (V. Chever et al., submitted; Matthes et al. 1996; Simonin et al. 1998; Zhu et al. 1999; Filliol et al. 2000). In contrast, brains from at least one strain of

Penk mutant mice show significant increases in mu and delta binding in regions thought to mediate the emotional aspect of opioid function such as the central amygdala nucleus for mu receptors and the ventral pallidum for delta receptors (Brady et al. 1999). There are no apparent behavioral manifestations of receptor upregulation in analgesic systems, however, since both basal analgesia as well as morphine dose–response curves are unchanged in enkephalin mutant mice (Nitsche et al. 2002). Analysis of other ligand mutants is more limited, although either mu, delta, and kappa agonist-stimulated [^{35}S]GTPγS binding or total opioid binding were unchanged in Pdyn KO mice (Wang et al. 2001) and βend mutants (Slugg et al. 2000), respectively.

In conclusion, significant regulatory interactions within the opioid system have thus far only been observed in the Penk mutant mice. Other changes may also occur in functionally associated systems, as illustrated by subtle modifications in orphanin FQ/nociceptin binding in individual DOR-1 and KOR-1 but not MOR-1 mutant mice (Slowe et al. 2001) as well as triple KO mice (Clarke et al. 2002). Since adaptations could conceivably extend to unexpected or uncharacterized genes, gene and protein profiling of opioid system mutant mice will ultimately be needed to provide an accurate assessment of compensatory change. The identification and extent of these changes represent a necessary component of characterizing the mutant mice.

3
Basal Behavioral Phenotypes

Since all opioid receptor and ligand KO mice are viable and generally exhibit minimal alterations in other opioid systems, behavior can be constructively examined in the absence of any known major alterations in these other systems. Baseline phenotypes of several behavioral systems have been reported. Generally, systems examined include those where exogenous opiate administration has previously been demonstrated to alter a behavior, which in turn has raised the question of whether the endogenous opioid system also provides significant regulation of a specific behavior. If the endogenous system in fact contributes to a behavior, changes from wild-type should be observed following baseline measurements. Altered responses of mutant mice in nociception (summarized in Table 1), locomotion and emotional/stress tests have indicated significant roles of the endogenous system. Other behaviors are also introduced below and have also been recently reviewed (Kieffer and Gaveriaux-Ruff 2002).

It is important to realize that many of these initial reports have utilized mice of mixed genetic background. Most studies have attempted to minimize the effect of genetic variation by using mice from heterozygous mating, but it is conceivable that genetic variation has obscured identification of some significant differences or, alternatively, led to some of the interlab variability observed if small numbers of mice have been tested. End points being measured certainly reflect contributions from non-opioid systems and behavioral phenotyping using recently developed standardized test batteries (Brown et al. 2000) can be ex-

Table 1 Nociceptive alterations in opioid-system knockout mice

Modality	MOR-1	DOR-1	KOR-1	β End	Penk	Pdyn
Thermal pain	No change in TI[2] Increase in TF[1] No change or increase in HP[1,2,8] Increase in PT[11]	No change in TI or HP[3] No change in TF[10]	No change in TI or HP[4,16]		No change in TF[6,15] Increase in HP[6]	Increase in TF[11] No change in HP, PT or TI[7,11]
Mechanical pain	No change in VF[12]	No change in TP[3]	No change in TP[4]			No change in VF[11]
Chemical pain	Reduction in W[13]	No change in W[3] No change in EF[3,10] No change in LF[10]	Increase in W[4] No change in EF[4]		Reduction in EF[6] Reduction in EF[6]	No change in EF[11] No change in EF[11] Increase in LF[11]
Inflammatory pain	Faster recovery from hyperalgesia in CFA[9]					
Stress-induced analgesia	Reduction[14]			Reduction[5]	No change[6]	

CFA, complete Freund's adjuvant; EF, early phase of formalin; HP, hot plate; late phase of formalin; PT, plantar test; R, rotarod; TF, tail flick; TI, tail immersion; TP, tail pressure; VF mechanical stimulation using von Frey filaments; W, acetic acid writhing.

References: 1. Sora et al. (1997); 2. Matthes et al. (1996); 3. Filliol et al. (2000); 4. Simonin et al. (1998); . Rubinstein et al. (1996); 6. Konig et al. (1996); 7. Zimmer et al. (2001); 8. Matthes et al. (1998); 9. Qiu et al. (2000); 10. Zhu et al. (1999); 11. Wang et al. (2001); 12. Fuchs et al. (1999); 13. Sora et al. (1999); 14. LaBuda et al. (2000); 15. Nitsche et al. (2002); 16. Chever et al. (submitted).

pected to provide additional information that minimizes these effects. Since different genetic backgrounds may impact the contribution of a specific opioid component to a specific behavior, one can anticipate that analysis of different inbred strains containing opioid system mutations will add to the results summarized below.

3.1
Pain Perception

Perhaps the most important recognized function of the opioid system is to modulate pain perception. Exogenous mu, delta, and kappa opioid agonists all produce analgesia and, in addition, an endogenous opioid tone has been proposed to regulate nociceptive information (Ossipov 1997). To evaluate the proposed tonic effects of the opioid system in pain perception, nociceptive thresholds have been examined in KO mice using a wide variety of pain models. Several acute painful stimuli, as well as intermediate and chronic pain models, have been tested (see Table 1 with references). Strain background may influence nociceptive thresholds (Mogil et al. 1999) and detection of more subtle but nonetheless significant differences may accompany testing of single and combinatorial mutants on different inbred backgrounds.

Several tests, including radiant heat-tail flick, warm water tail immersion, hot plate, and the plantar test, have all been used to determine the basal sensitivity of mice to thermal pain. DOR-1- and KOR-1-deficient mice do not exhibit any alteration in the perception of noxious heat. In contrast, MOR-1 mutant mice showed increased sensitivity in three different responses to heat, suggesting the existence of an MOR-mediated contribution to thermal nociception. Triple KO mice on a mixed outbred background also show decreased latencies in radiant heat testing (Clarke et al. 2002). No change in baseline sensitivity to thermal pain was reported in mice devoid of β-endorphin. Penk and Pdyn mutant mice showed increase pain sensitivity in the hot plate and tail flick tests, respectively, though a second Penk strain showed no different in long-latency radiant heat testing (Nitsche et al. 2002). There is a tendency for mice lacking either MOR or Penk genes to show a similar phenotype, suggesting a ligand–receptor interaction.

Responses to mechanical pain, determined by response to pressure, was unaltered in MOR-1, DOR-1, KOR-1, and Pdyn mutants (Simonin et al. 1998; Fuchs et al. 1999; Filliol et al. 2000; Wang et al. 2001) while other mutant strains have not been tested. Sensitivity to chemical pain has been assessed alternatively by measuring writhes after acetic acid injection or paw licking and lifting shortly after formalin injection. DOR-1 and Pdyn mutant mice showed no difference in response to chemical pain. Mice lacking KOR-1 showed a strong increase in writhes following acetic acid, which is consistent with previous antagonist treatments and indicates a tonic inhibitory role of kappa receptors in the perception of visceral pain. Paradoxically, MOR-1 mutants displayed decreased nociceptive responses in response to acetic acid (Sora et al. 1999), as did Penk mutant mice following formalin injection, but it is interesting that MOR-1 and Penk mutants again have similar responses.

Inflammation induces long-lasting pain and both the nervous system and immune cells may produce opioid peptides that induce analgesia after release at inflammatory sites (Stein et al. 2001). MOR mutant animals were analyzed for inflammatory hyperalgesia following complete Freund adjuvant (CFA) administration but the mutant mice unexpectedly recovered more rapidly from CFA-induced hyperalgesia than wild-type. This recovery was blocked by the delta-selective antagonist naltrindole, and MOR-1 KO mice were also more responsive to delta agonist analgesia (see Table 3 and Sect. 4.2), suggesting that delta receptor activity was augmented in these mice under conditions of persistent pain (Qiu et al. 2000). Pdyn mutant mice showed mild hyperalgesia in the late phase of the formalin test, suggesting that endogenous dynorphins produce some analgesia during inflammation.

Pdyn mice have been analyzed in a model of persistent neuropathic pain (Wang et al. 2001). While Pdyn KO and wild-type mice initially showed similar responses following spinal nerve ligation, both thermal and mechanical sensitivities remained elevated in wild-type mice for several days after responses of Pdyn KO mice had returned to baseline. Together with upregulation of dynorphin expression that also occurs following ligation, these data indicate that pronociceptive activity of dynorphin in the maintenance of neuropathic pain.

To summarize, the nociceptive responses measured thus far in opioid system KO mice indicate that most mutants contribute to basal pain sensitivity with deletion of an opioid receptor or peptide generally increasing sensitivity to acute noxious stimuli. This finding is consistent with antagonist studies, although the possibility that basal activation of receptors such as MOR-1 may produce nociceptive tone in the absence of ligand has yet to be rigorously explored on a ligand-deficient mutant background. The genetic approach therefore confirms the existence of an antinociceptive endogenous opioid tone. Importantly, since alterations exhibited by a given mutant differ among different nociceptive assays, each opioid system component appears to contribute to different modalities that mediate pain. Ideally, parallel studies in several KO models on inbred backgrounds that differ in nociceptive parameters should ultimately produce a clearer picture of respective contributions of each receptor and ligand in both acute and chronic models of pain.

3.2
Locomotion

Exogenous opioid agonists and antagonists have produced variable and inconsistent effects on locomotory behavior (see Vaccarino and Kastin 2000). Opioid system KO mice have thus represented an important new tool with which to assess this behavior, but have thus far provided results both consistent with and in conflict with prior studies. Basal locomotor activity of several MOR-1 mutant strains has thus been reported as either unchanged or slightly reduced (Matthes et al. 1996; Sora et al. 1997; Tian et al. 1997; Becker et al. 2000) with the variation possibly depending on the experimental conditions or genetic background. When observed, however, the decreased locomotion of the MOR-1 KO suggests that endogenous mu systems positively regulate locomotion. This pattern is consistent with observations that activation of MOR-1 by exogenous morphine produces a hyperlocomotion response. These findings from MOR-1 mutants generally support the likelihood that mu receptor activation, whether by exogenous or endogenous opiates, promotes locomotion.

In contrast to MOR-1 KO hypolocomotion, DOR-1 deficient animals instead show significant hyperlocomotion, which suggests that endogenous delta receptors tonically inhibit locomotion (Filliol et al. 2000). This result contrasts with pharmacologic data indicating that both mu and delta agonists increase locomotion (see Cowan 1993). Possibly the previously described hyperlocomotor activity of delta agonists could be mediated by mu receptor activation, as discussed above. Alternatively, as yet unidentified compensatory mechanisms may have developed in the absence of delta receptors to produce the observed increased locomotion.

Unlike the MOR-1 and DOR-1 KO mice, locomotory activity in KOR-1 mutant mice is unchanged (Simonin et al. 1998), though even here there is some inconsistency with pharmacologic studies in which activation of the kappa receptor by exogenous opioids decreased locomotion (Pfeiffer et al. 1986). The lack of altered locomotion in the KOR-1 mutants suggests a low contribution of kappa systems to control this behavior or, alternatively, compensatory mechanisms that cancel each other's effects.

Analysis of basal locomotion in opioid peptide KO mice has been more limited. βEnd and Pdyn mice showed normal locomotory activity. Penk animals displayed reduced locomotion in the open-field assay, which potentially results as a downstream consequence of increased anxiety (Konig et al. 1996). Since hypolocomotion in the MOR-1 KO was not associated with increased anxiety (Filliol et al. 2000), these two aspects of behavioral responses for mu receptors can be genetically dissociated. Thus, since the locomotory patterns of MOR-1 and Penk mice are similar, this result suggests that MOR-1 activation by endogenous Penk-derived peptides tonically stimulates locomotion.

3.3
Emotional/Stress Responses

A role for endogenous opioids contributing to an "emotional tone" remains relatively unexplored, but initial results from KO strains indicate that pharmacologic reevaluation of opioid effects on anxiety-related processes (Naber 1993) is warranted. All three subclasses of opioid receptor-deficient mice have recently been compared to wild-type mice using several models of anxiety or depression (Filliol et al. 2000). The results indicated that MOR-1 and DOR-1 KO animals differed not only from littermate controls, but also from each other. Thus while MOR-1 KO mice were less anxiogenic, DOR-1 mice showed increased anxiety in several tests. KOR-1 mutant mice did not show any alteration, suggesting that kappa receptors may not tonically contribute to these behaviors.

As with locomotor activity, discussed above, this pattern does not confirm predictions from pharmacologic studies, which would have expected similar effects of mu and delta receptor KO on these behaviors. Since DOR-1 mutant mice have consistently displayed anxiogenic and depressive-like responses, the endogenous activity of delta receptors may normally limit these behaviors. Thus, delta agonists may have the potential to treat affective disorders (Baamonde et al. 1992; Tejedor-Real et al. 1998).

The emotional responses of mice lacking βend or Penk have also been analyzed. While the βend mice did not show any alteration in anxiety, both strains of Penk mutant mice display increased responses in different anxiety-evoking environments (Konig et al. 1996; Ragnauth et al. 2001). Male mice were also more responsive in a model of aggressive behavior (Konig et al. 1996), while female mice exhibited a greater response in a fear conditioning paradigm (Ragnauth et al. 2001). These data suggest that endogenous enkephalins could lower exaggerated or depressive-like responses to challenging environmental cues. These data, combined with the DOR-1 phenotype described above, indicate that preproenkephalin-derived peptides contribute to these behaviors at least partially through delta receptors.

Stress responses have also begun to be explored in opioid system KO mice. Exposure to stress is itself sufficient to induce analgesia, which can often be partially reversed by opioid antagonists. Thus, release of endogenous opioid peptides has been proposed to mediate this "stress-induced" analgesia or SIA. Interestingly, the first reported phenotype for an opioid system KO was the absence of opioid SIA that accompanies deletion of β-EP (Rubinstein et al. 1996). Since naloxone-reversible SIA could not be obtained in wild-type control mice using the hot plate test, the more sensitive abdominal constriction assay was used to demonstrate that SIA was essentially completely abolished in mutant mice under conditions that produced strong analgesia in control mice. Paradoxically, and still unexplained, naloxone itself produced analgesia in the βend mutant mice, a phenomenon that may reflect its function as an inverse agonist at basally active receptors. Thus far no change in Penk KO SIA has been detected using the hot plate assay following either forced swim in warm conditions, which would maximize opioid-dependent SIA, or cold water, in which only partially opioid-dependent SIA would be detected (Konig et al. 1996). Just one study has attempted to identify the receptor(s) mediating the β-EP-dependent SIA, presumably because of the high variability of measuring this response, which is extremely sensitive to both background and paradigm. In this case, MOR-1-deficient mice displayed no change in SIA soon after stress, but less SIA than wild-type mice 15 min after stress, implicating mu receptors in the late phase of SIA (LaBuda et al. 2000). Since treatment with the delta antagonist naltrindole further reduced SIA in the MOR-1 mutant mice, a role for delta receptors has also been suggested.

3.4
Baseline Differences in Other Behaviors

3.4.1
Respiration

One major clinically relevant consequence of opioid administration is its depressive effect on respiration (Shook et al. 1990). Since mu agonists elicit analgesia exclusively through MOR-1, analysis of several respiratory parameters has been extensively studied only in MOR-1 KO but very few effects have been detected. MOR-1 KO mice, for example, show normal respiratory frequency, minute volume, and inspiratory time while at rest (Matthes et al. 1998; Morin-Surun et al. 2001) and do not exhibit any changes in response to hyperoxia (high O_2), hypoxia (low O_2), or hypercapnia (CO_2) (Morin-Surun et al. 2001). Breathing frequency is only slightly increased (15%) while the hypercapnic response is unchanged (Dahan et al. 2001).

3.4.2
Reproduction

The endogenous opioid system has been proposed to affect reproduction by regulating gonadotropin-releasing hormone and luteinizing hormone levels (Almeida 1993). Most initial descriptions of several MOR-1-deficient lines did not report any deficit in fecundity of either males or females or any impairment of maternal behavior (Matthes et al. 1996; Sora et al. 1997; Loh et al. 1998; Schuller et al. 1999). One more-detailed study did find a series of alterations in male MOR-1 KO mice that included deficiencies in mating behavior as well as sperm count and motility (Tian et al. 1997). The direction of these responses toward a less reproductive state was unexpected, since morphine and other exogenous opioids generally inhibit several reproductive parameters (Vaccarino and Kastin 2000). Reproductive behaviors in which Penk had been implicated, such as lordotic behavior, were surprisingly unchanged in Penk mutant mice (Ragnauth et al. 2001), while some other findings such as the increased litter size reported in KOR-1-deficient mice (Simonin et al. 1998) bear further study. Generally, while detailed studies of reproductive functions in several mutants remain to be reported, the apparently normal fertility of triple KO mice indicates that severe depletion of the endogenous opioid system is not incompatible with fecundity.

3.4.3
Hematology–Immunology

Many immune functions are altered by opioid treatment (e.g., see Eisenstein and Hilburger 1998; Sharp et al. 1998) but the mechanisms underlying this response remain controversial. Some studies propose that immune effects of opioids are mediated by receptors other than the classical opioid receptors (Stefano et al. 1996) and, in any case, the molecular identity of immune system opioid receptors remains elusive. Since the consequences of exogenous opioid administration are inconsistent, genetic models have provided an alternative tool to investigate the complex modulation of immune responses by endogenous and exogenous opioids.

The results so far have indicated modest effects of opioid mutants on the immune system with functional consequences still unclear. The number of bone marrow progenitor cells are higher in MOR-1 mutant mice, for example, suggesting that endogenous mu receptor activation plays a role in hematopoiesis, but paradoxically there is no change in mature circulating blood cell numbers (Tian et al. 1997). Two studies have reported effects of MOR-1 ablation on thymocyte populations. One reported no difference in the weight of the thymus, but a decrease in MOR-1 KO thymocyte proliferation in vitro (Roy et al. 1998), while another demonstrated that in vitro chemotactic migration of immature T cells, predominantly highly immature CD4$^-$ CD8$^-$ T cells, was reduced in MOR-1 KO mice (McCarthy et al. 2001). These effects might be expected to alter T cell maturation in vivo.

Nonetheless, the most thorough comparison of immune parameters in wild-type and MOR-1 KO mice has not yet revealed any major in vivo consequences of MOR-1 mutation. Parameters such as thymus and spleen cell-type histology, T lymphocyte distribution in the thymus, B and T cell distribution in the spleen, natural killer activity, mitogen-induced T and B cell proliferation in vitro as well as basal immunoglobulin levels in vivo were unchanged in MOR-1 KO mice (Gaveriaux-Ruff et al. 1998). While these baseline parameters are unchanged, effects typically elicited by morphine on immune system function are abolished, as are other morphine responses. Other minor effects of mutation of other system components on immune function have recently been reviewed elsewhere (Kieffer and Gaveriaux-Ruff 2002).

4
Opioid Pharmacology in Opioid System Mutant Mice

The remainder of this review will analyze the responses of opioid system KO mice to exogenous opiates. Prior to the cloning of opioid receptors, enormous effort was directed to developing specific mu, delta, and kappa ligands to analyze the endogenous opioid system. While the pharmacologic activities exhibited by these synthetic compounds have provided much of the current knowledge of opioid receptor function, mice lacking opioid receptors provide ideal models to confirm the specificity of these compounds. Theoretically, the biologic activities of highly selective mu, delta, and kappa agonists and antagonists should be abolished in mice lacking the MOR-1, DOR-1, and KOR-1 genes, respectively, while any residual activity could represent cross-activation of non-mutated receptors. The combination of classic pharmacology with contemporary genetics has now provided new information on both the specificity of compounds for specific receptors as well as the consequences of the activation elicited by these compounds in vivo.

The mutant mice also can be used to explore the action of compounds thought not to act directly on the opioid system. As one example, the analgesic cimetidine, a serotonergic receptor antagonist, was still able to elicit analgesia in the absence of several individual opioid receptors, demonstrating that this analgesia was indeed independent of the opioid system action (Hough et al. 2000). Additional responses of opioid system KO mice to non-opioid drugs has been reviewed elsewhere (Kieffer and Gaveriaux-Ruff 2002)

4.1
Effects of Mu Agonists

After production of the first MOR-1 KO mouse strain, the action of the proto-type opioid morphine was examined in detail. Several independent MOR-1-null strains have since been produced which permit similar experiments to be performed independently in several laboratories. Data from all these morphine-treated MOR-1-deficient mice have proved surprisingly clear-cut in that all studies agree that none of the pharmacologic activities of morphine observed in wild-type mice can be detected in mice lacking MOR-1 (see Table 2). In particular, analgesia elicited by morphine is absent in all the MOR-1 mutant mice not only at doses that produces maximal analgesia in wild-type mice but also at doses several fold higher than ED50 values, while analgesic effects are unaffected in DOR-1 and KOR-1 mutants. This finding indicates that possible in vivo binding of morphine to delta and kappa receptors, which would reflect binding detected in vitro, cannot activate any detectable analgesic response. Activation of the reward and dependence pathways, a second major action of morphine, was also abolished in MOR-1 mutant mice.

Recently, the ability of the general opioid antagonist naloxone to induce place aversion has also been shown to be MOR-1 dependent (Skoubis et al. 2001) and thus may reflect inhibition of tonically active MOR-1 in vivo. Interestingly, morphine appears to be aversive in self-administration experiments on MOR-1 KOs (Becker et al. 2000), potentially reflecting in vivo kappa receptor activation. Such a possibility can be tested directly using the combinatorial KO mice described above. All other acute morphine effects examined, such as respiratory depression, inhibition of gastrointestinal transit, and increased production of stress hormones, do not occur in MOR-1 mice. Given these results, it is not surprising that responses to chronic morphine administration, such as naloxone-precipitated withdrawal, upregulation of adenylyl cyclase activity (Matthes et al. 1996), and downregulation of brain dynamin (Noble et al. 2000), are also abolished. The genetic approach, therefore, has unambiguously demonstrated that MOR-1-derived receptors are essential for all the biologic activities elicited by morphine under standard experimental conditions.

Several morphine-elicited effects are clearly independent of DOR-1 and KOR-1; for example, identical dose–response curves for morphine analgesia are

Table 2 In vivo responses to morphine in mice lacking opioid system components

Responses	MOR-1[−/−]	DOR-1[−/−]	KOR-1[−/−]	Penk[−/−]
Analgesia	Abolished[1–6,20]	Maintained[7]	Maintained[8]	Maintained[18]
Tolerance to morphine analgesia		Abolished[7]		Abolished[18]
Hyperlocomotion	Abolished[9–11]			
Reward	Abolished[1,10]		Maintained[8]	
Self-administration	Abolished[10,11]			
Withdrawal	Abolished[1,10]	Maintained[18]	Reduced[8]	Maintained[18]
Respiratory depression	Abolished[12,13]			
Inhibition of GI transit	Abolished[14,19]			
Inhibition of VD twitch	Abolished[15]			
Immunosuppression	Abolished[16,17,a]			

GI, gastrointestinal; VD, vas deferens.

[a] Some parameters were maintained in a paradigm using morphine pellets.

References: 1. Matthes et al. (1996); 2. Sora et al. (1997); 3. Loh et al. (1998); 4. Schuller et al. (1999); 5. Sora et al. (1999); 6. Fuchs et al. (1999); 7. Zhu et al. (1999); 8. Simonin et al. (1998); 9. Tian et al. (1997); 10. Sora et al. (2001); 11. Becker et al. (2000); 12. Matthes et al. (1998); 13. Dahan et al. (2001); 14. Roy et al. (1998); 15. Maldonado et al. (2001); 16. Gaveriaux-Ruff et al. (1998); 17. Roy et al. (1998); 18. Nitscheet al. (2002); 19. King et al. (2002); 20. Nieland et al. (2002).

exhibited by both KOR-1- and DOR-1-deficient mice (Zhu et al. 1999; Slugg et al. 2000). These findings indicate that morphine does not require DOR-1 or KOR-1 for full activity, despite the fact that morphine selectivity is relatively low for MOR-1 in vitro and in vivo (see Matthes et al. 1998). Since both analgesic and undesirable effects of MOR-1 appear to be coordinately activated, MOR-1 itself will be difficult to target therapeutically, though perhaps divergent signaling pathways downstream mediating these effects can be identified and utilized.

It is also clear, however, that morphine activates pathways where downstream requirements for delta and kappa receptors have been revealed by mutational analysis (Table 2). For example, morphine withdrawal is significantly, though not dramatically, attenuated in KOR-1 mutant mice. Perhaps more significantly, analgesic tolerance to morphine is completely abolished in the DOR-1 mutant, and it will be of interest to determine whether MOR desensitization exhibited by different brain regions following chronic morphine (Sim et al. 1996) is differentially altered in DOR-1 mice. Thus both KOR-1 and DOR-1 receptors, although not directly activated by morphine, nevertheless contribute to pathways that are initiated by binding of morphine to MOR-1.

Recent work has attempted to determine whether endogenous opioid peptides could function as ligands for cognate receptors in these processes. While the Pdyn KO has not been tested in morphine withdrawal, the Pdyn mutation has no effect on tetrahydrocannabinol (THC) withdrawal (Zimmer et al. 2001). In contrast, mutation of Penk, like mutation of DOR-1, also completely blocks morphine tolerance in a daily injection paradigm (Nitsche et al. 2002). The simplest explanation for this result is that Penk, which is released following morphine treatment, activates DOR-1 in the pathway leading to morphine tolerance. Interestingly, in both DOR-1 and Penk mutants, morphine dependence as assessed by global withdrawal score is not altered, which has provided the clearest separation of these processes to date (Nitsche et al. 2002).

Use of heterozygous mice can provide information about the effect of decreasing receptor number by 50% (Zhu et al. 1999; Sora et al. 2001). Analysis of such mice showed that morphine-induced analgesia (see also Schuller et al. 1999), locomotory activity, and self-administration were all reduced in heterozygous animals, suggesting little mu receptor reserve for these responses. Decreases in spinal DPDPE analgesia were also found in heterozygous DOR-1 KO mice (Zhu et al. 1999). In contrast morphine analgesic tolerance and morphine dependence were unchanged, indicating that 50% of MOR-1 receptors are sufficient to elicit the long-term effects of morphine. The DOR-1 and Penkrequirements for tolerance are also markedly dependent on gene dosage, with morphine tolerance dramatically reduced in each heterozygous strain (Nitsche et al. 2002).

The effects of multiple other mu agonists in addition to morphine have been examined in MOR-1-deficient mice. Several studies have indicated that heroin (Kitanaka et al. 1998; Maldonado unpublished) and morphine-6-glucuronide (M6G) (Kitanaka et al. 1998; Loh et al. 1998; Maldonado unpublished), a major morphine metabolite in humans, do not elicit analgesia in MOR-1 KO mice, extending the previous morphine data to close morphine derivatives. In contrast, however, one study has indicated that heroin and M6G analgesia were present in exon 1 but not exon 2 MOR-deficient mice, suggesting the possible existence of MOR-1 splice variants that mediate this analgesia (Schuller et al. 1999); the functional relevance of specific variants to this process remains to be established. M6G can also inhibit GI transit in both exon 1 and exon 2 MOR-1 KO (M.A. King, submitted; Malonado, Pintar, Kieffer, unpublished). This effect is naltrexone sensitive at least in both the exon 1 MOR-1 KO as well as in triple KOs (M.A. King et al., submitted). Analgesic effects of the clinically relevant compound methadone, as well as the highly mu-specific agonists endomorphin-1 and -2 are abolished in MOR-1 KO mice, as are all activities of DAMGO including electrophysiologic responses of PAG neurons lacking MOR-1 (Loh et al. 1998; Connor et al. 1999; Mizoguchi et al. 1999; Schuller et al. 1999; Maldonado et al. 2001; Morin-Surun et al. 2001), while activity of [DMT1 DALDE, another mu-specific agonist is retained (Neilan et al. 2003). Together, the data indicate that MOR-1 mediates the main biologic activities of most mu agonists.

Ligand mutants have primarily been examined only for morphine responsiveness and in dependence/reward paradigms. Expression of morphine analgesia, hyperlocomotion, reward, and withdrawal were unchanged in the Pdyn mutant (Zimmer et al. 2001), indicating that major morphine effects do not require the presence of endogenous prodynorphin peptides. These data may implicate a constitutively active KOR-1 receptor in the aspects of withdrawal that are attenuated in this mutant. Systemic morphine analgesia was unchanged in both the absence of βend (Rubinstein et al. 1996) and Penk (Nitsche et al. 2002) while subtle modifications were noted when morphine was administered to βend KO mice i.c.v. or i.t. (Mogil et al. 2000). The participation of β-EP and Penk in food reward, using an operant conditioning paradigm, has also been demonstrated (Hayward et al. 2002), and it will be of interest to see if this response is MOR-1 dependent.

4.2
Effects of Delta Agonists

Functional interactions between mu and delta receptors not only in vitro but also in vivo have been suggested by prior pharmacologic studies (Rothman 1993; Traynor and Elliott 1993). Since the delta receptor remains a potential therapeutic target (Rapaka and Porreca 1991; Dondio 1997), studies on the activity of delta agonists in MOR-1-deficient mice have been of much interest. The data to date are summarized in Table 3 and remain an interesting area where the mutational analysis, like the pharmacology, has indicated a great deal of complexity.

Several delta agonists have been used to evaluate delta analgesia in MOR-1-deficient mice but with a wide range of results. Deltorphinand DPDPE, for example, have been reported to range from ineffective to fully effective in producing antinociception in thermal pain assays, depending on the test or route of administration. In particular, supraspinal delta analgesia is diminished while spinal analgesia is unaffected. DPDPE and SNC-80 analgesia were also decreased in models of mechanical pain and visceral chemical nociception. Finally, several non-analgesic effects of deltorphin (such as respiratory depression, reward, and physical dependence) are absent in the MOR-1 mutant following supraspinal administration (Hutcheson et al. 2001). Together these data at present strongly indicate that delta agonists require mu receptors to be fully active. One possible explanation is that delta compounds partially cross-react with mu receptors. However, no decreases in delta binding have been detected in the MOR-1 KO, which would be expected if traditional cross-occupancy were mediating these delta effects and, moreover, acute mu antagonist treatment does not alter delta analgesia (Suh and Tseng 1990). Alternatively, the absence of MOR-1 during development could prevent delta analgesic circuitry from maturing normally in vivo, and thus constitute the mu requirement for full delta analgesic activity.

Complementary studies examining delta agonist activities in mice lacking DOR-1 have also produced interesting results. DPDPE and deltorphin analgesia in the tail flick test following intrathecal administration are markedly reduced in the DOR-1 mutant, which is consistent with the maintenance of delta intrathecal analgesia in MOR-1 KO. The antinociceptive action of DPDPE in the formalin test is also abolished in DOR-1 KO mice, as are convulsions elicited by both SNC-80 and BW373U86. Together these data show clear DOR-1 receptor-mediated activities of delta agonists. Surprisingly, however, deltorphin and DPDPE continued to elicit analgesia in the DOR-1 mutants when the compounds were injected i.c.v., suggesting that supraspinal analgesia elicited by

Table 3 In vivo responses to kappa opioid agonists in mice lacking opioid receptors

Opioid	Responses	MOR[−/−]	DOR[−/−]	KOR[−/−]
Kappa agonists				
U50,488H	Thermal pain: spinal analgesia	Maintained[1,2,3]	Maintained[6]	Abolished[7]
	Thermal pain: supraspinal nalgesia	Maintained[1,2]		Abolished[7]
	Peripheral analgesia			Abolished[9]
	Visceral pain: analgesia	Maintained[4]		
	Mechanical pain: analgesia	Maintained[5]		
	Hypolocomotion			Reduced[7]
	Dysphoria			Reduced[7]
	Respiratory depression	Maintained[1]		
U69,593	CFA inflammatory pain: antihyperalgesia	Maintained[8]		

CFA, complete Freund's adjuvant.
Note: Spinal analgesia reflects physiological events that occur mainly at spinal cord level (tail-flick and tail-immersion tests). Supraspinal analgesia involves integrated responses (hot plate).
References: 1. Matthes et al. (1998); 2. Loh et al. (1998); 3. Schuller et al. (1999); 4. Sora et al. (1999); 5. Fuchs et al. (1999); 6. Zhu et al. (1999); 7. Simonin et al. (1998); 8. Qiu et al. (2000); 9. Chever et al. (2002).

these two compounds can utilize receptors other than DOR-1. While MOR-1 could be considered a possible candidate mediating this analgesia, DPDPE analgesia in DOR-1 KO mice is unaffected by antagonist treatments that are sufficient to block completely morphine action. Additional evidence that a distinct mechanism underlies this "delta-like" analgesia is that a striking increase in the analgesic potency of BW373U86 is also observed in DOR-1-deficient mice, suggesting a compensatory upregulation (or unmasking) of a second delta-like system. Thus data from both MOR-1 and DOR-1 KO mice suggest developmental modifications in the KO animals that become apparent at the behavioral level but are not readily discerned by binding or signaling studies (see Sect. 2.3).

4.3
Effects of Kappa Agonists

The in vivo responses of KOR-1 opioid receptor-deficient mice to kappa agonists, unlike the MOR-1 and DOR-1 KO, have been consistent with the pharmacologic predictions (see Table 4 and references therein). The analgesic action of U50,488H, studied in many different models, is abolished in KOR-deficient mice following all routes of administration, while it is maintained in MOR-1- and DOR-1-deficient mice. While two additional major effects of U50,488H, hypolocomotion and dysphoria, are dramatically reduced in KOR-1 KO mice, U50,488H respiratory depression and U69,593 antihyperalgesic responses are unchanged in the MOR-1 mutant, while the analgesic actions of both delta and mu agonists are unaffected by KOR-1 KO mice. Taken together, the genetic data indicate that compounds demonstrating kappa selectivity in vitro also retain

Table 4 In vivo responses to delta opioid agonists in mice lacking opioid receptors

Opioid	Responses	MOR$^{-/-}$	DOR$^{-/-}$	KOR$^{-/-}$
Delta agonists				
DPDPE	Thermal pain: spinal analgesia	Decreased[1,8] Maintained[2,3]	Reduced[6]	
	Thermal pain: supraspinal analgesia	Abolished[9] Decreased[8] Maintained[1,2]	Maintained[6]	
	Formalin chemical pain: analgesia		Abolished[6]	
	Mechanical pain: analgesia	Abolished[5]		
	Tolerance to analgesic effect		Abolished[6]	
	CFA inflammatory pain: antihyperalgesia	Increased[7]		
Deltorphin-II	Thermal pain: spinal analgesia	Decreased[1] Maintained[8]	Reduced[6]	
	Thermal pain: supraspinal analgesia	Maintained[1,8]	Maintained[6]	
	CFA inflammatory pain: antihyperalgesia	Increased[7]		
	Respiratory depression	Abolished[1]		
	Reward	Abolished[10]		
	Physical dependence	Abolished[10]		
SNC80	Visceral pain: analgesia	Abolished[4]		
	Convulsions		Abolished[11]	
BW373U86	Thermal pain: spinal analgesia		Increased[6]	
	Convulsions		Abolished[11]	

CFA, complete Freund's adjuvant.
Note: Spinal analgesia reflects physiological events that occur mainly at spinal cord level (tail-flick and tail-immersion tests). Supraspinal analgesia involves integrated responses (hot plate).
References: 1. Matthes et al. (1998); 2. Loh et al. (1998); 3. Schuller et al. (1999); 4. Sora et al. (1999); 5. Fuchs et al. (1999); 6. Zhu et al. (1999); 7. Qiu et al. (2000); 8. Hosohata et al. (2000); 9. Sora et al. (1997); 10. Hutcheson et al. (2001); 11. Broom et al. (2002).

that selectivity in standard in vivo experimental conditions. The kappa analgesic system function thus appears to function largely, if not completely, independently from mu and delta receptors systems.

U50,488H analgesia and hypolocomotion are also unchanged in the Pdyn mutant, suggesting that preprodynorphin-derived peptides generally do not participate in analgesia produced by exogenous kappa opioid compounds (Zimmer et al. 2001) and also indicating that any alteration in KOR-1 receptor number in the absence of Pdyn does not produce any detectable alterations in behavioral responses analyzed thus far.

4.4
Summary of Opioid Pharmacology

The application of pharmacologic agents to the opioid system has begun to illuminate several issues. Proposed receptor actions of several compounds have been confirmed and genetic evidence for functional interactions between opioid receptor subclasses have been obtained. MOR-1 KO strains have provided both clear-cut and more complex results. MOR-1-encoded receptors mediate a wide array of biologic events (see Sect. 4.1) that reflect the well-known pharmacologic profile of opiates either used clinically (morphine, fentanyl, methadone) or abused (heroin). Activation of KOR-1 evokes analgesia, hypolocomotion, and dysphoria, while activation of DOR-1 not only produces analgesia but also is required for morphine tolerance. Several lines of genetic evidence suggest that interactions between mu and delta systems may underlie several behavioral responses that remain poorly understood at the biochemical level. In contrast, the kappa system appears to act independently of the mu and delta system, general consistent with the pharmacologic predictions. Thus, genetic analysis has established that each receptor protein has a distinct role in both endogenous behavior (see "Basal Behavioral Phenotypes" above) and following responses to exogenous opiates (this section).

4.5
Non-classical Opioid Responses

The relationship between the multiple opioid receptor subtypes described pharmacologically and the three identified receptor genes remains a matter of some debate (Pasternak 1993; Gaveriaux-Ruff and Kieffer 1999). Since triple opioid receptor KO mice are viable, they have already become extremely valuable tools to possibly identify uncloned or unidentified opioid-like receptors that may mediate some of the responses discussed above as well as to explore "non-classical" opioid pharmacology. Triple KO mice have already been used to both clarify to some degree the identity of kappa-2 receptor sites as well as provide insight into "non-opioid" actions of naltrindole. Kappa-2 sites have classically been defined by labeling with the non-selective compound [^{3}H] bremazocine in the presence of excess cold DAMGO (mu), DPDPE (delta), and CI-977 (kappa-1). Since no selective ligand for kappa-2 sites has been made available, the nature of kappa-2 receptors has remained elusive. To clarify the contribution of the traditional opioid receptors to kappa-2 sites, [^{3}H] bremazocine binding was quantified in brain membranes from single opioid receptor-deficient mice, as well as the triple mutant. The data indicated most importantly that [^{3}H] bremazocine binding was totally absent from the triple KO mice (Simonin et al. 2001; Clarke et al. 2002). These studies demonstrate that all kappa-2 sites can be accounted for by a combination of [^{3}H] bremazocine binding to the three known opioid receptor proteins.

The immunosuppressive activity of the delta "*selective*" antagonist naltrindole in an vitro model of the graft rejection process has also been examined. Naltrindole as well as two structurally related derivatives showed the expected inhibitory effect in cells not only from wild-type mice but also from DOR-1 KO and triple opioid receptor KO as well (Gaveriaux-Ruff et al. 2001). This result clearly indicates that another molecular target should be identified to explain this intriguing biologic activity of the prototypic delta antagonist.

Other unexpected opioid receptor sites remain to be clarified at the molecular level. The triple KO mice can be used to investigate, for example, the multiplicity of β-endorphin binding and effects (Narita and Tseng 1998) as well as the DPDPE and BW373U86 responses observed so far in DOR-1 KO mice. Finally, though naloxone and naltrexone have been widely used to define opioid effects, early evidence for non-opioid activities of these agents has been described (Sawynok et al. 1979; Gold 1982) and can now be re-evaluated using triple KO mice.

5
Prospectus

Opioid system ligand and receptor-null mice have already provided important findings concerning the role of each component of the opioid system in mouse physiology as well as a the respective contributions of MOR-1, DOR-1, and KOR-1 to exogenous opiates. Baseline phenotypes of these mice have identified specific roles for individual receptors and ligands in specific pain modalities, emotional behaviors, and stress responses. The analysis of drug effects has identified MOR-1 as critical for multiple actions of morphine, while DOR-1 and KOR-1 remain potential targets for analgesia as well as higher-order behavioral abnormalities.

While many results have confirmed genetically the prior understanding of opioid action, most findings have nonetheless strengthened and extended the traditional pharmacologic view as well as opened novel areas of research. For example, while the genetic identification of the DOR-1 requirement for morphine tolerance was not entirely unexpected based on prior results, a role in dependence thus far not supported genetically could also have been expected. The extension of this finding to uncover the Penk requirement for morphine tolerance has identified a potential ligand/receptor necessary for tolerance and has opened a line of study to identify anatomical pathways mediating this response. Additional data suggest other ligand/receptors relationships in several independent pathways, such as MOR/Penk interaction in the regulation of locomotion, sensitivity to thermal pain and response to chemical pain, and the involvement of the DOR/Penk genes in anxiety-related behaviors, as well as morphine tolerance and a role for MOR/βend in stress-induced analgesia. The opposite responses exhibited by DOR-1- and MOR-1-deficient mice in several stress and anxiety behaviors were unexpected, clearly identifying a fertile area of study.

Some unexpected results from the study of analgesics have also emerged. Examples include retention of delta-like analgesia in the DOR-1 mutant (Zhu et al. 1999) and the reduced, rather than enhanced, perception of chemical pain in MOR-1 (Sora et al. 1997) and Penk (Konig et al. 1996). One possible explanation for these and other data is that adaptations have occurred in mutant mice to compensate for the absent gene and contribute to the unexpected responses. Genomic and proteomic phenotyping of these mutant strains, both under basal conditions and following drug treatment, is currently underway in several laboratories and can be expected to add considerably to our understanding the nature of any adaptations that accompany opioid system mutation.

Finally, additional genetic approaches are now well-established and can be expected to complement and extend traditional KO approaches as they are applied to the opioid system. Use of conditional mutations of opioid system components, for example, can be expected to help define opioid receptor circuitry both spatially and temporally, while knock-in approaches to introduce mutations that modify, rather than inactivate, opioid receptor function should help identify signaling pathways that mediate specific downstream opioid receptor activities. This next generation of mutant strains, coupled with knowledge of molecular adaptations, can be expected to further enhance the molecular and anatomical understanding of opioid system function that has already benefited from the fusion of pharmacology and genetics.

Acknowledgements. The authors are pleased to thank Michael Ansonoff for critical reading of the manuscripts. The authors also wish to acknowledge the support of the NIH (DA-09040, DA-15237 and DA-08622), the Human Frontier Science Program RG0011/2000-B, the INSERM, the Université Louis Pasteur, the Association de la Recherche pour le Cancer, the Institut UPSA de la Douleur, and the Mission Interministérielle de Lutte contre la Drogue et la Toxicomanie for support of original work performed in their laboratories.

References

Almeida, O.F.X. 1993. Opioids and the neuroendocrine control of reproduction. *In* Opioids II Vol. 104/II. Vol. 104. A. Hertz, editor. Springer Verlag: Berlin. 497–524

Baamonde, A., V. Dauge, M. Ruiz-Gayo, I.G. Fulga, S. Turcaud, M.C. Fournie-Zaluski, and B.P. Roques (1992) Antidepressant-type effects of endogenous enkephalins protected by systemic RB 101 are mediated by opioid delta and dopamine D1 receptor stimulation Eur J Pharmacol 216:157–66

Becker, A., G. Grecksch, R. Brodemann, J. Kraus, B. Peters, H. Schroeder, W. Thiemann, H.H. Loh, and V. Hollt (2000) Morphine self-administration in mu opioid receptor-deficient mice Naunyn Schmiedebergs Arch Pharmacol 361:584–9

Brady, L.S., M. Herkenham, R.B. Rothman, J.S. Partilla, M. Konig, A.M. Zimmer, and A. Zimmer (1999) Region-specific up-regulation of opioid receptor binding in enkephalin knockout mice Brain Res Mol Brain Res 68:193–7

Broom, D.C., J.F. Nitsche, J.E. Pintar, K.C. Rice, J.H. Woods, and J.R. Traynor (2002) Comparison of receptor mechanisms and efficacy requirements for delta-agonist-induced convulsive activity and antinociception in mice J Pharmacol Exp Ther 303:723–9

Brown, R.E., L. Stanford, and H.M. Schellinck (2000) Developing standardized behavioral tests for knockout and mutant mice Ilar J 41:163–74

Chen, H., V.S. Seybold, and H.H. Loh (2000) An autoradiographic study in mu-opioid receptor knockout mice Brain Res Mol Brain Res 76:170–2

Chever, V., J. Zhang, T. Czyzyk, M.A. King, J. Moron, G.W. Pasternak, J.E. Pintar, and T. Shipperberg (submitted) Nociceptin analgesia is reduced and the behavioral and neurochemical effects of cocaine are increased in a novel strain of kappa opioid receptor (KOR-1) KO mice

Clarke S., T. Czyzyk, M. Ansonoff, J.F. Nitsche, M.S. Hsu, L. Nilsson, K. Larsson, A. Borsodi, G. Toth, R. Hill, I. Kitchen, and J.E. Pintar (2002) Autoradiography of opioid and ORL1 ligands in opioid receptor triple knockout mice Eur J Neurosci 16:1705–12

Connor, M., A. Schuller, J.E. Pintar, and M.J. Christie (1999) Mu-opioid receptor modulation of calcium channel current in periaqueductal grey neurons from C57B16/J mice and mutant mice lacking MOR-1 Br J Pharmacol 126:1553–8

Corbett, A.D., Paterson, S. J. and Kosterlitz, H. W. (1993) Selectivity of ligands for opioid receptors. *In* Opioids I Vol. 104/I. Vol. 104/I. A. Hertz, editor. Springer-Verlagp: Berlin. 645–673

Cowan. (1993) Effects of opioids on the spontaneous behaviour of animals. *In* Opioids II Handbook of Experimental Pharmacology Vol. 104/II. Vol. 104/I. A. Hertz, editor. Springer Verlag: Berlin. 393–414

Dahan, A., E. Sarton, L. Teppema, C. Olievier, D. Nieuwenhuijs, H.W. Matthes, and B.L. Kieffer (2001) Anesthetic potency and influence of morphine and sevoflurane on respiration in mu-opioid receptor knockout mice Anesthesiology 94:824–32

Darland, T., M.M. Heinricher, and D.K. Grandy (1998) Orphanin FQ/nociceptin: a role in pain and analgesia, but so much more Trends Neurosci 21:215–21

Dondio, G., Ronzoni, S. and Petrilla, P. (1997) Non-peptide delta opioid agonists and antagonists. Exp. Opin. Ther. Pat. 7:1075–1098

Eisenstein, T.K., and M.E. Hilburger (1998) Opioid modulation of immune responses: effects on phagocyte and lymphoid cell populations J Neuroimmunol 83:36–44

Filliol, D., S. Ghozland, J. Chluba, M. Martin, H.W. Matthes, F. Simonin, K. Befort, C. Gaveriaux-Ruff, A. Dierich, M. LeMeur, O. Valverde, R. Maldonado, and B.L. Kieffer (2000) Mice deficient for delta- and mu-opioid receptors exhibit opposing alterations of emotional responses Nat Genet 25:195–200

Fuchs, P.N., C. Roza, I. Sora, G. Uhl, and S.N. Raja (1999) Characterization of mechanical withdrawal responses and effects of mu-, delta- and kappa-opioid agonists in normal and mu-opioid receptor knockout mice Brain Res 821:480–6

Gaveriaux-Ruff, C., D. Filliol, F. Simonin, H.W. Matthes, and B.L. Kieffer (2001) Immunosuppression by delta-opioid antagonist naltrindole: delta- and triple mu/delta/kappa-opioid receptor knockout mice reveal a nonopioid activity J Pharmacol Exp Ther 298:1193–8

Gaveriaux-Ruff, C., and B.L. Kieffer. 1999. Opioid receptors: gene structure and function. *In* Opioids in pain control: Basic and clinical aspects,. C. Stein, editor. Cambridge University Press: Cambridge. 1–20

Gaveriaux-Ruff, C., H.W. Matthes, J. Peluso, and B.L. Kieffer (1998) Abolition of morphine-immunosuppression in mice lacking the mu-opioid receptor gene Proc Natl Acad Sci U S A 95:6326–30

Gold, M.S., Dackis, C.A., Pottash, A.L. Sternbach, H.H., Annitto, W.J., Martin, D., Dackis, M.P. (1982) Naltrexone, opiate addiction, and endorphins Med Res Rev 2:211–246

Goody, R.J., S.M. Oakley, D. Filliol, B.L. Kieffer, and I. Kitchen (2002) Quantitative autoradiographic mapping of opioid receptors in the brain of delta-opioid receptor gene knockout mice Brain Res 945:9–19

Hayward, M.D., and M.J. Low (1999) Targeted mutagenesis of the murine opioid system Results Probl Cell Differ 26:169–91

Hayward M.D., J.E. Pintar, and M.J. Low (2002) Selective reward deficit in mice lacking beta-endorphin and enkephalin J Neurosci 22:8251–8

Hosohata, Y., T.W. Vanderah, T.H. Burkey, M.H. Ossipov, C.J. Kovelowski, I. Sora, G.R. Uhl, X. Zhang, K.C. Rice, W.R. Roeske, V.J. Hruby, H.I. Yamamura, J. Lai, and F. Porreca (2000) delta-Opioid receptor agonists produce antinociception and [35S]GTPgammaS binding in mu receptor knockout mice Eur J Pharmacol 388: 241–8

Hough, L.B., J.W. Nalwalk, Y. Chen, A. Schuller, Y. Zhu, J. Zhang, W.M. Menge, R. Leurs, H. Timmerman, and J.E. Pintar (2000) Improgan, a cimetidine analog, induces morphine-like antinociception in opioid receptor-knockout mice Brain Res 880:102–8

Hutcheson, D.M., H.W. Matthes, E. Valjent, P. Sanchez-Blazquez, M. Rodriguez-Diaz, J. Garzon, B.L. Kieffer, and R. Maldonado (2001) Lack of dependence and rewarding effects of deltorphin II in mu-opioid receptor-deficient mice Eur J Neurosci 13:153–61

Jordan, B.A., and L.A. Devi (1999) G-protein-coupled receptor heterodimerization modulates receptor function Nature 399:697–700

Kieffer, B. (2000) Opioid receptors: from genes to mice. Pain 1:45–50

Kieffer, B.L. (1995) Recent advances in molecular recognition and signal transduction of active peptides: receptors for opioid peptides Cell Mol Neurobiol 15:615–35

Kieffer, B.L. (1999) Opioids: first lessons from knockout mice Trends Pharmacol Sci 20:19–26

Kieffer, B.L., and C. Gaveriaux-Ruff (2002) Exploring the opioid system by gene knockout Prog Neurobiol 66:285–306

King, M.A., A.G.S. Schuller, M.A. Ansonoff, A.H. Chang, T.A. Czyzyk, J.E. Pintar, and G.W. Pasternak (submitted) Naltrexone-reversible inhibition of GI transit by morphine-6-glucoronide in MOR-1, MOR/DOR-1 and MOR-1/DOR-1/KOR-1 mutant mice

Kitanaka, N., I. Sora, S. Kinsey, Z. Zeng, and G.R. Uhl (1998) No heroin or morphine 6beta-glucuronide analgesia in mu-opioid receptor knockout mice Eur J Pharmacol 355:R1–3

Kitchen, I., S.J. Slowe, H.W. Matthes, and B. Kieffer (1997) Quantitative autoradiographic mapping of mu-, delta- and kappa-opioid receptors in knockout mice lacking the mu-opioid receptor gene Brain Res 778:73–88

Konig, M., A.M. Zimmer, H. Steiner, P.V. Holmes, J.N. Crawley, M.J. Brownstein, and A. Zimmer (1996) Pain responses, anxiety and aggression in mice deficient in preproenkephalin Nature 383:535–8

LaBuda, C.J., I. Sora, G.R. Uhl, and P.N. Fuchs (2000) Stress-induced analgesia in mu-opioid receptor knockout mice reveals normal function of the delta-opioid receptor system Brain Res 869:1–5

Loh, H.H., H.C. Liu, A. Cavalli, W. Yang, Y.F. Chen, and L.N. Wei (1998) mu Opioid receptor knockout in mice: effects on ligand-induced analgesia and morphine lethality Brain Res Mol Brain Res 54:321–6

Maldonado, R., C. Severini, H.W. Matthes, B.L. Kieffer, P. Melchiorri, and L. Negri (2001) Activity of mu- and delta-opioid agonists in vas deferens from mice deficient in MOR gene Br J Pharmacol 132:1485–92

Matthes, H.W., R. Maldonado, F. Simonin, O. Valverde, S. Slowe, I. Kitchen, K. Befort, A. Dierich, M. Le Meur, P. Dolle, E. Tzavara, J. Hanoune, B.P. Roques, and B.L. Kieffer (1996) Loss of morphine-induced analgesia, reward effect and withdrawal symptoms in mice lacking the mu-opioid-receptor gene Nature 383:819–23

Matthes, H.W., C. Smadja, O. Valverde, J.L. Vonesch, A.S. Foutz, E. Boudinot, M. Denavit-Saubie, C. Severini, L. Negri, B.P. Roques, R. Maldonado, and B.L. Kieffer (1998) Activity of the delta-opioid receptor is partially reduced, whereas activity of the kappa-receptor is maintained in mice lacking the mu- receptor J Neurosci 18:7285–95

McCarthy, L., I. Szabo, J.F. Nitsche, J.E. Pintar, and T.J. Rogers (2001) Expression of functional mu-opioid receptors during T cell development J Neuroimmunol 114:173–80

Mizoguchi, H., M. Narita, D.E. Oji, C. Suganuma, H. Nagase, I. Sora, G.R. Uhl, E.Y. Cheng, and L.F. Tseng (1999) The mu-opioid receptor gene-dose dependent reductions in G-protein activation in the pons/medulla and antinociception induced by endomorphins in mu-opioid receptor knockout mice Neuroscience 94:203–7

Mogil, J.S., J.E. Grisel, M.D. Hayward, J.R. Bales, M. Rubinstein, J.K. Belknap, and M.J. Low (2000) Disparate spinal and supraspinal opioid antinociceptive responses in beta-endorphin-deficient mutant mice Neuroscience 101:709–17

Mogil, J.S., and G.W. Pasternak (2001) The molecular and behavioral pharmacology of the orphanin FQ/nociceptin peptide and receptor family Pharmacol Rev 53:381–415

Mogil, J.S., S.G. Wilson, K. Bon, S.E. Lee, K. Chung, P. Raber, J.O. Pieper, H.S. Hain, J.K. Belknap, L. Hubert, G.I. Elmer, J.M. Chung, and M. Devor (1999) Heritability of nociception I: responses of 11 inbred mouse strains on 12 measures of nociception Pain 80:67–82

Monory, K., M.C. Bourin, M. Spetea, C. Tomboly, G. Toth, H.W. Matthes, B.L. Kieffer, J. Hanoune, and A. Borsodi (2000) Specific activation of the mu opioid receptor (MOR) by endomorphin 1 and endomorphin 2 Eur J Neurosci 12:577–84

Morin-Surun, M.P., E. Boudinot, C. Dubois, H.W. Matthes, B.L. Kieffer, M. Denavit-Saubie, J. Champagnat, and A.S. Foutz (2001) Respiratory function in adult mice lacking the mu-opioid receptor: role of delta-receptors Eur J Neurosci 13:1703–10

Naber, D. 1993. Opioids in the etiology and treatment of psychiatric disorders. In Handbook Exp Pharm: Opioids II Vol. 104/II. A. Hertz, editor. Springer-Verlag: Berlin. 781–793

Narita, M., H. Mizoguchi, I. Sora, G.R. Uhl, and L.F. Tseng (1999) Absence of G-protein activation by mu-opioid receptor agonists in the spinal cord of mu-opioid receptor knockout mice Br J Pharmacol 126:451–6

Narita, M., and L.F. Tseng (1998) Evidence for the existence of the beta-endorphin-sensitive "epsilon- opioid receptor" in the brain: the mechanisms of epsilon-mediated antinociception Jpn J Pharmacol 76:233–53

Neilan C.L., M.A. King, G. Rossi, M. Ansonoff, J.E. Pintar, P.W. Schiller, and G.W. Pasternak (2003) Differential sensitivities of mouse strains to morphine and [Dmt(1)]DAL-DA analgesia. Brain Res 974:254–7

Nitsche J.F., and J.E. Pintar (2003) Opioid receptor-induced GTPgamma35S binding during mouse development. Dev Biol 253:99–108

Nitsche J.F., A.G. Schuller, M.A. King, M. Zengh, G.W. Pasternak, and J.E. Pintar (2002) Genetic dissociation of opiate tolerance and physical dependence in delta-opioid receptor-1 and preproenkephalin knock-out mice. J Neurosci 22:10906–13

Noble, F., M. Szucs, B. Kieffer, and B.P. Roques (2000) Overexpression of dynamin is induced by chronic stimulation of mu- but not delta-opioid receptors: relationships with mu-related morphine dependence Mol Pharmacol 58:159–66

Ossipov, M.H., Malan, T. P. J., Lai, J. and Porreca, F. 1997. Opioid Pharmacology of acute and chronic pain. In Handbook of Experimental Pharmacology Vol. 130,. A.D.a.J.M. Besson, editor. Springer Verlag: Berlin Heidelberg. 305–327

Pan, Y.X., J. Xu, L. Mahurter, E. Bolan, M. Xu, and G.W. Pasternak (2001) Generation of the mu opioid receptor (MOR-1) protein by three new splice variants of the Oprm gene Proc Natl Acad Sci U S A 98:14084–9

Park, Y., T. Ma, S. Tanaka, C. Jang, H.H. Loh, K.H. Ko, and I.K. Ho (2000) Comparison of G-protein activation in the brain by mu-, delta-, and kappa-opioid receptor agonists in mu-opioid receptor knockout mice Brain Res Bull 52:297–302

Pasternak, G.W. (1993) Pharmacological mechanisms of opioid analgesics Clin Neuropharmacol 16:1–18

Pfeiffer, A., V. Brantl, A. Herz, and H.M. Emrich (1986) Psychotomimesis mediated by kappa opiate receptors Science 233:774–6

Qiu, C., I. Sora, K. Ren, G. Uhl, and R. Dubner (2000) Enhanced delta-opioid receptor-mediated antinociception in mu-opioid receptor-deficient mice Eur J Pharmacol 387:163–9

Ragnauth, A., A. Schuller, M. Morgan, J. Chan, S. Ogawa, J. Pintar, R.J. Bodnar, and D.W. Pfaff (2001) Female preproenkephalin-knockout mice display altered emotional responses Proc Natl Acad Sci U S A 98:1958–63

Rapaka, R.S., and F. Porreca (1991) Development of delta opioid peptides as nonaddicting analgesics Pharm Res 8:1–8

Rios, C.D., B.A. Jordan, I. Gomes, and L.A. Devi (2001) G-protein-coupled receptor dimerization: modulation of receptor function Pharmacol Ther 92:71–87

Rothman, R.B., Holaday, J. W. and Porreca, F. 1993. Allosteric coupling among opioid receptors: Evidence for an opioid receptor complex. *In* Handbook of experimental Pharmacology, Opioids I Vol. 104/I. A. Hertz, editor. Springer-Verlag: Berlin. 217-237

Roy, S., R.A. Barke, and H.H. Loh (1998) MU-opioid receptor-knockout mice: role of mu-opioid receptor in morphine mediated immune functions Brain Res Mol Brain Res 61:190–4

Rubinstein, M., J.S. Mogil, M. Japon, E.C. Chan, R.G. Allen, and M.J. Low (1996) Absence of opioid stress-induced analgesia in mice lacking beta- endorphin by site-directed mutagenesis Proc Natl Acad Sci U S A 93:3995–4000

Sawynok, J., C. Pinsky, and F.S. LaBella (1979) On the specificity of naloxone as an opiate antagonist Life Sci 25:1621–32

Schuller, A.G., M.A. King, J. Zhang, E. Bolan, Y.X. Pan, D.J. Morgan, A. Chang, M.E. Czick, E.M. Unterwald, G.W. Pasternak, and J.E. Pintar (1999) Retention of heroin and morphine-6 beta-glucuronide analgesia in a new line of mice lacking exon 1 of MOR-1 Nat Neurosci 2:151–6

Sharifi, N., N. Diehl, L. Yaswen, M.B. Brennan, and U. Hochgeschwender (2001) Generation of dynorphin knockout mice Brain Res Mol Brain Res 86:70–5

Sharp, B.M., S. Roy, and J.M. Bidlack (1998) Evidence for opioid receptors on cells involved in host defense and the immune system J Neuroimmunol 83:45–56

Shook, J.E., W.D. Watkins, and E.M. Camporesi (1990) Differential roles of opioid receptors in respiration, respiratory disease, and opiate-induced respiratory depression Am Rev Respir Dis 142:895–909

Sim, L.J., D.E. Selley, S.I. Dworkin, and S.R. Childers (1996) Effects of chronic morphine administration on mu opioid receptor- stimulated [35S]GTPgammaS autoradiography in rat brain J Neurosci 16:2684–92

Simonin, F., S. Slowe, J.A. Becker, H.W. Matthes, D. Filliol, J. Chluba, I. Kitchen, and B.L. Kieffer (2001) Analysis of [3H]bremazocine binding in single and combinatorial opioid receptor knockout mice Eur J Pharmacol 414:189–95

Simonin, F., O. Valverde, C. Smadja, S. Slowe, I. Kitchen, A. Dierich, M. Le Meur, B.P. Roques, R. Maldonado, and B.L. Kieffer (1998) Disruption of the kappa-opioid receptor gene in mice enhances sensitivity to chemical visceral pain, impairs pharmacological actions of the selective kappa-agonist U-50,488H and attenuates morphine withdrawal Embo J 17:886–97

Skoubis, P.D., H.W. Matthes, W.M. Walwyn, B.L. Kieffer, and N.T. Maidment (2001) Naloxone fails to produce conditioned place aversion in mu-opioid receptor knock-out mice Neuroscience 106:757–63

Slowe, S.J., S. Clarke, I. Lena, R.J. Goody, R. Lattanzi, L. Negri, F. Simonin, H.W. Matthes, D. Filliol, B.L. Kieffer, and I. Kitchen (2001) Autoradiographic mapping of the opioid receptor-like 1 (ORL1) receptor in the brains of mu-, delta- or kappa-opioid receptor knockout mice Neuroscience 106:469–80

Slowe, S.J., F. Simonin, B. Kieffer, and I. Kitchen (1999) Quantitative autoradiography of mu-,delta- and kappa1 opioid receptors in kappa-opioid receptor knockout mice Brain Res 818:335–45

Slugg, R.M., M.D. Hayward, O.K. Ronnekleiv, M.J. Low, and M.J. Kelly (2000) Effect of the mu-opioid agonist DAMGO on medial basal hypothalamic neurons in beta-endorphin knockout mice Neuroendocrinology 72:208–17

Sora, I., G. Elmer, M. Funada, J. Pieper, X.F. Li, F.S. Hall, and G.R. Uhl (2001) Mu opiate receptor gene dose effects on different morphine actions: evidence for differential in vivo mu receptor reserve Neuropsychopharmacology 25:41–54

Sora, I., X.F. Li, M. Funada, S. Kinsey, and G.R. Uhl (1999) Visceral chemical nociception in mice lacking mu-opioid receptors: effects of morphine, SNC80 and U-50,488 Eur J Pharmacol 366:R3–5

Sora, I., N. Takahashi, M. Funada, H. Ujike, R.S. Revay, D.M. Donovan, L.L. Miner, and G.R. Uhl (1997) Opiate receptor knockout mice define mu receptor roles in endogenous nociceptive responses and morphine-induced analgesia Proc Natl Acad Sci U S A 94:1544–9

Stefano, G.B., B. Scharrer, E.M. Smith, T.K. Hughes, Jr., H.I. Magazine, T.V. Bilfinger, A.R. Hartman, G.L. Fricchione, Y. Liu, and M.H. Makman (1996) Opioid and opiate immunoregulatory processes Crit Rev Immunol 16:109–44

Stein, C., H. Machelska, W. Binder, and M. Schafer (2001) Peripheral opioid analgesia Curr Opin Pharmacol 1:62–5

Suh, H.H., and L.F. Tseng (1990) Different types of opioid receptors mediating analgesia induced by morphine, DAMGO, DPDPE, DADLE and beta-endorphin in mice Naunyn Schmiedebergs Arch Pharmacol 342:67–71

Tejedor-Real, P., J.A. Mico, C. Smadja, R. Maldonado, B.P. Roques, and J. Gilbert-Rahola (1998) Involvement of delta-opioid receptors in the effects induced by endogenous enkephalins on learned helplessness model Eur J Pharmacol 354:1–7

Tian, M., H.E. Broxmeyer, Y. Fan, Z. Lai, S. Zhang, S. Aronica, S. Cooper, R.M. Bigsby, R. Steinmetz, S.J. Engle, A. Mestek, J.D. Pollock, M.N. Lehman, H.T. Jansen, M. Ying, P.J. Stambrook, J.A. Tischfield, and L. Yu (1997) Altered hematopoiesis, behavior, and sexual function in mu opioid receptor-deficient mice J Exp Med 185:1517–22

Traynor, J.R., and J. Elliott (1993) delta-Opioid receptor subtypes and cross-talk with mu-receptors Trends Pharmacol Sci 14:84–6

Vaccarino, A.L., and A.J. Kastin (2000) Endogenous opiates: 1999 Peptides 21:1975–2034

Wang, Z., L.R. Gardell, M.H. Ossipov, T.W. Vanderah, M.B. Brennan, U. Hochgeschwender, V.J. Hruby, T.P. Malan, Jr., J. Lai, and F. Porreca (2001) Pronociceptive actions of dynorphin maintain chronic neuropathic pain J Neurosci 21:1779–86

Yaswen, L., N. Diehl, M.B. Brennan, and U. Hochgeschwender (1999) Obesity in the mouse model of pro-opiomelanocortin deficiency responds to peripheral melanocortin Nat Med 5:1066–70

Zaki, P.A., E.J. Bilsky, T.W. Vanderah, J. Lai, C.J. Evans, and F. Porreca (1996) Opioid receptor types and subtypes: the delta receptor as a model Annu Rev Pharmacol Toxicol 36:379–401

Zhu, Y., M.S. Hsu, and J.E. Pintar (1998) Developmental expression of the mu, kappa, and delta opioid receptor mRNAs in mouse J Neurosci 18:2538–49

Zhu, Y., M.A. King, A.G. Schuller, J.F. Nitsche, M. Reidl, R.P. Elde, E. Unterwald, G.W. Pasternak, and J.E. Pintar (1999) Retention of supraspinal delta-like analgesia and loss of morphine tolerance in delta opioid receptor knockout mice Neuron 24:243–52

Zhu, Y., and J.E. Pintar (1998) Expression of opioid receptors and ligands in pregnant mouse uterus and placenta Biol Reprod 59:925–32

Zimmer, A., E. Valjent, M. Konig, A.M. Zimmer, P. Robledo, H. Hahn, O. Valverde, and R. Maldonado (2001) Absence of delta −9-tetrahydrocannabinol dysphoric effects in dynorphin- deficient mice J Neurosci 21:9499–505

Part 4
Cardiovascular System

Transgenic Mouse Models of Cardiovascular Function and Disease

B. C. Blaxall[2] · W. J. Koch[1]

[1] Department of Surgery, Duke University Medical Center, Durham, NC, 27710, USA
e-mail: koch0002@mc.duke.edu
[2] Division of Cardiology, Center for Cellular and Molecular Cardiology University
of Rochester Medical Center, Rochester, NY, 14642, USA

Abstract Transgenic mouse technology, coupled with cardiac-specific promoters and complex measurements of murine myocardial function and hemodynamics, have played an important role in expanding our knowledge regarding adrenergic receptors and downstream components of their signal transduction cascade in both normal and diseased heart function. Herein we discuss the results and implications of overexpression or ablation of several adrenergic receptors and/or downstream effectors in their G protein signaling pathway to further delineate their potential roles in both normal and diseased heart function. Finally, we discuss a number of mouse models of heart failure, and how they can act as important "in vivo reaction vessels" to identify and test specific genes/hypotheses which may lead to novel therapeutics for heart disease.

Keywords Heart failure · Adrenergic receptor · G protein · Kinase · Signaling · Transgenic · Knockout

1
Introduction

1.1
Adrenergic Receptor Signaling in the Heart

Description and functional distinction of adrenergic receptors was first reported by Ahlquist (1948), demonstrating a rank order of response to sympathomimetic agents for what were then termed α- and β-adrenergic receptors (α-ARs and β-ARs, respectively). These receptors belong to the superfamily of seven transmembrane-spanning receptors that activate heterotrimeric guanine nucleotide binding proteins (G proteins), also known as G protein-coupled receptors (GPCRs) (Caron and Lefkowitz 1993). In the myocardium, both α-ARs and β-ARs are expressed, where they mediate several physiological aspects of cardiac function via stimulation by the endogenous sympathetic neurotransmitters epinephrine and norepinephrine (Koch et al. 2000).

To date, three subtypes of β-ARs have been identified, namely β_1-, β_2-, and β_3-ARs. In the heart, the β_1-AR is the predominant sub-type, comprising 75%–80% of cardiac β-ARs, with the remaining 20%–25% of thought to be β_2-ARs (Brodde 1993), although recent evidence suggests the presence of β_3-ARs in the myocardium (Gauthier et al. 1996). Both β_1- and β_2-ARs couple to adenylyl cyclase in the heart through the stimulatory G protein, $G\alpha_s$, increasing cyclic adenosine monophosphate (cAMP) and thus leading to enhanced chronotropy and inotropy via calcium entry and release from intracellular stores (Bristow et al. 1989). Recent data also describe the interesting finding that, under certain conditions, β_2-ARs can couple to the inhibitory G protein, $G\alpha_i$ (Daaka et al. 1997; Xiao et al. 1999).

The α-ARs (both α_1- and α_2-ARs) are also expressed in the myocardium, particularly α_{1a}-, α_{1b}-, and α_{1c}-ARs, albeit to a much lesser extent than the β-ARs, at a ratio of 10:1 of β-ARs to α-ARs (Hoffman and Lefkowitz 1996). These receptors primarily couple to the G protein $G\alpha_q$, which in turn activates phospholipase C (PLC), leading to an increase in the second messengers inositol triphosphate (IP3) and diacylglycerol (DAG), thus enhancing intracellular calcium and activating protein kinase C (PKC) (Exton 1985). Of the three α-AR isoforms, the presence of α_{1a}- and α_{1b}-AR isoforms has been confirmed in the myocardium (Knowlton et al. 1993). The role of these α-ARs, as well as other $G\alpha_q$-coupled receptors have been implicated in both myocyte growth and hypertrophy (Simpson 1983; Dostal and Baker 1998).

Stimulation of either α_1- or β-ARs leads to dissociation of the heterotrimeric G proteins into their $G\alpha$ and $G\beta\gamma$ subunits, which can each propagate signals within the cell by modulating the activity of one or more effector molecules, as described above, such as adenylyl cyclases, phospholipases, and ion channels (Clapham and Neer 1997). In turn, the activity of these effector enzymes and channels regulates the production of second messenger molecules, which elicit cellular responses by activating different signaling pathways (Rockman et al. 2002).

Importantly, signaling through GPCRs, including the ARs, is under tight regulatory control, the most rapid form being targeted intracellular phosphorylation of activated receptors leading to G protein uncoupling, a process termed desensitization. Activation of protein kinase A (PKA) or PKC via signaling through these receptors results in receptor phosphorylation, a process known as heterologous (or non-agonist-specific) desensitization. In contrast, the most rapid form of regulatory control, which is agonist-specific, or homologous desensitization, involves targeted phosphorylation of agonist-occupied receptors by GPCR kinases (GRKs). This leads to rapid association of a second molecule, β-arrestin, with the phosphorylated receptors, which leads to uncoupling of the receptor from G proteins (Lefkowitz 1998). Several GPCRs are expressed in the heart, including the β-ARs, which are responsible for increasing both rate and force of contraction (Bristow et al. 1990; Brodde 1993). Therefore, tight regulation of the myocardial G protein signaling pathways is critical for maintenance of normal cardiac function. For example, in several cardiovascular diseases, where myocardial β-AR signaling and responsiveness is attenuated, increased expression and activity of the β-AR kinase (βARK1, also known as GRK2) has been described (Ungerer et al. 1993; Ungerer et al. 1996). Experimental animal models of heart failure have also shown increased expression and activity of both βARK1 (Anderson et al. 1999; Choi et al. 1997; Maurice et al. 1999) and GRK5 (Ping et al. 1997).

The seven members of the GRK family (GRK1–7) are all serine/threonine kinases that phosphorylate agonist-occupied or stimulated GPCRs (Lefkowitz 1998; Pitcher et al. 1998). With the exception of GRK1 (almost exclusively retinal expression) and GRK4 (found almost exclusively in testes, vasculature, and certain brain regions), the GRKs are expressed in all tissues, including the heart (Pitcher et al. 1998). In the heart, βARK1 is the primary GRK, although GRK3 (also known as βARK2), GRK5, and GRK6 are also found in the myocardium (Inglese et al. 1993; Iaccarino et al. 1998). Long-term exposure (i.e., hours) to agonist can also lead to internalization and inactivation of the receptor, mediated in part by both GRKs and β-arrestins (Laporte et al. 2000). The internalization process may also stimulate other signaling intracellular signaling cascades, such as various mitogen-activated protein kinase (MAPK) pathways.

Although there is some diversity within the GRK family, they all require targeting to the plasma membrane for functional activation. Many of the GRKs are constitutively localized to the plasma membrane, including GRK4, GRK5, and GRK6. In the case of βARK1 (GRK2) and GRK3, these kinases are primarily cytosolic, and are translocated to the plasma membrane following agonist stimulation of the cognate receptor, where they associate directly with membrane-bound G$\beta\gamma$ and are stabilized thereby direct interactions with the plasma membrane (Pitcher et al. 1992; Koch et al. 1993). Importantly, the activity of βARK1 can be inhibited by expression of a peptide inhibitor of the carboxyl-terminal 194 amino acid G$\beta\gamma$-binding and pleckstrin homology domain (βARKct) that competes with endogenous βARK1 for G$\beta\gamma$-mediated translocation (Pitcher et al. 1992; Koch et al. 1993; Koch et al. 1995), which is discussed below in greater detail.

1.2
Adrenergic Signaling in Heart Disease

In general, increased workload following myocardial injury results in the physiological response of cardiac hypertrophy, which can lead to contractile dysfunction and ultimately heart failure (Anversa et al. 1985; Harding et al. 1995; Gidh-Jain et al. 1998; Towbin and Bowles 2002). Numerous alterations in AR signaling have been associated with the progression of heart failure. In the early development of heart failure, the sympathetic nervous system responds by increasing adrenergic drive to enhance contractility. One of the results of this increased AR agonism is β-AR down-regulation and desensitization, as initially described by Bristow et al. (1982). There appears to be sub-type specific down-regulation of the β_1-ARs; however, both remaining β_1- and β_2-ARs are substantially uncoupled from G proteins and desensitized (Bristow et al. 1989), a process mediated in part by enhanced levels of myocardial βARK1 (Ungerer et al. 1994) and Gα_i (Feldman et al. 1988). The reduction of cardiac β_1-ARs leads to a notably different ratio of β_1-, β_2-, and α_1-ARs, and when coupled to altered AR signaling, may contribute to altered cardiac function. These disruptions in signaling may also lead to enhanced coupling of receptors to other signaling pathways involved in hypertrophic responses and ventricular remodeling (including promotion of cell survival and apoptosis), such as the MAPK and phospotidylinositol-3-kinase (PI3K) cascades (Daaka et al. 1997; Zhu et al. 2001).

With specific regard to the hypertrophic response , several GPCRs have been implicated. Gα_q-coupled receptors (such as α_1-ARs, angiotensin and endothelin receptors) have been shown to activate hypertrophic MAPK pathways (Sugden 2001). In vitro experiments have also suggested a pivotal role of α_1-ARs in promoting cardiomyocyte hypertrophy (Knowlton et al. 1993), which can lead to contractile dysfunction that ultimately results in heart failure (Harding et al. 1995). Furthermore, up-regulation of Gα_q and PLC was found in the border zones of myocardial infarction, suggesting that these signaling molecules/pathways play an important role in the surviving myocytes (Ju et al. 1998), although it is not established whether this is adaptive or maladaptive.

In this chapter, we will discuss how transgenic mouse technology, coupled with cardiac-specific promoters and complex measurements of murine myocardial function and hemodynamics, has played an important role in enhancing our knowledge regarding adrenergic receptors and downstream components of their signal transduction cascade in both normal and diseased heart function. In addition, we will discuss transgenic mice with overexpression of α_{1b}-ARs, $G\alpha_q$, or a peptide inhibitor of $G\alpha_q$ to further delineate their potential roles in both hypertrophy and heart failure. Finally, we will discuss a number of mouse models of heart failure, and how they can act as important "in vivo reaction vessels" to identify and test specific genes/hypotheses which may lead to novel therapeutics for heart disease.

2
Mouse Models of Adrenergic Receptor Signaling

The development and use of genetically engineered mice, which can provide targeted (over-) expression or "knockout" of specific genes, coupled with sophisticated physiological methods of measuring cardiovascular function and hemodynamics, has provided a powerful set of tools to study the regulation of cardiac contractility. Transgenic mouse studies of myocardial function were revolutionized by description of the α-myosin heavy chain (α-MHC) promoter, as this promoter is cardiac-specific and is not significantly active until the perinatal period, bypassing potential developmental effects of transgene expression (Subramaniam et al. 1991). Using this promoter, several GPCRs, including the β_1-, β_2-, and α_1-ARs, have been overexpressed in mouse myocardium, resulting in dramatically different phenotypes, indicating a fundamental difference in their signaling and function in the heart. For a summary of α-AR and β-AR transgenic animal models, please see summary Tables 1, 2, and 3 in the chapter by Engelhardt and Hein (this volume).

2.1
β-AR Signaling

2.1.1
β-AR Overexpression

Overexpression of the dominant cardiac β-AR subtype, the β_1-AR, at levels of 5- to 15-fold leads to a phenotype of dilated cardiomyopathy even in young mice, and is similar to resultant pathology from chronic exposure to catecholamines (Engelhardt et al. 1999). In another study, overexpression of the β_1-AR at levels greater than 20-fold resulted in similar pathology and diminished cardiac function, and also demonstrating an increase in myofibrillar disarray, fibrosis, and apoptosis (Bisognano et al. 2000).

   In contrast to the β_1-AR, several studies have demonstrated that overexpression of the β_2-AR at levels up to 200-fold higher than endogenous expression have not resulted in any significant cardiac pathology in mice, which are instead characterized by enhanced biochemical and in vivo cardiac function (Milano et al. 1994; Liggett et al. 2000). Interestingly, in mice with very high overexpression

(~200-fold), baseline cardiac function was equal to or greater than normal litter-mate control (NLC) cardiac function in response to the β-AR agonist isoproter-enol. Furthermore, there was no increase in contractility in the β_2-AR overex-pressing mice in response to treatment with the β-AR agonist isoproterenol. In addition to their enhanced cardiac function, these mice demonstrate enhanced myocardial relaxation accompanied by down-regulation of a sarcoplasmic retic-ulum calcium regulatory protein, phospholamban (PLB) (Rockman et al. 1996). Transgenic expression of very high levels of β_2-AR (i.e., >300-fold) results in a rapid and progressive cardiomyopathic phenotype, consistent with the patho-logical toxicity of chronic β-AR agonist stimulation (Liggett et al. 2000). In transgenic mice with such dramatic overexpression of the endogenous protein, it is difficult to determine whether the effects are due specifically to the protein itself, or simply due to the fact that extreme overexpression of any protein can produce pathophysiological effects, as was the case for cardiac overexpression of green fluorescent protein (Huang et al. 2000).

2.1.2
β-AR Gene Ablation

The role of β-ARs in cardiac function has been further delineated by gene "knockout" experiments, which have been eloquently detailed in a recent review (Rohrer 1998). Ablation of the β_1-AR in mice generally leads to embryonic le-thality, with the majority of mice homozygous for gene disruption dying in ute-ro (Rohrer 1998). If these mice are outbred, embryonic mortality can be re-duced. The surviving mice have normal resting heart rate and blood pressure; however, despite the presence of β_2-ARs in these mouse hearts, they do not re-spond to β-AR agonist stimulation. In contrast, the β_2-AR knockout mice are viable and apparently healthy. Only during the stress of exercise is a physiologi-cal consequence observed, and this is a result of alterations in vascular tone and energy metabolism (Chruscinski et al. 1999). These results suggest that under endogenous conditions the β_2-AR does not play a major role in cardiac func-tion.

These data suggest that the β_1-AR is the predominant mediator of catechol-amine-induced chronotropy and inotropy in the mouse heart. They further demonstrate that stimulation of β_1-ARs, as compared to β_2-ARs, have distinctly different effects in the myocardium. This functional difference may be due, at least in part, to the ability of the cardiac β_2-ARs to couple to both $G\alpha_s$ and $G\alpha_i$, whereas cardiac β_1-ARs appear to only couple to $G\alpha_s$. Interestingly, overexpres-sion of $G\alpha_s$ also leads to cardiac pathology (Iwase et al. 1996, 1997), indicating similarity of these mice with β_1- but not β_2-AR overexpression. Dual coupling of the β_2-AR to both $G\alpha_s$ and $G\alpha_i$ may provide the mechanism by which β_2-ARs elicit survival responses, while stimulation of β_1-ARs activates only apoptotic pathways (Communal et al. 1999; Zhu et al. 2001). However, overstimulation of the $G\alpha_i$ pathway may also be detrimental to cardiac function. This was indirectly demonstrated in conditional expression in the adult mouse heart of a $G\alpha_i$-cou-

Table 1 Transgenic models with altered expression of G proteins or adenylyl cyclase (AC)

Gene	Model	Phenotype	Reference(s)
Gαs	α-MHC	Increased heart rate, mortality, LV dilation; decreased ejection fraction	Iwase et al. 1996, 1997
Gαi-coupled ligand-specific opioid receptor	α-MHC, conditional Tet system	Conductance abnormalities and lethal cardiomyopathy	Redfern et al. 2000
Gαq	α-MHC	Hypertrophy, enhanced heart rate, myocyte size, HF gene expression; depressed fractional shortening, at baseline and in response to dobutamine	D'Angelo et al. 1997
		Hypertrophy, functional decompensation	Sakata et al. 1998
Gql (peptide inhibitor of Gαq)	α-MHC	Reduced hypertrophy following trans-aortic constriction	Akhter et al. 1997
CAM Gαq	α-MHC	Embryonic lethal. In utero hypertrophy followed by apoptosis	Adams et al. 1998
		Hypertrophy and ventricular dilation	Mende et al. 1998, 2001
AC V	α-MHC	Increased heart rate and ractional shortening, with no enhanced response to β-AR stimulation	Tepe et al. 1999; Ostram et al. 2000
AC VI	α-MHC	Increased heart rate, fractional shortening, and response to β-AR stimulation	Gao et al. 1998; Roth et al. 1999

pled, ligand-specific opioid receptor, where stimulation of the receptor and hence the Gα$_i$ pathway led to cardiac conductance abnormalities and a lethal cardiomyopathy (Redfern et al. 2000).

Of further interest, overexpression of the calcium-inhibitable adenylyl cyclases (ACs) found in the heart (AC V and VI) led to varying cardiac phenotypes (Table 1). Overexpression of AC V in the heart resulted in increased heart rate and fractional shortening at baseline, although there was no in vivo hemodynamic response (heart rate and contractility) to isoproterenol infusion, suggesting that AC V does not stoichiometrically constrain cardiomyocyte β-AR signaling (Tepe et al. 1999; Ostrom et al. 2000). Conversely, overexpression of AC VI in myocytes appeared to enhance not only baseline activity, but also β-AR signaling in response to isoproterenol (Gao et al. 1998). Further studies in AC VI transgenic mice cross-bred with a mouse model of heart failure revealed similar data (Roth et al. 1999).

2.2
α-AR Signaling in Heart Failure

As stated above, the α_1-ARs have been linked to the development of myocardial hypertrophy and heart failure, in that signaling through α_1-ARs (particularly in cell culture) or other receptors coupled to the $G\alpha_q$/PLC signaling pathway (i.e., angiotensin II AT1 or endothelin) have been implicated in pressure and/or volume overload-induced hypertrophy (Simpson 1983; Knowlton et al. 1993; Dostal and Baker 1998). Due to the peripheral vascular effects of α-AR agonist administration, which can induce myocardial hypertrophy, it has been difficult to specifically delineate the direct effect of cardiac α_1-ARs in the development of hypertrophy.

2.2.1
α_{1b}-AR Overexpression

To address the cardiac-specific role of the α_1-ARs, transgenic mouse models have been developed that overexpress the α_{1b}-AR, either in its wild-type form or as a constitutively active mutant (CAM), using the α-MHC promoter (Milano et al. 1994; Akhter et al. 1997). When the CAM α_{1b}-AR is targeted to the myocardium of transgenic mice, the adult hearts are significantly hypertrophied, with ventricular myocyte size increasing by 62% (Milano et al. 1994). Therefore, continued signaling through CAM α_{1b}-ARs expressed only in the heart can indeed induce ventricular hypertrophy independent of peripheral vascular effects. These mice also demonstrate other properties associated with ventricular hypertrophy, such as increased expression of atrial natriuretic factor (ANF) and enhanced signaling through the $G\alpha_q$/PLC pathway, such as significantly elevated basal levels of myocardial DAG and IP_3 (Milano et al. 1994; Harrison et al. 1998).

In two separate lines of transgenic mice expressing wild-type α_{1b}-ARs in the heart at greater than 40-fold over baseline, basal myocardial α_1-AR signaling, as measured by DAG accumulation, was significantly increased to levels similar to those found in the CAM α_{1b}-AR mice (Akhter et al. 1997). However, in contrast to the CAM α_{1b}-AR mice, the hearts of the wild-type α_{1b}-AR overexpressors did not develop hypertrophy, despite significant elevation of ANF expression (Akhter et al. 1997). Interestingly, in the wild-type α_{1b}-AR animals, response to the β-AR agonist isoproterenol was significantly depressed (Akhter et al. 1997; Lemire et al. 1998). Two mechanisms for this diminished β-AR response in vivo resulting from wild-type α_{1b}-AR overexpression have been discovered. First, overexpressed α_{1b}-ARs appear to also couple to $G\alpha_i$, which could negatively impinge on β-AR signaling through AC (Akhter et al. 1997). Second, as a result of enhanced $G\alpha_q$/PLC activity in these mice, myocardial PKC activity is increased (Lemire et al. 1998), PKC being an enzyme which can phosphorylate and activate βARK1 (Chuang et al. 1995). Indeed, βARK1 activity was enhanced in these mice, leading to enhanced βARK1-mediated desensitization of the β-AR (Akhter et al. 1997).

In follow-up studies, overexpression of the wild-type α_{1b}-AR has been demonstrated to result in dilated cardiomyopathy and premature death (Grupp et al. 1998; Lemire et al. 2001). This phenotype also occurred in rapid fashion in these mice when chronically stimulated with the α_1-AR agonist phenylephrine (Iaccarino et al. 2001). Furthermore, the mice demonstrate diminished sarco(endo)plasmic reticulum calcium ATPase (SERCA2) and endogenous α-MHC levels, and enhanced ANF and β-MHC, consistent with the phenotype (Lemire et al. 2001). These mice raise the important issue of integration site upon transgenesis and that of mouse background strain, both factors which can significantly affect the resultant mouse phenotype. However, further discussion of these issues is beyond the scope of this chapter.

2.2.2
α_{1b}-AR Knockout Animals

To further delineate the important role of the α_{1b}-AR in the cardiovascular system, a gene targeting approach has been used to develop α_{1b}-AR knockout mice (Cavalli et al. 1997). Homozygous knockout of the gene resulted in a 74% reduction of α_1-AR radioligand binding, indicating that indeed the α_{1b}-AR is the primary α_1-AR isoform expressed in the mouse heart. The homozygous mice also have significantly blunted blood pressure response to phenylephrine, and isolated aortic rings recapitulate this data, suggesting the important role of α_{1b}-ARs (as well as the previously documented role of α_{1a}-ARs) in mediating blood pressure elevation in response to α_1-AR stimulation in vivo (Cavalli et al. 1997).

2.3
Myocardial Gα_q Signaling and Inhibition

As described above, it has been well documented, particularly in vitro, that activation of Gα_q signaling through α_1-ARs, angiotensin II (AT1) and endothelin receptors can lead to hypertrophy, potentially through different mechanisms. To address the role of Gα_q in this process, two transgenic mouse models have been developed and tested: cardiac-targeted inhibition or overexpression of Gα_q. Experiments in our laboratory initially documented that in vivo activation of Gα_q is a final common trigger of ventricular hypertrophy in response to pressure overload (Akhter et al. 1997). In summary, a peptide inhibitor targeted to the receptor-Gα_q interface was expressed in transgenic mouse hearts using the α-MHC promoter. This inhibitory peptide is targeted to the carboxyl-terminal 54 amino acids of the Gα_q (GqI) that interacts with the activated Gα_q-coupled receptor. In vitro experiments documented that this peptide inhibitor can selectively block Gα_q-coupled signaling, and in vivo it significantly attenuated ventricular hypertrophy in response to transverse aortic constriction (TAC) and pressure overload (Akhter et al. 1997). This strategy demonstrates the importance of cardiac $G\alpha_q$ signaling in vivo in isolation of vascular effects.

Another approach to address $G\alpha_q$ signaling specifically in the heart was to derive mice with cardiac-targeted overexpression of $G\alpha_q$. The first description of these mice demonstrated that $G\alpha_q$ overexpression at more than fourfold resulted in hypertrophy, including increased heart weight and myocyte size, along with increased levels of canonical heart failure marker (fetal) genes, such as ANF, β-MHC, and α-skeletal actin, and decreased β-AR responsiveness (D'Angelo et al. 1997). Furthermore, they had decreased cardiac function at baseline and in response to dobutamine. At higher levels of $G\alpha_q$ overexpression, some of the mice developed biventricular failure, pulmonary congestion, and early mortality (D'Angelo et al. 1997). Further studies using similar mice have demonstrated that superimposition of hemodynamic stress via TAC (pressure overload) in the $G\alpha_q$ mice exacerbates hypertrophy to an eccentric hypertrophy that leads to rapid functional decompensation (Sakata et al. 1998). Finally, expression of a CAM $G\alpha_q$ led to enhanced hypertrophy and increased apoptosis, both in vitro and in vivo. In vivo, the CAM $G\alpha_q$ resulted in embryonic lethality due to cardiac hypertrophy followed by significant apoptosis, and overexpression of higher levels of the wild-type $G\alpha_q$ led to enhanced hypertrophy and apoptosis in adult mice (Adams et al. 1998). Transient expression of a CAM $G\alpha_q$ (and subsequent activation of PLC) also led to cardiac hypertrophy and dilation detectable long after the transient initial stimulus is no longer detectable, both at lower and higher levels of transient expression (Mende et al. 1998, 2001). These experiments further demonstrate the important role that $G\alpha_q$ may play in the development and progression of hypertrophy, and they also raise the important question of enhanced apoptosis in cardiomyopathy.

3
Mouse Models of GRK Expression and/or Activity

In addition to altering myocardial AR to directly study their effects on cardiac function, important information has been gathered using genetic manipulation of downstream signaling molecules, particularly the GRKs (Table 2). The majority of this work has focused on βARK1 (GRK2), which, as stated above, is the primary GRK family member expressed in the heart. Experiments have also been carried out to determine potential functional overlap of the activity of these GRKs in vivo.

3.1
Genetic Manipulation of Myocardial βARK1 Activity

The activity of βARK1 has been manipulated in transgenic mouse hearts using the α-MHC promoter to drive expression of either βARK1 or a cognate peptide inhibitor (βARKct), which acts by competing with endogenous βARK for $G\beta\gamma$-mediated translocation (Koch et al. 1995). Cardiac-targeted βARK1 overexpres-

Table 2 Transgenic models with altered expression of G protein-coupled receptor kinases (GRKs)

Gene	Model	Phenotype	Reference
βARK1	α-MHC	Decreased response to β-AR and angiotensin II AT1 receptor stimulation	Koch et al. 1995; Rockman et al. 1998
βARKct	α-MHC	Enhanced response to β-AR receptor stimulation	Koch et al. 1995
βARKct	Cardiac ankyrin repeat protein (CARP)	No expression in adult mouse unless given myocardial stress: enhanced response to β-AR stimulation following trans-aortic constriction (and thus βARKct expression), no effect on hypertrophy	Manning et al. 2000
βARKct/βARK1	α-MHC/ α-MHC	Restored cardiac function at baseline and in response to β-AR agonist stimulation	Akhter et al. 1999
βARK1$^{-/-}$	Targeted deletion	Embryonic lethal, cardiac malformation	Jaber et al. 1996
βARK1$^{+/-}$	Targeted deletion	Heterozygote of βARK1 targeted deletion, similar function to βARKct animals above	Rockman et al. 1998
βARK1$^{+/-}$ and βARKct	Mating of two lines	Augmentation of cardiac function beyond that of βARK1$^{+/-}$ or βARKct alone	Rockman et al. 1998
GRK5	α-MHC	Reduced response to β-AR stimulation, no effect on angiotensin II AT1 receptor stimulation	Rockman et al. 1996
GRK3	α-MHC	Reduced response to thrombin receptor stimulation, no change in response to β-AR or angiotensin II AT1 receptor stimulation	Iaccarino et al. 1998

sion or βARKct expression result in reciprocally regulated in vivo cardiac physiology. In transgenic mice overexpressing a myocardial targeted βARK1, cardiac β-AR response to isoproterenol was significantly decreased, as were cardiac responses to angiotensin II (Koch et al. 1995; Rockman et al. 1998). Conversely, transgenic mice expressing the βARKct demonstrated enhanced basal cardiac function and response to isoproterenol (Koch et al. 1995). Subsequently, direct evidence that the mechanism responsible for the phenotype in these mice was βARKct inhibition of $G_{\beta\gamma}$-mediated βARK1 activity was reported by our laboratory using hybrid transgenic mice, where βARKct expression in conjunction with βARK1 overexpression restored normal cardiac function (that had previously been attenuated as a result of βARK1 overexpression) (Akhter et al. 1999). The reciprocal nature of this physiology has been documented both in vivo, as well as in vitro with culture cardiac myocytes from βARK1 and βARKct mice (Koch et al. 1995; Korzick et al. 1997). These data indicate the critical role of βARK1 for the regulation of normal cardiac function.

Genetic ablation of βARK1 further demonstrated the important role of βARK1 in cardiovascular development, regulation, and function. Homozygous knockout was embryonic lethal resulting from severe cardiac malformations, with lethality varying from embryonic day 7.5 to 15, and abnormalities found in all mice from embryonic day 11 onward (Jaber et al. 1996). The cardiac malformation is representative of "thin myocardium syndrome" seen in the targeted inactivation/ablation of several transcription factors (Rossant 1996). Data from these knockout mice suggest an important role for βARK1 in normal heart development (Jaber et al. 1996). Heterozygous βARK1 mice have no developmental cardiac abnormalities and age normally (Rockman et al. 1998). Recently, we demonstrated that these heterozygous mice have cardiac function and contractility similar to the βARKct mice. Furthermore, heterozygous βARK mice with concurrent cardiac βARKct expression demonstrate even further augmentation of cardiac function (Rockman et al. 1998). These data suggest that regulation of cardiac βARK1 expression and activity are crucial in the maintenance of normal cardiac function, and have important implications in the setting of heart disease.

3.2
Cardiac Specificity of GRK3 and GRK5

In the family of six known GRKs, four appear to be expressed in the myocardium: GRK2, GRK3, GRK5, and GRK6. Study of these kinases in vitro suggested there was functional overlap of the myocardial GRKs for GPCR substrates. Although these kinases share substantial homology and functional overlap in vitro, studies of their function using transgenic mice has revealed numerous differences in vivo, including experiments described above for βARK1 and βARKct. Transgenic mice overexpressing GRK5 in myocardium were the first to demonstrate in vivo GRK substrate selectivity, in that GRK5 attenuated signaling in response to isoproterenol, but had no effect on cardiac signaling in response to angiotensin II (Rockman et al. 1996). Further evidence of in vivo GRK substrate selectivity in the heart was found in transgenic mice overexpressing GRK3, which demonstrated no effect on signaling following isoproterenol or angiotensin II (Iaccarino et al. 1998). However, the GRK3 mice had significantly decreased response to a thrombin receptor agonist as determined by analysis of MAPK signaling following thrombin receptor agonist, demonstrating that GRK3 was indeed active in these mice (Iaccarino et al. 1998). Desensitization of thrombin receptor signaling via GRK3 corroborated previous in vitro data (Ishii et al. 1994).

3.3
Delineation of GRK Specificity in Hybrid α_{1b}-AR Transgenic Mice

Subsequent studies of hybrid transgenic mice expressing cardiac targeted α_{1b}-AR in conjunction with each of the three cardiac GRKs further demonstrated in vivo GRK substrate selectivity (Eckhart et al. 2000). Signaling via the α_{1b}-AR as assessed by myocardial DAG content was attenuated by GRK3, but was unaffected by GRK2 or GRK5. Hypertrophy and ANF expression were induced by a CAM α_{1b}-AR; however, both of these measures were attenuated in mice overexpressing either GRK3 or GRK5, but not GRK2 (Eckhart et al. 2000). Thus, while GRK2 appears to be the primary GRK for in vivo regulation of β-AR signaling in the heart, the homologous GRK3 appears to be selectively involved in α_{1b}-AR and thrombin receptor regulation, while GRK5 activity toward these receptor substrates is mixed.

3.4
Role of βARK1 in Hypertrophy

Cardiac hypertrophy is an initially adaptive response to increased cardiac load (Grossman et al. 1975); however, it has become clear that sustained cardiac hypertrophy is maladaptive and can lead to decompensated heart failure (Lorell 1997). As described above, GPCR signaling, particularly through $G\alpha_q$, appears to play an obligatory role in the initiation of hypertrophy in response to increased cardiac load (Akhter et al. 1997). However, recent evidence also demonstrates functional abnormalities in β-AR signaling in cardiac models of hypertrophy (Bohm et al. 1994). Following TAC, β-ARs are desensitized concomitant with a threefold increase in βARK1 (Choi et al. 1997). Interestingly, it appears that the β-ARs and βARK1 are not playing a role in the initiation of hypertrophy per se, since TAC in βARKct mice resulted in similar levels of hypertrophy (Choi et al. 1997). However, the β-AR desensitization following TAC was completely reversed in the βARKct animals, suggesting that the β-AR desensitization was secondary to the development of hypertrophy.

To study the role of βARK1 inhibition in hypertrophy, βARKct was targeted to the hearts of mice under control of a promoter (cardiac ankyrin repeat protein, or CARP) that is normally functional only during development and during the first 2–3 weeks of life (Manning et al. 2000). These mice were viable and completely normal, and we documented loss of βARKct expression after 2–3 weeks of life (Manning et al. 2000). Interestingly, CARP expression, similar to other fetal genes such as ANF, can be activated in the adult heart by stress. Following TAC, an induction of βARKct expression in the heart was seen, and similar to findings in other mouse models of heart failure rescued by βARKct described below, resulted in enhanced β-AR responsiveness and reversal of β-AR desensitization during pressure overload (Manning et al. 2000). However, cardiac hypertrophy following TAC was not attenuated, confirming that βARK1 and GRK activity do not play a role in the cardiac hypertrophic response .

Levels of βARK1 expression have also been investigated in other mouse models of hypertrophy. Interestingly, βARK1 is not elevated in a $p21^{ras}$ overexpression mouse model of hypertrophy (Choi et al. 1997). Furthermore, although both isoproterenol and phenylephrine treatment result in similar levels of hypertrophy in mice, βARK1 expression was only enhanced following treatment with the β-AR agonist isoproterenol, data which was corroborated with in vitro experiments using isolated cardiac myocytes (Iaccarino et al. 1999). These data demonstrate that increased βARK1 expression and activity is not a generalized characteristic of all forms of hypertrophy. They also demonstrate that if hypertrophy is mediated through sympathetic activity, elevated βARK1 expression is mediated strictly through activation of β-ARs and not α_1-ARs, reinforcing the hypothesis that βARK1 is critically involved in the pathogenesis of β-AR dysfunction in heart failure. Importantly, chronic β-AR blockade with agents such as carvedilol, a β-AR antagonist used successfully in the treatment of heart failure (Packer et al. 1996; Packer et al. 2001), decreases the expression and activity of βARK1 in the hearts of mice (Iaccarino et al. 1998). Thus, decreased βARK1 and the resultant resensitization of cardiac β-AR signaling may represent a possible mechanism for the beneficial effect seen in β-AR blockade treatment of heart failure. To support this hypothesis, potential synergy of βARKct and β-AR blockade therapy in the treatment of heart failure has been recently demonstrated (Harding et al. 2001), and will be discussed in more detail below.

4
Mouse Models of Heart Failure and Rescue

An increasing number of genetic mouse models of heart failure and cardiomyopathy are being described, often discovered serendipitously following knockout or overexpression of a particular gene (Table 3). Often, these mouse models closely recapitulate many of the aspects of human heart failure, such as hypertrophy, dilation, and aberrations of the β-AR signaling system such as receptor down-regulation, desensitization, and enhanced βARK activity and expression (Rockman et al. 2002). These mouse models provide powerful tools to investigate the ability of other specific gene modulations to "rescue" the heart failure phenotype. For the sake of this chapter, we will only discuss those models of heart failure in which the phenotype has been alleviated by other genetic manipulations. These include: (1) knockout of the muscle LIM-domain protein (MLP), a cytoarchitectural protein and conserved regulator of myogenic differentiation (Arber et al. 1997); (2) cardiac-targeted overexpression of calsequestrin (CSQ), a high capacity calcium binding protein (Cho et al. 1999); (3) cardiac-targeted overexpression of a mutant form of the α-MHC gene (HCM) (mutation expressed is associated with human hypertrophic cardiomyopathy) (Freeman et al. 2001); and the cardiac-specific $G\alpha_q$ overexpressing mouse, as described above (D'Angelo et al. 1997).

4.1
Therapeutic Potential of βARKct

To determine the role that βARK and its inhibition may play in the development and potential rescue of any heart failure phenotype, cardiac targeted βARKct mice have been mated with the MLP, CSQ, and HCM mice (Rockman et al. 1998; Freeman et al. 2001; Harding et al. 2001). Strikingly, in each of these mouse models, cardiac-specific βARKct expression resulted in prevention of progressive deterioration in cardiac function, prevention of hypertrophy, improved ex-

Table 3 Transgenic models of heart failure and its phenotypic rescue

Gene	Model	Phenotype	Reference
Models of heart failure			
MLP$^{-/-}$	Targeted deletion	Hypertrophy followed by progressive dilated cardiomyopathy, disruption of cardiomyocyte cytoarchitecture	Arber et al. 1997
CSQ	α-MHC	Premature death (~14 weeks), hypertrophy, decreased calcium release, increased βARK1, decreased β-AR density and response to stimulation	Jones et al. 1998; Cho et al. 1999
Mutant α-MHC (HCM)	α-MHC	Hypertrophic cardiomyopathy, ncluding hypertrophy, dilation, and elevated βARK1 expression; phenotype much worse in males than females	Freeman et al. 1999
Gαq	α-MHC	Hypertrophy, enhanced heart rate, myocyte size, HF gene expression; depressed fractional shortening, at baseline and in response to dobutamine	D'Angelo et al. 1997
Models of phenotypic rescue of heart failure			
βARKct with MLP$^{-/-}$, CSQ, HCM	Mating of separate lines	Improvement of cardiac function, prevention of hypertrophy, enhanced exercise tolerance, restoration of β-AR signaling, reversal of HF marker gene expression, enhanced survival (synergistic enhancement of survival with β-AR blockade)	Rockman et al. 1998; Harding et al. 2001; Freeman et al. 2001
β2-AR with HCM	Mating of two lines	Initial enhancement of cardiac function, followed by decreased fractional shortening, and 50% early mortality at 8 months; no prevention of hypertrophy	Freeman et al. 2001
β2-AR with Gαq	Mating of two lines	*At low levels of β2-AR overexpression:* prevention of hypertrophy, restored baseline cardiac function, reversal of heart failure gene expression. *At high levels of β2-AR overexpression:* further deterioration of cardiac function.	Dorn et al. 1999
AC VI with Gαq	Mating of two lines	Improvement in cardiac function, enhanced response to β-AR stimulation	Roth et al. 1999
PLB$^{-/-}$ with MLP$^{-/-}$	Mating of two lines	Normalized cardiac function and heart failure marker gene expression, enhanced myocyte contractility	Minamisawa et al. 1999
PLB$^{-/-}$ with HCM	Mating of two lines	Normalization of heart failure marker gene expression with no phenotypic rescue of heart failure	Freeman et al. 2001

ercise tolerance, correction of aspects of classical β-AR receptor signaling dysfunction as described above, normalized expression of heart failure marker genes, and where assessed, markedly improved survival (Rockman et al. 1998; Freeman et al. 2001; Harding et al. 2001). Furthermore, combination of β-blocker therapy (metoprolol) and βARKct expression was synergistic in improving survival (Harding et al. 2001). These data are particularly interesting given the clinical promise of β-blocker therapy in individuals with chronic heart failure (CIBIS-II 1999; MERIT-HF 1999; Packer et al. 1996; Packer et al. 2001). Importantly, studies from our laboratory have also shown that chronic β-AR blockade by carvedilol decreases the expression of βARK1 in the heart and reduces cardiac GRK activity (Iaccarino et al. 1998). Furthermore, recent data from our laboratory suggest that βARKct not only rescues the cardiac phenotype of the MLP mice, but also appears to normalize the cardiac gene expression profile, as determined by oligonucleotide microarray analysis of gene expression (Blaxall et al. 2000). As an interesting aside, β_2-AR overexpression was unable to rescue the cardiac phenotype in MLP knockout mice (Rockman et al. 1998). In larger animal models of heart failure, adenoviral-mediated delivery of βARKct also enhances cardiac function, normalizes β-AR signaling, delays the hemodynamic onset of heart failure, and reverses the development of heart failure following myocardial infarction (Akhter et al. 1997; White et al. 2000; Shah et al. 2001).

Mechanism of action for the βARKct appears to be inhibition of the G$\beta\gamma$-βARK1 interaction; however, it is possible that βARKct may also affect other G$\beta\gamma$-dependent cell processes which may contribute to the extraordinary rescue of numerous animal models of heart failure by βARKct. Other documented biological interactions potentially inhibited by βARKct include PI3K (Naga Prasad et al. 2001) and $I_{K,ACh}$ channels (Clapham and Neer 1997); however, contribution of these effects, if any, to the salutary effects of βARKct remains to be determined. Moreover, since we have found that βARK1 can desensitize other GPCR systems in the heart (i.e., angiotensin II AT1), the therapeutic benefit of the βARKct may also involve enhanced signaling through other GPCRs. These non-β-AR effects of the βARKct are subjects of ongoing investigations.

4.2
Rescue of Mouse Models of Heart Failure by Other Genetic Alterations

Moderate overexpression of the β_2-AR in the cardiac-targeted Gα_q overexpressor mice rescued the hypertrophy and basal ventricular function, and normalized expression of ANF and α-skeletal actin (Dorn et al. 1999). Interestingly, high-level overexpression of the β_2-AR (>200-fold) in these mice resulted in a worsening of the cardiac phenotype (Dorn et al. 1999). Also of note is that cardiac overexpression of βARKct in the Gα_q mice had no effect on the phenotype (Dorn et al. 1999), which may be because there is no elevation of βARK1 in the Gα_q mice, contrary to what is found in the other mouse models of heart failure where βARKct has been tested, as described above. Finally, using the Gα_q mice, overexpression of myocardial AC VI also resulted in improved cardiac function and responsiveness to β-AR stimulation (Roth et al. 1999).

Regulation of intracellular calcium concentration remains an intensive focus of investigation, particularly with regard to the sarcoplasmic reticulum calcium regulatory protein SERCA2a and its inhibitor, phospholamban (PLB). Together, these proteins are involved in intracellular calcium release and reuptake in excitation–contraction coupling. Several studies have shown a disruption in the stoichiometry of these molecules in advanced heart failure. Recently, ablation of PLB was shown to normalize cardiac function and gene expression (reduced ANF, α-skeletal actin, β-MHC) in the MLP mouse model of dilated cardiomyopathy (Minamisawa et al. 1999). Furthermore, inhibition of the PLB/SERCA2a interaction by adenoviral-mediated delivery of a PLB point mutation resulted in enhanced myocyte contractility (Minamisawa et al. 1999).

Finally, seminal experiments were recently performed to assess the individual ability of β_2-AR, βARKct, and PLB to rescue the HCM mouse model of heart failure (Freeman et al. 2001). In these mice, β_2-AR overexpression initially showed enhanced cardiac function, however by 8 months, there was significant reduction of fractional shortening and nearly 50% mortality. In contrast, the PLB knockout and βARKct-expressing mice showed normal fractional shortening throughout the 12-month study period. Furthermore, neither β_2-AR overexpression or PLB ablation could abate the onset hypertrophy, whereas βARKct prevented the development of hypertrophy. PLB knockout mice showed the greatest reduction in β-MHC expression, whereas βARKct resulted in the greatest reduction of ANF and α-skeletal actin expression. In summary, these experiments indicate that βARKct is the most favorable chronic rescue of the HCM mice examined in this study (Freeman et al. 2001).

5
Conclusions

In summary, transgenic mice to date have allowed us to determine specific in vivo cardiac adrenergic signaling and kinase activity. These mice have also provided us with a valuable tool to determine viable targets for rescuing a heart failure phenotype. Their contribution to the development of novel therapies has been and will continue to be crucial to the investigation of cardiovascular disorders.

References

Adams, J. W., Sakata, Y., Davis, M. G., Sah, V. P., Wang, Y., Liggett, S. B., Chien, K. R., Brown, J. H., and Dorn, G. W., 2nd (1998). Enhanced Gαq signaling: a common pathway mediates cardiac hypertrophy and apoptotic heart failure. Proc Natl Acad Sci USA 95, 10140-5.

Ahlquist, R. (1948). A study of the adrenotropic receptors. Am J Physiol 153, 586-600.

Akhter, S. A., Milano, C. A., Shotwell, K. F., Cho, M. C., Rockman, H. A., Lefkowitz, R. J., and Koch, W. J. (1997). Transgenic mice with cardiac overexpression of α1B-adrenergic receptors. In vivo α1-adrenergic receptor-mediated regulation of β-adrenergic signaling. J Biol Chem 272, 21253-9.

Akhter, S. A., Skaer, C. A., Kypson, A. P., McDonald, P. H., Peppel, K. C., Glower, D. D., Lefkowitz, R. J., and Koch, W. J. (1997). Restoration of β-adrenergic signaling in failing cardiac ventricular myocytes via adenoviral-mediated gene transfer. Proc Natl Acad Sci USA 94, 12100-5.

Akhter, S. A., Eckhart, A. D., Rockman, H. A., Shotwell, K., Lefkowitz, R. J., and Koch, W. J. (1999). In vivo inhibition of elevated myocardial β-adrenergic receptor kinase activity in hybrid transgenic mice restores normal β- adrenergic signaling and function [see comments]. Circulation 100, 648-53.

Anderson, K. M., Eckhart, A. D., Willette, R. N., and Koch, W. J. (1999). The myocardial β-adrenergic system in spontaneously hypertensive heart failure (SHHF) rats. Hypertension 33, 402-7.

Anversa, P., Loud, A. V., Levicky, V., and Guideri, G. (1985). Left ventricular failure induced by myocardial infarction. I. Myocyte hypertrophy. Am J Physiol 248, H876-82.

Arber, S., Hunter, J. J., Ross, J., Jr., Hongo, M., Sansig, G., Borg, J., Perriard, J. C., Chien, K. R., and Caroni, P. (1997). MLP-deficient mice exhibit a disruption of cardiac cytoarchitectural organization, dilated cardiomyopathy, and heart failure. Cell 88, 393-403.

Bisognano, J. D., Weinberger, H. D., Bohlmeyer, T. J., Pende, A., Raynolds, M. V., Sastravaha, A., Roden, R., Asano, K., Blaxall, B. C., Wu, S. C., Communal, C., Singh, K., Colucci, W., Bristow, M. R., and Port, D. J. (2000). Myocardial-directed overexpression of the human β1-adrenergic receptor in transgenic mice. J Mol Cell Cardiol 32, 817-30.

Blaxall, B. C., Lefkowitz, R. J., and Koch, W. J. (2000). Differential patterns of gene expression in the development and rescue of mouse heart failure. Circulation 102, II-30.

Bohm, M., Moll, M., Schmid, B., Paul, M., Ganten, D., Castellano, M., and Erdmann, E. (1994). β-adrenergic neuroeffector mechanisms in cardiac hypertrophy of renin transgenic rats. Hypertension 24, 653-62.

Bristow, M. R., Ginsburg, R., Minobe, W., Cubicciotti, R. S., Sageman, W. S., Lurie, K., Billingham, M. E., Harrison, D. C., and Stinson, E. B. (1982). Decreased catecholamine sensitivity and β-adrenergic-receptor density in failing human hearts. N Engl J Med 307, 205-11.

Bristow, M. R., Hershberger, R. E., Port, J. D., Minobe, W., and Rasmussen, R. (1989). β1- and β2-adrenergic receptor-mediated adenylate cyclase stimulation in nonfailing and failing human ventricular myocardium. Mol Pharmacol 35, 295-303.

Bristow, M. R., Hershberger, R. E., Port, J. D., Gilbert, E. M., Sandoval, A., Rasmussen, R., Cates, A. E., and Feldman, A. M. (1990). β-adrenergic pathways in nonfailing and failing human ventricular myocardium. Circulation 82, I12-25.

Brodde, O. E. (1993). β-adrenoceptors in cardiac disease. Pharmacol Ther 60, 405-30.

Caron, M. G., and Lefkowitz, R. J. (1993). Catecholamine receptors: structure, function, and regulation. Recent Prog Horm Res 48, 277-90.

Cavalli, A., Lattion, A. L., Hummler, E., Nenniger, M., Pedrazzini, T., Aubert, J. F., Michel, M. C., Yang, M., Lembo, G., Vecchione, C., Mostardini, M., Schmidt, A., Beermann, F., and Cotecchia, S. (1997). Decreased blood pressure response in mice deficient of the α1b- adrenergic receptor. Proc Natl Acad Sci USA 94, 11589-94.

Cho, M. C., Rapacciuolo, A., Koch, W. J., Kobayashi, Y., Jones, L. R., and Rockman, H. A. (1999). Defective β-adrenergic receptor signaling precedes the development of dilated cardiomyopathy in transgenic mice with calsequestrin overexpression. J Biol Chem 274, 22251-6.

Choi, D. J., Koch, W. J., Hunter, J. J., and Rockman, H. A. (1997). Mechanism of β-adrenergic receptor desensitization in cardiac hypertrophy is increased β-adrenergic receptor kinase. J Biol Chem *272*, 17223-9.

Chruscinski, A. J., Rohrer, D. K., Schauble, E., Desai, K. H., Bernstein, D., and Kobilka, B. K. (1999). Targeted disruption of the β2 adrenergic receptor gene. J Biol Chem *274*, 16694-700.

Chuang, T. T., LeVine, H., 3rd, and De Blasi, A. (1995). Phosphorylation and activation of β-adrenergic receptor kinase by protein kinase C. J Biol Chem *270*, 18660-5.

CIBIS-II (1999). The Cardiac Insufficiency Bisoprolol Study II (CIBIS-II): a randomised trial. Lancet *353*, 9-13.

Clapham, D. E., and Neer, E. J. (1997). G protein beta gamma subunits. Annu Rev Pharmacol Toxicol *37*, 167-203.

Communal, C., Singh, K., Sawyer, D. B., and Colucci, W. S. (1999). Opposing effects of β1- and β2-adrenergic receptors on cardiac myocyte apoptosis : role of a pertussis toxin-sensitive G protein. Circulation *100*, 2210-2.

Daaka, Y., Luttrell, L. M., and Lefkowitz, R. J. (1997). Switching of the coupling of the β2-adrenergic receptor to different G proteins by protein kinase A. Nature *390*, 88-91.

D'Angelo, D. D., Sakata, Y., Lorenz, J. N., Boivin, G. P., Walsh, R. A., Liggett, S. B., and Dorn, G. W., 2nd (1997). Transgenic Gαq overexpression induces cardiac contractile failure in mice. Proc Natl Acad Sci USA *94*, 8121-6.

Dorn, G. W., 2nd, Tepe, N. M., Lorenz, J. N., Koch, W. J., and Liggett, S. B. (1999). Low- and high-level transgenic expression of β2-adrenergic receptors differentially affect cardiac hypertrophy and function in Gαq- overexpressing mice. Proc Natl Acad Sci USA *96*, 6400-5.

Dostal, D. E., and Baker, K. M. (1998). Angiotensin and endothelin: messengers that couple ventricular stretch to the Na+/H+ exchanger and cardiac hypertrophy. Circ Res *83*, 870-3.

Eckhart, A. D., Duncan, S. J., Penn, R. B., Benovic, J. L., Lefkowitz, R. J., and Koch, W. J. (2000). Hybrid transgenic mice reveal in vivo specificity of G protein-coupled receptor kinases in the heart. Circ Res *86*, 43-50.

Engelhardt, S., Hein, L., Wiesmann, F., and Lohse, M. J. (1999). Progressive hypertrophy and heart failure in β1-adrenergic receptor transgenic mice. Proc Natl Acad Sci USA *96*, 7059-64.

Exton, J. H. (1985). Mechanisms involved in α-adrenergic phenomena. Am J Physiol *248*, E633-47.

Feldman, A. M., Cates, A. E., Veazey, W. B., Hershberger, R. E., Bristow, M. R., Baughman, K. L., Baumgartner, W. A., and Van Dop, C. (1988). Increase of the 40,000-mol wt pertussis toxin substrate (G protein) in the failing human heart. J Clin Invest *82*, 189-97.

Freeman, K., Colon-Rivera, C., Olsson, M. C., Moore, R. L., Weinberger, H. D., Grupp, I. L., Vikstrom, K. L., Iaccarino, G., Koch, W. J., and Leinwand, L. A. (1999). Progression from hypertrophic to dilated cardiomyopathy in mice that express a mutant myosin transgene. Am J Physiol Heart Circ Physiol *280*, H151-9.

Freeman, K., Lerman, I., Kranias, E. G., Bohlmeyer, T., Bristow, M. R., Lefkowitz, R. J., Iaccarino, G., Koch, W. J., and Leinwand, L. A. (2001). Alterations in cardiac adrenergic signaling and calcium cycling differentially affect the progression of cardiomyopathy. J Clin Invest *107*, 967-74.

Gao, M., Ping, P., Post, S., Insel, P. A., Tang, R., and Hammond, H. K. (1998). Increased expression of adenylylcyclase type VI proportionately increases β-adrenergic receptor-stimulated production of cAMP in neonatal rat cardiac myocytes. Proc Natl Acad Sci USA *95*, 1038-43.

Gauthier, C., Tavernier, G., Charpentier, F., Langin, D., and Le Marec, H. (1996). Functional β3-adrenoceptor in the human heart. J Clin Invest *98*, 556-62.

Gidh-Jain, M., Huang, B., Jain, P., Gick, G., and El-Sherif, N. (1998). Alterations in cardiac gene expression during ventricular remodeling following experimental myocardial infarction. J Mol Cell Cardiol 30, 627-37.

Grossman, W., Jones, D., and McLaurin, L. P. (1975). Wall stress and patterns of hypertrophy in the human left ventricle. J Clin Invest 56, 56-64.

Grupp, I. L., Lorenz, J. N., Walsh, R. A., Boivin, G. P., and Rindt, H. (1998). Overexpression of α1B-adrenergic receptor induces left ventricular dysfunction in the absence of hypertrophy. Am J Physiol 275, H1338-50.

Harding, S. E., MacLeod, K. T., Davies, C. H., Wynne, D. G., and Poole-Wilson, P. A. (1995). Abnormalities of the myocytes in ischaemic cardiomyopathy. Eur Heart J 16 Suppl I, 74-81.

Harding, V. B., Jones, L. R., Lefkowitz, R. J., Koch, W. J., and Rockman, H. A. (2001). Cardiac βARK1 inhibition prolongs survival and augments β–blocker therapy in a mouse model of severe heart failure. Proc Natl Acad Sci USA 98, 5809-14.

Harrison, S. N., Autelitano, D. J., Wang, B. H., Milano, C., Du, X. J., and Woodcock, E. A. (1998). Reduced reperfusion-induced Ins(1,4,5)P3 generation and arrhythmias in hearts expressing constitutively active α1B-adrenergic receptors. Circ Res 83, 1232-40.

Hoffman, B. B., and Lefkowitz, R. J. (1996). . In Goodman and Gilman's The Pharmacological Basis of Therapeutics, J. G. Hardman, A. G. Gilman and L. E. Limbird, eds. (New York: McGraw-Hill), pp. 199-248.

Huang, W. Y., Aramburu, J., Douglas, P. S., and Izumo, S. (2000). Transgenic expression of green fluorescence protein can cause dilated cardiomyopathy. Nat Med 6, 482-3.

Iaccarino, G., Dolber, P. C., Lefkowitz, R. J., and Koch, W. J. (1999). β-adrenergic receptor kinase-1 levels in catecholamine-induced myocardial hypertrophy: regulation by β- but not α1-adrenergic stimulation. Hypertension 33, 396-401.

Iaccarino, G., Keys, J. R., Rapacciuolo, A., Shotwell, K. F., Lefkowitz, R. J., Rockman, H. A., and Koch, W. J. (2001). Regulation of myocardial βARK1 expression in catecholamine-induced cardiac hypertrophy in transgenic mice overexpressing α1B- adrenergic receptors. J Am Coll Cardiol 38, 534-40.

Iaccarino, G., Rockman, H. A., Shotwell, K. F., Tomhave, E. D., and Koch, W. J. (1998). Myocardial overexpression of GRK3 in transgenic mice: evidence for in vivo selectivity of GRKs. Am J Physiol 275, H1298-306.

Iaccarino, G., Tomhave, E. D., Lefkowitz, R. J., and Koch, W. J. (1998). Reciprocal in vivo regulation of myocardial G protein-coupled receptor kinase expression by β-adrenergic receptor stimulation and blockade. Circulation 98, 1783-9.

Inglese, J., Freedman, N. J., Koch, W. J., and Lefkowitz, R. J. (1993). Structure and mechanism of the G protein-coupled receptor kinases. J Biol Chem 268, 23735-8.

Ishii, K., Chen, J., Ishii, M., Koch, W. J., Freedman, N. J., Lefkowitz, R. J., and Coughlin, S. R. (1994). Inhibition of thrombin receptor signaling by a G-protein coupled receptor kinase. Functional specificity among G-protein coupled receptor kinases. J Biol Chem 269, 1125-30.

Iwase, M., Bishop, S. P., Uechi, M., Vatner, D. E., Shannon, R. P., Kudej, R. K., Wight, D. C., Wagner, T. E., Ishikawa, Y., Homcy, C. J., and Vatner, S. F. (1996). Adverse effects of chronic endogenous sympathetic drive induced by cardiac Gsα overexpression. Circ Res 78, 517-24.

Iwase, M., Uechi, M., Vatner, D. E., Asai, K., Shannon, R. P., Kudej, R. K., Wagner, T. E., Wight, D. C., Patrick, T. A., Ishikawa, Y., Homcy, C. J., and Vatner, S. F. (1997). Cardiomyopathy induced by cardiac Gsα overexpression. Am J Physiol 272, H585-9.

Jaber, M., Koch, W. J., Rockman, H., Smith, B., Bond, R. A., Sulik, K. K., Ross, J., Jr., Lefkowitz, R. J., Caron, M. G., and Giros, B. (1996). Essential role of β-adrenergic receptor kinase 1 in cardiac development and function. Proc Natl Acad Sci USA 93, 12974-9.

Ju, H., Zhao, S., Tappia, P. S., Panagia, V., and Dixon, I. M. (1998). Expression of Gqα and PLC-β in scar and border tissue in heart failure due to myocardial infarction. Circulation 97, 892-9.

Knowlton, K. U., Michel, M. C., Itani, M., Shubeita, H. E., Ishihara, K., Brown, J. H., and Chien, K. R. (1993). The α1A-adrenergic receptor subtype mediates biochemical, molecular, and morphologic features of cultured myocardial cell hypertrophy. J Biol Chem 268, 15374-80.

Koch, W. J., Inglese, J., Stone, W. C., and Lefkowitz, R. J. (1993). The binding site for the βγ subunits of heterotrimeric G proteins on the β-adrenergic receptor kinase. J Biol Chem 268, 8256-60.

Koch, W. J., Rockman, H. A., Samama, P., Hamilton, R. A., Bond, R. A., Milano, C. A., and Lefkowitz, R. J. (1995). Cardiac function in mice overexpressing the β-adrenergic receptor kinase or a βARK inhibitor. Science 268, 1350-3.

Koch, W. J., Lefkowitz, R. J., and Rockman, H. A. (2000). Functional consequences of altering myocardial adrenergic receptor signaling. Annu Rev Physiol 62, 237-60.

Korzick, D. H., Xiao, R. P., Ziman, B. D., Koch, W. J., Lefkowitz, R. J., and Lakatta, E. G. (1997). Transgenic manipulation of β-adrenergic receptor kinase modifies cardiac myocyte contraction to norepinephrine. Am J Physiol 272, H590-6.

Laporte, S. A., Oakley, R. H., Holt, J. A., Barak, L. S., and Caron, M. G. (2000). The interaction of β-arrestin with the AP-2 adaptor is required for the clustering of β2-adrenergic receptor into clathrin-coated pits. J Biol Chem 275, 23120-6.

Lefkowitz, R. J. (1998). G protein-coupled receptors. III. New roles for receptor kinases and β-arrestins in receptor signaling and desensitization. J Biol Chem 273, 18677-80.

Lemire, I., Allen, B. G., Rindt, H., and Hebert, T. E. (1998). Cardiac-specific overexpression of α1BAR regulates βAR activity via molecular crosstalk. J Mol Cell Cardiol 30, 1827-39.

Lemire, I., Ducharme, A., Tardif, J. C., Poulin, F., Jones, L. R., Allen, B. G., Hebert, T. E., and Rindt, H. (2001). Cardiac-directed overexpression of wild-type α1B-adrenergic receptor induces dilated cardiomyopathy. Am J Physiol Heart Circ Physiol 281, H931-8.

Liggett, S. B., Tepe, N. M., Lorenz, J. N., Canning, A. M., Jantz, T. D., Mitarai, S., Yatani, A., and Dorn, G. W., 2nd (2000). Early and delayed consequences of β2-adrenergic receptor overexpression in mouse hearts: critical role for expression level. Circulation 101, 1707-14.

Lorell, B. H. (1997). Transition from hypertrophy to failure. Circulation 96, 3824-7.

Manning, B. S., Shotwell, K., Mao, L., Rockman, H. A., and Koch, W. J. (2000). Physiological induction of a β-adrenergic receptor kinase inhibitor transgene preserves β-adrenergic responsiveness in pressure-overload cardiac hypertrophy. Circulation 102, 2751-7.

Maurice, J. P., Shah, A. S., Kypson, A. P., Hata, J. A., White, D. C., Glower, D. D., and Koch, W. J. (1999). Molecular β-adrenergic signaling abnormalities in failing rabbit hearts after infarction. Am J Physiol 276, H1853-60.

Mende, U., Kagen, A., Cohen, A., Aramburu, J., Schoen, F. J., and Neer, E. J. (1998). Transient cardiac expression of constitutively active Gαq leads to hypertrophy and dilated cardiomyopathy by calcineurin-dependent and independent pathways. Proc Natl Acad Sci USA 95, 13893-8.

Mende, U., Semsarian, C., Martins, D. C., Kagen, A., Duffy, C., Schoen, F. J., and Neer, E. J. (2001). Dilated cardiomyopathy in two transgenic mouse lines expressing activated G protein αq: lack of correlation between phospholipase C activation and the phenotype. J Mol Cell Cardiol 33, 1477-91.

MERIT-HF (1999). Effect of metoprolol CR/XL in chronic heart failure: Metoprolol CR/XL Randomised Intervention Trial in Congestive Heart Failure (MERIT-HF). Lancet 353, 2001-7.

Milano, C. A., Allen, L. F., Rockman, H. A., Dolber, P. C., McMinn, T. R., Chien, K. R., Johnson, T. D., Bond, R. A., and Lefkowitz, R. J. (1994). Enhanced myocardial function in transgenic mice overexpressing the β2-adrenergic receptor. Science *264*, 582-6.

Milano, C. A., Dolber, P. C., Rockman, H. A., Bond, R. A., Venable, M. E., Allen, L. F., and Lefkowitz, R. J. (1994). Myocardial expression of a constitutively active α1B-adrenergic receptor in transgenic mice induces cardiac hypertrophy. Proc Natl Acad Sci USA *91*, 10109-13.

Minamisawa, S., Hoshijima, M., Chu, G., Ward, C. A., Frank, K., Gu, Y., Martone, M. E., Wang, Y., Ross, J., Jr., Kranias, E. G., Giles, W. R., and Chien, K. R. (1999). Chronic phospholamban-sarcoplasmic reticulum calcium ATPase interaction is the critical calcium cycling defect in dilated cardiomyopathy. Cell *99*, 313-22.

Naga Prasad, S. V., Barak, L. S., Rapacciuolo, A., Caron, M. G., and Rockman, H. A. (2001). Agonist-dependent recruitment of phosphoinositide 3-kinase to the membrane by β-adrenergic receptor kinase 1. A role in receptor sequestration. J Biol Chem *276*, 18953-9.

Ostrom, R. S., Post, S. R., and Insel, P. A. (2000). Stoichiometry and compartmentation in G protein-coupled receptor signaling: implications for therapeutic interventions involving G(s). J Pharmacol Exp Ther *294*, 407-12.

Packer, M., Bristow, M. R., Cohn, J. N., Colucci, W. S., Fowler, M. B., Gilbert, E. M., and Shusterman, N. H. (1996). The effect of carvedilol on morbidity and mortality in patients with chronic heart failure. U.S. Carvedilol Heart Failure Study Group. N Engl J Med *334*, 1349-55.

Packer, M., Coats, A. J., Fowler, M. B., Katus, H. A., Krum, H., Mohacsi, P., Rouleau, J. L., Tendera, M., Castaigne, A., Roecker, E. B., Schultz, M. K., and DeMets, D. L. (2001). Effect of carvedilol on survival in severe chronic heart failure. N Engl J Med *344*, 1651-8.

Ping, P., Anzai, T., Gao, M., and Hammond, H. K. (1997). Adenylyl cyclase and G protein receptor kinase expression during development of heart failure. Am J Physiol *273*, H707-17.

Pitcher, J. A., Inglese, J., Higgins, J. B., Arriza, J. L., Casey, P. J., Kim, C., Benovic, J. L., Kwatra, M. M., Caron, M. G., and Lefkowitz, R. J. (1992). Role of beta gamma subunits of G proteins in targeting the β-adrenergic receptor kinase to membrane-bound receptors. Science *257*, 1264-7.

Pitcher, J. A., Freedman, N. J., and Lefkowitz, R. J. (1998). G protein-coupled receptor kinases. Annu Rev Biochem *67*, 653-92.

Redfern, C. H., Degtyarev, M. Y., Kwa, A. T., Salomonis, N., Cotte, N., Nanevicz, T., Fidelman, N., Desai, K., Vranizan, K., Lee, E. K., Coward, P., Shah, N., Warrington, J. A., Fishman, G. I., Bernstein, D., Baker, A. J., and Conklin, B. R. (2000). Conditional expression of a Gi-coupled receptor causes ventricular conduction delay and a lethal cardiomyopathy. Proc Natl Acad Sci USA *97*, 4826-31.

Rockman, H. A., Choi, D. J., Rahman, N. U., Akhter, S. A., Lefkowitz, R. J., and Koch, W. J. (1996). Receptor-specific in vivo desensitization by the G protein-coupled receptor kinase-5 in transgenic mice. Proc Natl Acad Sci USA *93*, 9954-9.

Rockman, H. A., Hamilton, R. A., Jones, L. R., Milano, C. A., Mao, L., and Lefkowitz, R. J. (1996). Enhanced myocardial relaxation in vivo in transgenic mice overexpressing the β2-adrenergic receptor is associated with reduced phospholamban protein. J Clin Invest *97*, 1618-23.

Rockman, H. A., Chien, K. R., Choi, D. J., Iaccarino, G., Hunter, J. J., Ross, J., Jr., Lefkowitz, R. J., and Koch, W. J. (1998). Expression of a β-adrenergic receptor kinase 1 inhibitor prevents the development of myocardial failure in gene-targeted mice. Proc Natl Acad Sci USA *95*, 7000-5.

Rockman, H. A., Choi, D. J., Akhter, S. A., Jaber, M., Giros, B., Lefkowitz, R. J., Caron, M. G., and Koch, W. J. (1998). Control of myocardial contractile function by the level of β- adrenergic receptor kinase 1 in gene-targeted mice. J Biol Chem 273, 18180-4.

Rockman, H. A., Koch, W. J., and Lefkowitz, R. J. (2002). Seven-transmembrane-spanning receptors and heart function. Nature 415, 206-12.

Rohrer, D. K. (1998). Physiological consequences of β-adrenergic receptor disruption. J Mol Med 76, 764-72.

Rossant, J. (1996). Mouse mutants and cardiac development: new molecular insights into cardiogenesis. Circ Res 78, 349-53.

Roth, D. M., Gao, M. H., Lai, N. C., Drumm, J., Dalton, N., Zhou, J. Y., Zhu, J., Entrikin, D., and Hammond, H. K. (1999). Cardiac-directed adenylyl cyclase expression improves heart function in murine cardiomyopathy. Circulation 99, 3099-102.

Sakata, Y., Hoit, B. D., Liggett, S. B., Walsh, R. A., and Dorn, G. W., 2nd (1998). Decompensation of pressure-overload hypertrophy in Gαq- overexpressing mice. Circulation 97, 1488-95.

Shah, A. S., White, D. C., Emani, S., Kypson, A. P., Lilly, R. E., Wilson, K., Glower, D. D., Lefkowitz, R. J., and Koch, W. J. (2001). In vivo ventricular gene delivery of a β-adrenergic receptor kinase inhibitor to the failing heart reverses cardiac dysfunction. Circulation 103, 1311-6.

Simpson, P. (1983). Norepinephrine-stimulated hypertrophy of cultured rat myocardial cells is an α1 adrenergic response. J Clin Invest 72, 732-8.

Subramaniam, A., Jones, W. K., Gulick, J., Wert, S., Neumann, J., and Robbins, J. (1991). Tissue-specific regulation of the alpha-myosin heavy chain gene promoter in transgenic mice. J Biol Chem 266, 24613-20.

Sugden, P. H. (2001). Signalling pathways in cardiac myocyte hypertrophy. Ann Med 33, 611-22.

Tepe, N. M., Lorenz, J. N., Yatani, A., Dash, R., Kranias, E. G., Dorn, G. W., 2nd, and Liggett, S. B. (1999). Altering the receptor-effector ratio by transgenic overexpression of type V adenylyl cyclase: enhanced basal catalytic activity and function without increased cardiomyocyte β-adrenergic signalling. Biochemistry 38, 16706-13.

Towbin, J. A., and Bowles, N. E. (2002). The failing heart. Nature 415, 227-33.

Ungerer, M., Bohm, M., Elce, J. S., Erdmann, E., and Lohse, M. J. (1993). Altered expression of β-adrenergic receptor kinase and β1- adrenergic receptors in the failing human heart [see comments]. Circulation 87, 454-63.

Ungerer, M., Parruti, G., Bohm, M., Puzicha, M., DeBlasi, A., Erdmann, E., and Lohse, M. J. (1994). Expression of β-arrestins and β-adrenergic receptor kinases in the failing human heart. Circ Res 74, 206-13.

Ungerer, M., Kessebohm, K., Kronsbein, K., Lohse, M. J., and Richardt, G. (1996). Activation of β-adrenergic receptor kinase during myocardial ischemia. Circ Res 79, 455-60.

White, D. C., Hata, J. A., Shah, A. S., Glower, D. D., Lefkowitz, R. J., and Koch, W. J. (2000). Preservation of myocardial β-adrenergic receptor signaling delays the development of heart failure after myocardial infarction. Proc Natl Acad Sci USA 97, 5428-33.

Xiao, R. P., Avdonin, P., Zhou, Y. Y., Cheng, H., Akhter, S. A., Eschenhagen, T., Lefkowitz, R. J., Koch, W. J., and Lakatta, E. G. (1999). Coupling of β2-adrenoceptor to Gi proteins and its physiological relevance in murine cardiac myocytes. Circ Res 84, 43-52.

Zhu, W. Z., Zheng, M., Koch, W. J., Lefkowitz, R. J., Kobilka, B. K., and Xiao, R. P. (2001). Dual modulation of cell survival and cell death by β2-adrenergic signaling in adult mouse cardiac myocytes. Proc Natl Acad Sci USA 98, 1607-12.

Renin-Angiotensin System/Blood Pressure Control

M. Bader

Max-Delbrück-Center for Molecular Medicine (MDC),
Robert-Rössle-Strasse 10, 13092 Berlin-Buch, Germany
e-mail: mbader@mdc-berlin.de

Abstract The control of blood pressure is achieved by a complex interplay of several hormonal systems acting either in an endocrine manner or locally in tissues such as brain, vessels, and kidney in a paracrine or autocrine manner. Because of the complexity of the cardiovascular system and its regulation, the study of these processes has been by and large limited to the whole organismic level. Thus, transgenic technology has been of the highest importance in recent years to assist in the discovery of the role of specific gene products in cardiovascular regulation . This review summarizes such findings about peptide systems involved in blood pressure control with a major emphasis on the renin–angiotensin system, which cardiovascularly may be the most relevant system. Also, transgenic animals with targeted genetic alterations in the synthesis or action of kinins, endothelins, natriuretic peptides, as well as adrenomedullin and the calcitonin gene-related peptide (CGRP) are described. For the renin–angiotensin system, all components have been deleted by gene targeting. Whenever angiotensin II synthesis or action was completely blunted, such as by the deletion of renin, angiotensinogen, angiotensin-converting enzyme, or the angiotensin II AT1 receptor, the mice showed very low blood pressure, kidney dysmorphology, and a high mortality. In contrast, most transgenic rat or mouse models overexpressing renin or angiotensinogen became hypertensive. Transgenic rats with reduced angiotensinogen in the brain are hypotensive and accordingly mice with enhanced angiotensin II generation in the central nervous system exhibited increased blood pressure, supporting an important role of the central renin–angiotensin system in cardiovascular control. Mice lacking endothelins or its receptors revealed functions of these peptides going beyond blood pressure regulation and implicating the endothelin system in the development of neural crest-derived cells. Novel transgenic technologies such as inducible conditional gene targeting will help to further this knowledge and to design new therapeutic strategies.

Keywords Renin · Angiotensins · Kinins · Endothelins · Natriuretic peptides · Adrenomedullin · CGRP · Transgenic · Gene targeting · Animal models

1
Introduction

The control of blood pressure is achieved by a complex interplay of several hormonal systems acting either in an endocrine manner or locally in tissues such as brain, vessels, and kidney in a paracrine or autocrine manner. Because of the complexity of the cardiovascular system and its regulation, the study of these processes has been by and large limited to the whole organismic level. Thus, transgenic technology has been of highest importance in recent years for discovering the role of specific gene products in cardiovascular regulation (Bader et al. 2000; Sigmund 2001; Doan et al. 2001). The expression of numerous genes has been altered by genetic manipulation in rats and mice. Rat would be the preferable model for such studies since this species has been used for decades in the physiological analysis of the cardiovascular system. Numerous experimental and genetic models for cardiovascular diseases such as hypertension exist in rat, in contrast to mouse, in which important experimental tools have just been developed. However, despite considerable efforts, it is not yet possible to establish gene targeting technology in rat. Therefore, mouse has also become the most frequently used model for transgenic studies of blood pressure control. Nevertheless, transgenic rats are among the models which have had the greatest impact on our understanding of these physiological processes (Mullins et al. 1990; Ganten et al. 1992; Schinke et al. 1996).

The renin–angiotensin system (RAS) is only one of numerous hormonal systems involved in blood pressure regulation. Some other very important systems are described in other chapters of this book, including the adrenergic and cholinergic system, nitric oxide, and steroid hormones. This review will focus on peptide systems involved in blood pressure control with a major emphasis on the renin–angiotensin system, which may cardiovascularly be the most relevant system. Also summarized are the findings obtained in transgenic animals with targeted genetic alterations in the synthesis or action of kinins, endothelins, natriuretic peptides, as well as adrenomedullin and the calcitonin gene-related peptide (CGRP) (Table 1).

2
Renin–Angiotensin System

The RAS generates peptide hormones with considerable impact on cardiovascular regulation and with great etiologic and therapeutic significance for cardiovascular diseases. Generation of active angiotensin peptides is achieved by a small number of proteins all of which have been overexpressed, as well as inactivated, by transgenic technology (Fig. 1). Renin was discovered by Tigerstedt and Bergman more than 100 years ago (Tigerstedt and Bergman 1898) and is generated by juxtaglomerular cells of the kidney. It cleaves its only substrate angiotensinogen, synthesized mainly in the liver, resulting in the liberation of the inactive decapeptide angiotensin I. The active peptide angiotensin II is generated by proteolytic ablation of the two carboxyterminal amino acids of angiotensin I primarily by the endothelium-associated angiotensin-converting enzyme (ACE). Angiotensin II elicits its effects via two different receptor subtypes, AT1 and AT2. AT1 is expressed in all main target organs such as the kidney, heart, brain, adrenal cortex, and vessel wall and represents the receptor responsible for most actions of the peptide. AT2 is mainly restricted to embryogenesis, certain brain regions, and the adrenal medulla, but it is also present at low levels in the heart, kidney, and vessel wall. In addition to the circulating RAS, angiotensin generation is observed in single organs such as the brain, heart, kidney, and adrenal gland from locally expressed or plasma-derived precursors. The physiological relevance of these tissue renin–angiotensin systems represent a major focus of transgenic models.

2.1
General Overexpression or Depletion

2.1.1
Angiotensinogen

The first transgenic model with alteration in angiotensinogen expression was a mouse overexpressing the rat gene under the control of the mouse metallothionein promoter (Ohkubo et al. 1990). Although exhibiting high levels of circulating angiotensin II, these mice were normotensive. Subsequently, the angiotensinogen genes of rats (Kimura et al. 1992) and humans (Takahashi et al. 1991; Ganten et al. 1992; Yang et al. 1994) have been expressed in transgenic mice (Takahashi et al. 1991; Yang et al. 1994) and rats (Ganten et al. 1992) under the

Table 1 Genetically modified animal models in blood pressure research. The species of the transgenic animal is noted last, e.g., (rat), if other animals than mice were examined

Altered component	Phenotype	Reference(s)
Renin-angiotensin system		
Loss of function		
Angiotensinogen	Hypotension, kidney pathomorphology and dysfunction, low survival rate	Tanimoto et al. 1994; Kim et al. 1995; Niimura et al. 1995
Angiotensinogen, brain-specific antisense inhibition (rat)	Hypotension, diabetes insipidus, altered circadian rhythm regulation of blood pressure	Schinke et al. 1999; Baltatu et al. 2001
Angiotensinogen, liver- and brain-specific rescue	Hypertension, normal kidney morphology	Kang et al. 2002
Angiotensinogen, fat-specific rescue	Normotension, normal kidney morphology, increased fat mass	Massiera et al. 2001
Angiotensinogen, kidney-specific rescue	Hypotension, kidney pathomorphology and dysfunction, low survival rate	Ding et al. 2001
Ren-2	No cardiovascular effects	Sharp et al. 1996
Ren-1[d]	Hypotension in females	Bertaux et al. 1997; Clark et al. 1997; Pentz et al. 2001
Ren-1[c]	Hypotension, kidney pathomorphology and dysfunction	Yanai et al. 2000
ACE	Hypotension, kidney pathomorphology and dysfunction, male sterility	Krege et al. 1995, 1997; Carpenter et al. 1996
ACE, membrane-bound form	Hypotension, kidney pathomorphology and dysfunction	Esther et al. 1997
ACE, ubiquitous rescue by testis-ACE	No cardiovascular effects, fertile	Cole et al. 2002; Kessler et al. 2002
ACE, testis-specific rescue by testis-ACE	Hypotension, kidney pathomorphology and dysfunction, fertile	Ramaraj et al. 1998
ACE, testis-specific rescue by endothelial ACE	Hypotension, kidney pathomorphology and dysfunction, male sterility	Kessler et al. 2000
AT1A	Hypotension, protection from renal and cardiac damage	Ito et al. 1995; Matsusaka et al. 1995; Sugaya et al. 1995
AT1B	No cardiovascular effects	Chen et al. 1997
AT1A/AT1B	Hypotension, kidney pathomorphology and dysfunction	Oliverio et al. 1998; Tsuchida et al. 1998
AT2	Higher sensitivity to angiotensin-II pressor effect	Hein et al. 1995; Ichiki et al. 1995
mas protooncogene	Altered variability of cardiovascular parameters	Walther et al. 1998, 2000

Table 1 (continued)

Altered component	Phenotype	Reference(s)
Gain of function		
Angiotensinogen	Hypertension, end-organ damage	Kimura et al. 1992; Kang et al. 2002
Angiotensinogen, kidney-specific promoter	hypertension	Davisson et al. 1999
Angiotensinogen, heart-specific promoter	Cardiac hypertrophy	Mazzolai et al. 1998, 2000
Angiotensinogen, fat-specific promoter	Hypertension, increased fat mass	Massiera et al. 2001
Ren-2 (rat)	Hypertension, end-organ damage	Mullins et al. 1990
Ren-2 prorenin, liver-specific promoter (rat)	Hypertension, end-organ damage	Veniant et al. 1996
Ren-2, inducible promoter (rat)	Inducible hypertension and vascular injury	Kantachuvesiri et al. 2001
Human renin/angiotensinogen (rat)	Hypertension, end-organ damage	Ganten et al. 1992; Luft et al. 1999
Human renin/angiotensinogen	Hypertension	Fukamizu et al. 1993; Merrill et al. 1996; Sinn et al. 1999
Human renin/angiotensinogen, brain-specific promoter	Hypertension, increased salt appetite	Morimoto et al. 2001, 2002
ACE, heart-specific promoter (rat)	Exaggerated heart hypertrophy induction	Tian et al. 1996
Chymase, inducible, vessel-specific promoter	Hypertension, smooth muscle proliferation	Ju et al. 2001
AT1, heart-specific promoter	Cardiac hypertrophy	Hein et al. 1997; Paradis et al. 2000
AT1, heart-specific promoter (rat)	Exaggerated heart hypertrophy induction	Hoffmann et al. 2001
AT1, brain-specific promoter	No cardiovascular effects	Lazartigues et al. 2002
AT2, heart-specific promoter	Lower sensitivity to angiotensin-II pressor effect	Masaki et al. 1998
AT2, vessel-specific promoter	Normotension, no hypertensive effect of angiotensin II	Tsutsumi et al. 1999
Angiotensin-II liberating protein, heart-specific promoter	Normotension, normal cardiac size, cardiac fibrosis	van Kats et al. 2001
Kallikrein-kinin system		
Loss of function		
Tissue kallikrein	Dilated cardiomyopathy	Meneton et al. 2001
B1	Attenuation of hypotension after endotoxin-induced shock, reduced angiogenesis	Pesquero et al. 2000; Emanueli et al. 2002

Table 1 (continued)

Altered component	Phenotype	Reference(s)
B2	Salt-sensitive hypertension (?), dilated cardiomyopathy	Borkowski et al. 1995; Alfie et al. 1996; Madeddu et al. 1997; Cervenka et al. 1999; Milia et al. 2001
Gain of function		
Tissue allikrein	Hypotension	Wang et al. 1994
Tissue kallikrein (rat)	Hypotension, cardioprotection	Pinto et al. 2000; Silva et al. 2000
B2	Hypotension	Wang et al. 1997
Endothelin-system		
Loss of function		
ET-1	+/-: Elevated blood pressure; -/-: lethality and malformations of craniofacial tissues	Kurihara et al. 1994
ET-3	Megacolon, early death	Baynash et al. 1994
ET_A	Cranial and cardiac neural crest defects	Clouthier et al. 1998
ET_B	Megacolon, early death	Baynash et al. 1994; Hosoda et al. 1994
ET_B, nervous system rescue	Salt-sensitive hypertension	Gariepy et al. 2000
ET_A/ET_B	Lethality (cardiac failure): $ET_A^{+/-}/ET_B^{-/-}$: 20%; $ET_A^{-/-}/ET_B^{+/-}$: 33%; $ET_A^{-/-}/ET_B^{-/-}$: 100%	Yanagisawa et al. 1998
ECE-1	Craniofacial and cardiac abnormalities	Yanagisawa et al. 1998
Gain of function		
ET-1	Kidney damage, normotension	Hocher et al. 1997
ET-2 (rat)	Kidney damage, normotension	Hocher et al. 1996
Natriuretic peptides		
Loss of function		
ANP	Salt-sensitive hypertension	John et al. 1995
CNP	Skeletal abnormalities, dwarfism	Chusho et al. 2001
NPR-A	Hypertension	Lopez et al. 1995; Oliver et al. 1998
NPR-A, smooth-muscle-specific	Normotension, blunted ANP response	Holtwick et al. 2002

Table 1 (continued)

Altered component	Phenotype	Reference(s)
NPR-C	Hypotension	Matsukawa et al. 1999
Gain of function		
ANP	Hypotension	Steinhelper et al. 1990
BNP	Hypotension	Ogawa et al. 1994
Others		
Loss of function		
NEP	Hypertension	Lu et al. 1997
CGRP	Hypertension (?)	Lu et al. 1999; Gangula et al. 2000; Oh-hashi et al. 2001
Adrenomedullin	Embryonic lethality; +/−: hypertension	Shindo et al. 2001
Gain of function		
Adrenomedullin, endothelial	Hypotension	Shindo et al. 2000

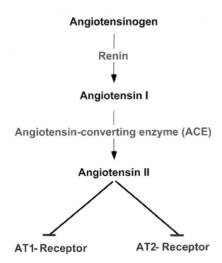

Fig. 1 The renin–angiotensin system. For description see text

control of their own regulatory sequences. The only reported transgenic mouse among these with a cardiovascular phenotype also carried the rat angiotensinogen gene, but this time under the control of its own regulatory sequences (Kimura et al. 1992). These animals developed high blood pressure and the typical signs of end-organ damage also observed in human hypertensives, such as cardiac hypertrophy and renal fibrosis (Kang et al. 2002).

All rodents transgenic for human angiotensinogen remained normotensive even though some of them exhibit very high levels of the human protein in plasma (Takahashi et al. 1991; Yang et al. 1994; Ganten et al. 1992). The same was true for all animals carrying the human reningene as transgene (Fukamizu et al. 1989; Ganten et al. 1992; Sigmund et al. 1992; Thompson et al. 1996; Sinn et al. 1999). These findings corroborated previous biochemical studies showing that human renin and angiotensinogen do not interact with their rodent counterparts (Oliver and Gross 1966). Because of this species specificity of the enzyme-substrate reaction, only double transgenic mice and rats carrying both the human renin and angiotensinogen genes as transgenes became hypertensive (Fukamizu et al. 1993; Thompson et al. 1996; Merrill et al. 1996; Bohlender et al. 1997; Sinn et al. 1999). These "humanized" rodent models independently developed by several groups are useful tools to study the local production and action of angiotensin II in tissues eliciting end-organ damage (Luft et al. 1999). They are also useful to test human renin inhibitors, which because of species specificity cannot be tested in normal rodents (Ganten et al. 1992; Mervaala et al. 1999). Besides this, such animals may help to elucidate the cause of specific forms of pregnancy-induced hypertension (Takimoto et al. 1996; Bohlender et al. 2000).

Mice carrying zero to four alleles of angiotensinogen were produced in a gene-titration experiment (Kim et al. 1995). Circulating angiotensinogen levels as well as blood pressure correlated strongly with the gene dose, supporting the

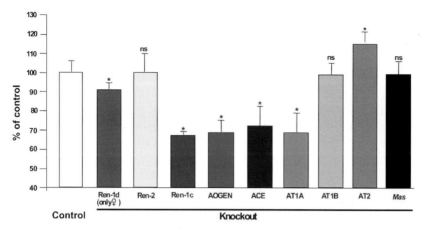

Fig. 2 Blood pressure in mice lacking components of the renin–angiotensin system. References for each animal model are cited in the text. The value of control mice was set as 100%. *Asterisk*, significantly different from control mice; *ns*, not significantly different from control mice

important role of this protein in blood pressure regulation at least in rodents. Very low blood pressure levels (Fig. 2) and morphological alterations in the kidney characterized by atrophy of the renal papilla and renovascular hyperplasia were detected in angiotensinogen knockout mice independently produced by three groups (Tanimoto et al. 1994; Kim et al. 1995; Niimura et al. 1995). Depending on the genetic background, targeted ablation of this protein even led to a lethal phenotype, the cause of which has not yet been clarified. The lethal phenotype as well as the kidney abnormalities were rescued by re-expressing angiotensinogen either in the liver and brain (Kang et al. 2002) or in adipose tissue with spillover into the circulation (Massiera et al. 2001) but not by angiotensin restoration exclusively in kidney (Ding et al. 2001).

2.1.2
Renin

The most frequently used transgenic model for studying the RAS has been a rat carrying one of the two murine renin genes, *Ren-2* [TGR(mREN2)27] (Mullins et al. 1990). These animals developed severe hypertension and cardiovascular hypertrophy despite low levels of circulating angiotensin II. However, the generation of this peptide was massively enhanced in several tissues, like adrenal gland and brain. These changes as well as the very high circulating levels of prorenin, the inactive precursor of renin, may contribute to the hypertensive phenotype of TGR(mREN2)27; however, its etiology is not yet completely clarified. Veniant et al. (1996) have shown that prorenin when expressed in the liver of transgenic rats by using the α_1-antitrypsin promoter and upon reaching similarly high circulating levels, can cause a comparable degree of cardiovascular hypertrophy than is observed in TGR(mREN2)27, probably because it can be activated in peripheral tissues. The same group has developed a transgenic rat model with inducible hypertension by expressing the *Ren-2* gene under the control of a cytochrome P450 promoter which can be induced in the liver by treatment of the animals with a xenobiotic drug (Kantachuvesiri et al. 2001). After application of the drug, the upregulated prorenin and renin levels lead to an increase in blood pressure and vascular injury. Others have presented evidence that elevated angiotensin levels in the brain, kidney, and adrenal gland of TGR(mREN2)27 also play important roles in the development of hypertension (Peters et al. 1993; Senanayake et al. 1994; Tokita et al. 1994; Campbell et al. 1995).

Overexpression of the human renin gene did not cause any cardiovascular alterations in rodents because of species specificity of the renin–angiotensinogen reaction (see above) (Fukamizu et al. 1989; Ganten et al. 1992; Sigmund et al. 1992; Thompson et al. 1996; Sinn et al. 1999).

All murine renin genes have been separately inactivated by gene targeting. *Ren-2* knockout mice were healthy and normotensive (Fig. 2), only exhibiting increased active renin and reduced prorenin levels in plasma (Sharp et al. 1996). Animals lacking *Ren-1*^{d} have been produced by three groups (Bertaux et al. 1997; Clark et al. 1997; Pentz et al. 2001). While the resulting animals were normotensive in one experiment (Bertaux et al. 1997), the other reports showed morphological alterations in the kidney exemplified by a lack of secretory granules in the juxtaglomerular cells and a hypertrophy of the macula densa as well as enhanced circulating prorenin levels and slightly reduced blood pressure (Clark et al. 1997; Pentz et al. 2001). The quite mild phenotype of both knockout models contends in favor of a high redundancy of the two renin genes (i.e., the presence of one gene can largely compensate for the lack of the other). In fact, when embryonic stem (ES) cells from a mouse strain carrying only one renin gene (*Ren-1*^{c}) were used for renin gene targeting, mice resulted with the same cardiovascular phenotype as angiotensinogen knockout animals (Fig. 2) (Yanai et al. 2000). Mice deficient for both renin genes in a two renin-gene strain have been generated by the Cre-lox technology (Rajewsky et al. 1996) but their cardiovascular phenotype has not yet been reported (Matsusaka et al. 2000).

2.1.3
ACE

ACE is expressed in two different isoforms from one gene, the full-length endothelial form and a testicular form derived from an intragenic promoter in intron 12 of the ACE gene.

Mice with zero to four alleles of ACE have been generated (Krege et al. 1997). Blood pressure is directly correlated with the amount of alleles, while the salt-induced pressure response is inversely related to the number of ACE gene copies (Krege et al. 1997; Carlson et al. 2002). Using three-copy animals, it was shown that the development of diabetic nephropathy is dependent upon at least a modest increase in blood pressure (Huang et al. 2001). Mice completely deficient for ACE are hypotensive (Fig. 2) and exhibit kidney abnormalities and reduced viability comparable to angiotensinogen knockout animals (Krege et al. 1995; Carpenter et al. 1996; Esther et al. 1996). The same phenotype was shown for mice in which only the membrane anchor of the ACE protein was deleted by knockout technology (Esther et al. 1997). These animals still have normal circulating ACE levels but lack the membrane-bound form, which according to this report is the only isoform of the enzyme which is functionally important in the cardiovascular system. Accordingly, expression of the testicular membrane-bound isoform of ACE in non-testicular organs—in particular in the kidney—rescues the phenotype of ACE knockout mice (Cole et al. 2002; Kessler et al. 2002). Exclusive transgenic expression of testicular ACE in testis does not cure the cardiovascular phenotype of ACE knockout mice (Ramaraj et al. 1998). However, it rescues male infertility, which is also observed in these mice (Krege et al. 1995). In contrast, the endothelial form of the enzyme when expressed in the testis is ineffective in this respect (Kessler et al. 2000). Thus, the testicular form of ACE performs an essential but as-yet-undefined function in male fertility, probably independent of angiotensin generation.

2.1.4
Angiotensin Receptors

Several groups have inactivated AT1 receptors by gene targeting in mice (Ito et al. 1995; Sugaya et al. 1995; Matsusaka et al. 1996; Chen et al. 1997). These studies are hampered by the existence of two different genes coding for AT1 receptors in rodents, AT1A and AT1B. The knockout experiments revealed that the AT1A receptor is the more important isoform for cardiovascular regulation as AT1A-deficient mice became significantly hypotensive (Ito et al. 1995; Sugaya et al. 1995; Matsusaka et al. 1996), whereas mice lacking AT1B were without obvious phenotype (Fig. 2) (Chen et al. 1997). However, in contrast to angiotensinogen knockout mice, kidney morphology was normal in AT1A-deficient animals, indicating that AT1B can partially complement the functions of AT1A (Oliverio et al. 1998a). Not surprising was the fact that double knockout animals for both receptors showed the same severe phenotype as mice lacking angiotensinogen, renin, or ACE(Oliverio et al. 1998b; Tsuchida et al. 1998). In the brain, the two AT1 subtypes seem to fulfill different tasks: AT1A is responsible for the blood pressure elevating effects of central angiotensin II while AT1B mediates its thirst-generating action (Davisson et al. 2000).

The AT2 receptor has also been independently inactivated by two groups (Hein et al. 1995; Ichiki et al. 1995). Besides behavioral and neuromorphological (Bohlen und Halbach et al. 2001) abnormalities, AT2 deficiency results in a slightly increased blood pressure (Fig. 2), a more pronounced pressor and antinatriuretic response to angiotensin II infusions and an enhanced cardiac hypertrophic response to DOCA-salt hypertension, corroborating the antagonism between AT1 and AT2 (Ichiki et al. 1995; Siragy et al. 1999; Gross et al. 2000a,b). These effects are partly due to an upregulation of AT1 receptors in cardiovascular organs of AT2-deficient mice (Tanaka et al. 1999; Gross et al. 2000a, 2001).

On the other hand, Ichihara et al. (2001) have recently shown that angiotensin-induced cardiac hypertrophy and fibrosis is dependent on the presence of AT2 receptors. The reason for this obvious contradiction is yet unresolved.

The *mas* protooncogene modulates angiotensin signaling by an up-to-now unknown mechanism (Jackson et al. 1988; von Bohlen und Halbach et al. 2000). Mice lacking this gene have normal blood pressure (Fig. 2) but the variability of cardiovascular parameters is markedly altered (Walther et al. 1998, 2000).

2.2
Brain-Specific Overexpression or Depletion

Transgenic mice with overexpression of the human RAS in several tissues (Merrill et al. 1996) or in the brain alone become hypertensive (Morimoto et al. 2001, 2002). In these models, the high blood pressure can be reduced by intracerebroventricular injection of the angiotensin II receptor AT1 antagonist, losartan, suggesting that the brain RAS is a major determinant of hypertension. Part of the effect seems to be mediated by vasopressin, since intravenous injection of a V1 receptor antagonist also attenuates the hypertensive phenotype. In contrast, ganglion blockade has no specific effect, indicating that the sympathetic nervous system is not primarily involved in this central angiotensin action.

Mice overexpressing the AT1A receptor in neurons by using the neuron-specific enolase promoter remain normotensive but are very sensitive to intracerebroventricular injections of losartan, indicating that blood pressure in this model is balanced by the baroreflex (Lazartigues et al. 2002).

Very recently, a transgenic mouse was presented with eight times more angiotensin II in the brain but normal levels in the circulation (Lochard et al. 2003). The peptide is liberated during secretion from an artificial chimeric protein (Methot et al. 1997) expressed under the control of the brain-specific glial fibrillary acidic protein (GFAP) promoter. Additionally, these animals are hypertensive.

The hypertension developed by transgenic rats carrying the mouse *Ren-2* gene, TGR(mREN2)27 (Mullins et al. 1990), is partially dependent on expression of the transgene in the brain. These animals generate up to tenfold more angiotensin II in the central nervous system than control rats (Senanayake et al. 1994). When they are anesthetized by chloralose-urethane, blood pressuredrops to normal arguing in favor of a neurogenic cause of their hypertension (Diz et al. 1998). Furthermore, when the central angiotensin generation in TGR(mREN2)27 is blunted by crossbreeding with transgenic rats exhibiting a brain-specific deficiency in angiotensinogen [TGR(ASrAOGEN)], a significant reduction in blood pressure is observed (Schinke et al. 1999).

The aforementioned transgenic rat model, TGR(ASrAOGEN), has provided numerous insights in the functionality of the brain RAS. These rats carry a transgene expressing an antisense RNA against angiotensinogen specifically in the brain under the control of the GFAP promoter (Schinke et al. 1999). This causes a reduction of local angiotensinogen levels by 90% without affecting the circulating RAS. The rats are slightly hypotensive and exhibit reduced vasopressin levels in the circulation, again supporting a central involvement of angiotensin II in vasopressin secretion. Furthermore, they show an increased baroreflex sensitivity due to an imbalance of the parasympathetic and sympathetic nervous system (Baltatu et al. 2001). Together with the findings that TGR(mREN2)27 (Borgonio et al. 2001) and mice expressing the human RAS (Davisson et al. 1998) exhibit a decreased baroreflex sensitivity these data characterize central angiotensin as a relevant moderator of the baroreflex.

Central angiotensin is also significantly involved in cardiovascular rhythm control. Renin overexpression in TGR(mREN2)27 (Lemmer et al. 1993), as well as low-dose peripheral infusions of angiotensin II in normal rats (Baltatu et al. 2001) cause an inversion of the circadian blood pressure rhythm. This effect of increased peripheral angiotensin II is absent in TGR(ASrAOGEN) (Baltatu et al. 2001). Thus, peripheral angiotensin II requires central angiotensin II as a mediator of the rhythm shift. In this respect, melatonin is a candidate downstream effector of central angiotensin because its synthesis is attenuated in TGR(ASrAOGEN) (Baltatu et al. 2002). Since only the rhythm of blood pressure but not of heart rate is altered by angiotensin II, the peptide does not appear to affect the main oscillator in the suprachiasmatic nucleus, but seems to affect its output pathways or its synchronization with peripheral oscillators in cardiovascular organs.

In contrast to the cardiovascular actions of central angiotensin II, its role in thirst and drinking remains controversial. TGR(ASrAOGEN), in which the expression of AT1 receptors is increased in the brain, the drinking response to injected angiotensin II is also augmented (Monti et al. 2001). However, mice with a permanent increase in brain angiotensin by local activation of the human RAS or liberation from a chimeric protein (Lochard et al. 2003; Morimoto et al. 2001) show normal water intake. Thus, acute elevation of central angiotensin II levels induce thirst, but chronic overproduction may be compensated by other mechanisms regulating drinking behavior.

2.3
Kidney-Specific Overexpression or Depletion

In addition to the brain, the locally generated angiotensin in the kidney is also relevant for blood pressure regulation. The Sigmund group (Davisson et al. 1999; Ding et al. 2001) recently showed that overexpression of human angiotensinogen in the kidney, in the presence of ubiquitously expressed human renin without spillover of angiotensin II into the circulation, leads to hypertension. The importance of local angiotensin generation in end-organs has been confirmed in a hybrid mouse model carrying a rat angiotensinogen transgene on a knockout background (Kang et al. 2002). These animals became hypertensive due to the exclusive expression of angiotensinogen in the liver and brain. However, due to the absence of local angiotensinogen synthesis in the kidney and heart, end-organ damage was attenuated.

2.4
Heart- and Vessel-Specific Overexpression or Depletion

Mice expressing angiotensinogen only in the heart remained normotensive but nevertheless developed cardiac hypertrophy, indicating that the local formation of angiotensin II induces cardiac damage independent of blood pressure elevation (Mazzolai et al. 1998, 2000). On the other hand, transgenic mice that generate angiotensin II from the aforementioned chimeric protein (Methot et al. 1997) exclusively in the heart do not develop hypertrophy unless spillover of the peptide into the circulation raises blood pressure (van Kats et al. 2001). Cardiac fibrosis is, however, detected in all angiotensinogen-transgenic mice, independent of hypertension, suggesting a direct effect of cardiac angiotensin II on this parameter.

Transgenic rats overexpressing ACE predominantly in the heart have been produced (Tian et al. 1996). In spite of very high levels of ACE activity in the heart, there are no morphological alterations of this organ unless it is pressure-overloaded by aortic banding. This treatment results in a significantly higher hypertrophic response in the ACE-transgenic rats than in control animals, supporting the important role of angiotensin II in this process as postulated earlier by pharmacological and transgenic studies.

Transgenic animal models overexpressing AT1 receptors in the heart have been reported by the use of the α-myosin-heavy chain promoter (Hein et al. 1997; Paradis et al. 2000; Hoffmann et al. 2001). However, the phenotypes of the transgenic animals generated were dramatically different. Mouse models exhibit a drastic cardiac hypertrophy and die within several days (Hein et al. 1997) or months (Paradis et al. 2000) of age. Rats appear absolutely normal unless the heart is pressure-overloaded by aortic banding which, as for the ACE-transgenic rats, leads to a more pronounced hypertrophy than in control animals (Hoffmann et al. 2001). The difference might be related to a differential sensitivity of mouse and rat hearts for angiotensin II effects.

When the AT2 receptor is overexpressed in the heart, the resulting transgenic mice show no obvious morphological alterations, but they are less sensitive to angiotensin II-induced blood pressure elevation, indicating that the AT2 receptor counteracts the AT1 receptor, at least in this respect (Masaki et al. 1998; Sugino et al. 2001). The possible mechanism of AT2 action involves activation of kinins as has been shown in another transgenic mouse model overexpressing the AT2 receptor in vascular smooth muscle cells (Tsutsumi et al. 1999). These animals did not increase blood pressure after angiotensin II infusion due to a counterregulatory hypotensive action of the transgenic AT2 receptor via bradykinin and NO.

Vascular smooth muscle overexpression of rat vascular chymase, an enzyme that like ACE metabolizes angiotensin I to II, caused hypertension and smooth muscle cell proliferation in transgenic mice (Ju et al. 2001). The authors used a tetracycline-regulated transgene (Kistner et al. 1996), allowing them to switch on and off transgene expression by doxycycline application. These animals un-

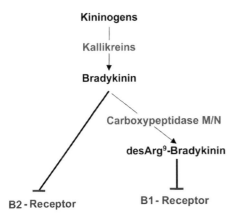

Kininogens

Kallikreins

Bradykinin

Carboxypeptidase M/N

desArg⁹-Bradykinin

B2 - Receptor   **B1 - Receptor**

Fig. 3 The kallikrein-kinin system. For description see text

derscored the possible importance of chymases for pathophysiological angiotensin II generation.

3
Kallikrein-Kinin System

Kinins are peptides with multiple actions in the cardiovascular and immune systems that are derived from precursors, kininogens, by the action of specific proteases, kallikreins, and interact with two different receptors, B1 and B2 (Fig. 3) (Pesquero and Bader 1998). Transgenic animals overexpressing tissue kallikrein (Wang et al. 1994; Silva et al. 2000) or the B2 receptor (Wang et al. 1997) became hypotensive, whereas mice deficient for the B2 receptor developed salt-sensitive hypertension; however, the latter effect remains controversial in the literature (Borkowski et al. 1995; Alfie et al. 1996; Madeddu et al. 1997; Cervenka et al. 1999; Milia et al. 2001). Mice lacking either tissue kallikrein (Meneton et al. 2001) or the B2 receptor (Emanueli et al. 1999) produce a dilated cardiomyopathy later in life, while tissue kallikrein transgenic rats are protected from ischemic and hypertrophic cardiac damage (Pinto et al. 2000; Silva et al. 2000). Tissue kallikrein may be responsible for the flow-induced dilation of arteries, which is particularly important for coronary perfusion (Bergaya et al. 2001). These results substantiate the notion based on pharmacological findings that kinins counteract the actions of angiotensin II and have profound cardioprotective effects. In addition, the marked beneficial actions of ACE inhibitors in cardiovascular diseases may be attributed not only to their inhibitory effects on angiotensin II generation but also to the blockade of bradykinin degradation elicited by these drugs.

Mice deficient for the B1 receptor have recently been generated in our laboratory (Pesquero et al. 2000). While basic blood pressure is normal in this model, the hypotensive response to bacterial lipopolysaccharide is attenuated, corrobo-

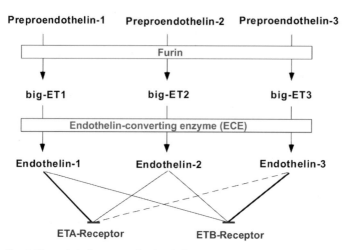

Fig. 4 The endothelin system. For description see text

rating an important role for the B1 receptor in inflammatory processes. Furthermore, these mice exhibit alterations in pain transmission and angiogenesis (Pesquero et al. 2000; Araujo et al. 2001; Ferreira et al. 2001; Emanueli et al. 2002). Nevertheless the results show, that this receptor is not of prime importance for normal blood pressure regulation.

4
Endothelin System

The endothelin (ET) family consists of three isopeptides (ET-1, -2, and -3) predominantly produced by endothelial and vascular smooth muscle cells (Fig. 4). ET-1 is one of the most potent vasoconstrictors known to date. Synthesis of all 21 amino-acid peptide isoforms occurs via precursors, the preproendothelins. Proteolytic processing by furin leads to the big-ETs consisting of 37 to 41 amino acids with low biological activity. Finally, endothelin-converting enzymes (ECEs) convert big-ETs to the active peptides ET-1, ET-2, and ET-3. The different endothelins show distinct affinities to the receptors of the system: while the ETA receptor binds ET-1, the ETB receptor has equal affinity to all three peptides. Surprisingly, transgenic animals overexpressing the human ET-1 and ET-2 isoforms were normotensive, but presented glomerulosclerosis and other renal modifications (Hocher et al. 1996, 1997).

In 1994, Kurihara and colleagues (Kurihara et al. 1994) published the first successful knockout of a component of the ET system. This group reported a slight elevation of blood pressure in heterozygous ET1 knockout mice versus wildtype. Once again, this was in contrast to the expected hypotension. This may be due to upregulated renal sympathetic nerve activity in these mice (Ling et al. 1998). Complete deletion of any component of the endothelin system results in embryonic or early postnatal lethality. Mice lacking ET1 or ETA die at birth from respiratory failure and morphological abnormalities of craniofacial tissues and organs derived from the pharyngeal arch (Kurihara et al. 1994; Clouthier et al. 1998). Knockout mice for ET3 and ETB succumb from megacolon at 3–6 weeks of age (Baynash et al. 1994; Hosoda et al. 1994) and ECE1-deficient animals show a combination of both phenotypes (Yanagisawa et al. 1998). Therefore, blood pressure regulatory functions of the endothelin system have not been studied in knockout models. However, rescue of the ETB-deficient mice and rats by expression of the receptor in the mesenteric nervous system yielded viable animals still lacking ETB in other organs (Gariepy et al. 1998; Ohuchi et al. 1999). These animals exhibit salt-sensitive hypertension, supporting a primary role of this receptor subtype in renal physiology (Gariepy et al. 2000). Mice lacking ET-1 just in endothelial cells which were generated by Cre-lox mediated tissue-specific gene targeting (Rajewsky et al. 1996) show reduced blood pressure, indicating a tonic blood pressure-regulating activity of this peptide in the vasculature (Kedzierski and Yanagisawa 2001).

5
Natriuretic Peptides

Three natriuretic peptides have been described, ANP, BNP, and CNP, probably liberated by the recently discovered protease corin (Yan et al. 2000; Wu et al. 2002) from distinct precursors, and they interact with three receptors NPR-A, NPR-B, and NPR-C (Fig. 5). ANP and BNP signal via NPR-A and CNP via NPR-B (Lopez et al. 1997). All three peptides bind to NPR-C, which is thought to act as a clearance receptor with little defined signaling function. Mice overexpressing ANP (Steinhelper et al. 1990) or BNP (Ogawa et al. 1994) became hypotensive and accordingly, NPR-A-deficient animals developed hypertension (Lopez et al. 1995; Oliver et al. 1998). ANP knockout mice (John et al. 1995) were also hypertensive, although only under a high-salt diet, indicating that BNP might partially compensate for the lack of ANP, when the animals are on a normal diet. Mice lacking NPR-C in accordance with a clearance function of this receptor

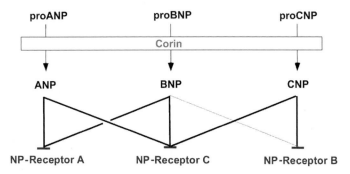

Fig. 5 The natriuretic peptide system. For description see text

show decreased blood pressure (Matsukawa et al. 1999). In the kidney, natriuretic peptides may counteract the RAS since mice overexpressing BNP are protected from renal injury induced by angiotensin II (Suganami et al. 2001). Recently, a vascular smooth muscle-specific knockout of NPR-A was reported (Holtwick et al. 2002). These animals were normotensive but showed a blunted hypotensive response to ANP infusion. Furthermore, acute volume expansion leads to hypertension in these mice since the counterregulatory effect of increased ANP is lacking. These mice show that NPR-A in vessels is not important for baseline blood pressure regulation, but becomes essential in pathophysiological situations of cardiac overload.

CNPknockout mice exhibit dwarfism and most of them die early from skeletal abnormalities (Chusho et al. 2001). Therefore, the cardiovascular function of CNP has not been studied. Furthermore, no transgenic models have yet been described for NPR-B and corin.

6
Neutral Endopeptidase

Neutral endopeptidase 24.11 (NEP) is an enzyme involved in the degradation of numerous cardiovascular peptides, such as angiotensin, bradykinin, endothelin, and natriuretic peptides. NEP-deficient mice develop hypertension with an up-to-now unknown etiology not based on the actions of bradykinin, NO, and circulating ANP (Lu et al. 1997).

7
CGRP and Adrenomedullin

Calcitonin gene-related peptide (CGRP) contains 37 amino acids and is encoded by the transcript of the calcitonin/CGRP gene. It is expressed in cells of the central and peripheral nervous system including neurons innervating the vascular wall and has receptors present in the media and intima of vessels. The cardiovascular phenotype of CGRP-deficient mice is controversial since two groups found an increase in blood pressure (Gangula et al. 2000; Oh-hashi et al. 2001) and one did not observe any difference (Lu et al. 1999). Oh-hashi et al. (2001) explain the hypertensive effect of the CGRP deletion by an increased activity of the sympathetic nervous system without distinguishing between central and peripheral effects.

Adrenomedullin is a 52 amino-acid peptide with a ring structure and structural homology to CGRP. It is generated by endothelial cells and has potent vasodilatory activity. Overexpression of this peptide in the vessel wall of transgenic mice by the use of the preproendothelin promoter led to a significant reduction in blood pressure (Shindo et al. 2000). Adrenomedullin-deficient mice are not viable due to a developmental abnormality of the vasculature (Shindo et al. 2001). However, heterozygous mice, in which one adrenomedullin allele is missing, are hypertensive, corroborating the importance of this peptide for blood pressure regulation (Shindo et al. 2001).

8
Conclusions

The described genetically modified animal models have already gained relevant evidence for the role of specific gene products in cardiovascular regulation and disease pathogenesis. Novel transgenic technologies such as inducible transgene expression (Kistner et al. 1996), conditional gene targeting (Rajewsky et al. 1996), and the development of gene-targeting technology for species other than mice (Brenin et al. 1997; Chesne et al. 2002) will help to further this knowledge and to design new therapeutic strategies.

References

Alfie ME, Yang XP, Hess F, Carretero OA (1996) Salt-sensitive hypertension in bradykinin B2 receptor knockout mice. Biochem Biophys Res Commun 224:625–630

Araujo RC, Kettritz R, Fichtner I, Paiva AC, Pesquero JB, Bader M (2001) Altered neutrophil homeostasis in kinin B1 receptor-deficient mice. Biol Chem 382:91–95

Bader M, Bohnemeier H, Zollmann FS, Lockley-Jones OE, Ganten D (2000) Transgenic animals in cardiovascular disease research. Exp Physiol 85:713–731

Baltatu O, Afeche SC, Jose dos Santos SH, Campos LA, Barbosa R, Michelini LC, Bader M, Cipolla-Neto J (2002) Locally synthesized angiotensin modulates pineal melatonin generation. J Neurochem 80:328–334

Baltatu O, Janssen BJ, Bricca G, Plehm R, Monti J, Ganten D, Bader M (2001) Alterations in blood pressure and heart rate variability in transgenic rats with low brain angiotensinogen. Hypertension 37:408–413

Baynash AG, Hosoda K, Giaid A, Richardson JA, Emoto N, Hammer RE, Yanagisawa M (1994) Interaction of endothelin-3 with endothelin-B receptor is essential for development of epidermal melanocytes and enteric neurons. Cell 79:1277–1285

Bergaya S, Meneton P, Bloch-Faure M, Mathieu E, Alhenc-Gelas F, Levy BI, Boulanger CM (2001) Decreased flow-dependent dilation in carotid arteries of tissue kallikrein-knockout mice. Circ Res 88:593–599

Bertaux F, Colledge WH, Smith SE, Evans M, Samani NJ, Miller CC (1997) Normotensive blood pressure in mice with a disrupted renin Ren- 1d gene. Transgenic Res 6:191–196

Bohlen und Halbach O., Walther T, Bader M, Albrecht D (2001) Genetic deletion of angiotensin AT2 receptor leads to increased cell numbers in different brain structures of mice. Regul Pept 99:209–216

Bohlender J, Fukamizu A, Lippoldt A, Nomura T, Dietz R, Menard J, Murakami K, Luft FC, Ganten D (1997) High human renin hypertension in transgenic rats. Hypertension 29:428–434

Bohlender J, Ganten D, Luft FC (2000) Rats transgenic for human renin and human angiotensinogen as a model for gestational hypertension. J Am Soc Nephrol 11:2056–2061

Borgonio A, Pummer S, Witte K, Lemmer B (2001) Reduced baroreflex sensitivity and blunted endogenous nitric oxide synthesis precede the development of hypertension in TGR(mREN2)27 rats. Chronobiol Int 18:215–226

Borkowski JA, Ransom RW, Seabrook GR, Trumbauer M, Chen H, Hill RG, Strader CD, Hess JF (1995) Targeted disruption of a B2 bradykinin receptor gene in mice eliminates bradykinin action in smooth muscle and neurons. J Biol Chem 270:13706–13710

Brenin DR, Bader M, Hübner N, Levan G, Iannaccone PM (1997) Rat embryonic stem cells: A progress report. Transplantation Proc 29:1761–1765

Campbell DJ, Rong P, Kladis A, Rees B, Ganten D, Skinner SL (1995) Angiotensin and bradykinin peptides in the TGR(mRen-2)27 rat. Hypertension 25:1014–1020

Carlson SH, Oparil S, Chen YF, Wyss JM (2002) Blood pressure and NaCl-sensitive hypertension are influenced by angiotensin-converting enzyme gene expression in transgenic mice. Hypertension 39:214–218

Carpenter C, Honkanen AA, Mashimo H, Goss KA, Huang P, Fishman MC, Asaad M, Dorso CR, Cheung H (1996) Renal abnormalities in mutant mice. Nature 380:292–292

Cervenka L, Harrison-Bernard LM, Dipp S, Primrose G, Imig JD, El-Dahr SS (1999) Early onset salt-sensitive hypertension in bradykinin B2 receptor null mice. Hypertension 34:176–180

Chen X, Li W, Yoshida H, Tsuchida S, Nishimura H, Takemoto F, Okubo S, Fogo A, Matsusaka T, Ichikawa I (1997) Targeting deletion of angiotensin type 1B receptor gene in the mouse. Am J Physiol 272: F299-F304

Chesne P, Adenot PG, Viglietta C, Baratte M, Boulanger L, Renard JP (2002) Cloned rabbits produced by nuclear transfer from adult somatic cells. Nat Biotechnol 20:366–369

Chusho H, Tamura N, Ogawa Y, Yasoda A, Suda M, Miyazawa T, Nakamura K, Nakao K, Kurihara T, Komatsu Y, Itoh H, Tanaka K, Saito Y, Katsuki M, Nakao K (2001) Dwarfism and early death in mice lacking C-type natriuretic peptide. Proc Natl Acad Sci U S A 98:4016–4021

Clark AF, Sharp MGF, Morley SD, Fleming S, Peters J, Mullins JJ (1997) Renin-1 is essential for normal renal juxtaglomerular cell granulation and macula densa morphology. J Biol Chem 272:18185–18190

Clouthier DE, Hosoda K, Richardson JA, Williams SC, Yanagisawa H, Kuwaki T, Kumada M, Hammer RE, Yanagisawa M (1998) Cranial and cardiac neural crest defects in endothelin-A receptor- deficient mice. Development 125:813–824

Cole J, Quach dL, Sundaram K, Corvol P, Capecchi MR, Bernstein KE (2002) Mice lacking endothelial angiotensin-converting enzyme have a normal blood pressure. Circ Res 90:87–92

Davisson RL, Ding Y, Stec DE, Catterall JF, Sigmund CD (1999) Novel mechanism of hypertension revealed by cell-specific targeting of human angiotensinogen in transgenic mice. Physiol Genomics 1:3-9

Davisson RL, Oliverio MI, Coffman TM, Sigmund CD (2000) Divergent functions of angiotensin II receptor isoforms in the brain. J Clin Invest 106:103–106

Davisson RL, Yang G, Beltz TG, Cassell MD, Johnson AK, Sigmund CD (1998) The brain renin–angiotensin system contributes to the hypertension in mice containing both the human renin and human angiotensinogen transgenes. Circ Res 83:1047–1058

Ding Y, Stec DE, Sigmund CD (2001) Genetic evidence that lethality in angiotensinogen-deficient mice is due to loss of systemic but not renal angiotensinogen. J Biol Chem 276:7431–7436

Diz DI, Westwood B, Bosch SM, Ganten D, Ferrario C (1998) NK1 receptor antagonist blocks angiotensin II responses in renin transgenic rat medulla oblongata. Hypertension 31:473–479

Doan TN, Gletsu N, Cole J, Bernstein KE (2001) Genetic manipulation of the renin–angiotensin system. Curr Opin Nephrol Hypertens 10:483–491

Emanueli C, Bonaria SM, Stacca T, Pintus G, Kirchmair R, Isner JM, Pinna A, Gaspa L, Regoli D, Cayla C, Pesquero JB, Bader M, Madeddu P (2002) Targeting kinin B(1) receptor for therapeutic neovascularization. Circulation 105:360–366

Emanueli C, Maestri R, Corradi D, Marchioni R, Minasi A, Tozzi MG, Salis MB, Straino S, Capogrossi MC, Olivetti G, Madeddu P (1999) Dilated and failing cardiomyopathy in bradykinin B(2) receptor knockout mice. Circulation 100:2359–2365

Esther CR, Marino EM, Howard TE, Machaud A, Corvol P, Capecchi MR, Bernstein KE (1997) The critical role of tissue angiotensin-converting enzyme as revealed by gene targeting in mice. J Clin Invest 99:2375–2385

Esther CR, Jr., Howard TE, Marino EM, Goddard JM, Capecchi MR, Bernstein KE (1996) Mice lacking angiotensin-converting enzyme have low blood pressure, renal pathology, and reduced male fertility. Lab Invest 74:953–965

Ferreira J, Campos MM, Pesquero JB, Araujo RC, Bader M, Calixto JB (2001) Evidence for the participation of kinins in Freund's adjuvant-induced inflammatory and nociceptive responses in kinin B(1) and B(2) receptor knockout mice. Neuropharmacology 41:1006–1012

Fukamizu A, Seo MS, Hatae T, Yokoyama M, Nomura T, Katsuki M, Murakami K (1989) Tissue-specific expression of the human renin gene in transgenic mice. Biochem Biophys Res Commun 165:826–832

Fukamizu A, Sugimura K, Takimoto E, Sugiyama F, Seo MS, Takahashi S, Hatae T, Kajiwara N, Yagami K, Murakami K (1993) Chimeric renin–angiotensin system demonstrates sustained increase in blood pressure of transgenic mice carrying both human renin and human angiotensinogen genes. J Biol Chem 268:11617–11621

Gangula PR, Zhao H, Supowit SC, Wimalawansa SJ, Dipette DJ, Westlund KN, Gagel RF, Yallampalli C (2000) Increased blood pressure in alpha-calcitonin gene-related peptide/calcitonin gene knockout mice. Hypertension 35:470–475

Ganten D, Wagner J, Zeh K, Bader M, Michel J-B, Paul M, Zimmermann F, Ruf P, Hilgenfeldt U, Ganten U, Kaling M, Bachmann S, Fukamizu A, Mullins JJ, Murakami K (1992) Species specificity of renin kinetics in transgenic rats harboring the human renin and angiotensinogen genes. Proc Natl Acad Sci USA 89:7806–7810

Gariepy CE, Ohuchi T, Williams SC, Richardson JA, Yanagisawa M (2000) Salt-sensitive hypertension in endothelin-B receptor-deficient rats. J Clin Invest 105:925–933

Gariepy CE, Williams SC, Richardson JA, Hammer RE, Yanagisawa M (1998) Transgenic expression of the endothelin-B receptor prevents congenital intestinal aganglionosis in a rat model of Hirschsprung disease. J Clin Invest 102:1092–1101

Gross V, Milia AF, Plehm R, Inagami T, Luft FC (2000a) Long-term blood pressure telemetry in AT2 receptor-disrupted mice. J Hypertens 18:955–961

Gross V, Schunck WH, Honeck H, Milia AF, Kargel E, Walther T, Bader M, Inagami T, Schneider W, Luft FC (2000b) Inhibition of pressure natriuresis in mice lacking the AT2 receptor. Kidney Int 57:191–202

Gross V, Walther T, Milia AF, Walter K, Schneider W, Luft FC (2001) Left ventricular function in mice lacking the AT2 receptor. J Hypertens 19:967–976

Hein L, Barsh GS, Pratt RE, Dzau VJ, Kobilka BK (1995) Behavioural and cardiovascular effects of disrupting the angiotensin II type-2 receptor in mice. Nature 377:744–747

Hein L, Stevens ME, Barsh GS, Pratt RE, Kobilka BK, Dzau VJ (1997) Overexpression of angiotensin AT1 receptor transgene in the mouse myocardium produces a lethal phenotype associated with myocyte hyperplasia and heart block. Proc Natl Acad Sci USA 94:6391–6396

Hocher B, Liefeldt L, Thone-Reineke C, Orzechowski HD, Distler A, Bauer C, Paul M (1996) Characterization of the renal phenotype of transgenic rats expressing the human endothelin-2 gene. Hypertension 28:196–201

Hocher B, Thone-Reineke C, Rohmeiss P, Schmager F, Slowinski T, Burst V, Siegmund F, Quertermous T, Bauer C, Neumayer HH, Schleuning WD, Theuring F (1997) Endothelin-1 transgenic mice develop glomerulosclerosis, interstitial fibrosis, and renal cysts but not hypertension. J Clin Invest 99:1380–1389

Hoffmann S, Krause T, van Geel PP, Willenbrock R, Pagel I, Pinto YM, Buikema H, Van Gilst WH, Lindschau C, Paul M, Inagami T, Ganten D, Urata H (2001) Overexpression of the human angiotensin II type 1 receptor in the rat heart augments load induced cardiac hypertrophy. J Mol Med 79:601–608

Holtwick R, Gotthardt M, Skryabin B, Steinmetz M, Potthast R, Zetsche B, Hammer RE, Herz J, Kuhn M (2002) Smooth muscle-selective deletion of guanylyl cyclase-A prevents the acute but not chronic effects of ANP on blood pressure. Proc Natl Acad Sci U S A 99:7142–7147

Hosoda K, Hammer RE, Richardson JA, Baynash AG, Cheung JC, Giaid A, Yanagisawa M (1994) Targeted and natural (piebald-lethal) mutations of endothelin-B receptor gene produce megacolon associated with spotted coat color in mice. Cell 79:1267–1276

Huang W, Gallois Y, Bouby N, Bruneval P, Heudes D, Belair MF, Krege JH, Meneton P, Marre M, Smithies O, Alhenc-Gelas F (2001) Genetically increased angiotensin I-converting enzyme level and renal complications in the diabetic mouse. Proc Natl Acad Sci U S A 98:13330–13334

Ichihara S, Senbonmatsu T, Price E, Jr., Ichiki T, Gaffney FA, Inagami T (2001) Angiotensin II type 2 receptor is essential for left ventricular hypertrophy and cardiac fibrosis in chronic angiotensin II-induced hypertension. Circulation 104:346–351

Ichiki T, Labosky PA, Shiota C, Okuyama S, Imagawa Y, Fogo A, Niimura F, Ichikawa I, Hogan BL, Inagami T (1995) Effects on blood pressure and exploratory behaviour of mice lacking angiotensin II type-2 receptor. Nature 377:748–750

Ito M, Oliverio MI, Mannon PJ, Best CF, Maeda N, Smithies O, Coffman TM (1995) Regulation of blood pressure by the type 1A angiotensin II receptor gene. Proc Natl Acad Sci USA 92:3521–3525

Jackson TR, Blair AC, Marshall J, Goedert M, Hanley MR (1988) The mas oncogene encodes an angiotensin receptor. Nature 335:437–440

John SW, Krege JH, Oliver PM, Hagaman JR, Hodgin JB, Pang SC, Flynn TG, Smithies O (1995) Genetic decreases in atrial natriuretic peptide and salt-sensitive hypertension. Science 267:679–681

Ju H, Gros R, You X, Tsang S, Husain M, Rabinovitch M (2001) Conditional and targeted overexpression of vascular chymase causes hypertension in transgenic mice. Proc Natl Acad Sci U S A 98:7469–7474

Kang N, Walther T, Tian XL, Bohlender J, Fukamizu A, Ganten D, Bader M (2002) Reduced hypertension-induced end-organ damage in mice lacking cardiac and renal angiotensinogen synthesis. J Mol Med., 80:359–366

Kantachuvesiri S, Fleming S, Peters J, Peters B, Brooker G, Lammie AG, McGrath I, Kotelevtsev Y, Mullins JJ (2001) Controlled hypertension, a transgenic toggle switch reveals differential mechanisms underlying vascular disease. J Biol Chem 276:36727–36733

Kedzierski RM, Yanagisawa M (2001) Endothelin system: the double-edged sword in health and disease. Annu Rev Pharmacol Toxicol 41:851–876

Kessler SP, Gomos JB, Scheidemantel TS, Rowe TM, Smith HL, Sen GC (2002) The germinal isozyme of angiotensin-converting enzyme can substitute for the somatic isozyme in maintaining normal renal structure and functions. J Biol Chem 277:4271–4276

Kessler SP, Rowe TM, Gomos JB, Kessler PM, Sen GC (2000) Physiological non-equivalence of the two isoforms of angiotensin- converting enzyme. J Biol Chem 275:26259–26264

Kim H-S, Krege JH, Kluckman KD, Hagaman JR, Hodgin JB, Best CF, Jennette JC, Coffman TM, Maeda N, Smithies O (1995) Genetic control of blood pressure and the angiotensinogen locus. Proc Natl Acad Sci USA 92:2735–2739

Kimura S, Mullins JJ, Bunnemann B, Metzger R, Hilgenfeldt U, Zimmermann F, Jacob H, Fuxe K, Ganten D, Kaling M (1992) High blood pressure in transgenic mice carrying the rat angiotensinogen gene. EMBO J 11:821–827

Kistner A, Gossen M, Zimmermann F, Jerecic J, Ullmer C, Lubbert H, Bujard H (1996) Doxycycline-mediated quantitative and tissue-specific control of gene expression in transgenic mice. Proc Natl Acad Sci USA 93:10933–10938

Krege JH, John SW, Langenbach LL, Hodgin JB, Hagaman JR, Bachman ES, Jennette JC, O'Brien DA, Smithies O (1995) Male-female differences in fertility and blood pressure in ACE- deficient mice. Nature 375:146–148

Krege JH, Kim HS, Moyer JS, Jennette JC, Peng L, Hiller SK, Smithies O (1997) Angiotensin-converting enzyme gene mutations, blood pressures, and cardiovascular homeostasis. Hypertension 29:150–157

Kurihara Y, Kurihara H, Suzuki H, Kodama T, Maemura K, Nagai R, Oda H, Kuwaki T, Cao W-H, Kamada N, Jishage K, Ouchi Y, Azuma S, Toyoda Y, Ishikawa T, Kumada M, Yazaki Y (1994) Elevated blood pressure and craniofacial abnormalities in mice deficient in endothelin-1. Nature 368:703–710

Lazartigues E, Dunlay SM, Loihl AK, Sinnayah P, Lang JA, Espelund JJ, Sigmund CD, Davisson RL (2002) Brain-selective overexpression of angiotensin (AT1) receptors causes enhanced cardiovascular sensitivity in transgenic mice. Circ Res 90:617–624

Lemmer B, Mattes A, Böhm M, Ganten D (1993) Circadian blood pressure variation in transgenic hypertensive rats. Hypertension 22:97–101

Ling GY, Cao WH, Onodera M, Ju KH, Kurihara H, Kurihara Y, Yazaki Y, Kumada M, Fukuda Y, Kuwaki T (1998) Renal sympathetic nerve activity in mice: comparison between mice and rats and between normal and endothelin-1 deficient mice. Brain Res 808:238–249

Lochard N, Silversides DW, van Kats JP, Mercure C, Reudelhuber TL (2003) Brain-specific restoration of angiotensin II corrects renal defects seen in angiotensinogen-deficient mice. J Biol Chem 278:2184–2189

Lopez MJ, Garbers DL, Kuhn M (1997) The guanylyl cyclase-deficient mouse defines differential pathways of natriuretic peptide signaling. J Biol Chem 272:23064–23068

Lopez MJ, Wong SKF, Kishimoto I, Dubois S, Mach V, Friesen J, Garbers DL, Beuve A (1995) Salt-resistant hypertension in mice lacking the guanylyl cyclase-A receptor for atrial natriuretic peptide. Nature 378:65–68

Lu B, Figini M, Emanueli C, Geppetti P, Grady EF, Gerard NP, Ansell J, Payan DG, Gerard C, Bunnett N (1997) The control of microvascular permeability and blood pressure by neutral endopeptidase. Nat Med 3:904–907

Lu JT, Son YJ, Lee J, Jetton TL, Shiota M, Moscoso L, Niswender KD, Loewy AD, Magnuson MA, Sanes JR, Emeson RB (1999) Mice lacking alpha-calcitonin gene-related peptide exhibit normal cardiovascular regulation and neuromuscular development. Mol Cell Neurosci 14:99–120

Luft FC, Mervaala E, Müller DN, Gross V, Schmidt F, Park JK, Schmitz C, Lippoldt A, Breu V, Dechend R, Dragun D, Schneider W, Ganten D, Haller H (1999) Hypertension-induced end-organ damage : A new transgenic approach to an old problem. Hypertension 33:212–218

Madeddu P, Varoni MV, Palomba D, Emanueli C, Demontis MP, Glorioso N, Dessi Fulgheri P, Sarzani R, Anania V (1997) Cardiovascular phenotype of a mouse strain with disruption of bradykinin B2-receptor gene. Circulation 96:3570–3578

Masaki H, Kurihara H, Yamaki A, Inomata N, Nozawa Y, Mori Y, Murasawa S, Kizima K, Maruyama M, Horiuchi M, Dzau VJ, Takahashi H, Iwasaka T, Inada M, Matsubara H (1998) Cardiac-specific overexpression of angiotensin II AT2 receptor causes attenuated response to AT1 receptor-mediated pressor and chronotropic effects. J Clin Invest 101:527–535

Massiera F, Bloch-Faure M, Ceiler D, Murakami K, Fukamizu A, Gasc JM, Quignard-Boulange A, Negrel R, Ailhaud G, Seydoux J, Meneton P, Teboul M (2001) Adipose angiotensinogen is involved in adipose tissue growth and blood pressure regulation. FASEB J 15:2727–2729

Matsukawa N, Grzesik WJ, Takahashi N, Pandey KN, Pang S, Yamauchi M, Smithies O (1999) The natriuretic peptide clearance receptor locally modulates the physiological effects of the natriuretic peptide system. Proc Natl Acad Sci U S A 96:7403–7408

Matsusaka T, Kon V, Takaya J, Katori H, Chen X, Miyazaki J, Homma T, Fogo A, Ichikawa I (2000) Dual renin gene targeting by Cre-mediated interchromosomal recombination. Genomics 64:127–131

Matsusaka T, Nishimura H, Utsunomiya H, Kakuchi J, Niimura F, Inagami T, Fogo A, Ichikawa I (1996) Chimeric mice carrying 'regional' targeted deletion of the angiotensin type 1a receptor gene. Evidence against the role for local angiotensin in the *in vivo* feedback regulation of renin synthesis in juxtaglomerular cells. J Clin Invest 98:1867–1877

Mazzolai L, Nussberger J, Aubert JF, Brunner DB, Gabbiani G, Brunner HR, Pedrazzini T (1998) Blood pressure-independent cardiac hypertrophy induced by locally activated renin–angiotensin system. Hypertension 31:1324–1330

Mazzolai L, Pedrazzini T, Nicoud F, Gabbiani G, Brunner HR, Nussberger J (2000) Increased cardiac angiotensin II levels induce right and left ventricular hypertrophy in normotensive mice. Hypertension 35:985–991

Meneton P, Bloch-Faure M, Hagege AA, Ruetten H, Huang W, Bergaya S, Ceiler D, Gehring D, Martins I, Salmon G, Boulanger CM, Nussberger J, Crozatier B, Gasc JM, Heudes D, Bruneval P, Doetschman T, Menard J, Alhenc-Gelas F (2001) Cardiovascular abnormalities with normal blood pressure in tissue kallikrein-deficient mice. Proc Natl Acad Sci U S A 98:2634–2639

Merrill DC, Thompson MW, Carney CL, Granwehr BP, Schlager G, Robillard JE, Sigmund CD (1996) Chronic hypertension and altered baroreflex responses in transgenic mice containing the human renin and human angiotensinogen genes. J Clin Invest 97:1047–1055

Mervaala EM, Müller DN, Park JK, Schmidt F, Lohn M, Breu V, Dragun D, Ganten D, Haller H, Luft FC (1999) Monocyte infiltration and adhesion molecules in a rat model of high human renin hypertension. Hypertension 33:389–395

Methot D, Lapointe MC, Touyz RM, Yang XP, Carretero OA, Deschepper CF, Schiffrin EL, Thibault G, Reudelhuber TL (1997) Tissue targeting of angiotensin peptides. J Biol Chem 272:12994–12999

Milia AF, Gross V, Plehm R, Silva JA, Jr., Bader M, Luft FC (2001) Normal blood pressure and renal function in mice lacking the bradykinin B(2) receptor. Hypertension 37:1473–1479

Monti J, Schinke M, Böhm M, Ganten D, Bader M, Bricca G (2001) Glial angiotensinogen regulates brain angiotensin II receptors in transgenic rats TGR(ASrAOGEN) Am J Physiol Regul Integr Comp Physiol 280: R233-R240

Morimoto S, Cassell MD, Beltz TG, Johnson AK, Davisson RL, Sigmund CD (2001) Elevated blood pressure in transgenic mice with brain-specific expression of human angiotensinogen driven by the glial fibrillary acidic protein promoter. Circ Res 89:365–372

Morimoto S, Cassell MD, Sigmund CD (2002) The brain renin–angiotensin system in transgenic mice carrying a highly regulated human renin transgene. Circ Res 90:80–86

Mullins JJ, Peters J, Ganten D (1990) Fulminant hypertension in transgenic rats harbouring the mouse Ren-2 gene. Nature 344:541–544

Niimura F, Labosky PA, Kakuchi J, Okubo S, Yoshida H, Oikawa T, Ichiki T, Naftilan AJ, Fogo A, Inagami T, Hogan BLM, Ichikawa I (1995) Gene targeting in mice reveals a requirement for angiotensin in the development and maintenance of kidney morphology and growth factor regulation. J Clin Invest 96:2947–2954

Ogawa Y, Itoh H, Tamura N, Suga S, Yoshimasa T, Uehira M, Matsuda S, Shiono S, Nishimoto II, Nakao K (1994) Molecular cloning of the complementary DNA and gene that encode mouse brain natriuretic peptide and generation of transgenic mice that over-express the brain natriuretic peptide gene. J Clin Invest 93:1911–1921

Oh-hashi Y, Shindo T, Kurihara Y, Imai T, Wang Y, Morita H, Imai Y, Kayaba Y, Nishimatsu H, Suematsu Y, Hirata Y, Yazaki Y, Nagai R, Kuwaki T, Kurihara H (2001) Elevated sympathetic nervous activity in mice deficient in alphaCGRP. Circ Res 89:983–990

Ohkubo H, Kawakami H, Kakehi Y, Takumi T, Arai H, Yokota Y, Iwai M, Tanabe Y, Masu M, Hata J, Iwao H, Okamoto H, Yokoyama M, Nomura T, Katsuki M, Nakanishi S (1990) Generation of transgenic mice with elevated blood pressure by introduction of the rat renin and angiotensinogen genes. Proc Natl Acad Sci USA 87:5153–5157

Ohuchi T, Kuwaki T, Ling GY, Dewit D, Ju KH, Onodera M, Cao WH, Yanagisawa M, Kumada M (1999) Elevation of blood pressure by genetic and pharmacological disruption of the ETB receptor in mice. Am J Physiol 276: R1071-R1077

Oliver PM, John SW, Purdy KE, Kim R, Maeda N, Goy MF, Smithies O (1998) Natriuretic peptide receptor 1 expression influences blood pressures of mice in a dose-dependent manner. Proc Natl Acad Sci USA 95:2547–2551

Oliver WJ, Gross F (1966) Unique specificity of mouse angiotensinogen to homologous renin. Proc Soc Exp Biol Med 122:923–926

Oliverio MI, Kim HS, Ito M, Le T, Audoly L, Best CF, Hiller S, Kluckman K, Maeda N, Smithies O, Coffman TM (1998b) Reduced growth, abnormal kidney structure, and type 2 (AT2) angiotensin receptor-mediated blood pressure regulation in mice lacking both AT1A and AT1B receptors for angiotensin II. Proc Natl Acad Sci USA 95:15496–15501

Oliverio MI, Madsen K, Best CF, Ito M, Maeda N, Smithies O, Coffman TM (1998a) Renal growth and development in mice lacking AT1A receptors for angiotensin II. Am J Physiol 274: F43-F50

Paradis P, Dali-Youcef N, Paradis FW, Thibault G, Nemer M (2000) Overexpression of angiotensin II type I receptor in cardiomyocytes induces cardiac hypertrophy and remodeling. Proc Natl Acad Sci USA 97:931–936

Pentz ES, Lopez ML, Kim HS, Carretero O, Smithies O, Gomez RA (2001) Ren1d and Ren2 cooperate to preserve homeostasis: evidence from mice expressing GFP in place of Ren1d. Physiol Genomics 6:45–55

Pesquero JB, Araujo RC, Heppenstall PA, Stucky CL, Silva JA, Jr., Walther T, Oliveira SM, Pesquero JL, Paiva AC, Calixto JB, Lewin GR, Bader M (2000) Hypoalgesia and altered inflammatory responses in mice lacking kinin B1 receptors. Proc Natl Acad Sci U S A 97:8140–8145

Pesquero JB, Bader M (1998) Molecular biology of the kallikrein-kinin system: from structure to function. Braz J Med Biol Res 31:1197–1203

Peters J, Münter K, Bader M, Hackenthal E, Mullins JJ, Ganten D (1993) Increased adrenal renin in transgenic hypertensive rats, TGR(mREN2)27, and its regulation by cAMP, angiotensin II, and calcium. J Clin Invest 91:742–747

Pinto YM, Bader M, Pesquero JB, Tschöpe C, Scholtens E, Van Gilst WH, Buikema H (2000) Increased kallikrein expression protects against cardiac ischemia. FASEB J 14:1861–1863

Rajewsky K, Gu H, Kühn R, Betz UA, Müller W, Roes J, Schwenk F (1996) Conditional gene targeting. J Clin Invest 98:600–603

Ramaraj P, Kessler SP, Colmenares C, Sen GC (1998) Selective restoration of male fertility in mice lacking angiotensin- converting enzymes by sperm-specific expression of the testicular isozyme. J Clin Invest 102:371–378

Schinke M, Baltatu O, Böhm M, Peters J, Rascher W, Bricca G, Lippoldt A, Ganten D, Bader M (1999) Blood pressure reduction and diabetes insipidus in transgenic rats deficient in brain angiotensinogen. Proc Natl Acad Sci USA 96:3975–3980

Schinke M, Böhm M, Bricca G, Ganten D, Bader M (1996) Permanent inhibition of angiotensinogen synthesis by antisense RNA expression. Hypertension 27:508–513

Senanayake P, Moriguchi A, Kumagai H, Ganten D, Ferrario CM, Brosnihan KB (1994) Increased expression of angiotensin peptides in the brain of transgenic hypertensive rats. Peptides 15:919–926

Sharp MG, Fettes D, Brooker G, Clark AF, Peters J, Fleming S, Mullins JJ (1996) Targeted inactivation of the Ren-2 gene in mice. Hypertension 28:1126–1131

Shindo T, Kurihara H, Maemura K, Kurihara Y, Kuwaki T, Izumida T, Minamino N, Ju KH, Morita H, Oh-hashi Y, Kumada M, Kangawa K, Nagai R, Yazaki Y (2000) Hypotension and resistance to lipopolysaccharide-induced shock in transgenic mice overexpressing adrenomedullin in their vasculature. Circulation 101:2309–2316

Shindo T, Kurihara Y, Nishimatsu H, Moriyama N, Kakoki M, Wang Y, Imai Y, Ebihara A, Kuwaki T, Ju KH, Minamino N, Kangawa K, Ishikawa T, Fukuda M, Akimoto Y, Kawakami H, Imai T, Morita H, Yazaki Y, Nagai R, Hirata Y, Kurihara H (2001) Vascular abnormalities and elevated blood pressure in mice lacking adrenomedullin gene. Circulation 104:1964–1971

Sigmund CD (2001) Genetic manipulation of the renin–angiotensin system: targeted expression of the renin–angiotensin system in the kidney. Am J Hypertens 14:33S-37S

Sigmund CD, Jones CA, Kane CM, Wu C, Lang JA, Gross KW (1992) Regulated tissue- and cell-specific expression of the human renin gene in transgenic mice. Circ Res 70:1070–1079

Silva JA, Jr., Araujo RC, Baltatu O, Oliveira SM, Tschöpe C, Fink E, Hoffmann S, Plehm R, Chai KX, Chao L, Chao J, Ganten D, Pesquero JB, Bader M (2000) Reduced cardiac hypertrophy and altered blood pressure control in transgenic rats with the human tissue kallikrein gene. FASEB J 14:1858–1860

Sinn PL, Davis DR, Sigmund CD (1999) Highly regulated cell type-restricted expression of human renin in mice containing 140- or 160-kilobase pair P1 phage artificial chromosome transgenes. J Biol Chem 274:35785–35793

Siragy HM, Inagami T, Ichiki T, Carey RM (1999) Sustained hypersensitivity to angiotensin II and its mechanism in mice lacking the subtype-2 (AT2) angiotensin receptor. Proc Natl Acad Sci U S A 96:6506–6510

Steinhelper ME, Cochrane KL, Field LJ (1990) Hypotension in transgenic mice expressing atrial natriuretic factor fusion genes. Hypertension 16:301–307

Suganami T, Mukoyama M, Sugawara A, Mori K, Nagae T, Kasahara M, Yahata K, Makino H, Fujinaga Y, Ogawa Y, Tanaka I, Nakao K (2001) Overexpression of brain natriuretic peptide in mice ameliorates immune- mediated renal injury. J Am Soc Nephrol 12:2652–2663

Sugaya T, Nishimatsu S, Tanimoto K, Takimoto E, Yamagishi T, Imamura K, Goto S, Imaizumi K, Hisada Y, Otsuka A, Uchida H, Sugiura M, Fukuta K, Fukamizu A, Murakami K (1995) Angiotensin II type 1a receptor-deficient mice with hypotension and hyperreninemia. J Biol Chem 270:18719–18722

Sugino H, Ozono R, Kurisu S, Matsuura H, Ishida M, Oshima T, Kambe M, Teranishi Y, Masaki H, Matsubara H (2001) Apoptosis is not increased in myocardium overexpressing type 2 angiotensin II receptor in transgenic mice. Hypertension 37:1394–1398

Takahashi S, Fukamizu A, Hasegawa T, Yokoyama M, Nomura T, Katsuki M, Murakami K (1991) Expression of the human angiotensinogen gene in transgenic mice and transfected cells. Biochem Biophys Res Commun 180:1103–1109

Takimoto E, Ishida J, Sugiyama F, Horiguchi H, Murakami K, Fukamizu A (1996) Hypertension induced in pregnant mice by placental renin and maternal angiotensinogen. Science 274:995–998

Tanaka M, Tsuchida S, Imai T, Fujii N, Miyazaki H, Ichiki T, Naruse M, Inagami T (1999) Vascular response to angiotensin II is exaggerated through an upregulation of AT1 receptor in AT2 knockout mice. Biochem Biophys Res Commun 258:194–198

Tanimoto K, Sugiyama F, Goto Y, Ishida J, Takimoto E, Yagami K, Fukamizu A, Murakami K (1994) Angiotensinogen-deficient mice with hypotension. J Biol Chem 269:31334–31337

Thompson MW, Smith SB, Sigmund CD (1996) Regulation of human renin mRNA expression and protein release in transgenic mice. Hypertension 28:290–296

Tian X-L, Costerousse O, Urata H, Franz W-M, Paul M (1996) A new transgenic rat model overexpressing human angiotensin-converting enzyme in the heart. Hypertension 28:520

Tigerstedt R, Bergman PG (1898) Niere und Kreislauf. Arch Physiol 8:223–271

Tokita Y, Franco-Saenz R, Mulrow PJ, Ganten D (1994) Effects of nephrectomy and adrenalectomy on the renin–angiotensin system on transgenic rats TGR(mRen2)27. Endocrinology 134:253–257

Tsuchida S, Matsusaka T, Chen X, Okubo S, Niimura F, Nishimura H, Fogo A, Utsunomiya H, Inagami T, Ichikawa I (1998) Murine double nullizygotes of the angiotensin type 1A and 1B receptor genes duplicate severe abnormal phenotypes of angiotensinogen nullizygotes. J Clin Invest 101:755–760

Tsutsumi Y, Matsubara H, Masaki H, Kurihara H, Murasawa S, Takai S, Miyazaki M, Nozawa Y, Ozono R, Nagakawa K, Miwa T, Kawada N, Mori Y, Shibasaki Y, Tanaka Y, Fujiyama S, Koyama Y, Fujiyama A, Takahashi H, Iwasaka T (1999) Angiotensin II type 2 receptor overexpression activates the vascular kinin system and causes vasodilation. J Clin Invest 104:925–935

van Kats JP, Methot D, Paradis P, Silversides DW, Reudelhuber TL (2001) Use of a biological peptide pump to study chronic peptide hormone action in transgenic mice. Direct and indirect effects of angiotensin II on the heart. J Biol Chem 276:44012–44017

Veniant M, Menard J, Bruneval P, Morley S, Gonzales MF, Mullins J (1996) Vascular damage without hypertension in transgenic rats expressing prorenin exclusively in the liver. J Clin Invest 98:1966–1970

von Bohlen und Halbach O, Walther T, Bader M, Albrecht D (2000) Interaction between Mas and the angiotensin AT1 receptor in the amygdala. J Neurophysiol 83:2012–2021

Walther T, Balschun D, Voigt J-P, Fink H, Zuschratter W, Birchmeier C, Ganten D, Bader M (1998) Sustained long-term potentiation and anxiety in mice lacking the Mas protooncogene. J Biol Chem 273:11867–11873

Walther T, Wessel N, Kang N, Sander A, Tschöpe C, Malberg H, Bader M, Voss A (2000) Altered heart rate and blood pressure variability in mice lacking the Mas protooncogene. Braz J Med Biol Res 33:1-9

Wang DZ, Chao L, Chao J (1997) Hypotension in transgenic mice overexpressing human bradykinin B2 receptor. Hypertension 29:488–493

Wang J, Xiong W, Yang Z, Davis T, Dewey MJ, Chao J, Chao L (1994) Human tissue kallikrein induces hypotension in transgenic mice. Hypertension 23:236–243

Wu F, Yan W, Pan J, Morser J, Wu Q (2002) Processing of Pro-atrial Natriuretic Peptide by Corin in Cardiac Myocytes. J Biol Chem 277:16900–16905

Yan W, Wu F, Morser J, Wu Q (2000) Corin, a transmembrane cardiac serine protease, acts as a pro-atrial natriuretic peptide-converting enzyme. Proc Natl Acad Sci U S A 97:8525–8529

Yanagisawa H, Yanagisawa M, Kapur RP, Richardson JA, Williams SC, Clouthier DE, de Wit D, Emoto N, Hammer RE (1998) Dual genetic pathways of endothelin-mediated intercellular signaling revealed by targeted disruption of endothelin converting enzyme-1 gene. Development 125:825–836

Yanai K, Saito T, Kakinuma Y, Kon Y, Hirota K, Taniguchi-Yanai K, Nishijo N, Shigematsu Y, Horiguchi H, Kasuya Y, Sugiyama F, Yagami K, Murakami K, Fukamizu A (2000) Renin-dependent cardiovascular functions and renin-independent blood-brain barrier functions revealed by renin-deficient mice. J Biol Chem 275:5-8

Yang G, Merrill DC, Thompson MW, Robillard JE, Sigmund CD (1994) Functional expression of the human angiotensinogen gene in transgenic mice. J Biol Chem 269:32497–32502

Lipoprotein Transport

H. H. Bock · P. May · J. Herz

Department of Molecular Genetics, University of Texas Southwestern Medical Center,
5323 Harry Hines Boulevard, Dallas, TX 75390-9046, USA
e-mail: Joachim.Herz@UTSouthwestern.edu

Abstract Transgenic animals have become an important tool that has helped to shape our current understanding of the mechanisms of lipoprotein metabolism. They have also proved invaluable for the evaluation of therapeutic strategies directed against disorders of lipid homeostasis and related diseases such as atherosclerosis, obesity, and Alzheimer's disease. In this chapter, we will briefly outline the biochemical and physiological basis of cellular and systemic lipoprotein metabolism and review selected examples how genetically modified animals have aided us in dissecting the molecular function of the genes that regulate lipoprotein transport in the context of the whole organism.

Keywords Lipoprotein · Lipid metabolism · Atherosclerosis · Endocytosis ·
Lipase · Apoprotein · Cholesterol · Vascular wall · Apolipoprotein

Abbreviations

ABCA1	ATP-binding cassette, sub-family A (ABC1), member 1
ACAT (1/2)	Acyl coenzyme A: cholesterol acyltransferase types 1 and 2
Apo	Apolipoprotein
Apobec	ApoB mRNA editing complex
ARH	Autosomal-recessive hypercholesterolemia
CE	Cholesteryl ester
CETP	Cholesteryl ester transfer protein
Chol	Cholesterol
FFA	Free fatty acids
FH	Familial hypercholesterolemia
HDL	High-density lipoprotein
HL/HTGL	Hepatic lipase
IDL	Intermediate-density lipoprotein
LCAT	Lecithin–cholesterol acyltransferase
LDL	Low-density lipoprotein
LDLR	LDL receptor
LPL	Lipoprotein lipase
LRP	Low-density lipoprotein receptor-related protein
LXR (α/β)	Liver X receptor (α/β)
Ox-LDL	Oxidized LDL
MTP	Microsomal transfer protein
PL	Phospholipids
PLTP	Phospholipid transfer protein
SR-A	Scavenger receptor class A
SR-B1	Scavenger receptor class B type I
TG	Triglycerides
VLDL	Very low-density lipoprotein

1
Lipoprotein Metabolism and Human Disease

Transgenic animals have become an important tool that has helped to shape our
current understanding of the mechanisms of lipoprotein metabolism. They have
also proved invaluable for the evaluation of therapeutic strategies directed
against disorders of lipid homeostasis and related diseases such as atherosclerosis, obesity, and Alzheimer's disease. In this chapter, we will briefly outline the
biochemical and physiological basis of cellular and systemic lipoprotein metabolism and review selected examples how genetically modified animals have aided us in dissecting the molecular function of the genes that regulate lipoprotein

transport in the context of the whole organism. (For a summary of all the animal models currently available for the study of lipid metabolism, see Table 1.)

1.1
Overview: Lipoprotein Metabolism

Lipid transport in plasma and extracellular fluids (Fig. 1) is mediated by lipoproteins, large spherical particles which contain unesterified and esterified cholesterol, triglycerides, and phospholipids as major lipid components. A family of proteins, the apolipoproteins, cover the surface of lipoprotein particles. They mediate not only the solubilization and transport of hydrophobic lipids in the aqueous environment but also play important roles in the cellular uptake and metabolism of lipoproteins. According to their physicochemical properties, lipoproteins have been classified into chylomicrons, very low-density lipoproteins (VLDL), intermediate-density lipoproteins (IDL), low-density lipoproteins (LDL), and high-density lipoproteins (HDL).

Apolipoprotein B (for review, see Davidson and Shelness 2000) exists in two major forms: ApoB-100 is exclusively secreted by the liver and constitutes the major apolipoprotein of LDL, IDL, and VLDL, whereas apoB-48, synthesized by the intestinal mucosa, is necessary for the assembly of chylomicrons. It lacks the LDL receptor-binding domain present in apoB-100. Apolipoprotein A-I, A-II, and A-IV are found primarily in HDL and are derived from different genes. A fourth apoA-gene, apolipoprotein A-V, was discovered only recently by genomic cross-species comparison and implied in regulation of plasma triglyceride levels using transgene and knockout approaches (Pennacchio et al. 2001). This study represents a paradigm for the combined use of transgenic, genomic, and classical biochemical techniques to reveal novel aspects of lipoprotein metabolism. ApoC-I, apoC-II, and apoC-III are present in all lipoprotein classes (though only traces are detected in LDL) and are mainly involved in triglyceride metabolism. ApoE, which is found in all major lipoprotein classes except LDL, is secreted primarily by the liver, but can be synthesized by other cell types, including macrophages and glial cells in the brain (Mahley and Rall 2000). It binds to all core family members of the LDL receptor gene family and is present in three major isoforms (apoE2, apoE3, and apoE4) in humans, which in turn differ from each other only by one or two amino acids. The individual apoE alleles are genetically associated with different risks for the development of atherosclerosis as well as Alzheimer's disease, suggesting a possible link between lipoprotein metabolism and neurodegenerative disease.

1.1.1
Transport and Metabolism of Dietary and Endogenous Lipids

Dietary lipids are incorporated into nascent chylomicrons, which are essentially triglyceride droplets secreted by the intestinal mucosa, containing apoB-48 and apolipoproteins A-I, A-II, and A-IV as well as free cholesterol and phospho-

Table 1 Genetically modified animal models in lipid research. For transgenic animals, e.g., Tg(h)ApoAI, Tg(h)ApoAI (rat), first the species from which the transgene is taken is mentioned, e.g., human (h), then the name of the transgene follows. The species of the transgenic animal is noted last, e.g., rat, if animals other than mice were examined. Tissue specificity of targeted gene disruptions is noted in brackets after the gene name if applicable

Altered component	Phenotype	Reference(s)
I. Apolipoproteins		
ApoAI		
Tg(h)AI	HDL (smaller type) and HDL–Chol elevated, posttranscriptional down-regulation of mouse ApoAI	J Biol Chem 264:6488 (1989); PNAS 88:434 (1991)
Tg(h)AI (rat)	Elevated HDL, down-regulation of rat ApoAI	Transgenic Res 1:142 (1992)
Tg(h)AI (rabbit)	Decreased diet-induced atherosclerosis	Circulation 94:713 (1996)
Tg(h)AI/ApoE$^{-/-}$	Decreased susceptibility to atherosclerosis	J Clin Invest 94:899 (1994)
ApoAI$^{-/-}$	Decreased HDL, decreased plasma cholesterol	PNAS 89:7134 (1992)
ApoAI$^{-/-}$/Tg(h)B	Hypertriglyceridemia, increased atherosclerosis	J Lipid Res 39:313 (1998)
ApoAII		
Tg(h)AII	Decreased LCAT activity	J Biol Chem 271:6720 (1996)
Tg(h)AII/ApoE$^{-/-}$	Features of combined familial hyperlipidemia	J Lipid Res 41:1328 (2000)
Tg(m)AII	Elevated HDL–Chol, increased atherosclerosis	Science 261:469 (1993)
ApoAII$^{-/-}$	Elevated HDL–Chol, increased remnant clearance	PNAS 93:14788 (1996)
ApoAIV		
Tg(m)AIV	Elevated HDL, reduced aortic lesions	J Clin Invest 99:1906 (1997)
Tg(h)AIV	Protection against atherosclerosis	Science 273:966 (1996)
ApoAIV$^{-/-}$	Reduced HDL levels	J Lipid Res 38:1782 (1997)
ApoAV		
Tg(h)AV	Decreased triglyceride levels	Science 294:169 (2001)
ApoV$^{-/-}$	Hypertriglyceridemia	Science 294:169 (2001)
ApoB		
Tg(h)B	Messenger RNA for human ApoB is edited by mouse apobec, elevated LDL–Chol, diet-induced atherosclerosis	J Biol Chem 268:23747 (1993); Curr Opin Lipidol 5:94 (1994); J Clin Invest 95:2246 (1995)
Tg(h)B/Tg(h)(a)	Increased atherosclerosis in comparison to wildtype and monotransgenic mice	J Clin Invest 92:3029 (1993); J Clin Invest 96:1639 (1995)

Table 1 (continued)

Altered component	Phenotype	Reference(s)
Tg(m)B	Increased LDL, decreased HDL	McCormick
Tg(h)B (rabbit)	Increased LDL, decreased HDL	Arterioscler Thromb Vasc Biol 15:1889 (1995) PNAS 92:1774 (1995)
ApoB−/−	Embryonic lethality, heterozygotes exhibit reduced plasma cholesterol	J Clin Invest 96:2932 (1995)
Tg(h)ApoB/ApoB−/−	Lack of intestinal ApoB, malabsorption of fat and fat-soluble vitamins, lipid accumulation in enterocytes due to absent chylomicron synthesis	
ApoB48/48-knock-in	Increased LDL-Chol, hypertriglyceridemia	PNAS 93:6393 (1996)
ApoB100/100-knock-in	Decreased LDL-Chol, hypotriglyceridemia	PNAS 93:6393 (1996)
ApoB70-knock-in	Reduced beta-lipoproteins, plasma cholesterol and triglycerides; exencephalus and hydrocephalus	PNAS 90:2389 (1993)
Ad(rat)apobec (rabbit)	Editing of ApoB mRNA in rabbit liver	Hum Gene Ther 7:39 (1996)
Ad-apobec/LDLR−/− (rabbit)	Amelioration of hypercholesterolemia	Hum Gene Ther 7:943 (1996); J Lipid Res 37:2001 (1996)
Ad-apobec (dominant negative)	Inhibition of hepatic apobec-1, increased LDL	J Biol Chem 272:1456 (1997)
Tg(rabbit)apobec-1 (mouse and rabbit)	Reduced LDL, hepatic dysplasia, high rates of hepatocellular carcinoma	PNAS 92:8483 (1995)
apobec-1−/−	No apoB48, normal serum cholesterol and triglycerides, LDL fraction increased, HDL–Chol reduced	J Biol Chem 271:9887 (1996); PNAS 93:7154 (1996)
Apo(a) Tg(h)apo(a)	No association of apo(a) with mouse LDL, but association with injected human LDL, increased atherosclerosis susceptibility	J BiolChem 267:24369 (1992); Nature 360:670 (1992)
ApoC Tg(h)CI	Combined hyperlipidemia	J Clin Invest 98:846 (1996)
ApoCI−/−	Increased response to cholesterol feeding, impaired hepatic uptake of VLDL remnants	Biochem J 305 (Pt 3):905 (1995); Biochem J 321 (Pt 2):445 (1997)
Tg(h)ApoCII	Hypertriglyceridemia	J Clin Invest 93:1683 (1994)

Table 1 (continued)

Altered component	Phenotype	Reference(s)
Tg(h)ApoCIII	Hypertriglyceridemia, reduced remnant clearance, which is correctable by hApoE overexpression	J Biol Chem 269:2324 (1994)
Tg(h)ApoCIII/LDLR$^{-/-}$	Elevated VLDL, elevated LDL, increased susceptibility to atherosclerosis	Science 275:391 (1997)
ApoCIII$^{-/-}$	Hypotriglyceridemia, enhanced triglyceride lipolysis by LPL	J Biol Chem 269:23610 (1994); J Lipid Res 42:1578 (2001)
Tg(h)CIV	Hypertriglyceridemia	J Lipid Res 37:1510 (1996)
ApoE		
Tg(h)ApoE	Accumulation of human ApoE in plasma	J Biol Chem265:14709 (1990)
Tg(h)ApoE2	Hypolipidemia (intermediate transgene expression), hyperlipidemia (high expression)	J Biol Chem271:29146 (1996)
Tg(h)ApoE3Leiden	Hypercholesterolemia, hypertriglyceridemia	J Biol Chem268:10540 (1993)
Tg(h)ApoE4	Increased ApoE, rapid chylomicron clearance	Arterioscler Thromb 14:1542 (1994)
Tg(rat)ApoE	Reduction in plasma lipoproteins (not HDL), resistance against diet-induced hypercholesterolemia	PNAS 89:1750 (1992)
ApoE$^{-/-}$	Severe hypercholesterolemia and atherosclerosis	Cell 71:343 (1992)
Ad(h)ApoE/ApoE$^{-/-}$	ApoE3 and E4 (not E2) ameliorate hypercholesterolemia, all increase HDL levels	J Clin Invest 100:107 (1997)
Tg(h)ApoE(macrophages)/ApoE$^{-/-}$	Reduction of atherosclerosis	J Clin Invest 96:2170 (1995)
ApoE*3/4 humanized-knock-in	Hypercholesterolemia in knock-in mice with humanized apoE genes: human APOE*4>APOE*3>murine apoE	J Biol Chem 272:17972 (1997)
ApoE*2 humanized-knock-in	Type III hyperlipoproteinemia and spontaneous atherosclerosis	J Clin Invest 103:1579 (1999); J Clin Invest 102:130 (1998)
II. Receptors		
LDLR Gene Family		
Tg(h)LDLR	Absence of LDL	Science 239:1277 (1988)
LDLR$^{-/-}$	Hypercholesterolemia, elevated LDL and IDL	J Clin Invest 92:883 (1993)
LRP$^{-/-}$	Embryonic lethality	Cell 71:411 (1992)
TgMX1Cre/LRP$^{lox/lox}$	Accumulation of cholesterol-rich remnant proteins	J Clin Invest 101:689 (1998)
RAP$^{-/-}$	Reduced LRP activity	PNAS 92:4537 (1995)

Table 1 (continued)

Altered component	Phenotype	Reference(s)
Megalin−/−	Perinatal lethality, holoprosencephaly	PNAS 93:8460 (1996)
VLDLR−/−	Reduction in adipose tissue mass, resistance against obesity, cerebellar developmental defects	PNAS 92:8453 (1995); Arterioscler Thromb Vasc Biol 21:1488 (2001)
ApoER2−/−	Hippocampal developmental defects	Cell 97:689 (1999)
VLDLR−/−/LDLR−/−	Hypertriglyceridemia	J Lipid Res 41:2055 (2000)
VLDLR−/−/ApoER2−/−	Neural developmental defects	Cell 97:689 (1999)
Scavenger receptors		
Tg(h)SRA(bone marrow-derived cells)/ApoE−/−	Reduced serum cholesterol	Arterioscler Thromb Vasc Biol 20:2600 (2000)
SRAI/II−/−	80% reduced uptake of acetylated LDL, 30% reduced uptake of oxidized LDL by macrophages, normal hepatic clearance of modified cholesterol	J Biol Chem272:12938 (1997); J Clin Invest 100:244 (1997)
SRAI/II−/−/ApoE−/−	Reduced size of atherosclerotic lesions	Nature 386:292 (1997)
AdSRBI	Decreased plasma HDL, increased biliary cholesterol	Nature 387:414 (1997)
TgSRBI(liver)/LDLR+/−	Reduced LDL and VLDL levels, reduced diet-induced atherosclerosis	J Biol Chem 274:2366 (1999)
SRBI−/−	Hypercholesterolemia, defect erythrocyte maturation	Blood 99:1817 (2002)
SRBI−/−/ApoE−/−	Severe atherosclerosis, myocardial infarction, premature death	Circ Res 90:270 (2002)
TgCD36 (SHR)	Amelioration of insulin-resistance, reduced serum fatty acids	Nat Genet 27:156 (2001)
CD36−/−	Increased cholesterol and triglyceride levels	J Biol Chem274:19055 (1999)
CD36−/−/ApoE−/−	Reduced atherosclerosis	J Clin Invest 105:1049 (2000)
III. Enzymes and transporters		
Tg(h)HTGL	Decreased ApoB-containing and HDL lipoproteins, reduced diet-induced aortic cholesterol accumulation	J Biol Chem 273:1896 (1998); Biochim Biophys Acta 1392:276 (1998); J Biol Chem 269:16376 (1994)
Tg(h)HTGL (rabbit)	Reduced HDL, reduced IDL	PNAS 91:8724 (1994)
HTGL−/−	Increased total cholesterol, increased HDL	J Biol Chem 270:2974 (1995)

Table 1 (continued)

Altered component	Phenotype	Reference(s)
Tg(h)LPL	Resistance to diet-induced hypercholesterolemia and hypertriglyceridemia, decreased VLDL	J Biol Chem 268:17924 (1993); J Biol Chem 269:11417 (1994); J Biol Chem 269:18757 (1994)
TgLPL/ApoE⁻/⁻	Reduced diet-induced atherosclerosis in comparison to ApoE⁻/⁻	J Lipid Res 40:1677 (1999)
TgLPL/LDLR⁻/⁻	Reduced diet-induced atherosclerosis in comparison to LDLR⁻/⁻	PNAS 93:7242 (1996)
LPL⁻/⁻	Severe hypertriglyceridemia, reduced HDL, increased perinatal mortality	J Clin Invest 96:2555 (1995)
Tg(h)EL	Reduced HDL and ApoAI	Nat Genet 21:424 (1999)
Ad(h)ACAT-1/LDLR⁻/⁻	Increased hepatic cholesterol esterification and cholesterol synthesis, increased VLDL secretion	J Biol Chem 275:27005 (2000)
ACAT-1⁻/⁻	Reduced cholesterol esterification in adrenals and fibroblasts, normal esterification in liver	PNAS 93:14041 (1996)
ACAT-2⁻/⁻	Resistance to diet-induced hypercholesterolemia and gall-stone formation	Nat Med 6:1341 (2000)
ACAT1⁻/⁻/LDLR⁻/⁻	Increased atherosclerosis	J Clin Invest 107:163 (2001)
Tg(h)LCAT (rabbit)	Increased HDL, increased plasma cholesterol esterification rate, prevention of diet-induced atherosclerosis	J Biol Chem 271:4396 (1996); PNAS 93:11448 (1996)
Tg(h)LCAT	Increased HDL, enhanced diet-induced atherosclerosis	J Clin Invest 96:1440 (1995); J Lipid Res 38:813 (1997); Nat Med 3:744 (1997)
LCAT⁻/⁻	Decreased HDL, decreased ApoAI and AII, hypertriglyceridemia	J Biol Chem 272:7506 (1997); J Biol Chem 272:15777 (1997)
Tg(h)CETP/ApoE⁻/⁻	Increased cholesterol, increased atherosclerosis	Arterioscler Thromb Vasc Biol 19(4):1105 (1999)
Tg(h)CETP/LDLR⁻/⁻	Correction of dysfunctional HDL, reduced atherosclerosis	J Biol Chem 274:36912 (1999)
Tg(h)CETP/Tg(h)LCAT	Increased hepatic secretion of VLDL and ApoB	J Lipid Res 40:2134 (1999)
Ad(h)MTP	Strongly decreased VLDL assembly and ApoB100 secretion from liver	J Clin Invest 103:1287 (1999)
TgCre(liver)MTPˡᵒˣ/ˡᵒˣ		
MTP⁻/⁻	Embryonic lethality, no yolk sac lipoprotein synthesis, reduced ApoB secretion in heterozygotes	PNAS 95:8686 (1988)

Table 1 (continued)

Altered component	Phenotype	Reference(s)
Tg(h)PLTP	Increased antiatherogenic potential of HDL	Arterioscler Thromb Vasc Biol 20:1082 (2000)
PLTP−/−	Reduced HDL	J Clin Invest 103:907 (1999)
PLTP−/−/ApoE−/−	Reduced atherosclerosis	Nat Med 7:847 (2001)
Tg(h)ABCA1	Increased HDL, increased biliary cholesterol excretion, reduced atherosclerosis susceptibility, increased cholesterol efflux from macrophages	J Biol Chem 276:18046 (2001); J Biol Chem 276:33969 (2001); J Clin Invest 108:303 (2001)
ABCA1−/−	Absence of HDL and ApoAI, reduced cholesterol absorption, unimpaired hepatobiliary cholesterol transport, placental malformation, glomerulonephritis	PNAS 97:4245 (2000); Am J Pathol 157:1017 (2000); Gastroenterology 120:1203 (2001); J Clin Invest 108:843 (2001)

Ad, adenovirus; Chol, cholesterol; Cre, cre recombinase; EL, endothelial-derived lipase; h, human; m, mouse; RAP, receptor associated protein; SHR, spontaneously hypertensive rat; Tg, transgenic; other abbreviations are as introduced in text.
The list of references is incomplete due to space limitations. In addition, it was not possible to include all of the innumerous lipid metabolism related animal models created during the last years. This table is intended to give an overview about the different kinds of animal models used in the study of lipoprotein transport by selecting some representative models.

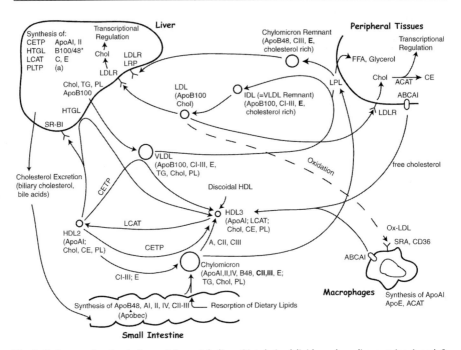

Fig. 1 Pathways of systemic lipoprotein metabolism. Diet-derived lipids and apolipoproteins A and C are added to nascent chylomicrons in enterocytes. They are secreted into the lymphatic system and reach the systemic circulation via the thoracic duct. Activated by apolipoprotein CII, endothelial-bound LPL hydrolyzes chylomicron triglycerides, thereby providing FFA as an energy substrate to peripheral tissues. The apoE-containing cholesterol-enriched chylomicron remnants are finally taken up by hepatocytes via LRP and LDLR. Endogenous lipids are assembled with apoB, apoCs, and apoE into VLDL by hepatocytes. Following their secretion into the circulation, they are also subject to lipolysis by LPL. In turn they develop to cholesterin-enriched VLDL remnants (*IDL*), which mature to LDL, the main cholesterol delivering lipoprotein. LDL is taken up via the LDLR by peripheral tissues or by hepatocytes. Modified, e.g., oxidized, LDL particles are taken up by macrophages via scavenger receptors. This process can lead to foam cell formation in the arterial vessel wall. Reverse cholesterol transport starts with the PLTP-assisted assembly of liver- or intestine-derived apoAI with phospholipids to discoidal pre-β-HDL in the circulation, which accepts cholesterol that is excreted from peripheral tissues via ABCA1. HDL cholesterol is taken up via SRBI by hepatocytes. Note that apoCs and E can also be transferred from HDL2 to VLDL, which delivers apoC to HDL3. CETP also transfers cholesterol esters to IDL. *ApoB48 is synthesized in mouse liver only. Human hepatocytes do no express the apoB mRNA editing complex and consequently contain only the full-length mRNA coding for apoB100

lipids. The triglyceride core of chylomicrons is hydrolyzed after the transfer of apoC-II, an activator of lipoprotein lipase, from HDL particles, giving rise to the so-called chylomicron remnants. Addition of apoE allows the binding and hepatic uptake of the chylomicron remnants by LDL receptors and the LDL-related receptor protein (LRP). The absorption of dietary lipids in the gut involves members of the ATP-binding cassette (ABC) family of transporters, the ABCG family members (reviewed by Schmitz et al. 2001) and ABCA1 (Repa et al. 2000).

Endogenously synthesized triglycerides and cholesterol are secreted by the liver as VLDL particles containing phospholipids and apoB-100, apolipoproteins C-I, C-II, and C-III as well as apoE. Exchange of apoproteins between the different classes of lipoprotein particles occurs to a substantial degree in plasma. Hydrolysis of the triglycerides by lipoprotein lipase and hepatic lipase converts VLDL into IDL and eventually to LDL. The removal of LDL from the plasma via receptor-mediated endocytosis occurs primarily in the liver and is dependent on the LDL receptor, a transmembrane glycoprotein that is expressed in virtually all cell types (Goldstein et al. 2001).

1.1.2
Reverse Cholesterol Transport

The liver is the only organ that catabolizes and excretes cholesterol to a significant extent. The net efflux of cholesterol from peripheral tissues to the liver ("reverse cholesterol transport") thus plays a major role in regulating the organism's cholesterol homeostasis.

In contrast to the apoB-containing lipoproteins, chylomicrons and VLDL, which are secreted as mature particles (reviewed by Kang and Davis 2000), HDL, the major lipoprotein involved in reverse cholesterol transport, is assembled mostly extracellularly. In the plasma, apoA-I, which is secreted by the liver or the small intestine, associates with phospholipids, which are generated during the lipolysis of triglyceride-rich lipoproteins. This process is facilitated by phospholipid transfer protein (PLTP). The resulting disk-shaped pre-β-HDL particles are acceptors for cellular phospholipid and cholesterol complexes. Their transfer to the HDL involves ABCA1, a member of the ABC superfamily of plasma membrane ATPases (Attie et al. 2001). Free cholesterol is esterified through the action of lecithin–cholesterol acyltransferase (LCAT), which promotes the formation of a stable cholesteryl ester-enriched lipoprotein particle called α-HDL. Scavenger receptors of the type B-I (SR-BI) mediate the "selective uptake" of HDL-derived cholesteryl esters by hepatocytes and steroidogenic tissues, but the precise molecular details of this process are still unclear (Krieger 1999; Silver and Tall 2001). However, in vitro SR-BI can also promote cholesterol efflux from cholesterol-laden cells to HDL. Inside the hepatocyte, HDL-derived cholesteryl esters are hydrolyzed by a neutral cholesteryl esterase, providing free cholesterol which can either be directly secreted into bile or catabolized to bile acids by the sequential action of members of the cytochrome P450 family of hydroxylases (Russell and Setchell 1992).

1.1.3
Intracellular Lipoprotein Metabolism

Prior to secretion as well as following cellular reuptake, a range of different enzymes act on lipoproteins. For instance, in contrast to the apoA-containing HDL, apoB-containing lipoproteins are generated exclusively intracellularly. The enzymatic activities of microsomal triglyceride transfer protein (MTP) and phospholipases are required for the assembly and secretion of VLDL particles and chylomicrons (Shelness and Sellers 2001). Following cellular reuptake, cholesteryl esters in the particles are hydrolyzed in the lysosome and free cholesterol is transported to cellular membranes by the NPC (Niemann-Pick Type C) transporters. Acyl coenzyme A:cholesterol acyltransferases (ACATs) are involved in intracellular cholesterol esterification and the loading of VLDL particles with cholesteryl esters. Transgenic animal models have contributed greatly to the elucidation of the role of these intracellular enzymes in normal physiology and under pathophysiological conditions.

1.2
Disorders of Lipoprotein Metabolism and Transport

Genetic abnormalities of lipoprotein metabolism can be divided into monogenic and polygenic disorders. Clinical consequences that arise from these defects include hyperlipidemias, atherosclerosis, coronary artery disease, lipid storage diseases, metabolic syndrome, gallstone disease, and even Alzheimer's disease. Immediate consequences, for instance, of hypertriglyceridemia (increased plasma triglyceride levels) may include acute pancreatitis. Lipid depositions in familial disorders such as Tangier disease or familial hypercholesterolemia can cause organ enlargement or cholesterol deposits in the skin and subcutaneous tissues (xanthomas). Clinically most relevant is the established role of disorders in lipoprotein metabolism and transport as an independent risk factor for the development of atherosclerosis (Wilson et al. 1998), a leading cause of death and disability in industrialized countries.

1.2.1
Hyperlipidemia

A common classification of primary hyperlipidemias (Fredrickson et al. 1967) is based on the isolated or combined occurrence of hypercholesterolemia and hypertriglyceridemia. Human genetic studies have identified gene defects underlying a number of these lipoprotein disorders (Breslow 2000). A classical example for a monogenic hyperlipoprotein disorder is familial hypercholesterolemia (FH), an autosomal co-dominant disorder that is generally caused by functional defects in the LDL receptor (Goldstein et al. 2001) and more rarely by mutations that affect the ability of its ligand, apoB-100, to bind to the LDL receptor [type B familial hypercholesterolemia (Innerarity et al. 1987)]. Other hyperlipidemias, such as the more common polygenic hypercholesterolemia, on the other hand, cannot be attributed to a single gene defect, and the availability of transgenic animal models has proved helpful in evaluating underlying candidate genes. Another example is type III hyperlipoproteinemia (dysbetalipoproteinemia), a combined hyperlipidemia, where a polymorphism at the *apoE* gene locus gives rise to an apoE isoforms that binds poorly to receptors (Mahley and Rall 2000).

1.2.2
Rare Lipoprotein Disorders

Autosomal-recessive disorders, which are usually rare and therefore epidemiologically of lesser importance, have nevertheless significantly contributed to our current concepts of lipoprotein metabolism. For instance, the study of cultured cells from patients suffering from Tangier disease, characterized by cholesteryl ester accumulation in macrophages, HDL deficiency, and premature coronary artery disease due to a defect in the ABCA1 transport protein (Oram and Lawn 2001), were pivotal in confirming the importance of apolipoproteins in cholesterol and phospholipid efflux and developing the concept of "reverse cholesterol transport."

1.2.3
Atherosclerosis

One of the consequences of abnormally elevated plasma lipoprotein levels is the development of vascular lesions in the form of atherosclerosis. This degenerative process of the vessel wall begins with fatty streak formation through accumulation and chemical modification of lipoproteins in the arterial wall, monocyte infiltration, and their transformation into foam cells by lipid uptake through LDL and scavenger receptors. The next stage is characterized by the development of a fibrous plaque with a central necrotic core which is covered by a cap of collagen and smooth muscle cells (Glass and Witztum 2001). Reverse cholesterol transport mediated by HDL mitigates and may even reverse this process of atheroma formation and is thought to be mainly responsible for the established inverse relationship between plasma HDL levels and the risk for coronary events (Barter and Rye 1996). However, atherosclerosis is a complex disease that is influenced by a multitude of internal (genetic) and external (environmental) factors. Animal models are indispensable for further insights into the mechanisms of its pathogenesis, since they allow one to conduct genetically defined, prospective studies within a reasonable time frame, in contrast to epidemiological studies in humans.

1.2.4
Dyslipidemia and Metabolic Syndrome

Insulin resistance combined with hyperinsulinemia, essential hypertension and obesity (commonly referred to as metabolic syndrome or syndrome X) is often associated with atherogenic dyslipidemia characterized by hypertriglyceridemia, low HDL, and small, dense LDL particles (Grundy 1998), probably primarily due to enhanced secretion of hepatic VLDL–triglyceride particles (Adeli et al. 2001). The metabolism of cholesterol, fatty acids, and glucose and their regulation by hormones and differential gene expression is tightly interwoven and still incompletely understood. Yet again, the ability to manipulate the genes that are involved in these processes in laboratory animals has become the driving force by which our understanding of these central biochemical pathways is now taking shape.

1.2.5
Gallstone Disease

A central step in the pathophysiology of cholesterol gallstone formation involves abnormal cholesterol transport, specifically the biliary hypersecretion of cholesterol compared to bile acids and phospholipids. The genetic basis for this complex disorder remains largely unknown (reviewed in Lammert et al. 2001). Transgenic animals, as well as inbred animals on gallstone susceptible and non-susceptible strain backgrounds, not only aid in the study of the clinical aspects of the disease itself, but more importantly, allow us to identify the genes that directly or indirectly contribute to it. An example of this is a recent report that showed that genetic deficiency in the cholesterol-esterifying enzyme ACAT2 completely protected mice from diet-induced gallstone formation (Buhman et al. 2000).

2
Animal Models for the Study of Lipoprotein Metabolism and Its Disorders

Many central aspects of lipoprotein transport and metabolism have been originally elucidated using in vitro or cell culture-based approaches. One of the most notable examples is the discovery of the LDL receptor pathway of receptor-mediated endocytosis (Brown and Goldstein 1986). However, a thorough understanding of the complex interactions of lipoproteins, their receptors and modifying enzymes which govern lipid homeostasis in vivo requires experimental systems that allow one to study these elements in a physiological context. Animal models have therefore proved to be indispensable as tools for basic research in lipoprotein metabolism and lipoprotein-related disorders, as well as to evaluate potential therapeutic strategies. In particular, the ability to generate transgenic and knockout animals has vastly accelerated the rate at which insights are currently gained into complex physiological processes, including the metabolism of lipoproteins.

2.1
Methods for Manipulating Genes in the Animal

The three most commonly used approaches to manipulate the expression of a gene of interest in a laboratory animal involve the overexpression of a transgene in the germline, the generation of knockout or knock-in animals, and the transfer of the exogenous gene to the intact animal, usually by means of recombinant, replication-defective viruses. The vast majority of mammalian animal models involve the mouse. The advantages of this species are (1) a rapid generation time of approximately three months, which allows for multi-generation, prospective studies within a reasonable time-frame, (2) the ability to maintain and interbreed relatively large populations of animals (up to several thousand individuals), and (3) the availability of efficient methods to precisely manipulate the genome of the animal in the germline. Genetic variability in different mutant mouse models may influence the observed phenotype (Sigmund 2000). These phenotypic differences between various inbred mouse strains have been used to genetically map atherosclerosis susceptibility loci (Paigen et al. 1987) and can be exploited to identify modifier genes for mutations on different genetic backgrounds. All of these approaches, isolated or in combination with each other, have been used to analyze the genetics, biochemistry, and physiology of lipoprotein metabolism. In the following we present a necessarily incomplete review of this field by selecting representative examples that in our opinion are particularly suited to illustrate different aspects of lipoprotein metabolism and also serve to highlight the power of the various approaches.

2.2
Manipulation of Lipoproteins

The polypeptides that are embedded within or that are associated with the surface of lipoprotein particles are called apoproteins. They vary greatly in size, ranging from less than 70 to more than 4,500 amino acids. The metabolically most important and consequently most extensively studied apoproteins are apoAI, AII, B48, B100, CI-III, apoE, and Lp(a). ApoAI and apoAII primarily determine the properties of HDL. ApoBs are the main structural components of VLDL, LDL and chylomicrons, and chylomicron remnants and are required for their assembly and secretion by the liver and the intestine. ApoB48 is a truncated version of apoB100 and a product of the same gene that is generated by RNA editing. ApoCs mainly regulate the activity of lipases that metabolize VLDLs and chylomicrons and modulate the ability of the particles to bind to remnant receptors (i.e., the LRP on the hepatocyte surface). ApoE is a small and mobile apoprotein that, like the C apoproteins, can readily exchange between different particles in the circulation. ApoE avidly binds to the LDL receptor and other members of the LDL receptor gene family, in particular the remnant receptor LRP. ApoE is required for the clearance of chylomicron remnants, since the apoB48 in the remnant lacks the necessary sequences for binding to the LDL receptor.

An extensive array of genetically altered mice has been created in which the wildtype genes for each of these apoproteins have been manipulated by overexpression or by gene knockout. In addition, numerous strains of mice have been created in which "humanized" versions of the genes have been inserted, or in which naturally occurring or experimentally designed mutations of these genes were expressed by conventional transgenic approaches, targeted insertion (knock-in) (Willems Van Dijk et al. 2000), or viral gene transfer. Bone-marrow transplantation with transgenic mice as donors or as recipients has been widely used to study the effect of macrophage gene expression, for example of apolipoprotein E (Linton et al. 1995) on lipoprotein metabolism and atherosclerotic lesion formation.

Notable examples are the transgenic expression of apoAII, which diminished the antiatherogenic properties of HDL (Warden et al. 1993), the generation of mice deficient in apoE (Plump et al. 1992; Zhang et al. 1992), which have been used to generate a multitude of animal models for the study of lipoprotein disorders, atherosclerosis, and neurodegeneration, or the overexpression of dominant negative forms of apoE that interfere with receptor binding of the lipoprotein particles (Groot et al. 1996). Farese and colleagues used homologous recombination to "knock in" a point mutation that altered the single nucleotide that is the target of the apoB editing complex (apobec) (Farese et al. 1996). Lp(a) is a lipoprotein that occurs only in humans, old-world primates, and the hedgehog (Hobbs and White 1999; Utermann 1999). It is derived from LDL and formed by the covalent linkage of one apo(a) moiety to the apoB100 in the LDL particle. The generation of transgenic mice that express human apoB100 and apo(a) has made the study of the biochemical and cell biological properties of this unusual lipoprotein possible (Linton et al. 1993).

2.3
Manipulation of Lipoprotein Receptors

The cellular uptake of lipoproteins circulating in the plasma and extracellular space is mediated by different classes of transmembrane receptors.

2.3.1
The LDL Receptor Gene Family

All members of the LDL receptor gene family are receptors for apoE (Herz and Bock 2002). However, only the LDL receptor and the LDL receptor-related protein (LRP) appear to play a major physiological role in the clearance of lipoproteins from the circulation. Nevertheless, the other members of the family may have roles in intercellular lipid transport, for instance in the brain, where apoE is secreted by astrocytes, while the receptors are primarily expressed by neurons.

In 1993, Ishibashi et al. generated a knockout mouse strain that lacks functional LDL receptors and therefore mimics the human genetic disease of familial hypercholesterolemia (Ishibashi et al. 1993). This mouse has found widespread application as a model system on which hyperlipidemia and the development of atherosclerosis, as well as the effect of atherosclerosis-susceptibility genes can be studied. In the same report it was demonstrated that adenoviral gene delivery could transiently reverse the hyperlipidemia that was caused by the inactivation of the LDL receptor inactivation in these mice. This provided a first rational basis for a causal therapy of human familial hypercholesterolemia by somatic gene therapy.

The LRP is highly expressed by hepatocytes. It is also structurally closely related to the LDL receptor. It was therefore proposed that both receptors may work together in the removal of chylomicron remnants from the circulation, a process that is largely unaffected by genetic defects of the LDL receptor. Unfortunately, conventional knockout mice for LRP that were initially generated primarily to address this question die early during embryonic development, indicating that LRP fulfills critical functions that go beyond simple roles in lipoprotein transport (Herz et al. 1992). Indeed, more than 30 distinct biological ligands are currently known that bind to LRP and that function in diverse biological processes (Herz and Strickland 2001), including the regulation of proteinase activity at the cell surface and the modulation of cellular signaling (Boucher et al. 2002). To address the function of LRP in chylomicron remnant metabolism it was thus necessary to use a conditional gene targeting approach. Inducible, tissue-specific, and quantitative disruption of the LRP gene in the liver using the Cre/loxP recombination system finally confirmed a physiological role of LRP as a hepatic chylomicron remnant receptor (Rohlmann et al. 1996; Rohlmann et al. 1998).

Megalin (gp330, LRP2), another member of the LDL receptor gene family, is expressed on the apical surface of resorptive epithelia of different organs, where it mediates the endocytic uptake of lipoproteins, vitamin-binding proteins, and other macromolecules (Nykjaer et al. 1999). Most megalin knockout mice die perinatally and display a complex phenotype including holoprosencephaly resulting from impaired neuroepithelial proliferation (Willnow et al. 1996). Because mice that lack either apoB or the microsomal lipid transfer protein (MTP) and are therefore unable to secrete large cholesterol-carrying lipoproteins also die early in utero, involving atrophy of their nervous system, it is possible that a defective maternal–fetal transport of lipoproteins and lipoprotein-bound nutrients is at least in part responsible for the megalin-deficient phenotype (Farese and Herz 1998).

The VLDL receptor (VLDLR) is another multifunctional member of the LDL receptor gene family, which is, however, expressed in non-hepatic tissues. A role in VLDL triglyceride metabolism was unmasked in VLDLR-deficient mice that also lacked LDL receptors (Tacken et al. 2000). VLDLR-deficient mice also show a reduction in adipose tissue mass (Frykman et al. 1995) and are resistant against obesity induced by dietary or genetic factors (Goudriaan et al. 2001), suggesting a role of the VLDL receptor in the delivery of triglycerides to peripheral tissues. Yet the VLDL receptor, in conjunction with its close relative, the ApoER2 also controls neuronal migration during embryonic brain development, a non-lipoprotein-dependent process that is regulated by the signaling ligand Reelin (Trommsdorff et al. 1999).

2.3.2
Scavenger Receptors

Scavenger receptors were originally narrowly defined as macrophage receptors that mediate the cellular uptake of chemically modified LDL by a mechanism different from the classical LDL receptor pathway, thereby promoting foam cell formation in the arterial wall. This type of scavenger receptor is now referred to as type A (SR-A). In the meantime, another type of scavenger receptor, type B (SR-BI, SR-BII), has been defined, which plays important physiological roles in the metabolism of high-density lipoproteins. Support for a proatherogenic role of SR-A, which is expressed as one of three isoforms generated by alternative splicing, came from mice with a targeted deletion of this gene, which displayed decreased degradation of modified LDL by peritoneal macrophages in vitro and a reduction in the size of atherosclerotic lesions on an apoE-knockout background (Suzuki et al. 1997).

SR-BI was identified as a receptor that mediates the selective uptake of HDL-derived cholesteryl ester, but not its protein components, mainly by hepatic and steroidogenic cells as part of a process named "reverse cholesterol transport" (Krieger 1999). Hepatic overexpression of SR-BI by adenovirus-mediated gene transfer (Kozarsky et al. 1997) decreased plasma HDL levels and increased biliary cholesterol, consistent with a model in which reverse cholesterol transport from peripheral tissues to the liver via HDL is followed by increased biliary cholesterol secretion. SR-BI-deficient mice have dysfunctional HDL particles that are larger than normal. Remarkably, mice lacking SR-BI as well as apoE, which makes these animals highly susceptible to the development of atherosclerotic lesions, develop severe occlusive coronary disease with myocardial infarction and premature death (Braun et al. 2002).

CD36, a related multifunctional class B scavenger receptor, was identified as a cellular long-chain fatty acid transporter. The elucidation of its physiological role in decreasing plasma triglyceride levels in spontaneously hypertensive rats (Pravenec et al. 1999; Pravenec et al. 2001) provides an excellent example for the use of transgenic rats as model organisms in lipid metabolism.

Whereas LDL receptor gene expression is regulated by a feedback mechanism involving transcriptional regulation by the sterol regulatory element binding proteins (SREBPs), CD36 expression in macrophages is regulated by a feedforward mechanism involving the ligand-dependent nuclear hormone receptors peroxisome proliferator-activated receptor (PPAR)γ and liver X receptor (LXR)α. Conditional disruption of the PPARγ gene in mice provided in vivo evidence for a critical role of this gene in controlling the expression of a network of genes involved in cholesterol and lipoprotein homeostasis (Akiyama et al. 2002).

2.4
Manipulation of Metabolizing Enzymes, Transport Proteins, and Chaperones

2.4.1
Enzymes and Transport Proteins

Cholesteryl ester transfer protein (CETP, also called lipid transfer protein I), facilitates the transfer of neutral lipids from HDL to apolipoprotein B-containing lipoproteins. Transgenic mice have been used to elucidate the physiological functions of this protein, which is normally not functional in rodents. Another enzyme that modulates cholesterol and phospholipids on high-density lipoproteins is lecithin–cholesterol acyltransferase (LCAT). Overexpression of CETP in an atherosclerosis-susceptible genetic background increased plasma cholesterol and was proatherogenic (Plump et al. 1999), whereas transgenic CETP reversed the development of atherosclerosis in LCAT-overexpressing mice (Foger et al. 1999). LCAT overexpression leads to increased HDL cholesterol and protects transgenic rabbits, which express functional CETP, from atherosclerosis (Hoeg et al. 1996).

Lipoprotein lipase (LPL) and hepatic lipase (HL) are members of the triacylglycerol lipase family. They act at the endothelial surfaces of extrahepatic and hepatic tissues and are not only the major lipolytic enzymes responsible for the hydrolysis of triglycerides and phospholipids, but can also actively participate in the cellular uptake of lipoproteins (Beisiegel et al. 1991). Capillaries of LPL-deficient mice are clogged with chylomicrons, contributing to their perinatal death. This phenotype can be rescued completely by muscle-specific overexpression of LPL (Weinstock et al. 1995). Santamarina-Fojo, Brewer, and colleagues reported adenoviral gene transfer of human hepatic lipase to the endothelium of HL-deficient mice, which corrected the lipoprotein abnormalities and demonstrated the feasibility of therapeutic replacement of endothelial-bound lipolytic enzymes through recombinant adenoviral vectors (Applebaum-Bowden et al. 1996). Jaye et al. (1999) cloned a novel endothelial-derived lipase (LIPG), which upon overexpression in mice, reduced plasma apoA-I and HDL levels.

ACAT is an enzyme involved in intracellular cholesterol esterification and storage (Rudel et al. 2001). Residual enzymatic activity in ACAT1-deficient mice (Accad et al. 2000) led to the identification of a second mammalian ACAT gene, which has a distinct expression pattern. ACAT2-knockout mice were resistant to diet-induced hypercholesterolemia and cholesterol gallstone formation, due to its role in intestinal cholesterol absorption (Buhman et al. 2000).

Deficiency in the heterodimeric MTP causes human abetalipoproteinemia. As conventional gene-targeting yielded a lethal phenotype, Raabe and colleagues (1999) used Cre-mediated recombination to obtain a liver-specific knockout and found that MTP is essential for VLDL assembly and apoB secretion by the liver and the yolk sac.

Inactivation of the Tangier disease gene ABCA1 gene in mice by homologous recombination resulted in complete absence of plasma HDL and its structural apolipoprotein apoA-I, mimicking a key feature of the human disease and underlining its function as a central player in "reverse cholesterol transport." In their knockout study, McNeish et al. (2000) used gene expression profiling to identify genes that are differentially regulated in these mice.

2.4.2
Chaperones and Intracellular Trafficking Proteins

The biosynthesis of some LDL receptor family members, in particular the LRP, requires the function of a specialized chaperone by the name of RAP (for receptor-associated protein) in the endoplasmic reticulum (ER). RAP normally prevents the premature association of coexpressed ligands with nascent receptors by generically blocking all binding sites on the receptors. Mice carrying a targeted disruption of the RAP gene are unable to produce normal amounts of the receptor, which instead accumulates in the form of misfolded, insoluble aggregates in the ER. RAP-deficient mice that also lacked functional LDL receptors accumulated large amounts of chylomicron remnants in their circulation (Willnow et al. 1995). In a converse experiment, Willnow et al. (1994) used adenoviral gene transfer to overexpress RAP in the liver of LDL receptor-deficient mice. Due to the high level of expression, RAP was secreted from the hepatocytes where it blocked the interaction of chylomicron remnants with the receptor. In this rare example, overexpression and gene knockout of the same protein had a similar loss of function effect, albeit by different mechanisms.

Garcia et al. (2001) recently reported on the identification of an autosomal gene that when defective results in a recessive form of hypercholesterolemia (ARH). The gene encodes a cytoplasmic protein that would be predicted to serve as an adaptor protein that regulates the endocytosis of the LDL receptor. An animal for ARH deficiency will be required to study the role of this protein in receptor trafficking and in the intracellular routing of endosomal vesicles.

3
Conclusions

The generation and evaluation of transgenic animals will continue to contribute invaluably to our understanding of lipoprotein metabolism and lipoprotein-related disorders. Novel genes involved in lipid homeostasis still await their characterization by gene targeting and overexpression in mice, such as the genes responsible for autosomal recessive hypercholesterolemia (ARH; Garcia et al. 2001) and sitosterolemia (ABCG5 and 8, (Hubacek et al. 2001)). Unanticipated roles for other well-known genes in lipoprotein metabolism will be revealed with the widespread use of more sophisticated gene manipulation techniques, and novel genes will likely continue to be identified for some time to come in large-scale genome mutation screens. Gene expression profiling is another promising application for genetically altered animals, which will help to unveil the complex transcriptional network that regulates the genes that are involved in lipoprotein metabolism and transport. Likewise, the continuing requirement for human disease models, which mimic clinical aspects of lipoprotein-related disorders in pharmacological research, will fuel the development of new animal models.

References

Accad, M., Smith, S. J., Newland, D. L., Sanan, D. A., King, L. E., Jr., Linton, M. F., Fazio, S., and Farese, R. V., Jr. (2000) Massive xanthomatosis and altered composition of atherosclerotic lesions in hyperlipidemic mice lacking acyl CoA:cholesterol acyltransferase 1. J Clin Invest 105, 711–9

Adeli, K., Taghibiglou, C., Van Iderstine, S. C., and Lewis, G. F. (2001) Mechanisms of hepatic very low-density lipoprotein overproduction in insulin resistance. Trends Cardiovasc Med 11, 170–6

Akiyama, T. E., Sakai, S., Lambert, G., Nicol, C. J., Matsusue, K., Pimprale, S., Lee, Y. H., Ricote, M., Glass, C. K., Brewer, H. B., Jr., and Gonzalez, F. J. (2002) Conditional disruption of the peroxisome proliferator-activated receptor gamma gene in mice results in lowered expression of ABCA1, ABCG1, and apoE in macrophages and reduced cholesterol efflux. Mol Cell Biol 22, 2607–19

Applebaum-Bowden, D., Kobayashi, J., Kashyap, V. S., Brown, D. R., Berard, A., Meyn, S., Parrott, C., Maeda, N., Shamburek, R., Brewer, H. B., Jr., and Santamarina-Fojo, S. (1996) Hepatic lipase gene therapy in hepatic lipase-deficient mice. Adenovirus-mediated replacement of a lipolytic enzyme to the vascular endothelium. J Clin Invest 97, 799–805

Attie, A. D., Kastelein, J. P., and Hayden, M. R. (2001) Pivotal role of ABCA1 in reverse cholesterol transport influencing HDL levels and susceptibility to atherosclerosis. J Lipid Res 42, 1717–26

Barter, P. J., and Rye, K. A. (1996) High density lipoproteins and coronary heart disease. Atherosclerosis 121, 1–12

Beisiegel, U., Weber, W., and Bengtsson-Olivecrona, G. (1991) Lipoprotein lipase enhances the binding of chylomicrons to low density lipoprotein receptor-related protein. Proc.Natl.Acad.Sci.USA 88, 8342–8346

Boucher, P., Liu, P., Gotthardt, M., Hiesberger, T., Anderson, R. G., and Herz, J. (2002) Platelet-derived Growth Factor Mediates Tyrosine Phosphorylation of the Cytoplasmic Domain of the Low Density Lipoprotein Receptor-related Protein in Caveolae. J Biol Chem 277, 15507–13

Braun, A., Trigatti, B. L., Post, M. J., Sato, K., Simons, M., Edelberg, J. M., Rosenberg, R. D., Schrenzel, M., and Krieger, M. (2002) Loss of SR-BI expression leads to the early onset of occlusive atherosclerotic coronary artery disease, spontaneous myocardial infarctions, severe cardiac dysfunction, and premature death in apolipoprotein E-deficient mice. Circ Res 90, 270–6

Breslow, J. L. (2000) Genetics of lipoprotein abnormalities associated with coronary artery disease susceptibility. Annu Rev Genet 34, 233–254

Brown, M. S., and Goldstein, J. L. (1986) A receptor-mediated pathway for cholesterol homeostasis. Science 232, 34–47

Buhman, K. K., Accad, M., Novak, S., Choi, R. S., Wong, J. S., Hamilton, R. L., Turley, S., and Farese, R. V., Jr. (2000) Resistance to diet-induced hypercholesterolemia and gallstone formation in ACAT2-deficient mice. Nat Med 6, 1341–7

Davidson, N. O., and Shelness, G. S. (2000) APOLIPOPROTEIN B: mRNA editing, lipoprotein assembly, and presecretory degradation. Annu Rev Nutr 20, 169–93

Farese, R., Veniant, M. M., Cham, C. M., Flynn, L. M., Pierotti, V., Loring, J. F., Traber, M., Ruland, S., Stokowski, R. S., Huszar, D., and Young, S. G. (1996) Phenotypic analysis of mice expressing exclusively apolipoprotein B48 or apolipoprotein B100. Proc Natl Acad Sci USA 93, 6393–8

Farese, R. V., Jr., and Herz, J. (1998) Cholesterol metabolism and embryogenesis. Trends Genet 14, 115–20

Foger, B., Chase, M., Amar, M. J., Vaisman, B. L., Shamburek, R. D., Paigen, B., Fruchart-Najib, J., Paiz, J. A., Koch, C. A., Hoyt, R. F., Brewer, H. B., Jr., and Santamarina-Fojo, S. (1999) Cholesteryl ester transfer protein corrects dysfunctional high density lipoproteins and reduces aortic atherosclerosis in lecithin cholesterol acyltransferase transgenic mice. J Biol Chem 274, 36912–20

Fredrickson, D. S., Levy, R. I., and Lees, R. S. (1967) Fat transport in lipoproteins–an integrated approach to mechanisms and disorders. N Engl J Med 276, 34–42, 94–103, 148–156, 215–225

Frykman, P. K., Brown, M. S., Yamamoto, T., Goldstein, J. L., and Herz, J. (1995) Normal plasma lipoproteins and fertility in gene-targeted mice homozygous for a disruption in the gene encoding very low density lipoprotein receptor. Proc Natl Acad Sci USA 92, 8453–7

Garcia, C. K., Wilund, K., Arca, M., Zuliani, G., Fellin, R., Maioli, M., Calandra, S., Bertolini, S., Cossu, F., Grishin, N., Barnes, R., Cohen, J. C., and Hobbs, H. H. (2001) Autosomal recessive hypercholesterolemia caused by mutations in a putative LDL receptor adaptor protein. Science 292, 1394–8

Glass, C. K., and Witztum, J. L. (2001) Atherosclerosis. The road ahead. Cell 104, 503–16

Goldstein, J. L., Hobbs, H. H., and Brown, M. S. (2001) Familial hypercholesterolemia. In Metabolic and Molecular Bases of Inherited Disease, C. R. Scriver, A. L. Beaudet, W. S. Sly, D. Valle, B. Childs, K. W. Kinzler and B. Vogelstein, eds. (New York: McGraw-Hill Publishing Company), pp. 2863–2913

Goudriaan, J. R., Tacken, P. J., Dahlmans, V. E., Gijbels, M. J., van Dijk, K. W., Havekes, L. M., and Jong, M. C. (2001) Protection from obesity in mice lacking the VLDL receptor. Arterioscler Thromb Vasc Biol 21, 1488–94

Groot, P. H., van Vlijmen, B. J., Benson, G. M., Hofker, M. H., Schiffelers, R., Vidgeon-Hart, M., and Havekes, L. M. (1996) Quantitative assessment of aortic atherosclerosis in APOE*3 Leiden transgenic mice and its relationship to serum cholesterol exposure. Arterioscler Thromb Vasc Biol 16, 926–33

Grundy, S. M. (1998) Hypertriglyceridemia, atherogenic dyslipidemia, and the metabolic syndrome. Am J Cardiol 81, 18B-25B

Herz, J., and Bock, H. H. (2002) Lipoprotein Receptors in the Nervous System. Ann. Rev. Biochem. in press

Herz, J., Clouthier, D. E., and Hammer, R. E. (1992) LDL receptor-related protein internalizes and degrades uPA-PAI-1 complexes and is essential for embryo implantation [published erratum appears in Cell 1993 May 7;73(3):428]. Cell 71, 411–21

Herz, J., and Strickland, D. K. (2001) LRP: a multifunctional scavenger and signaling receptor. J Clin Invest 108, 779–84

Hobbs, H. H., and White, A. L. (1999) Lipoprotein(a): intrigues and insights. Curr Opin Lipidol 10, 225–36

Hoeg, J. M., Santamarina-Fojo, S., Berard, A. M., Cornhill, J. F., Herderick, E. E., Feldman, S. H., Haudenschild, C. C., Vaisman, B. L., Hoyt, R. F., Jr., Demosky, S. J., Jr., Kauffman, R. D., Hazel, C. M., Marcovina, S. M., and Brewer, H. B., Jr. (1996) Overexpression of lecithin:cholesterol acyltransferase in transgenic rabbits prevents diet-induced atherosclerosis. Proc Natl Acad Sci USA 93, 11448–53

Hubacek, J. A., Berge, K. E., Cohen, J. C., and Hobbs, H. H. (2001) Mutations in ATP-cassette binding proteins G5 (ABCG5) and G8 (ABCG8) causing sitosterolemia. Hum Mutat *18*, 359–60

Innerarity, T. L., Weisgraber, K. H., Arnold, K. S., Mahley, R. W., Krauss, R. M., Vega, G. L., and Grundy, S. M. (1987) Familial defective apolipoprotein B-100: low density lipoproteins with abnormal receptor binding. Proc Natl Acad Sci USA *84*, 6919–23

Ishibashi, S., Brown, M. S., Goldstein, J. L., Gerard, R. D., Hammer, R. E., and Herz, J. (1993) Hypercholesterolemia in low density lipoprotein receptor knockout mice and its reversal by adenovirus-mediated gene delivery [see comments]. J Clin Invest *92*, 883–93

Jaye, M., Lynch, K. J., Krawiec, J., Marchadier, D., Maugeais, C., Doan, K., South, V., Amin, D., Perrone, M., and Rader, D. J. (1999) A novel endothelial-derived lipase that modulates HDL metabolism. Nat Genet *21*, 424–8

Kang, S., and Davis, R. A. (2000) Cholesterol and hepatic lipoprotein assembly and secretion. Biochim Biophys Acta *1529*, 223–30

Kozarsky, K. F., Donahee, M. H., Rigotti, A., Iqbal, S. N., Edelman, E. R., and Krieger, M. (1997) Overexpression of the HDL receptor SR-BI alters plasma HDL and bile cholesterol levels. Nature *387*, 414–7

Krieger, M. (1999) Charting the fate of the "good cholesterol": identification and characterization of the high-density lipoprotein receptor SR-BI. Annu Rev Biochem *68*, 523–58

Lammert, F., Carey, M. C., and Paigen, B. (2001) Chromosomal organization of candidate genes involved in cholesterol gallstone formation: a murine gallstone map. Gastroenterology *120*, 221–38

Linton, M. F., Atkinson, J. B., and Fazio, S. (1995) Prevention of atherosclerosis in apolipoprotein E-deficient mice by bone marrow transplantation. Science *267*, 1034–7

Linton, M. F., Farese, R. V., Jr., Chiesa, G., Grass, D. S., Chin, P., Hammer, R. E., Hobbs, H. H., and Young, S. G. (1993) Transgenic mice expressing high plasma concentrations of human apolipoprotein B100 and lipoprotein(a) J Clin Invest *92*, 3029–37

Mahley, R. W., and Rall, S. C., Jr. (2000) Apolipoprotein E: far more than a lipid transport protein. Annu Rev Genomics Hum Genet *1*, 507–37

McCormick, S. P., Ng, J. K., Cham, C. M., Taylor, S., Marcovina, S. M., Segrest, J. P., Hammer, R. E., Young, S. G. (1997) Transgenic mice expressing human ApoB95 and ApoB97. Evidence that sequences within the carboxyl-terminal portion of human apoB100 are important for the assembly of lipoprotein. J Biol Chem *272*, 23616–22

McNeish, J., Aiello, R. J., Guyot, D., Turi, T., Gabel, C., Aldinger, C., Hoppe, K. L., Roach, M. L., Royer, L. J., de Wet, J., Broccardo, C., Chimini, G., and Francone, O. L. (2000) High density lipoprotein deficiency and foam cell accumulation in mice with targeted disruption of ATP-binding cassette transporter-1. Proc Natl Acad Sci USA *97*, 4245–50

Nykjaer, A., Dragun, D., Walther, D., Vorum, H., Jacobsen, C., Herz, J., Melsen, F., Christensen, E. I., and Willnow, T. E. (1999) An endocytic pathway essential for renal uptake and activation of the steroid 25-(OH) vitamin D3. Cell *96*, 507–15

Oram, J. F., and Lawn, R. M. (2001) ABCA1. The gatekeeper for eliminating excess tissue cholesterol. J Lipid Res *42*, 1173–9

Paigen, B., Mitchell, D., Reue, K., Morrow, A., Lusis, A. J., and LeBoeuf, R. C. (1987) Ath-1, a gene determining atherosclerosis susceptibility and high density lipoprotein levels in mice. Proc Natl Acad Sci USA *84*, 3763–7

Pennacchio, L. A., Olivier, M., Hubacek, J. A., Cohen, J. C., Cox, D. R., Fruchart, J. C., Krauss, R. M., and Rubin, E. M. (2001) An apolipoprotein influencing triglycerides in humans and mice revealed by comparative sequencing. Science *294*, 169–73

Plump, A. S., Masucci-Magoulas, L., Bruce, C., Bisgaier, C. L., Breslow, J. L., and Tall, A. R. (1999) Increased atherosclerosis in ApoE and LDL receptor gene knock-out mice as a result of human cholesteryl ester transfer protein transgene expression. Arterioscler Thromb Vasc Biol *19*, 1105–10

Plump, A. S., Smith, J. D., Hayek, T., Aalto-Setälä, K., Walsh, A., Verstuyft, J. G., Rubin, E. M., and Breslow, J. L. (1992) Severe Hypercholesterolemia and Atherosclerosis in Apolipoprotein E-Deficient Mice Created by Homologous Recombination in ES Cells. Cell *71*, 343–353

Pravenec, M., Landa, V., Zidek, V., Musilova, A., Kren, V., Kazdova, L., Aitman, T. J., Glazier, A. M., Ibrahimi, A., Abumrad, N. A., Qi, N., Wang, J. M., St Lezin, E. M., and Kurtz, T. W. (2001) Transgenic rescue of defective Cd36 ameliorates insulin resistance in spontaneously hypertensive rats. Nat Genet *27*, 156–8

Pravenec, M., Zidek, V., Simakova, M., Kren, V., Krenova, D., Horky, K., Jachymova, M., Mikova, B., Kazdova, L., Aitman, T. J., Churchill, P. C., Webb, R. C., Hingarh, N. H., Yang, Y., Wang, J. M., Lezin, E. M., and Kurtz, T. W. (1999) Genetics of Cd36 and the clustering of multiple cardiovascular risk factors in spontaneous hypertension. J Clin Invest *103*, 1651–7

Raabe, M., Veniant, M. M., Sullivan, M. A., Zlot, C. H., Bjorkegren, J., Nielsen, L. B., Wong, J. S., Hamilton, R. L., and Young, S. G. (1999) Analysis of the role of microsomal triglyceride transfer protein in the liver of tissue-specific knockout mice. J Clin Invest *103*, 1287–98

Repa, J. J., Turley, S. D., Lobaccaro, J. A., Medina, J., Li, L., Lustig, K., Shan, B., Heyman, R. A., Dietschy, J. M., and Mangelsdorf, D. J. (2000) Regulation of absorption and ABC1-mediated efflux of cholesterol by RXR heterodimers. Science *289*, 1524–9

Rohlmann, A., Gotthardt, M., Hammer, R. E., and Herz, J. (1998) Inducible Inactivation of Hepatic LRP Gene By Cre-Mediated Recombination Confirms Role of LRP in Clearance of Chylomicron Remnants. J. Clin. Invest. *101*, 689–695

Rohlmann, A., Gotthardt, M., Willnow, T. E., Hammer, R. H., and Herz, J. (1996) Sustained somatic gene inactivation by viral transfer of Cre recombinase. Nature Biotechnology *14*, 1562–1565

Rudel, L. L., Lee, R. G., and Cockman, T. L. (2001) Acyl coenzyme A: cholesterol acyltransferase types 1 and 2: structure and function in atherosclerosis. Curr Opin Lipidol *12*, 121–7

Russell, D. W., and Setchell, K. D. (1992) Bile acid biosynthesis. Biochemistry *31*, 4737–49

Schmitz, G., Langmann, T., and Heimerl, S. (2001) Role of ABCG1 and other ABCG family members in lipid metabolism. J Lipid Res *42*, 1513–20

Shelness, G. S., and Sellers, J. A. (2001) Very-low-density lipoprotein assembly and secretion. Curr Opin Lipidol *12*, 151–7

Sigmund, C. D. (2000) Viewpoint: are studies in genetically altered mice out of control? Arterioscler Thromb Vasc Biol *20*, 1425–9

Silver, D. L., and Tall, A. R. (2001) The cellular biology of scavenger receptor class B type I. Curr Opin Lipidol *12*, 497–504

Suzuki, H., Kurihara, Y., Takeya, M., Kamada, N., Kataoka, M., Jishage, K., Ueda, O., Sakaguchi, H., Higashi, T., Suzuki, T., Takashima, Y., Kawabe, Y., Cynshi, O., Wada, Y., Honda, M., Kurihara, H., Aburatani, H., Doi, T., Matsumoto, A., Azuma, S., Noda, T., Toyoda, Y., Itakura, H., Yazaki, Y., Kodama, T., and et al. (1997) A role for macrophage scavenger receptors in atherosclerosis and susceptibility to infection. Nature *386*, 292–6

Tacken, P. J., Teusink, B., Jong, M. C., Harats, D., Havekes, L. M., van Dijk, K. W., and Hofker, M. H. (2000) LDL receptor deficiency unmasks altered VLDL triglyceride metabolism in VLDL receptor transgenic and knockout mice. J Lipid Res *41*, 2055–62

Trommsdorff, M., Gotthardt, M., Hiesberger, T., Shelton, J., Stockinger, W., Nimpf, J., Hammer, R. E., Richardson, J. A., and Herz, J. (1999) Reeler/Disabled-like disruption of neuronal migration in knockout mice lacking the VLDL receptor and ApoE receptor 2. Cell *97*, 689–701

Utermann, G. (1999) Genetic architecture and evolution of the lipoprotein(a) trait. Curr Opin Lipidol *10*, 133–41

Warden, C. H., Hedrick, C. C., Qiao, J. H., Castellani, L. W., and Lusis, A. J. (1993) Atherosclerosis in transgenic mice overexpressing apolipoprotein A-II. Science *261*, 469–72

Weinstock, P. H., Bisgaier, C. L., Aalto-Setala, K., Radner, H., Ramakrishnan, R., Levak-Frank, S., Essenburg, A. D., Zechner, R., and Breslow, J. L. (1995) Severe hypertriglyceridemia, reduced high density lipoprotein, and neonatal death in lipoprotein lipase knockout mice. Mild hypertriglyceridemia with impaired very low density lipoprotein clearance in heterozygotes. J Clin Invest *96*, 2555–68

Willems Van Dijk, K., Hofker, M. H., and Havekes, L. M. (2000) Use of transgenic mice to study the role of apolipoprotein E in lipid metabolism and atherosclerosis. Int J Tissue React *22*, 49–58

Willnow, T. E., Armstrong, S. A., Hammer, R. E., and Herz, J. (1995) Functional expression of low density lipoprotein receptor-related protein is controlled by receptor-associated protein in vivo. Proc Natl Acad Sci USA *92*, 4537–41

Willnow, T. E., Hilpert, J., Armstrong, S. A., Rohlmann, A., Hammer, R. E., Burns, D. K., and Herz, J. (1996) Defective forebrain development in mice lacking gp330/megalin. Proc Natl Acad Sci USA *93*, 8460–4

Willnow, T. E., Sheng, Z., Ishibashi, S., and Herz, J. (1994) Inhibition of hepatic chylomicron remnant uptake by gene transfer of a receptor antagonist. Science *264*, 1471–4

Wilson, P. W., D'Agostino, R. B., Levy, D., Belanger, A. M., Silbershatz, H., and Kannel, W. B. (1998) Prediction of coronary heart disease using risk factor categories. Circulation *97*, 1837–47

Zhang, S. H., Reddick, R. L., Piedrahita, J. A., and Maeda, N. (1992) Spontaneous hypercholesterolemia and arterial lesions in mice lacking apolipoprotein E. Science *258*, 468–471

Transgenic Animals of Enzymes and Receptors in Prostanoid Synthesis and Actions; Phenotypes and Implications in Drug Development

S. Narumiya

Department of Pharmacology, Kyoto University Faculty of Medicine,
Yoshida, Sakyo-ku, Kyoto 606-8501, Japan
e-mail: snaru@mfour.med.kyoto-u.ac.jp

Abstract Prostanoids, consisting of the prostaglandins (PGs) and the thromboxanes (TXs), are oxygenated products of C20 unsaturated fatty acids, and include PGD_2, PGE_2, $PGF_{2\alpha}$, PGI_2, and TXA_2. Precursor fatty acids such as arachidonic acid are liberated from the membrane phospholipids by the action of phospholipase A_2 (PLA_2) in response to various stimuli. Arachidonic acid thus liberated, for example, is metabolized to prostaglandin H_2 (PGH_2) by the actions of cyclooxygenase (COX), which is then converted to respective PGs by the respective PG synthases. There are two isoforms of cyclooxygenase known as COX-1 and COX-2. Because aspirin-like nonsteroidal anti-inflammatory drugs exert their actions by inhibiting COX and suppressing prostanoid production, prostanoids are believed to work in physiological and pathophysiological processes inhibited by these drugs such as inflammation, fever, and pain. Prostanoids are released outside of the cells immediately after synthesis, and exert their actions by binding to a G protein-coupled rhodopsin-type receptor on the surface of target cells. There are eight types and subtypes of the prostanoid receptors conserved in mammals from mouse to human. They are the PGD receptor, four subtypes of the PGE receptor, EP1, EP2, EP3, and EP4, the PGF receptor, PGI receptor, and TxA receptor. Genes for several enzymes in prostanoid synthesis such as PLA_2 and COX isoforms and genes for the eight types and subtypes of the prostanoid receptors were individually disrupted, and various phenotypes of these knockout mice have been reported. In addition, transgenic mice over-expressing a relevant gene and transfer of such a gene in experimental animals were also reported. In this article, we discuss the phenotypes of these animals in context of prostanoid actions under various physiological and pathophysiological conditions.

Keywords Prostanoid · Prostaglandin · Thromboxane · Phospholipase A_2 (PLA_2) · Cyclooxygenase (COX) · PGD_2 · PGE_2 · $PGF_{2\alpha}$ · PGI_2 · TXA_2 · DP · EP1 · EP2 · EP3 · EP4 · FP · IP · TP

Abbreviations

PLA_2	Phospholipase A_2
COX	Cyclooxygenase
NSAID	Nonsteroidal anti-inflammatory drug
PG	Prostaglandin
TX	Thromboxane
Apc	Adenomatous polyposis coli
ACTH	Adrenocorticotropic hormone
LPS	Lipopolysaccharide
IL	Interleukin
TNF	Tumor necrosis factor
OVA	Ovalbumin
NMDA	N-Methyl-D-aspartate
MCT	Monocrotaline

IBD   Inflammatory bowel disease
DSS   Dextran sodium sulfate
PTH   Parathyroid hormone

1
Introduction: Enzymes and Receptors in Prostanoid Synthesis and Actions

Prostanoids, consisting of the prostaglandins (PGs) and the thromboxanes (TXs), are cyclooxygenase products derived from C20 unsaturated fatty acids (Fig. 1). Precursor fatty acids include γ-homolinolenic acid, arachidonic acid, and 5,8,11,14,17-eicosapentaenoic acid, which are precursors for the series 1, 2, and 3 prostanoids containing the 13-*trans* double bond, the 5-*cis* and 13-*trans* double bonds, and the 5-*cis*, 13-*trans*, and 17-*cis* double bonds, respectively. Since arachidonic acid is the most abundant among these precursor fatty acids in most mammals, including humans, the series 2 prostanoids are predominantly formed in their bodies. These fatty acids are esterified to the *sn*-2 position of glycerophospholipids in cell membranes, and are liberated from the membrane phospholipids by the action of phospholipase A_2 in response to various physiological and pathological stimuli (Dennis 1997). There are several forms of phospholipase A_2, such as the Ca^{2+}-dependent cytosolic phospholipase A_2 ($cPLA_2$), the Ca^{2+}-independent phospholipase A_2 ($iPLA_2$), and several types of secretory phospholipase A_2 ($sPLA_2$). Among them, $cPLA_2$ is thought to be a dominant

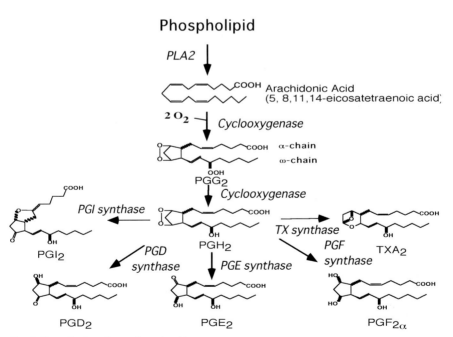

Fig. 1 Biosynthetic pathway of prostanoids

phospholipase A_2 involved in stimulus-induced liberation of arachidonic acid utilized for prostanoid synthesis, whereas $iPLA_2$ is thought to work primarily in cell membrane remodeling under the basal conditions (reviewed in Fitzpatrick and Soberman 2001). On the other hand, the $sPLA_2$ isozyme is induced and secreted under sustained and intense stimuli, and might serve in liberation of arachidonic acid in a paracrine amplification loop. Arachidonic acid thus liberated is metabolized to PGH_2 by the actions of cyclooxygenase, which is then converted to respective PGs by the respective PG synthases. There are two distinct isoforms of cyclooxygenase encoded by separate genes, COX-1 and COX-2 (Smith et al. 2000). The two COX isoforms are about 60% identical and 75% homologous in the amino acid sequence, and catalyze the reaction in a mechanistically similar fashion with about the same Km values for arachidonic acid. However, they quite differ in their expression and regulation. Whereas COX-1 is constitutively expressed in most tissues, COX-2 is undetectable under the basal conditions and induced dramatically in response to various physiological and pathological stimuli. Notably, the expression of COX-2, but not COX-1, is suppressed by glucocorticoids such as dexamethasone. As is well known, aspirin-like nonsteroidal anti-inflammatory drugs (NSAIDs) exert their pharmacological actions by inhibiting COX and suppressing prostanoid production, and COX-2-selective inhibitors have been developed recently to inhibit inflammatory prostanoid actions, while sparing constitutive prostanoid actions. The conversion of PGH_2 to PGD_2 is catalyzed by PGD synthase (Urade and Hayaishi 2000). There are two distinct types of PGD synthase. One is the lipocalin-type PGD synthase, which is localized in brain, ocular tissues, and male genital organs of various mammals. The other is hematopoietic PGD synthase, which is identical with the sigma class of glutathione S-transferase and is localized in antigen-presenting cells, mast cells, and megakaryocytes distributed in various peripheral tissues. Similarly, conversion of PGH_2 to PGE_2 is catalyzed by two distinct isoforms of PGE synthases. One is cPGE synthase (cPGES), that is constitutively expressed and present in the cytosolic fraction, and the other is the inducible, perinuclear membrane-bound form of PGE synthase (mPGES) (Jacobsson et al. 1999; Murakami et al. 2000; Tanioka et al. 2000). Like COX-2, the expression of mPGES is strongly induced by proinflammatory stimuli and is downregulated by anti-inflammatory glucocorticoids. Formation of the F-type PGs is performed by the action of PGF synthase, a cytosolic enzyme belonging to the aldo-keto reductase family (Suzuki et al. 1999). Conversion of PGH_2 to TXA_2 and PGI_2 is catalyzed by TX synthase and PGI synthase, respectively, both of which are hemoproteins belonging to the cytochrome P450 family and are reportedly localized in the endoplasmic reticulum and perinuclear membranes (Tanabe and Ullrich 1995).

Prostanoids thus formed are released outside of the cells immediately after synthesis. PGH_2, PGI_2, and TXA_2 are chemically unstable and are degraded into inactive products under physiological conditions, with half-lives of 30 s to a few minutes, respectively. Other PGs, although chemically stable, are metabolized quickly. For example, they are inactivated during a single passage through the

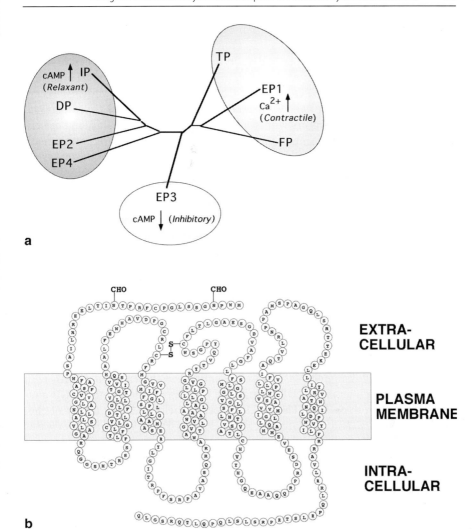

Fig. 2. a Prostanoid receptor family. **b** Membrane topology model for human TP

lung. It is believed therefore that prostanoids work locally, acting only in the vicinity of the site of their production. Prostanoids exert a variety of actions in various tissues and cells. The most typical actions are the relaxation and contraction of various types of smooth muscles. They also modulate neuronal activity by either inhibiting or stimulating neurotransmitter release, sensitizing sensory fibers to noxious stimuli, or inducing central actions such as fever generation and sleep induction. PGs also regulate secretion and motility in the gastrointestinal tract as well as transport of ions and water in the kidney. They are involved in apoptosis, cell differentiation, and oncogenesis. Prostanoids also regulate the activity of blood platelets both positively and negatively, and are involved in vascular homeostasis and hemostasis. Prostanoids exert these actions via membrane receptors on the surface of target cells (Narumiya et al. 1999). There is a family of eight types and subtypes of the prostanoid receptors conserved in mammals from mouse to human (Fig. 2). They are the PGD receptor (DP), four subtypes of the PGE receptor EP1, EP2, EP3, and EP4, the PGF receptor (FP), PGI receptor (IP) and TXA receptor (TP). They all are G protein-coupled rhodopsin-type receptors with seven transmembrane domains, and are encoded by different genes. Among them, the IP, DP, EP2, and EP4 receptors mediate a cyclic adenosine monophosphate (cAMP) rise and have been termed "relaxant" receptors. Likewise, the TP, FP, and EP1 receptors induce calcium mobilization and constitute a "contractile" receptor group. The remaining EP3 receptor mediates decreases in cAMP and has been termed the "inhibitory" receptor. However, the coupling of prostanoids with G protein-coupled signaling pathways may differ as a function of ligand concentration or structure. Then, why are there four subtypes of receptors for PGE_2 and only one type each for other prostanoids? The phylogenetic tree derived from amino acid sequence homologies indicates that the prostanoid receptors originated from the primitive PGE receptor from which the subtypes of the PGE receptor then evolved, and that receptors for other PGs and TX subsequently evolved from functionally related PGE receptor subtypes by gene duplication. In addition to this family of prostanoid receptors, there is a distinct type of PGD receptor termed "CRTH2" (Hirai et al. 2001). This receptor was originally cloned as an orphan receptor expressed in T helper (Th)2 lymphocytes, and has recently been shown to bind PGD_2 with an affinity as high as that of DP, though the binding profile to other PGD analogs differs from that of DP. The CRTH2 receptor belongs to the family of chemokine receptors, and mediates chemotaxis to PGD_2 of Th2 lymphocytes as well as eosinophils or basophils.

Of the enzymes involved in prostanoid synthesis, the genes for $cPLA_2$, COX-1, COX-2, and the lipocalin-type PGD synthase were individually disrupted. In addition, double-knockout mice deficient in both COX-1 and COX-2 were generated. No knockout mouse studies for other PG synthases such as PGE synthases, PGF synthase, PGI synthase, or TX synthase have yet been reported. On the other hand, transgenic mice over-expressing either the lipocalin-type PGD synthase or PGI synthase have been generated. The gene transfer experiments of PGI synthase in rats were also reported. The phenotypes of these knockout mice and transgenic animals are summarized in Table 1. As for the prostanoid receptor family, individual disruption of the genes for the eight types and subtypes of the receptors has been reported. One study also reported transgenic expression of TP in mice. No report is yet found on gene disruption of CRTH2. The phenotypes of knockout mice deficient in each of the eight types or subtypes of prostanoid receptors and TP-transgenic mice are summarized in Table 2. In this article, the phenotypes of these mice are discussed in context of prostanoid actions under various physiological and pathophysiological conditions.

Table 1 Transgenic animals of enzymes in prostanoid synthesis

Affected gene	Phenotype (references)
Knockout mouse with disruption of a gene or genes for:	
Cytosolic phospholipase A2	Parturition failure (Uozumi et al. 1997; Bonventre et al. 1997)
	Decreased production of eicosanoids and platelet activating factor by peritoneal macrophages stimulated either by LPS or A-23187 failure (Uozumi et al. 1997; Bonventre et al. 1997)
	Reduced eicosanoid synthesis from bone-marrow-derived mast cells (Nakatani et al. 2000; Fujishima et al. 1999)
	Reduced bronchoconstriction and airway hypersensitivity in OVA-induced systemic anaphylaxis (Uozumi et al. 1997)
	Reduced postischemic brain injury (Bonventre et al. 1997)
	Reduced acute lung injury induced by systemic LPS or acid aspiration (Nagase et al. 2000)
	Suppression of intestinal polyposis in $Apc^{\Delta716}$ mice (Takaku et al. 2000)
	Renal concentrating defect (Downey et al. 2001)
Cyclooxygenase-1	Reduced inflammatory swelling after arachidonic acid application (Langenbach et al. 1995)
	Decreased arachidonic acid-induced platelet aggregation (Langenbach et al. 1995)
	Reduced susceptibility to indomethacin-induced stomach ulceration (Langenbach et al. 1995)
	Augmented airway inflammation and sensitivity in OVA-induced allergic asthma model (Gavett et al. 1999)
	Increased susceptibility to dextran sodium sulfate-induced colitis (Morteau et al. 2000)
	Increased susceptibility to ischemic brain injury (Iadecola et al. 2001)
	Increased cardiac ischemia-reperfusion injury (Camitta et al. 2001)
	Decreased crypt cell survival in radiation injury (Houchen et al. 2000)
	Less acetic acid-induced writhing response (Ballou et al. 2000)
	Reduced polyp formation in Min mice (Chulada et al. 2000)
	Impaired transition of CD4$^-$CD8$^-$ double-negative to CD4$^+$CD8$^+$ double-positive thymocyte maturation (Rocca et al. 1999)
	Delayed onset of labor in parturition (Gross et al. 1998)

Table 1 (continued)

Affected gene	Phenotype (references)
Cyclooxygenase-2	Renal dysplasia (Dincuk et al. 1995; Morham et al. 1995)
	Myocardial fibrosis (Dincuk et al. 1995)
	Reduced LPS-induced hepatotoxicity (Dinchuk et al. 1995)
	Multiple female reproductive failures including ovulation, fertilization, implantation, and decidualization (Lim et al. 1997)
	Reduced intestinal polyp formation in $Apc^{\Delta716}$ mice (Ohshima et al. 1996)
	Reduced polyp formation in Min mice (Chulada et al. 2000)
	Enhanced allergic inflammation in OVA-induced allergic asthma model (weaker phenotype than COX-1-deicient mice) (Gavett et al. 1999)
	Increased susceptibility to dextran sodium sulfate-induced colitis (Morteau et al. 2000)
	Loss of febrile response to LPS and interleukin 1β (Li et al. 1999, 2001)
	Reduced osteoclast formation in culture (Okada et al. 2000)
	Reduced susceptibility to collagen-induced arthritis (Myers et al. 2000)
	Patent ductus arteriosus (35%) (Loftin et al. 2001)
	Reduced LPS-induced anorexia (Johnson et al. 2002)
	Increased toxicity and lethality in acetaminophen-induced liver injury (Reilly et al. 2001)
	Increased cardiac ischemia and reperfusion injury (Camitta et al. 2001)
	Reduced brain ischemic injury (Iadecola et al. 2001)
	Impaired renin production in response to ACE inhibition (Cheng et al. 2001)
	Impaired transition of $CD4^+CD8^+$ double-positive thymocytes to CD4 single-positive T cells (Rocca et al. 1999)
Combined Cox-1 and Cox-2	Patent ductus arteriosus (100% penetrance) (Loftin et al. 2001)
Lipocalin-type PGD synthase	Reduced mechanical allodynia induced by intrathecal injection of PGE_2 (Eguchi et al. 1999)
Transgenic mouse with overexpression of a gene for:	
Lipocalin-type PGD synthase	Enhanced airway inflammation in OVA-induced allergic asthma model (Fujitani et al. 2002)
	Induction of non-REM sleep by tail clipping (Pinzar et al. 2000)
PGI synthase	Suppression of development of hypoxic pulmonary hypertension (Geraci et al. 1999)
Human PGI synthase	Decreased lung tumorigenesis (Keith et al. 2002)
	Suppression of neointimal formation in carotid balloon injury in rat (Todaka et al. 1999)
	Amelioration of monocrotaline-induced pulmonary hypertension in rat (Nagaya et al. 2000)

Table 2 Transgenic mice of prostanoid receptors

Affected Gene	Phenotypes (references)
Knockout mouse with disruption of a gene for:	
DP	Decreased allergic responses in ovalbumin-induced bronchial asthma (Matsuoka et al. 2000) Impaired PGD_2-induced sleep (Mizoguchi et al. 2001)
E- P1	Decreased aberrant foci formation to azoxymethane (Watanabe et al. 1997) Deceased PGE_2-induced mechanical allodynia (Minami et al. 2001)
E- P2	Impaired ovulation and fertilization (Hizaki et al. 1999; Kennedy et al. 1999; Tilley et al. 1999) Salt-sensitive hypertension (Kennedy et al. 1999; Tilley et al. 1999) Vasopressor or impaired vasodepressor response to PGE_2 (Audoly et al. 1999; Zhang et al. 2000) Loss of bronchodilation to PGE_2 (Sheller et al. 2000) Impaired osteoclastogenesis in vitro (Li et al. 2000) Impaired amplification of COX and angiogenesis of intestinal polyps in $Apc^{\Delta716}$ mice (Sonoshita et al. 2001; Seno et al. 2002)
E- P3	Impaired febrile response to pyrogens (Ushikubi et al. 1998) Impaired duodenal bicarbonate secretion and mucosal integrity (Takeuchi et al. 1999) Enhanced vasodepressor response to PGE_2 (Audoly et al. 1999) Disappearance of indomethacin-sensitive urine diluting function (Fleming et al. 1998) Decreased acetic acid-induced writhing in endotoxin-pretreated mice (Ueno et al. 2001) Impaired PGE_2-induced potentiation of platelet activation (Ma et al. 2001; Fabre et al. 2001).
E- P4	Patent ductus arteriosus (Nguyen et al. 1997; Segi et al. 1998) Impaired vasodepressor response to PGE_2 (Audoly et al. 1999) Decreased inflammatory bone resorption (Miyaura et al. 2000; Sakuma et al. 2000) Lack of PGE_2-induced in vivo bone formation (Yoshida et al. 2002) Exaggerated dextran sodium sulfate-induced colitis (Kabashima et al. 2002) Decreased aberrant foci formation to azoxymethane (Mutoh et al. 2002)
FP	Loss of parturition (Sugimoto et al. 1997)
IP	Thrombotic tendency (Murata et al. 1997) Decreased inflammatory swelling (Murata et al. 1997; Ueno et al. 2000) Decreased acetic acid writhing (Murata et al. 1997) Enhanced cardiac ischemia-reperfusion injury (Xiao et al. 2001) Impaired adaptive gastric cytoprotection (Boku et al. 2001) Impaired capsaicin-induced gastric cytoprotection (Takeuchi et al. 2001) Enhanced pulmonary hypertension and vascular remodeling under chronic hypoxic conditions (Hoshikawa et al. 2001)
TP	Bleeding tendency and resistance to thromboembolism (Thomas et al. 1998)
Transgenic mouse with overexpression of a gene for:	
TP in vasculature	Intrauterine growth retardation of embryos (Rocca et al. 2000) Amplified proliferation in the balloon-induced vascular injury (Cheng et al. 2002)

2
Sickness Behaviors and Other Central Nervous System Actions

A systemic disease causes in patients general and characteristic central symptoms including fever generation, adrenocorticotropic hormone (ACTH) release, reduced locomotion, loss of social contact, anorexia, and increased sleep (Kent et al. 1992). These effects, collectively referred to as "sickness behaviors," can be reproduced experimentally in animals by treatment with sickness substances such as lipopolysaccharide (LPS) and inflammatory cytokines. Because administration of NSAIDs alleviates most of these behaviors, involvement of prostanoids in generation of these symptoms has been strongly suggested. However, little is known about molecular and neuronal mechanism underlying these behaviors.

2.1
Fever Generation

Fever is a representative component of the sickness behaviors. Both cellular components of infectious organisms, such as LPS, as well as by noninfectious inflammatory insults stimulate the production of cytokines such as interleukin (IL)-1, IL-6, and tumor necrosis factor (TNF)-α, that then work as endogenous pyrogens and stimulates the neural pathways that raise body temperature (Kluger 1991). Fever can be suppressed by NSAIDs, which indicates that PGs are important in fever generation. Li et al. (1999) examined the involvement of COX isoforms in fever generation by subjecting COX-1$^{-/-}$ and COX2$^{-/-}$ mice to LPS treatment. They found that COX-2$^{-/-}$ homozygous mice did not develop febrile response to LPS, while COX-1$^{-/-}$ mice exhibited about 1°C rise of core temperature within 1 h after LPS administration, as did wildtype mice. This group also reported loss of fever generation in COX-2$^{-/-}$ but not in COX-1$^{-/-}$ mice in response to IL-1β (Li et al. 2001). This is consistent with inhibition of fever generation by selective COX-2 inhibitors (Li et a. 1999). It is also known that pyrogens induce COX-2 expression in endothelial cells in the organum vasculosum laminae terminalis, a presumed site of pyrogen action (Cao et al. 1995). As to a prostanoid-mediating fever, PGE$_2$ has been strongly suspected, because PGE$_2$ injected into the brain induces fever in many species. Ushikubi et al. (1998) used mice lacking each subtype of the PGE receptor, EP1, EP2, EP3, and EP4, and examined their febrile responses to PGE$_2$, IL-1β, and LPS. They found that the EP3 receptor-deficient mice failed to show febrile responses to all of these stimuli. This study has thus clearly demonstrated that PGE$_2$ mediates fever generation in response to both exogenous and endogenous pyrogens by acting on the EP3 receptor. Recently, Ek et al. (2001) reported that the IL-1-induced induction of COX-2 in rat brain vascular cells is associated with upregulation of membrane-type PGE synthase (mPGES) mRNA. Yamagata et al. (2001) also reported LPS-induced induction of mPGES, and its colocalization with COX-2 in brain endothelial cells. These results suggest that mPGES may play an essential role in

PGE_2 production in fever generation. However, no knockout mice study on this enzyme has yet been reported.

2.2
Sleep Induction

PGD_2 is one of the major PGs in the brain and a potent endogenous sleep-promoting substance in rats and other mammals including humans (Urade and Hayaishi 2000). In the brain, the lipocalin-type PGD synthase is present in a high amount in the leptomeninges, and is thought responsible for production of PGD_2 in this organ. Indeed, transgenic mice over-expressing this type of PGD synthase were reported to show a marked increase in slow-wave sleep with concomitant increase in brain PGD_2 content, when stimulated by tail clipping (Pinzar et al. 2000). The PGD_2-induced sleep is apparently mediated by the DP receptor present also in leptomeninges. Mizoguchi et al. (2001) used DP-deficient mice and compared the effects of PGD_2 infusion into the lateral ventricle on sleep of wildtype and $DP^{-/-}$ mice. They found that, while the PGD_2 infusion significantly increased slow-wave sleep in wildtype mice, it did not change the amounts of slow-wave as well as paradoxical sleep in DP-deficient mice. These results clearly demonstrate that DP is crucially involved in the PGD_2-induced slow-wave sleep. PGD_2-induced sleep has been shown to be mediated by adenosine through the adenosine A_{2A} receptor system (Satoh et al. 1998). Consistently, Mizoguchi et al. demonstrated that the extracellular adenosine content is increased in the subarachnoid space after PGD_2 infusion in a DP-dependent manner. Interestingly, the baseline sleep–wake patterns were essentially identical between wildtype and DP-deficient mice, suggesting that the PGD_2-DP system may not be crucial for basal sleep–wake regulation. This system may be more likely involved in generation of pathological sleep. It was already reported that injection of IL-1β and TNF-α into the PGD_2-sensitive zone of the brain induces sleep in a COX-2-dependent manner (Terao et al. 1998). Overproduction of PGD_2 has been observed in some sleep disorders such as systemic mastocytosis and African sleeping sickness (Urade and Hayaishi 2000). Recently, a malaria parasite, *Plasmodium falciparum*, was reported to produce PGs, including PGD_2 in humans (Kilunga Kubata et al. 1998). Studies in mice deficient in the lipocalin-type PGD synthase (Eguchi et al. 1999) are expected to help clarify this issue further.

2.3
Other Sickness Behaviors

Anorexia is another behavior of sickness. Swiergiel and Dumm (2001) and Johnson et al. (2002) examined involvement of COX isozymes in elicitation of this behavior by using knockout mice deficient in either isoform. Both groups found that genetic disruption or pharmacological inhibition of COX-2 significantly attenuated anorexia induced in mice by LPS or IL-1, and partially prevented weight loss. However, the effect of COX-2 inhibition on anorexia remained partial, suggesting that the existence of both COX-dependent and COX-independent mechanisms in hypophagic response to sickness stimuli.

3
Inflammation and Pain

3.1
Inflammation

Local reddening, heat generation, swelling, and pain are classic signs of acute inflammation. Each of these symptoms, except pain, is caused by increased blood flow and vascular permeability with resultant edema. Previous studies suggested that PGs are primarily involved in vasodilation in the inflammatory process and synergize with other mediators such as histamine and bradykinin to cause an increase in vascular permeability and edema. Since the identification of COX-2 as an inducible COX isoform by various inflammatory stimuli, a significant number of studies have associated this isoform with the inflammatory processes. It was therefore surprising that the initial analyses of COX-$2^{-/-}$ mice showed unaltered inflammation in these mice in tests such as ear swelling by arachidonic acid or 12-O-tetradecanoylphorbol 13-acetate (TPA) and carrageenan-induced paw edema (Dinchuk et al. 1995; Morham et al. 1995). On the other hand, COX-$1^{-/-}$ mice showed reduced ear swelling to arachidonic acid but not to TPA (Langenbach et al. 1995). These results may be due to relatively short observation time after the stimuli, 1–2 h, 4–7 h, and 3 h after application of arachidonic acid, TPA, and carrageenan, respectively. Nonetheless, these studies suggest that COX-1 can contribute to inflammatory response, particularly in the acute phase, and that relative contribution of COX-1 and COX-2 may depend on the inflammatory stimuli, the time after insult, and the relative abundance of each isoform in involved tissues. For example, Langenbach et al. (1999) applied the air pouch model of inflammation to wildtype, COX-$1^{-/-}$, and COX-$2^{-/-}$ mice, and evaluated contribution of each COX isoform to the inflammatory process and the PG level at the inflammatory site. They reported that the PG level in the pouch was elevated 6 h after carrageenan injection, to which COX-1 and COX-2 contributed 25% and 75%, respectively. They further found that the cell infiltration at day 3 was reduced by 50% in COX-$2^{-/-}$ mice but only slightly in COX-$1^{-/-}$ mice, and the resolution of inflammation was delayed in COX-$2^{-/-}$ mice compared to wildtype or COX-$1^{-/-}$ animals. Similarly, Wallace et al. (1998) found in the paw edema model that the footpad swelling in wildtype mice had mostly subsided by 1 week after carrageenan treatment, while the swelling persisted in COX-$2^{-/-}$ mice with lymphocyte infiltration. These results indicate that both COX-1 and COX-2 contribute to PG production but their roles change during extension of inflammation. They further suggest that COX-2 has an additional role in the resolution or healing phase.

It has been previously shown that PGE$_2$ and PGI$_2$ are the potent prostanoids in causing vasodilation and that both of these PGs are present at high concentrations at sites of inflammation (Davies et al. 1984). Murata et al. (1997) used IP-deficient mice to test the role of PGI_2 in inflammatory swelling. They employed carrageenan-induced paw swelling as a model. In this model, swelling increased in a time-dependent manner up to 6 h after injection and was decreased by about 50% upon treatment with indomethacin. IP-deficient mice developed swelling only to a level comparable to that observed in indomethacin-treated wildtype mice, and indomethacin treatment of IP-deficient animals did not induce a further decrease in swelling. On the other hand, PGE_2 injected intradermally could synergize with bradykinin to induce increased vascular permeability in both wildtype and IP-deficient mice. These results indicate that PGI_2 and IP receptor work as the principal PG system mediating vascular changes in this model of inflammation. Whether PGI_2 and the IP receptor play a dominant role in any type of inflammation remains to be seen. An alternative and more likely possibility is that this system and the PGE_2 and EP receptor system are utilized in a context-dependent manner, i.e., one dependent on the stimulus, site, and time of inflammation, as seen for the case of COX isoforms. This point will likely be clarified by comparing responses in IP-deficient mice with those in mice deficient in each subtype of the EP receptors in various inflammation models.

3.2
Pain

The role of prostaglandins in inflammatory pain is also well accepted. This is due to the antinociceptive effects of aspirin-like drugs. Ballou et al. (2000) examined the contribution of COX-1 and COX-2 to pain sensation by subjecting mice deficient in either isoform to acetic acid writhing. They found that COX-$1^{-/+}$ heterozygous mutants showed decreased nociception and that an even greater decrease in COX-1-null mice. On the other hand, no decrease was found in COX-2-null mice, suggesting that only COX-1 plays a role in this type of nociception. However, this result may be taken with caution because an irritant, acetic acid, was injected into the abdomen of naive mice in this test (see below). It was documented in various model systems that PGs added exogenously are able to induce hyperalgesia, an increased sensitivity to a painful stimulus, or allodynia, a pain response to a usually nonpainful stimulus. These studies using exogenous PGs showed that PGE_2, PGE_1, and PGI_2 exert stronger effects than the other types of PG, indicating the involvement of EP or IP receptors in inducing inflammatory pain (Bley et al. 1998). The main site of hyperalgesic action of prostanoids lies in the periphery where prostaglandins are believed to sensitize the free ends of sensory neurons. The primary sensory afferents have their cell bodies in the dorsal root ganglion, and several types of prostanoid receptor mRNAs, including those of IP, EP1, EP3, and EP4, were found in neurons in the ganglion (Sugimoto et al. 1994; Oida et al. 1995). Murata et al. (1997) used IP receptor-deficient mice to address this issue. The IP$^{-/-}$ mice did not show any alteration in their nociceptive reflexes examined by hot plate and tail flick tests, indicating that PGI_2 is not involved in nociceptive neurotransmission at the spinal and supraspinal levels. On the other hand, when these mice were subjected to the acetic acid-induced writing test, they showed markedly decreased responses compared with control wildtype mice, and their responses were as low as those observed in control mice treated with indomethacin. Additionally, both PGE_2 and PGI_2 injected intraperitoneally induced modest writhing responses in wildtype mice, whereas IP-deficient mice showed responses only to PGE_2. These results indicate that the hyperalgesic response in this model is evoked by endogenous PGI_2 acting on the IP receptor in the peripheral end of nociceptive afferents. This study, together with other reports that PGI_2 or its agonists are more effective in eliciting nociception in several model systems, has led to the proposal that IP has a key role in facilitating the sensation of pain (Bley et al. 1998). Recently, however, we found that the receptors other than IP can also amplify pain sensations in a context-dependent manner. Ueno et al. (2001) pretreated $EP1^{-/-}$, $EP2^{-/-}$, $EP3^{-/-}$, $EP4^{-/-}$, $IP^{-/-}$, and wildtype mice with LPS and then examined their hyperalgesic responses to acetic acid administered i.p. Whereas $EP1^{-/-}$, $EP2^{-/-}$, and $EP4^{-/-}$ mice showed a similar enhanced writhing response as the wildtype mice, $IP^{-/-}$ and $EP3^{-/-}$ mice showed significant reductions. Thus, the nociception of the writhing response in non-treated mice is mediated mainly by the IP receptor, whereas in LPS-pretreated mice it is mediated by both IP and EP3 receptors. Probably consistent with this finding, two groups reported that a neutralizing monoclonal antibody against PGE_2 inhibits phenylbenzoquinone-induced writhing in mice and carrageenan induced paw hyperalgesia in rats to the same extent as indomethacin (Mnich et al. 1995; Portanova et al. 1996). It was also reported that the selective COX-2 inhibitor, celecoxib, but not selective COX-1 inhibitor, SC560, reduced carrageenan-induced paw hyperalgesia (Smith et al. 1998). These results indicate also the COX isoform involved in hyperalgesia can vary in a context-dependent manner.

In addition to these hyperalgesic actions in the periphery, PGs are also involved in augmenting processing of pain information in the spinal cord. For example, Minami et al. (1994) found that intrathecal injection of PGE_2 into mice induced allodynia; the mice showed squeaking, biting, and scratching in response to low-threshold stimuli. To characterize EP subtype(s) involved in PGE_2-induced allodynia, Minami et al. (2001) examined the response in the $EP1^{-/-}$ or $EP3^{-/-}$ mice. Intrathecal (i.t.) administration of PGE_2 (500 ng/kg) induced allodynia over the 50-min experimental period in the wildtype and the EP3-deficient mice, but not in the EP1-deficient mice, suggesting that the EP1 receptor is involved in the PGE_2-induced allodynia. Eguchi et al. (1999) examined further PGE_2-induced allodynia in mice deficient in lipocalin-type PGD synthase. They found that PGE_2-induecd allodynia was absent in these mice, and was recovered by the i.t. addition of PGD_2. Interestingly, the recovering effect of PGD_2 showed a bell-shaped dose–effect relationship, suggesting that PGD_2 exerts dual actions in elicitation of allodynia by PGE_2. The PGD synthase-deficient mice also exhibited loss of allodynia induced by i.t. injection of a γ-aminobutyric acid (GABA) antagonist, bicuculline, indicating that PGD_2 also mediated this type of allodynia.

4
Allergy and Immunity

4.1
Allergy

The type I allergic reaction (anaphylaxis) underlies the pathogenesis of bronchial asthma, atopic dermatitis, and anaphylactic shock. Affected individuals produce immunoglobulin (Ig)E antibodies to allergens such as those derived from house dust mites and plant pollens. Exposure to those allergens induces mast cell activation by antigen-antibody-mediated cross-linking of IgE receptors on their surface, which develops allergic reactions. The Th2 subset of T lymphocytes and their cytokines are critically involved in mediating IgE production as well as development of the diseases. In addition, various prostanoids, leukotrienes, and platelet-activating factor are produced in significant amounts by initial mast cell activation and during subsequent disease development. PGD_2 is the major prostanoid produced by mast cells in response to antigen challenge. The role and contribution of prostanoids in the type I allergic responses have been examined by subjecting transgenic mice for related enzymes and receptors. Uozumi et al. (1997) sensitized $cPLA_2^{-/-}$ mice with ovalbumin (OVA) and evoked systemic anaphylaxis in these mice by intravenous injection of OVA 18 days later. They found that both bronchoconstriction and airway hypersensitivity induced by OVA challenge were much reduced in $cPLA_2^{-/-}$ mice. This finding indicates that $cPLA_2$ is the major PLA_2 for production of various lipid mediators in allergy and plays a critical role in elicitation of allergic reactions. The same group (Nakatani et al. 2000) then used bone marrow-derived mast cells obtained from $cPLA_2^{-/-}$ mice and specifically examined involvement of $cPLA_2$ in lipid mediator release from mast cells. They found that antigen cross-linking of FcεRI on cells from $cPLA_2^{-/-}$ mice caused the release of only negligible amounts of arachidonic acid and its metabolites, PGD_2 and cysteinyl leukotrienes, indicating that $cPLA_2$ is indeed essential for production of these lipid mediators in activated mast cells. The same conclusion was obtained by another group in a different strain of $cPLA_2^{-/-}$ mice (Fujishima et al. 1999). The role of COX in type I allergy was also examined by OVA-sensitized knockout mice. There is a subset of patients with asthma in whom aspirin precipitates asthmatic attacks. Interestingly, these patients develop not only severe asthmatic attacks, but also other signs of immediate hypersensitivity such as rhinorrhea, conjunctival irritation, and flushing of head and neck. The existence of such a distinct clinical syndrome, called aspirin-induced asthma (Szczeklik et al. 1999), suggests that there should be a PG(s) negatively modulating type I allergic reactions. Gavett et al. (1999) examined this issue by subjecting $COX-1^{-/-}$ mice or $COX-2^{-/-}$ mice to OVA-induced allergic asthma. They sensitized these mice with intraperitoneal injection of OVA and then challenged them with inhalation of OVA aerosol. They found that both COX-1-deficient and COX-2-deficient mice exhibited enhanced allergic lung responses. These phenotypes are consistent with the findings in patients with aspirin-induced asthma. While some of the increased responses may be due to increased biosynthesis of leukotrienes in COX-deficient mice, increased allergic responses seen with both types of knock-out mice could not be explained by this hypothesis alone, and strongly suggest that both COX-1 and COX-2 products limit allergic lung inflammation. This study thus highlights the beneficial aspects of prostanoids in allergy. As described above, PGD_2 is a major PG produced by activated mast cells and is released in large amounts during asthmatic attacks in some population of patients. However, the role of PGD_2 in allergic asthma has remained unclear. If this PG were a part of protective PG system against allergy as discussed, disruption in the PGD_2 signaling would worsen the allergic reaction as seen in COX-deficient mice. Matsuoka et al. (2000) tested this issue by applying OVA-induced asthma model to DP-deficient mice. Sensitization and aerosol challenge of $DP^{-/-}$ mice with OVA induced increases in the serum concentration of IgE, similar to that found in wildtype mice. However, $DP^{-/-}$ mice did not develop asthmatic responses in this model; OVA-challenged $DP^{-/-}$ mice showed decreased concentrations of Th2-cytokines and a reduced extent of lymphocyte accumulation and eosinophil infiltration in the lung compared to the wildtype animals subjected to this model. Thus, it is apparent that PGD_2 functions as a mast cell-derived mediator to trigger asthmatic responses and not as a negative modulator. This conclusion was supported by the findings in mice overexpressing the lipocalin-type PGD synthase. These mice subjected to essentially the same protocol exhibited enhanced asthmatic response to OVA challenge. Thus, there is a discrepancy between the observation in COX-deficient mice and those obtained in $DP^{-/-}$ and PGD synthase transgenic mice. The most likely explanation for this discrepancy is that a PG other than PGD_2 works for negative modulation of allergy. The most likely candidate is PGE_2, because it has been known for some time that PGE_2 exerts anti-allergic effects in some contexts (see, for example, Raud et al. 1988). The identity of the EP receptor mediating this action remains to be clarified.

4.2
Immunity

While COX isoforms and prostanoid receptors such as EP, IP, and TP are widely expressed in cells of immunity and in vitro immunomodulatory actions of PGE_2 are well known, only a few reports are available that have dissected in vivo roles of prostanoids in immunity using transgenic animals. Rocca et al. (1999) used fetal thymic organ culture and examined effects on thymocyte differentiation of selective COX-1 or COX-2 inhibitors as well as disruption of a gene for either isoform. They found that COX-1 inhibitors, added to the culture, significantly suppressed transition of $CD4^-CD8^-$ double-negative thymocytes to $CD4^+CD8^+$ double-positive cells, while COX-2-selective inhibitors impaired the differentiation of $CD4^+CD8^+$ cells to $CD4^+$ single-positive T cells. The effect of the COX-2 inhibitors was reproduced in the thymus culture from $COX-2^{-/-}$ mice, and the suppression of the double-negative to double-positive cells was also noted, albeit weakly, in the thymi of COX-$1^{-/-}$ mice. They also reported that PGE analogs with the EP2 agonist activity could rescue the inhibition on CD4$^+$CD8$^+$ double-positive cell maturation by COX-1 inhibitors, and those with the EP1 agonist activity reversed the effects of COX-2 inhibitors. These results suggest that both COX isozymes and the PGE$_2$ signaling are required for the efficient maturation of the T cell lineage in fetal thymus.

Rheumatoid arthritis is a disease of immunological inflammation in which NSAIDs are widely used. One animal model for rheumatoid arthritis is the collagen-induced arthritis, in which immunization with type II collagen induces a polyarthritis in 2–4 weeks after immunization in susceptible animals through both T cell activation and the production of anti-collagen antibody. This model is quite sensitive to NSAID treatment. Myers et al. (2000) applied this model to COX-$1^{-/-}$ or COX-$2^{-/-}$ mice and examined the roles of COX isoforms in the development of arthritis. The development of arthritis was greatly suppressed both clinically and histologically in COX-$2^{-/-}$ mice. COX-$2^{-/-}$ mice not only showed marked suppression in production of anti-collagen antibodies, but also did not develop arthritis even when anti-collagen antibodies were passively transferred. On the other hand, essentially no difference was noted in development of arthritis between wildtype and COX-$1^{-/-}$ mice. These results indicate that COX-2 works critically in this model in elicitation of both immune and inflammation responses. Interestingly, these authors found upregulation of production of cytokines such as lymphotoxin (LT)β, TNF-α, and transforming growth factor (TGF)-β in splenocytes from immunized COX-$1^{-/-}$ and COX-$2^{-/-}$ mice, suggesting modulatory action of PGs in production of these cytokines. This is consistent with a recent report by Shinomiya et al. (2001).

They found that indomethacin upregulates and PGE$_2$ or an IP agonist downregulates the production of TNF-α in peritoneal macrophages stimulated with zymosan. They then used various type-selective compounds and mice deficient in EP subtype or IP, and found that this modulation of TNF-α production is elicited redundantly by EP2, EP4, and IP receptors through an increase in cAMP. Intriguingly, the apparently identical mechanisms work to suppress IL-10 production. Thus, indomethacin decreases, and signaling through EP2, EP4, and IP increases production of this anti-inflammatory cytokine. Interestingly, IL-10 suppresses induction of COX-2 in LPS-treated spleen cells, and thereby decreases the production of PGs (Berg et al. 2001).

5
Cardiovascular Homeostasis

5.1
Thrombosis, Hemostasis, and Blood Pressure

Most PGs elicit contractile and/or relaxant activities on vascular smooth muscles in vitro and in vivo. In particular, PGI$_2$ and TXA$_2$, produced abundantly by vascular endothelial cells and platelets, respectively, are a potent vasodilator and vasoconstrictor, respectively. PGE_2 also exerts either contraction or relaxation of blood vessels dependent on the EP receptor subtypes (see below). However, mice deficient in $cPLA_2$, one of the COX isoforms, or any of the eight types of prostanoid receptors do not show abnormality in blood pressure or develop spontaneous vascular accidents such as thrombosis under the basal conditions. For example, Murata et al. (1997) found that while $IP^{-/-}$ mice lacked the hypotensive response to the synthetic IP agonist cicaprost, their basal blood pressure and heart rate were not different from those of control animals. This is probably because the prostanoid system does not work constitutively in cardiovascular regulation but more likely works on demand in response to local stimuli. This kind of role is quite important to maintain vascular homeostasis locally. Because PGI_2 and TXA_2 act oppositely on platelets and blood vessels, it has been suggested that a balance between the PGI_2 and TXA_2 systems is important to prevent thrombosis and vasospasm while performing efficient hemostasis. A study on $IP^{-/-}$ mice (Murata et al. 1997) indeed showed that, while they develop and age normally, they show an enhanced thrombotic tendency when endothelial damage is evoked. These findings confirmed the long-standing role of PGI_2 as an endogenous anti-thrombotic agent and suggest that this anti-thrombotic system is activated in response to vascular injury to attenuate its effects. Consistently, the increased production of PGI_2 by gene transfer of PGI synthase at the site of balloon injury was reported to prevent restenosis of rat carotid artery (Todaka et al. 1999). In contrast to PGI_2, TXA_2 has been implicated in thrombosis and hemostasis on the basis of its pro-aggregatory and vasocontractile activities. Indeed, TP-deficient mice showed increased bleeding tendencies and were resistant to cardiovascular shock induced by intravenous infusion of a TP agonist, U-46619, and arachidonic acid (Thomas et al. 1998). Cheng et al. (2002) recently examined the interplay between IP and TP signaling in cardiovascular homeostasis. They subjected $IP^{-/-}$ mice and $TP^{-/-}$ mice to balloon catheter-induced vascular injury model, and found that the IP deficiency increased and TP-deficiency decreased injury-induced vascular proliferation and platelet activation. They further showed that the augmented response in $IP^{-/-}$ mice was abolished in mice deficient in both IP and TP. The authors concluded that PGI_2, through its action on IP, modulates platelet–vascular interactions in vivo and specifically limits the response to TXA_2. In addition to PGI_2 and TXA_2, PGE_2 is also known to act on blood platelets and potentiate aggregation response. However, the identity of receptor mediating this PGE_2 action and its pathophysiological significance remains unknown. Using mice deficient in each EP subtype, Fabre et al. (2001) and Ma et al. (2001) identified that EP3 mediates this potentiation by PGE_2. They further showed that $EP3^{-/-}$ mice exhibited decreased response in the arachidonic acid-induced thrombosis models. In addition, Ma et al., but not Fabre et al., found that the bleeding time was significantly prolonged in $EP3^{-/-}$ mice. These findings suggest that this PGE_2 action may play a role in vascular homeostasis in vivo.

PGE$_2$ also elicits contractile and/or relaxant responses when tested on vascular smooth muscles in vitro. These PGE$_2$ actions that are not obviously seen in vivo in wildtype animals become evident in mice deficient in each EP subtype. For example, Kennedy et al. (1999) administered PGE$_2$ and PGE analogs intravenously into EP2$^{-/-}$ mice and found that PGE$_2$ or a mixed EP1/3 agonist, sulprostone, evoked considerable hypertension, while an EP2 agonist, butaprost, failed to induce a transient hypotension seen in wildtype mice. The authors suggested that the absence of the EP2 receptor abolishes the ability of the mouse vasculature to vasodilate in response to PGE$_2$ and unmasks the contractile response mediated via the vasoconstrictor EP receptor(s). Interestingly, when fed a high-salt diet, the EP2-deficient mice develop significant hypertension with a concomitant increase in urinary excretion of PGE$_2$. These results indicate that PGE$_2$ is produced in the body in response to a high-salt diet and works to decrease blood pressure via the relaxant EP2 receptor, and that dysfunction of this pathway may be involved in the development of salt-sensitive hypertension. Recently, Audoly et al. (1999) compared the roles of individual EP receptors in males and females. They found that the relative contribution of each EP receptor subtype was strikingly different between males and females. In females, the EP2 and EP4 receptors mediate the major portion of the vasodepressor response to PGE$_2$. In males, the EP2 receptor has a modest role, and most of the vasodepressor effect is mediated by the phospholipase C-coupled EP1 receptor. In addition, in male mice the EP3 receptor actively opposes the vasodepressor actions of PGE$_2$. Thus, the hemodynamic actions of PGE$_2$ are mediated through complex interactions involving several EP subtypes, and the role of individual EP receptors in males differs dramatically from that in females.

5.2
Ischemic and Reperfusion Injury

Lack of prostanoid signaling appears to affect injuries by ischemia and post-ischemic reperfusion in various ways. Iadecola et al. (2001a,b) examined effects of the lack of COX-1 or COX-2 on ischemic brain injury by permanent occlusion of the left middle cerebral artery in COX-1$^{-/-}$ or COX-2$^{-/-}$ mice. Interestingly, deficiency of COX-1 significantly increased, and that of COX-2 significantly decreased the infarct volume as compared to that found in wildtype control mice. Monitoring of cerebral blood flow of these mice revealed that the blood flow at the periphery of ischemic area was significantly reduced in COX-1$^{-/-}$ mice. On the other hand, no alteration of blood flow was observed in COX-2$^{-/-}$ mice. They next microinjected N-methyl-D-aspartate (NMDA) directly into the cortex and examined the involvement of the NMDA-mediated cytotoxicity in elicitation of the phenotypes of COX-1 or COX-2 deficiency, because glutamate receptors play a critical role in the initiation of ischemic brain injury. NMDA caused the brain injury at the site of injection, and also induced local production of PGE$_2$. The size of the lesion was significantly suppressed in COX-2$^{-/-}$ mice or in wildtype mice treated with a COX-2 inhibitor, NS398. NS398 also suppressed the

NMDA-induced increase in PGE_2 production. On the other hand, the NMDA injection caused as much brain lesion in COX-1$^{-/-}$ mice as in wildtype control mice. These results indicate that in brain ischemia, COX-1-derived prostanoids work to limit an ischemia area by maintaining circulation around its periphery, while COX-2-derived prostanoids work to amplify NMDA receptor-mediated cytotoxicity. Brain ischemic injury was also caused by the middle cerebral artery occlusion in cPLA$_2$$^{-/-}$ mice (Bonventre et al. 1997). As observed in COX-2$^{-/-}$ mice, no difference in the cerebral blood flow was noted, either, between cPLA$_2$$^{-/-}$ mice and wildtype control mice, but protection of the similar extent as observed in COX-2$^{-/-}$ mice was obtained in cPLA$_2$$^{-/-}$ mice.

The roles of COX isoforms and receptors such as IP and TP were also examined in cardiac ischemia and reperfusion injury. Camitta et al. (2001) used perfusion of isolated heart in the Langendorff mode, and examined effects of ischemia on left ventricle function in COX-deficient mice. They found that disruption of either gene inhibited recovery of the ventricle function about 50% of that seen in wildtype heart, indicating that prostanoids derived from either COX isoform work to protect cardiac ischemic injury. Curiously, their results indicate that this protective effect was not exerted by prostanoids generated during ischemia and reperfusion but through long-term effects of prostanoids prior to the experiment. On the other hand, Xiao et al. (2001) examined cardiac ischemia–reperfusion injury both in vivo and ex vivo in mice deficient in IP or TP. In vivo they reperfused heart after transient occlusion of the left anterior descending coronary artery for 1 h and examined the size of myocardial infarct. They found a significant increase of the infarct in IP$^{-/-}$ mice compared to that found in wildtype mice, while there was no difference between wildtype and TP$^{-/-}$ mice. Similarly, the ex vivo heart perfusion experiment showed that the coronary flow and the developed cardiac tension were significantly suppressed in the heart from IP$^{-/-}$ mice. From these findings, the authors conclude that PGI_2 is apparently produced during cardiac ischemia and reperfusion and exerts a protective effect on cardiomyocytes independent of its effect on platelets and neutrophils.

5.3
Pulmonary Hypertension

Pulmonary hypertension is a disease in which the pulmonary vasculature undergoes extensive remodeling, leading to elevations in pulmonary artery pressure and pulmonary vascular resistance. While decreased prostacyclin formation has been found in the patients with pulmonary hypertension and in several animal models for this disease, the causative relation of this phenomenon remains unknown. Geraci et al. (1999) addressed this question by creating and subjecting transgenic mice with pulmonary overexpression of PGI synthase to the hypobaric hypoxic condition. They found that, while exposure to this condition for 5 weeks induced pulmonary hypertension in wildtype mice, the PGI synthase transgenic mice were apparently unaffected as evidenced by no elevation of pulmonary artery pressure and no hypertrophy of the pulmonary vessel wall. Involvement of impaired PGI_2 signaling in pathogenesis of pulmonary hypertension was further suggested by experiments with mice deficient in IP. Hoshikawa et al. (2001) exposed $IP^{-/-}$ mice to a hypobaric and hypoxic condition for 3 weeks and compared the development of pulmonary hypertension in these mice with that found in wildtype mice. They found that chronic hypoxic exposure induced more severe pulmonary hypertension in $IP^{-/-}$ mice as evidenced by increased right ventricular systolic pressure, resulting in more extensive right ventricle hypertrophy and vessel wall thickening. Protective effect of PGI_2 signaling in pulmonary hypertension was also noted in another model, that is, monocrotaline (MCT)-induced pulmonary hypertension. MCT, a toxic plant alkaloid, causes in rats delayed and progressive lung injury characterized by pulmonary vascular remodeling, pulmonary hypertension, and compensatory right heart hypertrophy (Schultze and Roth 1998). Endothelial cell dysfunction and thrombosis of the pulmonary microvasculature likely underlies the pathogenesis of MCT-induced pneumotoxicity. Nagaya et al. (2000) subjected rats transfected with a gene for human PGI synthase in the lung to MCT treatment, and examined the effect of overexpression of PGI synthase on development of pulmonary hypertension. They observed expression of PGI synthase, and, consequently, increased production of PGI_2 in the lung, significantly ameliorated development of pulmonary hypertension by MCT treatment, and improved survival of treated rats.

5.4
Closure of Ductus Arteriosus

At birth, with the commencement of respiration, mammals including humans undergo a dramatic change in their circulation, i.e., from the fetal circulation that shunts blood flow from the main pulmonary artery directly to the aorta via the ductus arteriosus, to the pulmonary circulation system of the neonate. This adaptive change is caused by the closure of the ductus. Maternal administration of NSAIDs induces contraction of the ductus in late-term fetuses, and administration of a vasodilator PG such as PGE_1 maintains the patency of the ductus in neonates. Thus, the patency of the ductus during the fetal period is believed to be maintained principally by the dilator effects of a prostaglandin, and its closure is induced by withdrawal of the dilator prostaglandins as well as active contraction exerted by an increased oxygen tension. Dilator prostanoid receptors such as IP and EP4 are present in the ductus, indicating that they work to maintain the ductus patency. Disruption of the mouse IP gene did not appear to cause any abnormality of the ductus (Murata et al. 1997). On the other hand, most EP4-deficient mice die within 3 days after birth, due to marked pulmonary congestion and heart failure (Nguyen et al 1997; Segi et al. 1998). Administration of indomethacin into maternal mice during late pregnancy did not induce the closure of the ductus in the EP4-deficient fetuses, indicating that the dilatory effect of PGE_2 on this vessel is mediated by the EP4 receptor. These results suggest a critical role for the EP4 receptor in the ductus and can be interpreted to mean that, in the absence of the EP4 receptor, a compensatory mechanism maintains ductus patency not only in the fetal period but also after birth. The role of COX isoforms on the patency of the ductus was also examined recently in mice deficient in either COX isozyme (Loftin et al. 2001). Typically, 35% of COX-2$^{-/-}$ mice die from patent ductus arteriosus within 48 h after birth, whereas no abnormality was found in COX-1$^{-/-}$ mice. The mortality of COX-2$^{-/-}$ mice increased to 79% when one copy of the COX-1 gene was disrupted, and 100% of the mice deficient in both isoforms die with patent ductus arteriosus within 12 h of birth. Thus, the phenotype observed in COX-deficient mice is quite similar to that found in EP4-deficient mice, and indicates the combined contribution of COX-1 and COX-2 to the normal function of the ductus by the PGE2–EP4 signaling. A small but significant difference in survival time and rate between EP4-deficeint mice and mice with combined disruption of COX-1 and COX-2 may suggest that additional prostanoid signaling plays a role in closure of the ductus. Interestingly no ductus phenotype has been reported in cPLA$_2$-deficient mice.

6
Kidney

Prostanoids regulates various functions of the kidney including renal blood flow, glomerular filtration rate, transports of solutes and water through the regulation of thick ascending limb function and antagonism against vasopressin action, and renin secretion in macula densa. Downey et al. (2001) examined the kidney function of cPLA$_2$$^{-/-}$ mice. They found that cPLA$_2$$^{-/-}$ mice did not show alteration in plasma sodium, potassium, creatinine concentrations, creatinine clearance, and fractional excretion of sodium and potassium under the basal conditions. However, these mice showed significantly lower urine osmolality under the basal condition as well as with water deprivation, indicating that they had a defect in urine concentration. This defect worsened with age of the animals, and injection of vasopressin into cPLA$_2$$^{-/-}$ mice during water deprivation did not rescue this phenotype. The authors found marked reduction in aquaporin-1 association with the membrane of proximal tubules of cPLA$_2$$^{-/-}$ mice, and suggested that the mislocalization of this water channel may be a cause of renal concentrating defect in cPLA$_2$$^{-/-}$ mice. Because PGE$_2$ inhibits sodium transport in ascending limb and antagonizes the action of vasopressin, its absence would result in excessive concentration of urine. Therefore, the phenotype of cPLA$_2$ appears opposite to that expected from inhibition of prostanoid action in the kidney tubules. Thus, the renal concentrating defect in cPLA$_2$$^{-/-}$ mice may be a consequence of inhibition of eicosanoids other than prostanoids or the secondary change caused by chronic prostanoid inhibition. In contrast to this relatively mild renal impairment in cPLA$_2$$^{-/-}$ mice, disruption of COX-2 gene caused marked renal dysplasia (Dinchuk et al. 1995; Morham et al. 1995). This dysplasia that begins around postnatal day 10 of COX-2$^{-/-}$ mice increases progressively with age, and results in profound diffuse cyst formation, outer glomerular hypoplasia, periglomerular fibrosis, inner cortical nephron hypertrophy, and diffuse interstitial fibrosis in adult mice (Norwood et al. 2000). As a result, the glomerular filtration rate was reduced by more than 50% and the serum urea and creatinine concentration was elevated in COX-2$^{-/-}$ mice compared to wildtype mice. This degenerative change of the kidney in COX-2$^{-/-}$ mice has made it difficult to evaluate the role of COX-2 in physiological regulation of various kidney functions. However, Cheng et al. (2001) circumvented this problem by using heterozygous COX-2$^{+/-}$ mice together with homozygous mutants, and examined the role of COX-2 in regulation of renin release. COX-2 is known to be expressed in macula densa during various high renin states. They found that COX-2 deficiency prevented the production of renin in response to inhibition of angiotensin-converting enzyme in a gene dose-dependent fashion, suggesting that COX-2 indeed is involved in stimulus-evoked renin release.

There are also reports analyzing kidney functions of mice deficient in prostanoid receptors. As described in the "Cardiovascular System" section above, EP2-deficient mice develop significant hypertension when fed a high-salt diet (Kenedy et al. 1999; Tilley et al. 1999). These animals as well as wildtype mice concomitantly excreted increased amounts of PGE$_2$ in urine (Kenndy et al. 1999). Because unmetabolized PGE$_2$ in the urine mostly reflects the PGE$_2$ production in the kidney medulla, these results indicate that PGE$_2$ produced in response to a high-salt diet may work locally in the kidney to adjust salt handling. Fleming et al. (1998) examined the role of EP3 in sodium and water handling in the kidney tubules in subjecting EP3$^{-/-}$ mice to vasopressin administration or water loading and deprivation. They found that, while EP3$^{-/-}$ mice showed impaired increase of urine osmolality that was found in wildtype mice after indomethacin treatment, they showed no alteration in concentration and dilution of urine in response to the above stimuli. While these results indicate that the EP3-mediated process is not critically involved in regulation of urine osmolality under these conditions, whether they indicate relatively little physiological role of prostanoids or involvement of prostanoid receptors other than EP3 in this type of regulation is not known.

7
Reproduction

Various reproductive effects of NSAIDs have long indicated that prostanoids critically work at multiple steps of pregnancy and parturition. Recent studies on various knockout mice deficient in enzymes and receptors for prostanoids have confirmed this long-standing speculation and provided deeper insights into their actions. First, there appeared multiple defects in reproduction in cPLA$_2$$^{-/-}$ mice (Bonventre et al. 1997; Uozumi et al. 1997). Female cPLA$_2$$^{-/-}$ mice become pregnant less frequently, and produce smaller litters. Their pregnancy often fails near the time of implantation, and when the pregnancy continues, the onset of labor is commonly delayed, resulting in production of dead pups. These findings indicate that a cPLA$_2$$^{-/-}$ mother has defects in ovulation, fertilization, implantation, and parturition. Pups near term in cPLA$_2$$^{-/-}$ mother can be rescued by Caesarian section and by administration of a progesterone antagonist RU486. This phenotype of delayed onset of labor in cPLA$_2^{-/-}$ female is similar to that observed in COX-1$^{-/-}$ mice and FP-deficient mice (see below), suggesting that cPLA$_2$ couples to COX-1 to produce PGF$_{2\alpha}$ to induce parturition at term. Similar to cPLA$_2^{-/-}$ mice, the presence of multiple defects in reproduction was also noted in mice deficient in COX isoforms. Interestingly, COX-1 and COX-2 have distinct roles in reproduction. While COX-1$^{-/-}$ females become pregnant normally and have a normal litter size, they show delayed parturition resulting in neonatal death (Gross et al. 1998). Bolus injection of PGF$_{2\alpha}$ at day 19.5 gestation can induce labor in the COX-1$^{-/-}$ mother and result in successful parturition of live pups. These results suggest that COX-1 is not involved in the early events of pregnancy but regulates the onset of labor by producing PGF$_{2\alpha}$. On the other hand, COX-2-deficient female mice showed multiple reproductive failures in early pregnancy (Dinchuk et al. 1995; Lim et al. 1997). Ovaries of null mice were small to a virtual absence of corpora lutea, though follicular development appeared normal. They ovulated fewer eggs on normal ovulation as well as on superovulation, and their fertilization rate was much reduced compared to that in wildtype mice. Furthermore, when wildtype blastocysts were transferred into uteri of day 4 pseudo-pregnant mice, they failed to implant in uteri of COX-2$^{-/-}$ mice. Thus, COX-2$^{-/-}$ females have defects in ovulation, fertilization, and implantation. Due to these defects, COX-2$^{-/-}$ females are largely infertile, but births, if present, occur normally.

The above findings thus suggest that PGs play essential roles in various steps of pregnancy, which have been addressed by analysis of mice deficient in prostanoid receptors. First, three groups reported failure in early pregnancy in EP2-deficient female mice (Hizaki et al. 1999; Kennedy et al. 1999; Tilley et al. 1999). They found that EP2-deficient female mice consistently deliver fewer pups than their wildtype counterparts irrespective of the genotypes of mating males. They detected slightly impaired ovulation and a dramatic reduction in fertilization in EP2-deficient mice. Hizaki et al. (1999) further found that this phenotype is due to impaired expansion of the cumulus of oophorus. Because the EP2 receptor and COX-2 are induced in the cumulus in response to gonadotropins, and PGE$_2$ can induce cumulus expansion by elevating cAMP, these authors proposed that the PGE$_2$ and EP2 receptor system works as a positive-feedback loop to induce the oophorus maturation required for fertilization during and after ovulation. Indeed, unovulated eggs were observed in the ovary at a higher rate in EP2-deficient mice. The next question is the identity and mechanism of prostanoid in the implantation process. Lim et al. (1997) found that the implantation/decidualization defect in COX-2$^{-/-}$ mice was partially rescued by the addition of either PGE$_2$ or a PGI analog or by treatment with cholera toxin, and suggested a role for PG receptors elevating cAMP level in the cell, such as EP2, EP4, or IP. Indeed, EP2 is highly induced in luminal epithelial cells during the peri-implantation period via a steroid-dependent pathway (Katsuyama et al. 1997; Lim et al. 1997). However, the uteri of EP2-deficient females appear normal in their ability to support implantation of wildtype embryos. One possibility is that EP4 expression in the luminal epithelium can compensate for the EP2 receptor in implantation. Recently, Lim et al. (1999) reported impaired implantation in COX-2-deficient mice, which was reversed by both PGI_2 analogs and an agonist for PPARδ, and proposed that COX-2-derived PGI_2 may participate in implantation through PPARδ. This interesting finding should be carefully interpreted and verified using PPARδ-deficient mice or PPARδ antagonists, particularly because the doses of PGI analogs used in this study were higher than those of PGI_2 under physiological conditions.

$PGF_{2\alpha}$ is accepted as an inducer of luteolysis in domestic animals such as sheep and cow, and has been implicated in parturition via its action as a strong uterotonic substance. However, the FP-deficient mice did not show any abnormalities in early pregnancy, and there were no changes in the estrous cycle. This may be because luteolysis is not required for entrance into a new estrous cycle in mice, and their ovaries contain corpora lutea from a few previous estrous cycles. Sugimoto et al. (1997) found that, despite no alteration in estrous cycle, FP-deficient mothers do not undergo parturition, apparently due to the lack of labor. They further found that FP-deficient mice do not undergo parturition even when given exogenous oxytocin and that they show no prepartum decline in progesterone. A reduction in progesterone levels by ovariectomy 24 h before term resulted in an upregulation of uterine receptors for oxytocin and normal parturition in FP-deficient mice. These experiments indicate that the luteolytic action of $PGF_{2\alpha}$ is required in mice to diminish progesterone levels and thus permit the initiation of labor. In addition to these studies using knockout mice, Rocca et al. (2000) over-expressed TP selectively in vascular tissues under the control of pre-proendothelin-1 promotor, and found that TP over-expression led to the intrauterine growth retardation of embryos in pregnant mothers. This growth retardation could be rescued by suppression of TXA_2 formation with indomethacin, suggesting that the augmented TXA_2 signaling indeed caused this condition. Their findings are quite implicative, because intrauterine growth retardation is commonly associated with maternal diabetes or cigarette smoking, both conditions known associated with increased TXA_2 biosynthesis.

8
Digestive System

8.1
Gastrointestinal Functions

The PGs are widely distributed in the digestive system and regulate a number of physiological processes including secretion of acid and mucus, motility, blood flow, water and electrolyte absorption, and epithelium proliferation. In addition, treatment with aspirin-like drugs is known to induce gastric erosion and ulcer, exacerbate intestinal inflammation, and reduce the risk of colorectal neoplasia, suggesting various roles of PGs in pathogenesis of these conditions. It has been hypothesized that the suppression of gastric COX-1 is critical for gastric erosion formation. From this hypothesis, it appears puzzling that mice deficient in COX-1 exhibit greatly reduced gastric PG synthesis but do not develop spontaneous gastric injury (Langenbach et a. 1995). Interestingly, these mice do develop gastric ulceration when exposed to indomethacin but with less sensitivity. These findings together with a recent pharmacological study comparing effects of COX-1-selective or COX-2-selective inhibition or inhibition of both COX isoforms (Wallace et al. 2000) suggest that inhibition of both COX-1 and COX-2 is required for NSAID-induced gastric damage. Another pharmacological study (Brzozwski et al. 1999) also indicated that both COX-1 and COX-2 are required for healing of gastric lesions induced by ischemia reperfusion. NSAID-induced damage in the stomach and duodenum can be prevented or ameliorated by administration of exogenous PGE_2. Takeuchi and collaborators (Kunikata et al. 2001) examined the identity of EP subtype(s) mediating this effect by using EP subtype-selective agonists and mice deficient in each EP subtype. They found that protection by PGE_2 against gastric damage was mimicked by agonists with EP1 selectivity, while that for the duodenum was mimicked by agonists with EP3 or EP4 selectivity. Consistently, the protective effect of PGE_2 for gastric lesion was not observed in $EP1^{-/-}$ mice, whereas that for duodenal ulcer was absent in $EP3^{-/-}$ mice. These results indicate different EP subtypes mediate protective effects of PGE_2 against NSAID-induced gastrointestinal ulceration, probably through different mechanisms. As a mechanism of the EP3 action in the duodenum, Takeuchi et al. (1999) found that EP3 but not EP1 is involved in acid-induced duodenal bicarbonate secretion, which is important in mucosal defense against acid injury. Another proposed effect of prostanoid for gastric damage is adaptive cytoprotection, a phenomenon in which exposure to mild irritants attenuates gastric damage by subsequent exposure to strong stimuli such as HCl/ethanol. Boku et al. (2001) performed perfusion of stomach with mildly hypertonic saline (1 M NaCl) and then exposed it to ethanol. The preperfusion increases generation of gastric PGE_2 and PGI_2 and reduces the extent of the subsequent ethanol-induced mucosal damage in wildtype mice. They found, however, that the preperfusion with 1 M NaCl to $IP^{-/-}$ mice did not elicit the protective effects seen in the wildtype mice. Their subsequent study revealed that endogenous PGI_2, but not PGE_2, had a role in adaptive cytoprotection of gastric mucosa through release of calcitonin gene-related peptide from sensory nerves. Takeuchi et al. (2001) also examined this issue in $IP^{-/-}$ mice, and reported that PGI_2 is involved critically in capsaicin-induced gastric cytoprotection. This may be consistent with the findings by Boku and colleagues. On the other hand, they found that adaptive cytoprotection by 20 mM taurocholate can be induced normally in $IP^{-/-}$ mice. These results may suggest the presence of different mechanisms for adaptive cytoprotection in response to different stimuli.

8.2
Intestinal Inflammation

Human inflammatory bowel disease (IBD), including Crohn's disease and ulcerative colitis, is a chronic, relapsing, and remitting condition of unknown origin that exhibits various features of immunological inflammation and affects at least one in 1,000 people in Western countries (Fiocchi 1998). IBD is characterized by inflammation in the large and/or small intestine associated with diarrhea, occult blood, abdominal pain, weight loss, anemia, and leukocytosis. Studies in humans have implicated impaired mucosal barrier function, pronounced innate immunity, production of proinflammatory and immunoregulatory cytokines, and the activation of $CD4^+$ T cells in the pathogenesis of IBD. One of the major risk factors triggering and worsening the disease is the administration of NSAIDs (Bjarnason et al. 1993), indicating that the COX inhibition has adverse effects on IBD. Morteau et al. (2000) addressed this issue by examining the susceptibility of mice deficient in either COX-1 or COX-2 to the dextran sodium sulfate (DSS)-induced intestinal inflammation, an animal model for IBD. They have challenged the two strains of mice together with wildtype control mice with either high (10%) or low (2.5%) dose of DSS. While mice with either mutation did not develop spontaneous intestinal inflammation without DSS, both developed severe colitis to a low-dose DSS that induced only marginal colitis in wildtype mice, and 50% of both types homozygous mutant mice died after 5 days of the high-dose DSS treatment. $COX-2^{-/-}$ mice appeared more susceptible than $COX-1^{-/-}$ mice, and showed more severe clinical symptoms and histological injury. These findings have clarified that both COX isoforms play a role in the defense of the intestinal mucosa, the inducible COX-2 being more active during inflammation. While this work verified the involvement of COX in the defense against intestinal inflammation and strongly indicates that COX-derived prostanoids work in this process, little is known about the identity of prostanoid and receptor involved in this process and their mode of actions. Kabashima et al. (2002) used mice deficient in each of the eight types and subtypes of prostanoid receptors, and addressed this issue again by examining their susceptibility to DSS treatment. They found that only EP4-deficient mice developed severe colitis with 3% DSS treatment. They confirmed this finding by reproducing this phenotype in wildtype mice by administration of an EP4-selective antagonist. They further found that the EP4 deficiency impaired mucosal barrier function, and induced epithelial loss, crypt damage, and accumulation of neutrophils and $CD4^+$ T cells in the colon. By DNA microarray, elevated expression of genes associated with immune response and reduced expression of genes with mucosal repair and remodeling were found in the colon of EP4-deficient mice. Based on these findings, they concluded that EP4 maintains intestinal homeostasis by preserving mucosal integrity and downregulating immune response.

The role of PGs in renewal and repair of gastrointestinal epithelium was also examined in a different setting. Houchen, Stenson, and Cohn (2000) applied γ-irradiation to $COX-1^{-/-}$ and $COX-2^{-/-}$ mice and examined apoptosis, stem cell survival in the crypt, and PG synthesis in the intestine. They found that the number of apoptotic cells in the crypt increased and the number of crypt with proliferating cells decreased significantly in COX-1$^{-/-}$ mice. On the other hand, the response of COX-2$^{-/-}$ mice to radiation injury was indistinguishable from that observed in wildtype mice. They also found that production of PGE$_2$ after irradiation was much reduced in the intestine of COX-1$^{-/-}$ mice but not in COX-2$^{-/-}$ mice, and administration of dimethyl-PGE$_2$ significantly suppressed apoptosis of crypt cells, while that of neutralizing anti-PGE$_2$ antibody significantly attenuated the number of surviving crypts. These results indicate that PGs, most likely PGE$_2$, work for protection of gastrointestinal mucosa against radiation injury, and suggest that the relative importance of COX-1 or COX-2 in epithelial wound repair may depend on the nature of the injury and the extent of inflammation accompanying the injury.

8.3
Intestinal Polyposis and Colon Cancer

The involvement of COX isoforms and their products in the development of colon cancer was first suggested by epidemiological studies in humans, and then by pharmacological experiments with rodents. In transgenic mice experiments, two mouse models for human familial adenomatous polyposis are employed. One is Min mice and the other is $Apc^{\Delta716}$ mice. Both have a truncation mutation in the Apc gene and develop polyposis by loss of heterozygosity in heterozygous mutants. The Taketo group (Oshima et al. 1996) constructed compound mice with $Apc^{\Delta716}$ and disruption of COX-2, and showed that disruption of the COX-2 gene reduces the number and size of the intestinal polyps dramatically. Inhibition of polyp formation in the $Apc^{\Delta716}$ mice was also observed upon treatment with a COX-2-selective inhibitor. These results suggested that COX-2 contributes to an early event of the tumorigenesis. This group also examined the role of cPLA$_2$ by constructing compound $Apc^{\Delta716}$ mice deficient in cPLA$_2$ (Takaku et al. 2000). They found that loss of cPLA$_2$ reduced the size of polyps in the small intestine of $Apc^{\Delta716}$ mice significantly, although it did not affect the number of the polyps. Disruption of the cPLA$_2$ gene did not influence the number and size of polyps in the colon either. These differences between $Apc^{\Delta716}/$ cPLA$_2$$^{-/-}$ and $Apc^{\Delta716}/$COX-2$^{-/-}$ mice led the authors to suggest that cPLA$_2$ plays a role in expansion of small intestine polyps, while other PLA$_2$s may be required for polyp generation and expansion in the colon. Indeed, they found overexpression of group X sPLA$_2$ in the colon of $Apc^{\Delta716}$ mice. The Taketo group further examined which type of prostanoid or prostanoid receptor mediates this action by making compound mice with $Apc^{\Delta716}$ mutation and a deletion of either EP1, EP2, or EP3 gene. Using this approach, Sonoshita et al. (2001) reported that homozygous disruption of the EP2 receptor in $Apc^{\Delta716}$ mice caused significant decreases in the number and size of the intestinal polyps, effects similar to those induced by the COX-2 gene disruption. As for the mechanism, they found that the increased PGE$_2$-EP2 receptor signaling amplifies COX-2 expression through a rise in the cellular cAMP level and stimulates the expression of vascular endothelial growth factor (VEGF) in the polyp stroma. Consistently, this group determined angiogenesis by the microvessel density and found that angiogenesis was seen in polyps of $Apc^{\Delta716}$ mice but not in mice with combined mutation in Apc and either of the COX-2 or EP2 gene (Seno et al. 2002). While these studies implicate COX-2, rather than COX-1, in colon carcinogenesis, a role of COX-1 in this process has also been suggested. Chulada et al. (2000) bred COX-1$^{-/-}$ mice or COX-2$^{-/-}$ to the Min mice, and examined the contribution of either COX isoform in colon carcinogenesis. Unexpectedly, they found disruption of either COX-1 or COX-2 reduced polyp formation by ~80% in Min mice. These results suggest that, although $Apc^{\Delta716}$ mice and Min mice have a similar truncation mutation in the Apc gene, the polyp formation in these mice may develop differently, and that COX-1 and COX-2 may contribute to colon carcinogenesis through different mechanisms. Such a situation may be reflected in the findings obtained in the third model of colon carcinogenesis, i.e., the azoxymethane-induced aberrant cryptic foci formation, which is also known to be sensitive to NSAIDs. Wakabayashi and collaborators (Watanabe et al. 1999; Mutoh et al. 2002) subjected mice deficient in each prostanoid receptor to this model, and examined the contribution of each prostanoid receptor in colon carcinogenesis. They found reduction in foci formation in both EP1$^{-/-}$ mice and EP4$^{-/-}$ mice but not in mice deficient in other receptors. In both cases, the number of foci was decreased to 50%–60% of the level of wildtype mice. They furthermore found that administration of an EP1-specific antagonist, ONO-8711, or an EP4 antagonist ONO-AE2-227, in the diet reduced the number and size of polyps in Min mice. An apparent discrepancy between their results and the findings by Taketo's group may indicate that the EP1 and EP4 pathway is linked preferentially to the COX-1 pathway, and are involved in the early phase of carcinogenesis, while the COX-2–EP2 pathway is required for promotion of carcinogenesis.

8.4
Drug-Induced Liver Injury

PGs added exogenously have been shown to be cytoprotective against hepatotoxic agents including LPS, D-galactosamine, carbon tetrachloride, and acetaminophen. Two studies have evaluated the role of endogenous prostanoids in elicitation of and cytoprotection against drug-induced hepatotoxicity by studying responses of COX-2$^{-/-}$ mice. Dinchuk et al. (1995) evoked liver injury in wildtype and COX-2$^{-/-}$ mice by treatment with LPS and D-galactosamine. They found that, while the serum TNF-α level was similarly elevated by this treatment in the two groups, elevation of serum levels of aminotransferase and aspartate aminotransferase were significantly suppressed in COX-2$^{-/-}$ mice compared to wildtype mice. These results suggest that COX-2-derived prostanoids contribute to exacerbate the hepatotoxicity under these conditions. On the other hand, Reilly et al. (2001) administered acetaminophen to wildtype, COX-1$^{-/-}$ and

COX-$2^{-/-}$ mice and compared the extent of hepatotoxicity induced by this drug. They found significantly more extensive liver necrosis, increased mortality, and higher serum aminotransferase level in COX-$2^{-/-}$ mice than wildtype or COX-$1^{-/-}$ mice. This phenotype was induced in wildtype mice by treatment with a COX-2-selective inhibitor, Celecoxib. Thus, COX-2 metabolites work oppositely in hepatotoxicity in the above two models, for exacerbation in the former and for protection in the latter. This difference most likely reflects mechanistic difference between the two models. Dissection of each mechanism may help us to develop a more efficient therapeutic strategy against hepatotoxicity induced by various agents.

9
Bone Metabolism

Bones undergo continuous destruction and renewal, a process termed bone remodeling. Bone resorption is carried out by osteoclasts, and bone formation by osteoblasts. These events are controlled by systemic humoral factors such as parathyroid hormone (PTH), estradiol, and vitamin D as well as by local cytokines such as IL-1β, IL-6, and insulin-like growth factor. Osteoclasts develop from precursor cells of macrophage lineage in the microenvironment of the bone. Factors such as PTH, vitamin D, IL-1, and IL-6 act first on osteoblasts to induce formation of the osteoclast differentiation factor named receptor activator of NFκB ligand (RANKL), which then stimulates the formation of mature osteoclasts from hematopoietic precursors by cell–cell interaction. Interestingly, these substances induce COX-2 in osteoblasts, and osteoclast induction by these substances is at least in part inhibited by aspirin-like drugs, and this impairment was rescued by the addition of PGE$_2$, indicating the role of COX and PGE$_2$ in this process (Tai et al. 1997). The role of COX-2 in this process was confirmed by Okada et al. (2000), who observed blunted (~30%–40%) osteoclast formation in response to vitamin D or PTH in hematopoietic precursors incubated with osteoblasts from COX-$2^{-/-}$ but not COX-$1^{-/-}$ mice. Sakuma et al. (2000) and Miyaura et al. (2000) reported impaired osteoclast formation in cells cultured from EP4-deficient mice. Sakuma et al. found that PGE$_2$-induced osteoclast formation was impaired in cultures of osteoblasts from EP4-deicient mice and osteoclast precursors from the spleen of wildtype mice. IL-1α, TNF-α, and basic fibroblast growth factor fail to induce osteoclast formation in these cultures. Miyaura et al. (2000) added PGE$_2$ to cultures of parietal bone from mice deficient in each of the PGE receptor subtype as well as wildtype mice and examined the bone resorptive activity of this PG by measuring Ca^{2+} released into the medium. They found that bone resorption by PGE$_2$ was much decreased in bones from EP4-deficient mice, which, on the other hand, showed an equal extent of response to dibutyryl cAMP added to the culture as the bones from control mice. These studies unequivocally establish the role of EP4 in mature osteoblasts, in induction of osteoclast differentiation factor, and in PGE$_2$-mediated bone resorption. On the other hand, Li et al. (2000) reported that the osteoclastogenic response to PGE_2, parathyroid hormone, and 1,25-dihydoxyvitamin D in vitro is reduced significantly in cultures of cells from EP2-deficient mice. This apparent discrepancy is likely to reflect redundant roles of the two relaxant PGE receptor subtypes. Sakuma et al. and Miyaura et al. found a small but significant PGE_2-dependent response in EP4-deficient mice, and Li et al. reported a further decrease in osteoclastogenesis when an EP4-selective antagonist was added to EP2-deficient cells. Such redundant actions of EP2 and EP4 were confirmed by Suzawa et al. (2000), who showed an additive effect of an EP2-selective agonist and an EP4-selective agonist in resorption of wildtype bone and the bone resorbing activity of an EP2 agonist in $EP4^{-/-}$ bone.

It has also been long known that in addition to bone resorption, PGE_2 added exogenously induces bone formation in vivo. However, its mechanism of action and its relation to the bone resorbing activity remain obscure. Recently, Yoshida et al. (2002) infused PGE_2 into the periosteal region of the femur of wildtype mice or mice deficient in each EP subtype using a mini-osmotic pump. After 6 weeks, the femur was isolated and bone formation was examined. Radiographic analysis revealed that PGE_2 induced extensive callus formation on the femur at the site of infusion in wildtype, EP1-, EP2-, and EP3-deficient mice. In contrast, no bone formation was detected radiographically in EP4-deficient mice. Consistently, bone formation was induced in wildtype mice by infusion of an EP4-selective agonist, but not by agonists specific for other EP subtypes. Yoshida et al. next used rats subjected to ovariectomy or immobilization, and examined the effects of the EP4-selective agonist on the bone loss induced by either condition. The addition of the EP4-selective agonist potently prevented the bone loss in both cases and restored the bone mass. Consistently, the histomorphometric analysis revealed that the density of osteoblasts lining the bone surface increased with the increase in the bone mass. Intriguingly, this analysis revealed that the total number of osteoclasts increased with the increase in new bone surface. These results suggest that EP4 is responsible for both bone resorption and bone formation induced by PGE_2 and that activation of EP4 in situ integrates these two actions for bone remodeling.

10
Conclusion

The phenotypes of the transgenic animals in prostanoid synthesis and action discussed above is summarized in Table 3. As seen in this table and as discussed above, the transgenic animal studies have revealed and are revealing what this family of pleiotropic substances actually do in the animal physiology and pathophysiology. These studies are providing significant information for development of new therapeutics that selectively stimulate or inhibit each prostanoid action. Indeed, some of the knockout mouse phenotypes have been confirmed and reproduced by the use of newly developed compounds selective to each enzyme or each type of receptor. The transgenic animal studies may also give us some indication as to the susceptibility of humans to certain diseases. The pheno-

Table 3 Pathophysiological phenotypes of transgenic animals of prostanoid synthesis and action

Pathophysiology	Transgenic animal	Phenotype	Reference(s)
Fever generation	COX-2$^{-/-}$	Loss of febrile response to LPS and interleukin 1β (no phenotype in COX-1$^{-/-}$)	Li et al. 1999, 2000
Sleep induction	EP3$^{-/-}$	Impaired febrile response to pyrogens	Ushikubi et al. 1998
	DP$^{-/-}$	Impaired PGD$_2$-induced sleep	Mizoguchi et al. 2001
	Lipocalin-type PGD synthase overexpression	Induction of non-REM sleep by tail clipping	Pinzar et al. 2000
Other sickness behaviors	COX-2$^{-/-}$	Reduced LPS-induced anorexia (no phenotype in COX-1$^{-/-}$)	Swiergiel 2001; Johnson et al. 2002
Inflammation	cPLA2$^{-/-}$	Decreased production of eicosanoids and platelet activating factor by peritoneal macrophages stimulated either by LPS or A-23187	Uozumi et al. 1997; Bonventre et al. 1997
		Reduced acute lung injury induced by systemic LPS or acid aspiration	Nagase et al. 2000
	COX-1$^{-/-}$	Reduced inflammatory swelling after arachidonic acid application	Langenbach et al. 1995
	COX-1$^{-/-}$ or COX-2$^{-/-}$	Time-dependent change in contribution of the two COX isoforms to inflammatory processes in the air pouch model	Langenbach et al. 1999
	COX-2$^{-/-}$	Persistent swelling and lymphocyte infiltration in carrageenan-induced paw edema	Wallace et al. 1998
	IP$^{-/-}$	Decreased inflammatory swelling	Murata et al. 1997; Ueno et al. 2000
Pain	COX-1$^{-/-}$	Less acetic acid-induced writhing response	Ballou et al. 2000
	IP$^{-/-}$	Decreased acetic acid writhing	Murata et al. 1997
	IP$^{-/-}$ and EP3$^{-/-}$	Decreased acetic acid-induced writhing in endotoxin-pretreated mice	Ueno et al. 2001
	Lipocalin-type PGD synthase$^{-/-}$	Reduced mechanical allodynia induced by intrathecal injection of PGE$_2$	Eguchi et al. 1999
	EP1$^{-/-}$	Deceased PGE$_2$-induced mechanical allodynia	Minami et al. 2001

Table 3 (continued)

Pathophysiology	Transgenic animal	Phenotype	Reference(s)
Allergy and immunity	cPLA2$^{-/-}$	Reduced eicosanoid synthesis from bone-marrow-derived mast cells	Fujishima et al. 1999; Nakatani et al. 2000
		Reduced bronchoconstriction and airway hypersensitivity in OVA-induced systemic anaphylaxis	Uozumi et al. 1997
	COX-1$^{-/-}$	Augmented airway inflammation and sensitivity in OVA-induced allergic asthma model	Gavett et al. 1999
	COX-2$^{-/-}$	Enhanced allergic inflammation in OVA-induced allergic asthma model (weaker phenotype than COX-1$^{-/-}$ mice)	Gavett et al. 1999
	DP$^{-/-}$	Decreased allergic responses in OVA-induced bronchial asthma	Matsuoka et al. 2000
	Lipocalin-type PGD synthase overexpression	Enhanced airway inflammation in OVA induced allergic asthma model	Fujitani et al. 2002
	COX-1$^{-/-}$	Impaired transition of CD4$^-$CD8$^-$ double-negative to CD4$^+$CD8$^+$ double-positive thymocyte maturation	Rocca et al. 1999
	COX-2$^{-/-}$	Impaired transition of CD4$^+$CD8$^+$ double-positive thymocytes to CD4 single-positive T cells	Rocca et al. 1999
	COX-2$^{-/-}$	Reduced susceptibility to collagen-induced arthritis	Myers et al. 2000
	EP2$^{-/-}$, EP4$^{-/-}$, IP$^{-/-}$	Impaired suppression of TNF-α production and impaired induction of IL-10 production	Shinomiya et al. 2001
Lung	EP2$^{-/-}$	Loss of bronchodilation PGE$_2$	Sheller et al. 2000
Cardiovascular system	COX-2$^{-/-}$	Myocardial fibrosis	Dinchuk et al. 1995

Table 3 (continued)

Pathophysiology	Transgenic animal	Phenotype	Reference(s)
Thrombosis, hemostasis, and blood pressure	COX-1$^{-/-}$	Decreased arachidonic acid-induced platelet aggregation	Langenbach et al. 1995
	EP3$^{-/-}$	Impaired PGE$_2$-induced potentiation of platelet activation.	Fabre et al. 2001; Ma et al. 2001
	IP$^{-/-}$	Thrombotic tendency	Murata et al. 1997
	TP$^{-/-}$	Bleeding tendency and resistance to thromboembolism	Thomas et al. 1998
	IP$^{-/-}$, TP$^{-/-}$	Increased and decreased stenosis in balloon catheter-induced vascular injury in IP$^{-/-}$ and TP$^{-/-}$ mice, respectively	Cheng et al. 2002
	PGI synthase (gene transfer)	Suppression of neointimal formation in carotid balloon injury	Todaka et al. 1999
	EP2$^{-/-}$	Salt-dependent hypertension	Kennedy et al. 1999; Tilley et al. 1999
	EP2$^{-/-}$	Vasopressor or impaired vasodepressor response to PGE$_2$	Audoly et al. 1999; Zhang et al. 2000
	EP3$^{-/-}$	Enhanced vasodepressor response to PGE$_2$	Audoly et al. 1999
	EP4$^{-/-}$	Impaired vasodepressor response to PGE$_2$	Audoly et al. 1999
Post ischemic injury: brain	cPLA2$^{-/-}$	Reduced postischemic brain injury	Bonventre et al. 1997
	COX-1$^{-/-}$	Increased susceptibility to ischemic brain injury	Iadecola et al. 2001
	COX-2$^{-/-}$	Reduced brain ischemic injury	Iadecola et al. 2001
Post ischemic injury: heart	COX-1$^{-/-}$	Increased cardiac ischemia-reperfusion injury	Camitta et al. 2001
	COX-2$^{-/-}$	Increased cardiac ischemia and reperfusion injury	Camitta et al. 2001
	IP$^{-/-}$	Enhanced cardiac ischemia-reperfusion injury	Xiao et al. 2001
Pulmonary hypertension	PGI synthase over-expression	Suppression of development of hypoxic pulmonary hypertension	Garaci et al. 1999
	PGI synthase (gene transfer)	Amelioration of monocrotaline-induced pulmonary hypertension	Nagaya et al. 2000
	IP$^{-/-}$	Enhanced pulmonary hypertension and vascular remodeling under chronic hypoxic conditions	Hoshikawa et al. 2001

Table 3 (continued)

Pathophysiology	Transgenic animal	Phenotype	Reference(s)
Patent ductus arteriosus	COX-2−/−	Patent ductus arteriosus (35%)	Loftin et al. 2001
	COX-1−/− and COX-2−/−	Patent ductus arteriosus (100% penetrance)	Loftin et al. 2001
	EP4−/−	Patent ductus arteriosus	Nguyen et al. 1997; Segi et al. 1998
Kidney	cPLA2−/−	Renal concentrating defect	Downey et al. 2001
	COX-2−/−	Renal dysplasia	Dincuk et al. 1995; Morham et al. 1995; Norwood et al. 2000
		Impaired renin production in response to ACE inhibition	Cheng et al. 2001
	EP2−/−	Salt-induced hypertension	Kennedy et al. 1999; Tilley et al. 1999
	EP3−/−	Disappearance of indomethacin-sensitive urine diluting function	Fleming et al. 1998
Reproduction	cPLA2−/−	Parturition failure	Bonventre et al. 1997; Uozumi et al. 1997
	COX-2−/−	Multiple female reproductive failures including ovulation, fertilization, implantation and decidualization	Lim et al. 1997
	EP2−/−	Impaired ovulation and fertilization	Hizaki et al. 1999; Kennedy et al. 1999; Tilley et al. 1999
	COX-1−/−	Loss of parturition	Gross et al. 1998
	FP−/−	Loss of parturition	Sugimoto et al. 1997
	TP overexpression in vasculature	Intrauterine growth retardation of embryos	Rocca et al. 2000

Table 3 (continued)

Pathophysiology	Transgenic animal	Phenotype	Reference(s)
Gastrointestinal functions	COX-1$^{-/-}$	Reduced susceptibility to indomethacin-induced stomach ulceration	Langenbach et al. 1995
	EP1$^{-/-}$	Impaired PGE$_2$-induced protection for NSAID-induced gastric damage	Kunikata et al. 2001
	EP3$^{-/-}$	Impaired PGE$_2$-induced protection for NSAID-induced duodenal damage	Kunikata et al. 2001
	EP3$^{-/-}$	Impaired duodenal bicarbonate secretion and mucosal integrity	Takeuchi et al. 1999
	IP$^{-/-}$	Impaired adaptive gastric cytoprotection	Boku et al. 2001
	IP$^{-/-}$	Impaired capsaicin-induced gastric cytoprotection	Takeuchi et al. 2001
Intestinal inflammation	COX-1$^{-/-}$	Increased susceptibility to dextran sodium sulfate–induced colitis	Morteau et al. 2000
		Decreased crypt cell survival in radiation injury	Houchen et al. 2000
	COX-2$^{-/-}$	Increased susceptibility to dextran sodium sulfate-induced colitis	Morteau et al. 2000
	EP4$^{-/-}$	Exaggerated dextran sodium sulfate-induced colitis	Kabashima et al. 2002
Intestinal polyposis	cPLA2$^{-/-}$	Suppression of intestinal polyposis in $Apc^{\Delta716}$ mice	Takaku et al. 2000
	COX-2$^{-/-}$	Reduced intestinal polyp formation in $Apc^{\Delta716}$ mice	Ohshima et al. 1996
	COX-1$^{-/-}$, COX-2$^{-/-}$	Reduced polyp formation in Min mice	Chulada et al. 2000
	EP2$^{-/-}$	Impaired auto-amplification of COX and angiogenesis of intestinal polyps in $Apc^{\Delta716}$ mice.	Sonoshita et al. 2001; Seno et al. 2002
	EP1$^{-/-}$	Decreased aberrant foci formation to azoxymethane	Watanabe et al. 1997
	EP4$^{-/-}$	Decreased aberrant foci formation to azoxymethane	Mutoh et al. 2002
Hepatotoxicity	COX-2$^{-/-}$	Reduced LPS-induced hepatotoxicity	Dinchuk et al. 1995
		Increased toxicity and lethality in acetaminophen-induced liver injury	Reilly et al. 2001

Table 3 (continued)

Pathophysiology	Transgenic animal	Phenotype	Reference(s)
Bone metabolism	$COX-2^{-/-}$	Reduced osteoclast formation in culture	Okada et al. 2000
	$EP2^{-/-}$	Impaired osteoclastogenesis in vitro	Li et al. 2000
	$EP4^{-/-}$	Decreased inflammation bone resorption	Sakuma et al. 2000; Miyaura et al. 2000
		Lack of PGE_2-induced in vivo bone formation	Yoshida et al. 2002

types in these mice certainly will facilitate a search for single nucleotide polymorphisms in the genes of the respective human enzymes and receptors as causative factors in related diseases. Elucidation and analysis of the complete human and mouse genome sequences may clarify these issues.

References

Audoly LP, Tilley SL, Goulet J, Key M, Nguyen M, Stock JL, McNeish JD, Koller BH, Coffman TM (1999) Identification of specific EP receptors responsible for the hemodynamic effects of PGE$_2$. Am J Physiol 277: H924–930

Ballou LR, Botting RM, Goorha S, Zhang J, Vane JR (2000) Nociception in cyclooxygenase isozyme-deficient mice. Proc Natl Acad Sci USA 97:10272–10276

Berg DJ, Zhang J, Lauricella DM, Moore SA (2001) IL-10 is a central regulator of cyclooxygense-2 expression and prostaglandin production. J Immunol 166:2674–2680

Bley KR, Hunter JC, Eglen RM, Smith JAM (1998) The role of IP prosanoid receptors in inflammatory pain. Trends Pharmacol Sci 19:141–147

Bjarnason I, Hayllar J, MacPherson AJ, Russell AS (1993) Side effects of nonsteroidal anti-inflammatory drugs on the small and large intestine in humans. Gastroenterology **104**: 1832–1847

Boku K, Ohno T, Saeki T, Hayashi H, Hayashi I, Katori M, Murata T, Narumiya S, Saigenji K, Majima M (2001) Adaptive cytoprotection mediated by prostaglandin I$_2$ is attributable to sensitization of CRGP-containing sensory nerves. Gastroenterology 120:134–14

Bonventre JV, Huang Z, Taheri MR, O'Leary E, Li E, Moskowitz MA, Sapirstein A (1997) Reduced fertility and postischaemic brain injury in mice deficient in cytosolic phospholipase A2. Nature 390:622–625

Brzozowski T, Konturek PC, Konturek SJ, Sliwowski Z, Drozdowicz D, Stachura J, Pajdo R, Hahn EG (1999) Role of prostaglandins generated by cyclooxygenase-1 and cyclooxygenase-2 in healing of ischemia-reperfusion-induced gastric lesions. Eur J Pharmacol 385:47–61

Camitta MG, Gabel SA, Chulada P, Bradbury JA, Langenbach R, Zeldin DC, Murphy E (2001) Cyclooxygenase-1 and −2 knockout mice demonstrate increased cardiac ischemia/reperfusion injury but are protected by acute preconditioning. Circulation 104:2453–2458

Cao C, Matsumura K, Yamagata K, Watanabe Y (1995) Induction by lipopolysaccharide of cyclooxygenase-2 mRNA in rat brain; its possible role in the febrile response. Brain Res 697:187–196

Cheng HF, Wang JL, Zhang MZ, Wang SW, McKanna JA, Harris RC (2001) Genetic deletion of COX-2 prevents increased renin expression in response to ACE inhibition. Am J Physiol Renal Physiol 280: F449–456

Cheng Y, Austin SC, Rocca B, Koller BH, Coffman TM, Grosser T, Lawson JA, FitzGerald GA (2002) Role of prostacyclin in the cardiovascular response to thromboxane A$_2$. Science 296: 539–541

Chulada PC, Thompson MB, Mahler JF, Doyle CM, Gaul BW, Lee C, Tiano HF, Morham SG, Smithies O, Langenbach R (2000) Genetic disruption of Ptgs-1, as well as Ptgs-2, reduces intestinal tumorigenesis in Min mice. Cancer Res 60:4705–4708

Davies P. Bailey PJ, Goldenberg MM, Ford-Hutchinson AW (1984) The role of arachidonic acid oxygenation products in pain and inflammation. Ann Rev Immunol 2:335–357

Dennis EA (1997) The growing phospholipase A2 superfamily of signal transduction enzymes. Trends Biochem Sci. 22:1–2

Dinchuk JE, Car BD, Focht RJ, Johnston JJ, Jaffee BD, Covington MB, Contel NR, Eng VM, Collins RJ, Czerniak PM, et al (1995) Renal abnormalities and an altered inflammatory response in mice lacking cyclooxygenase II. Nature 378:406–409

Downey P, Sapirstein A, O'Leary E, Sun TX, Brown D, Bonventre JV (2001) Renal concentrating defect in mice lacking group IV cytosolic phospholipase A2. Am J Physiol Renal Physiol 280: F607–618

Eguchi N, Minami T, Shirafuji N, Kanaoka Y, Tanaka T, Nagata A, Yoshida N, Urade Y, Ito S, Hayaishi O (1999) Lack of tactile pain (allodynia) in lipocalin-type prostaglandin D synthase-deficient mice. Proc Natl Acad Sci USA 96:726–730

Ek M (2001) Pathway across the blood-brain barrier. Nature 410:430–431

Fabre JE, Nguyen M, Athirakul K, Coggins K, McNeish JD, Austin S, Parise LK, FitzGerald GA, Coffman TM, Koller BH (2001) Activation of the murine EP3 receptor for PGE2 inhibits cAMP production and promotes platelet aggregation. J Clin Invest 107:603–610

Fiocchi C (1998) Inflammatory bowel disease: etiology and pathogenesis. *Gastroenterology.* **115:** 182–205

Fitzpatrick FA, Soberman R (2001) Regulated formation of eicosanoids. J Clin Invest 107:1347–1351

Fleming EF, Athirakul K, Oliverio MI, Key M, Goulet J, Koller BH, Coffman TM (1998) Urinary concentrating function in mice lacking EP3 receptors for prostaglandin E$_2$. Am J Physiol 275: F955–961

Fujishima H, Sanchez Mejia RO, Bingham CO, 3rd, Lam BK, Sapirstein A, Bonventre JV, Austen KF, Arm JP (1999) Cytosolic phospholipase A2 is essential for both the immediate and the delayed phases of eicosanoid generation in mouse bone marrow-derived mast cells. Proc Natl Acad Sci USA 96:4803–4807

Fujitani Y, Kanaoka Y, Aritake K, Uodome N, Okazaki-Hatake K, Urade Y (2002) Pronounced eosinophilic lung inflammation and Th2 cytokine release in human lipocalin-type prostaglandin D synthase transgenic mice. J Immunol 168:443–449

Gavett SH, Madison SL, Chulada PC, Scarborough PE, Qu W, Boyle JE, Tiano HF, Lee CA, Langenbach R, Roggli VL, Zeldin DC (1999) Allergic lung responses are increased in prostaglandin H synthase-deficient mice. J Clin Invest 104:721–732

Geraci MW, Gao B, Shepherd DC, Moore MD, Westcott JY, Fagan KA, Alger LA, Tuder RM, Voelkel NF (1999) Pulmonary prostacyclin synthase overexpression in transgenic mice protects against development of hypoxic pulmonary hypertension. J Clin Invest 103:1509–1515

Gross GA, Imamura T, Luedke C, Vogt SK, Olson LM, Nelson DM, Sadovsky Y, Muglia LJ (1998) Opposing actions of prostaglandins and oxytocin determine the onset of murine labor. Proc Natl Acad Sci USA 95:11875–11879

Hizaki H, Segi E, Sugimoto Y, Hirose M, Saji T, Ushikubi F, Matsuoka T, Noda Y, Tanaka T, Yoshida N, Narumiya S, Ichikawa A (1999) Abortive expansion of the cumulus and impaired fertility in mice lacking the prostaglandin E receptor subtype EP(2). Proc Natl Acad Sci USA 96:10501–10506

Hirai H, Tanaka K, Yoshie O, Ogawa K, Kenmotsu K, Takamori Y, Ichimasa M, Sugamura K, Nakamura, M, Takano, S, Nagata K (2001). Prostaglandin D$_2$ selectively induces chemotaxis in T helper type 2 cells, eosinophils, and basophils via seven-transmembrane receptor CRTH2. J Exp Med 193:255–261

Hoshikawa Y, Voelkel NF, Gesell TL, Moore MD, Morris KG, Alger LA, Narumiya S, Geraci MW (2001) Prostacyclin receptor-dependent modulation of pulmonary vascular remodeling. Am J Respir Crit Care Med 164:314–318

Houchen CW, Stenson WF, Cohn SM (2000) Disruption of cyclooxygenase-1 gene results in an impaired response to radiation injury. Am J Physiol Gastrointest Liver Physiol 279: G858–865

Iadecola C, Sugimoto K, Niwa K, Kazama K, Ross ME (2001a) Increased susceptibility to ischemic brain injury in cyclooxygenase-1-deficient mice. J Cereb Blood Flow Metab 21:1436–1441

Iadecola C, Niwa K, Nogawa S, Zhao X, Nagayama M, Araki E, Morham S, Ross ME (2001b) Reduced susceptibility to ischemic brain injury and N-methyl-D-aspartate-mediated neurotoxicity in cyclooxygenase-2-deficient mice. Proc Natl Acad Sci USA 98:1294–1299

Jakobsson PJ, Thoren S, Morgenstern R, Samuelsson B (1999) Identification of human prostaglandin E synthase: a microsomal, glutathione-dependent, inducible enzyme, constituting a potential novel drug target. Proc Natl Acad Sci USA 96:7220–7225

Johnson PM, Vogt SK, Burney MW, Muglia LJ (2002) COX-2 inhibition attenuates anorexia during systemic inflammation without impairing cytokine production. Am J Physiol Endocrinol Metab 282: E650–656

Kabashima K, Saji T, Murata T, Nagamachi M, Matsuoka T, Segi E, Tsuboi K, Sugimoto Y, Kobayashi T, Miyachi Y, Ichikawa A, Naumiya S (2002) The prostaglandin receptor EP4 suppresses colitis, mucosal damage and CD4 cell activation in the gut. J Clin Invest 109:883–893

Katsuyama M, Sugimoto Y, Morimoto K, Hasumoto K, Fukumoto M, Negishi M, Ichikawa A (1997) Distinct cellular localization of the messenger ribonucleic acid for prostaglandin E receptor subtypes in the mouse uterus during pseudopreganancy. Endocrinology 138:344–350

Kennedy CR, Zhang Y, Brandon S, Guan Y, Coffee K, Funk CD, Magnuson MA, Oates JA, Breyer MD, Breyer RM (1999) Salt-sensitive hypertension and reduced fertility in mice lacking the prostaglandin EP2 receptor. Nat Med 5:217–220

Kent S, Bluthé R-M, Kelley KW, Dantzer R (1992) Sickness behavior as a new target for drug development. Trends Pharmacol Sci 13: 24–28

Kilunga Kubata B, Eguchi N, Urade Y, Yamashita K, Mitamura T, Tai K, Hayaishi O, Horii T (1998) Plasmodium falciparum produces prostaglandins that are pyrogenic, somnogenic, and immunosuppressive substances in humans. J Exp Med 188: 1197–1202

Kluger MJ (1991) Fever: role of pyrogens and cryogens. Physiol Rev 71:93–127

Kunikata T, Araki H, Takeeda M, Kato S, Takeuchi K (2001) Prostaglandin E prevents indomethacin-induced gastric and intestinal damage through different EP receptor subtypes. J Physiol Paris 95:157–163

Langenbach R, Morham SG, Tiano HF, Loftin CD, Ghanayem BI, Chulada PC, Mahler JF, Lee CA, Goulding EH, Kluckman KD, et al (1995) Prostaglandin synthase 1 gene disruption in mice reduces arachidonic acid-induced inflammation and indomethacin-induced gastric ulceration. Cell 83:483–492

Langenbach R, Loftin C, Lee C, Tiano H (1999) Cyclooxygenase knockout mice: models for elucidating isoform-specific functions. Biochem Pharmacol 58:1237–1246

Li S, Wang Y, Matsumura K, Ballou LR, Morham SG, Blatteis CM (1999) The febrile response to lipopolysaccharide is blocked in cyclooxygenase-2(-/-), but not in cyclooxygenase-1(-/-) mice. Brain Res 825:86–94

Li X, Okada Y, Pilbeam CC, Lorenzo JA, Kennedy CR, Breyer RM, Raisz LG (2000) Knockout of the murine prostaglandin EP2 receptor impairs osteoclastogenesis in vitro. Endocrinology 141:2054–2061

Li S, Ballou LR, Morham SG, Blatteis CM (2001) Cyclooxygenase-2 mediates the febrile response of mice to interleukin-1beta. Brain Res 910:163-173

Lim H, Gupta RA, Ma WG, Paria BC, Moller DE, Morrow JD, DuBois RN, Trzaskos JM, Dey SK (1999) Cyclo-oxygenase-2-derived prostacyclin mediates embryo implantation in the mouse via PPARδ. . Genes Dev 13:1561–1574

Lim H, Paria BC, Das SK, Dinchuk JE, Langenbach R, Trzaskos JM, Dey SK (1997) Multiple female reproductive failures in cyclooxygenase 2-deficient mice. Cell 91:197–208

Loftin CD, Trivedi DB, Tiano HF, Clark JA, Lee CA, Epstein JA, Morham SG, Breyer MD, Nguyen M, Hawkins BM, Goulet JL, Smithies O, Koller BH, Langenbach R (2001) Failure of ductus arteriosus closure and remodeling in neonatal mice deficient in cyclooxygenase-1 and cyclooxygenase-2. Proc Natl Acad Sci USA 98:1059–1064

Ma H, Hara A, Xiao CY, Okada Y, Takahata O, Nakaya K, Sugimoto Y, Ichikawa A, Narumiya S, Ushikubi F (2001) Increased bleeding tendency and decreased susceptibility to thromboembolism in mice lacking the prostaglandin E receptor subtype EP3. Circulation 104:1176–1180

Matsuoka T, Hirata M, Tanaka H, Takahashi Y, Murata T, Kabashima K, Sugimoto Y, Kobayashi T, Ushikubi F, Aze Y, Eguchi N, Urade Y, Yoshida N, Kimura K, Mizoguchi A, Honda Y, Nagai H, Narumiya S (2000) Prostaglandin D_2 as a mediator of allergic asthma. Science 287:2013–2017

Minami T, Uda R, Horiguchi S, Ito S, Hyodo M, Hayaishi O (1994) Allodynia evoked by intrathecal administration of prostaglandin E_2 to conscious mice. Pain 57:217223

Minami T, Nakano H, Kobayashi T, Sugimoto Y, Ushikubi F, Ichikawa A, Narumiya S, Ito S (2001) Characterization of EP receptor subtypes responsible for prostaglandin E_2-induced pain responses by use of EP1 and EP3 receptor knockout mice. Br J Pharmacol 133:438–444

Mnich SJ, Veenhuizen AW, Monahan JB, Sheehan KCF, Lynch KR, Isakson PC, Portanova JP (1995) Characterization of a monoclonal antibody that neutralizes the activity of prostaglandin E_2. J Immunol 155:4437–4444

Miyaura C, Inada M, Suzawa T, Sugimoto Y, Ushikubi F, Ichikawa A, Narumiya S, Suda T (2000) Impaired bone resorption to prostaglandin E_2 in prostaglandin E receptor EP4-knockout mice. J Biol Chem 275:19819–19823

Mizoguchi A, Eguchi N, Kimura K, Kiyohara Y, Qu WM, Huang ZL, Mochizuki T, Lazarus M, Kobayashi T, Kaneko T, Narumiya S, Urade Y, Hayaishi O (2001) Dominant localization of prostaglandin D receptors on arachnoid trabecular cells in mouse basal forebrain and their involvement in the regulation of non-rapid eye movement sleep. Proc Natl Acad Sci USA 98:11674–11679

Morham SG, Langenbach R, Loftin CD, Tiano HF, Vouloumanos N, Jennette JC, Mahler JF, Kluckman KD, Ledford A, Lee CA, et al (1995) Prostaglandin synthase 2 gene disruption causes severe renal pathology in the mouse. Cell 83:473–482

Morteau O, Morham SG, Sellon R, Dieleman LA, Langenbach R, Smithies O, Sartor RB (2000) Impaired mucosal defense to acute colonic injury in mice lacking cyclooxygenase-1 or cyclooxygenase-2. J Clin Invest 105:469–478

Murakami M, Naraba H, Tanioka T, Semmyo N, Nakatani Y, Kojima F, Ikeda T, Fueki M, Ueno A, Oh S, Kudo I (2000) Regulation of prostaglandin E_2 biosynthesis by inducible membrane-associated prostaglandin E_2 synthase that acts in concert with cyclooxygenase-2. J Biol Chem. 275:32783–32792

Murata T, Ushikubi F, Matsuoka T, Hirata M, Yamasaki A, Sugimoto Y, Ichikawa A, Aze Y, Tanaka T, Yoshida N, Ueno A, Oh-ishi S, Narumiya S (1997) Altered pain perception and inflammatory response in mice lacking prostacyclin receptor. Nature 388:678–682

Mutoh M, Watanabe K, Kitamura T, Shoji Y, Takahashi M, Kawamori T, Tani K, Kobayashi M, Maruyama T, Kobayashi K, Ohuchida S, Sugimoto Y, Narumiya S, Sugimura T, Wakabayashi K (2002) Involvement of prostaglandin E receptor subtype EP4 in colon carcinogenesis. Cancer Res 62:28–32

Myers LK, Kang AH, Postlethwaite AE, Rosloniec EF, Morham SG, Shlopov BV, Goorha S, Ballou LR (2000) The genetic ablation of cyclooxygenase 2 prevents the development of autoimmune arthritis. Arthritis Rheum 43:2687–2693

Nagaya N, Yokoyama C, Kyotani S, Shimonishi M, Morishita R, Uematsu M, Nishikimi T, Nakanishi N, Ogihara T, Yamagishi M, Miyatake K, Kaneda Y, Tanabe T (2000) Gene transfer of human prostacyclin synthase ameliorates monocrotaline-induced pulmonary hypertension in rats. Circulation 102:2005–2010

Nakatani N, Uozumi N, Kume K, Murakami M, Kudo I, Shimizu T (2000) Role of cytosolic phospholipase A2 in the production of lipid mediators and histamine release in mouse bone-marrow-derived mast cells. Biochem J 352 Pt 2:311–317

Narumiya S, Sugimoto Y, Ushikubi F (1999) Prostanoid receptors: structures, properties, and functions. Physiol Rev 79:1193–1226

Nguyen M, Camenisch T, Snouwaert JN, Hicks E, Coffman TM, Anderson PA, Malouf NN, Koller BH (1997) The prostaglandin receptor EP4 triggers remodelling of the cardiovascular system at birth. Nature 390:78–81

Norwood VF, Morham SG, Smithies O (2000) Postnatal development and progression of renal dysplasia in cyclooxygenase-2 null mice. Kidney Int 58:2291–2300

Oida H, Namba T, Sugimoto Y, Ushikubi F, Ohishi H, Ichikawa A, Narumiya S (1995) In situ hybridization studies of prostacyclin receptor mRNA expression in various mouse organs. Br J Pharmacol 116:2828–2837

Okada Y, Lorenzo JA, Freeman AM, Tomita M, Morham SG, Raisz LG, Pilbeam CC (2000) Prostaglandin G/H synthase-2 is required for maximal formation of osteoclast-like cells in culture. J Clin Invest 105:823–832

Oshima M, Dinchuk JE, Kargman SL, Oshima H, Hancock B, Kwong E, Trzaskos JM, Evans JF, Taketo MM (1996) Suppression of intestinal polyposis in $Apc^{\Delta716}$ knockout mice by inhibition of cyclooxygenase 2 (COX-2). Cell 87:803–809

Pinzar E, Kanaoka Y, Inui T, Eguchi N, Urade Y, Hayaishi O (2000) Prostaglandin D synthase gene is involved in the regulation of non-rapid eye movement sleep. Proc Natl Acad Sci USA 97:4903–4907

Portanova JP, Zhang Y, Anderson GD, Masferrer SD, Seibert K, Gregory SA, Isakson PC (1996) Selective neutralization of prostaglandin E_2 blocks inflammation, hyperalgesia and interleukin 6 production in vivo. J Exp Med 184: 883–891

Raud JS, Dahlen E, Sydbom A, Lindbom L, Hedqvist P (1988) Enhancement of acute allergic inflammation by indomethacin is reversed by prostaglandin E_2: apparent correlation with in vivo modulation of mediator release. Proc Natl Acad Sci USA 85:2315–2319

Reilly TP, Brady JN, Marchick MR, Bourdi M, George JW, Radonovich MF, Pise-Masison CA, Pohl LR (2001) A protective role for cyclooxygenase-2 in drug-induced liver injury in mice. Chem Res Toxicol 14:1620–1628

Rocca B, Spain LM, Pure E, Langenbach R, Patrono C, FitzGerald GA (1999) Distinct roles of prostaglandin H synthases 1 and 2 in T-cell development. J Clin Invest 103:1469–1477

Rocca B, Loeb AL, Strauss JF, 3rd, Vezza R, Habib A, Li H, FitzGerald GA (2000) Directed vascular expression of the thromboxane A_2 receptor results in intrauterine growth retardation. Nat Med 6:219–221

Sakuma Y, Tanaka K, Suda M, Yasoda A, Natsui K, Tanaka I, Ushikubi F, Narumiya S, Segi E, Sugimoto Y, Ichikawa A, Nakao K (2000) Crucial involvement of the EP4 subtype of prostaglandin E receptor in osteoclast formation by proinflammatory cytokines and lipopolysaccharide. J Bone Miner Res 15:218–227

Satoh S, H. Matsumura H, Suzuki F, Hayaishi O (1996) Promotion of sleep mediated by the A_{2a}-adenosine receptor and possible involvement of this receptor in the sleep induced by prostaglandin D_2 in rats. Proc Natl Acad Sci USA 91:5980–5984

Schultze AE, Roth RA (1998) Chronic pulmonary hypertension-the monocrotaline model and involvement of the hemostatic system. J Toxicol Environ Health B Crit Rev 1:271–346

Sheller JR, Mitchell D, Meyrick B, Oates J, Breyer R (2000) EP2 receptor mediates bronchodilation by PGE_2 in mice. J Appl Physiol 88:2214–2218

Shinomiya S, Naraba H, Ueno A, Utsunomiya I, Maruyama T, Ohuchida S, Ushikubi F, Yuki K, Narumiya S, Sugimoto Y, Ichikawa A, Oh-ishi A (2001) Regulaiton of TNFα and interleukin-10 production by prostaglandin I_2 and E_2: studies with prostaglandin receptor-deficient mice and prostaglandin E-receptor subtype-specific synthetic agonists. Biochem Pharmacol 61:1153–1160

Segi E, Sugimoto Y, Yamasaki A, Aze Y, Oida H, Nishimura T, Murata T, Matsuoka T, Ushikubi F, Hirose M, Tanaka T, Yoshida N, Narumiya S, Ichikawa A (1998) Patent ductus arteriosus and neonatal death in prostaglandin receptor EP4-deficient mice. Biochem Biophys Res Commun 246:7-12

Seno H, Oshima M, Ishikawa TO, Oshima H, Takaku K, Chiba T, Narumiya S, Taketo MM (2002) Cyclooxygenase 2- and prostaglandin E_2 receptor EP2-dependent angiogenesis in Apc$^{\Delta716}$ mouse intestinal polyps. Cancer Res 62:506–511

Smith CJ, Zhang Y, Koboldt CM, Muhammad J, Zweifel BS, Shaffer A, Talley JJ, Masferrer JL, Seibert K, Isakson PC (1998) Pharmacological analysis of cyclooxygenase-1 in inflammation. Proc Natl Acad Sci USA 95:13313–13318

Smith WL, DeWitt DL, Garavito RM (2000) Cyclooxygenases; structural, cellular and molecular biology Annu Rev Biochem 69:149–182

Sonoshita M, Takaku K, Sasaki N, Sugimoto Y, Ushikubi F, Narumiya S, Oshima M, Taketo MM (2001) Acceleration of intestinal polyposis through prostaglandin receptor EP2 in Apc$^{\Delta716}$ knockout mice. Nat Med 7:1048–1051

Sugimoto Y, Shigemoto R, Namba T, Negishi M, Mizuno N, Narumiya S, Ichikawa A (1994) Distribution of the messenger RNA for the prostaglandin E receptor subtype EP_3 in the mouse nervous system. Neurosci 62:919–928

Sugimoto Y, Yamasaki A, Segi E, Tsuboi K, Aze Y, Nishimura T, Oida H, Yoshida N, Tanaka T, Katsuyama M, Hasumoto K, Murata T, Hirata M, Ushikubi F, Negishi M, Ichikawa A, Narumiya S (1997) Failure of parturition in mice lacking the prostaglandin F receptor. Science 277:681–683

Suzawa T, Miyaura C, Inada M, Maruyama T, Sugimoto Y, Ushikubi F, Ichikawa A, Narumiya S, Suda T (2000) The role of prostaglandin E receptor subtypes (EP1, EP2, EP3, and EP4) in bone resorption: an analysis using specific agonists for the respective EPs. Endocrinology 141:1554–1559

Suzuki T, Fujii Y, Miyano M, Chen LY, Takahashi T, Watanabe K (1999) cDNA cloning, expression, and mutagenesis study of liver-type prostaglandin F synthase. J Biol Chem 274:241–248

Swiergiel AH, Dunn AJ (2001) Cyclooxygenase 1 is not essential for hypophagic responses to interleukin-1 and endotoxin in mice. Pharmacol Biochem Behav 69:659–663

Szczeklik A, Stevenson, DD (1999) Aspirin-induced asthma: advances in pathogenesis and management. J Allergy Clin Immunol 104:5-13

Tai H, Miyaura C, C.C. Pilbeam CC, Tamura T, Ohsugi Y, Koshihara Y, Kubodera N, Kawaguchi H, Raisz LG, Suda T (1997) Transcriptional induction of cyclooxygenase-2 in osteoblasts is involved in interleukin-6-induced osteoclast formation. Endocrinology 138:2372–2379

Takaku K, Sonoshita M, Sasaki N, Uozumi N, Doi Y, Shimizu T, Taketo MM (2000) Suppression of intestinal polyposis in Apc$^{\Delta716}$ knockout mice by an additional mutation in the cytosolic phospholipase A2 gene. J Biol Chem 275:34013–34016

Takeuchi K, Ukawa H, Kato S, Furukawa O, Araki H, Sugimoto Y, Ichikawa A, Ushikubi F, Narumiya S (1999) Impaired duodenal bicarbonate secretion and mucosal integrity in mice lacking prostaglandin E-receptor subtype EP3. Gastroenterology 117:1128–1135

Takeuchi K, Kato S, Ogawa Y, Kanatsu K, Umeda M (2001) Role of endogenous prostacyclin in gastric ulcerogenic and healing responses—a study using IP-receptor knockout mice. J Physiol Paris 95:75–80

Tanabe T, Ullrich V (1995) Prostacyclin and thromboxane synthases. J Lipid Mediat Cell Signal 12:243–255

Tanioka T, Nakatani Y, Semmyo N, Murakami M, Kudo I (2000) Molecular identification of cytosolic prostaglandin E_2 synthase that is functionally coupled with cyclooxygenase-1 in immediate prostaglandin E_2 biosynthesis. J Biol Chem. 275:32775–32782

Terao A, Matsumura H, Saito M (1998) Interleukin-1 induces slow-wave sleep at the prostagalndin D_2-sensitive sleep-promoting zone in the rat brain. J Neurosci 18:6599–6607

Thomas DW, Mannon RB, Mannon PJ, Latour A, Oliver JA, Hoffman M, Smithies O, Koller BH, Coffman TM (1998) Coagulation defects and altered hemodynamic responses in mice lacking receptors for thromboxane A_2. J Clin Invest 102:1994–2001

Tilley SL, Audoly LP, Hicks EH, Kim HS, Flannery PJ, Coffman TM, Koller BH (1999) Reproductive failure and reduced blood pressure in mice lacking the EP2 prostaglandin E_2 receptor. J Clin Invest 103:1539–1545

Todaka T, Yokoyama C, Yanamoto H, Hashimoto N, Nagata I, Tsukahara T, Hara S, Hatae T, Morishita R, Aoki M, Ogihara T, Kaneda Y, Tanabe T (1999) Gene transfer of human prostacyclin synthase prevents neointimal formation after carotid balloon injury in rats. Stroke 30:419–426

Ueno A, Naraba H, Ikeda Y, Ushikubi F, Murata T, Narumiya S, Oh-ishi S (2000) Intrinsic prostacyclin contributes to exudation induced by bradykinin or carrageenin: a study on the paw edema induced in IP-receptor-deficient mice. Life Sci 66: PL155–160

Ueno A, Matsumoto H, Naraba H, Ikeda Y, Ushikubi F, Matsuoka T, Narumiya S, Sugimoto Y, Ichikawa A, Oh-ishi S (2001) Major roles of prostanoid receptors IP and EP3 in endotoxin-induce enhancement of pain perception. Biochem Pharmacol 62: 157–160

Uozumi N, Kume K, Nagase T, Nakatani N, Ishii S, Tashiro F, Komagata Y, Maki K, Ikuta K, Ouchi Y, Miyazaki J, Shimizu T (1997) Role of cytosolic phospholipase A2 in allergic response and parturition. Nature 390:618–622

Urade Y, Hayaishi O (2000) Biochemical, structural, genetic, physiological, and pathophysiological features of lipocalin-type prostaglandin D synthase. Biochim Biophys Acta 1482:259–271

Ushikubi F, Segi E, Sugimoto Y, Murata T, Matsuoka T, Kobayashi T, Hizaki H, Tuboi K, Katsuyama M, Ichikawa A, Tanaka T, Yoshida N, Narumiya S (1998) Impaired febrile response in mice lacking the prostaglandin E receptor subtype EP3. Nature 395:281–284

Watanabe K, Kawamori T, Nakatsugi S, Ohta T, Ohuchida S, Yamamoto H, Maruyama T, Kondo K, Ushikubi F, Narumiya S, Sugimura T, Wakabayashi K (1999) Role of the prostaglandin E receptor subtype EP1 in colon carcinogenesis. Cancer Res 59:5093–5096

Wallace JL, Bak A, McKnight W, Asfaha S, Sharkey KA, MacNaughton WK (1998) Cyclooxygenase 1 contributes to inflammatory responses in rats and mice: implications for gastrointestinal toxicity. Gastroenterology 115:101–109

Wallace JL, McKnight W, Reuter BK, Vergnolle N (2000) NSAID-induced gastric damage in rats: requirement for inhibition of both cyclooxygenase 1 and 2. Gastroenterology 119:706–714

Xiao CY, Hara A, Yuhki K, Fujino T, Ma H, Okada Y, Takahata O, Yamada T, Murata T, Narumiya S, Ushikubi F (2001) Roles of prostaglandin I_2 and thromboxane A_2 in cardiac ischemia-reperfusion injury: a study using mice lacking their respective receptors. Circulation 104:2210–2215

Yamagata K, Matsumura K, Inoue W, Shiraki T, Suzuki K, Yasuda S, Sugiura H, Cao C, Watanabe Y, Kobayashi S (2001) Coexpression of mirosomal-type prostaglandin E synthase with cyclooxygenase-2 in brain endothelial cells of rats during endotoxin-induced fever. J Neurosci 21:2669–2677

Yoshida K, Oida H, Kobayashi T, Maruyama T, Tanaka M, Katayama T, Yamaguchi K, Segi E, Tsuboyama T, Matsushita M, Ito K, Ito Y, Sugimoto Y, Ushikubi F, Ohuchida S, Kondo K, Nakamura T, Narumiya S (2002) Stimulation of bone formation and prevention of bone loss by prostaglandin E EP4 receptor activation. Proc Natl Acad Sci USA 99:4580–4585

Zhang Y, Guan Y, Schneider A, Brandon S, Breyer RM, Breyer MD (2000) Characterization of murine vasopressor and vasodepressor prostaglandin E_2 receptors. Hypertension 35:1129–1134

Coagulation and Fibrinolysis in Genetically Modified Mice

B. Isermann[1] · H. Weiler[2]

[1] Blood Research Institute, The Blood Center of Southeastern Wisconsin, Milwaukee,
WI 53226, USA
e-mail: bhisermann@bcsew.edu
[2] Department of Physiology, Medical College of Wisconsin, Milwaukee, WI 53226, USA
e-mail: hweiler@bcsew.edu

Abstract The hemostatic mechanism is based on the extraordinarily complex interactions of numerous cellular, biochemical, and physiological pathways. The ability to precisely alter the function of individual genes in the mouse genome has opened a new opportunity to dissect the specific role of individual factors in coagulation and fibrinolysis, and to design animal models of rare diseases resulting from defects in these pathways. This chapter attempts a synopsis of such animal models and their relevance for our understanding of the pathogenic mechanisms underlying vascular disease. Importantly, the analysis of genetically engineered animals has also yielded exciting insights into the function of coagulation and fibrinolysis in embryonic development. By default, this overview can just provide a snapshot of a rapidly developing field, but may provide valuable guidelines for designing further experiments.

Keywords Coagulation · Fibrinolysis · Hemostasis · Transgenic · Mice · Animal model · Gene targeting · Vascular disease · Embryonic development

1
Introduction: A summary of Blood Coagulation and Fibrinolysis

Blood coagulation is initiated when tissue factor (TF) binds plasma-derived factor VII (fVII) and activated fVII (fVIIa) (for an overview, see Fig. 1). The complex of TF and fVII/VIIa initiates the TF-dependent prothrombin activation through limited proteolysis of the coagulation factors IX and X. The TF-dependent initiation pathway of coagulation is regulated by the tissue factor pathway inhibitor (TFPI), which forms a ternary complex with fVIIa, fXa, and TF. Thus, the exposure of TF to plasma-derived coagulation components results in an initial, but timely limited activation of prothrombin.

Further generation of thrombin occurs in a TF-independent manner through a thrombin-dependent positive feedback activation of the coagulation fXI and the coagulation cofactors V and VIII. The latter two enhance the activation of fIX and fX about 1,000-fold. Akin to the function of TFPI in controlling TF-dependent thrombin generation, specific inhibitors regulate this thrombin dependent amplification pathway of coagulation. Antithrombin is a plasma serine protease inhibitor (serpin) that inactivates thrombin and coagulation factors Xa, IXa, XIa, and XIIa. The anticoagulant efficiency of antithrombin is enhanced in the presence of endothelial heparan sulfate or exogenous heparin. The serpin heparin cofactor II is a specific thrombin inhibitor, whose inhibitory activity is about 1,000-fold increased in the presence of heparin, heparan sulfate, or dermatan sulfate. The protein Z-dependent protease inhibitor (PZI) is a specific inhibitor for fXa, which requires the vitamin K-dependent cofactor protein Z (PZ) for full anticoagulant efficiency.

The endothelial transmembrane molecule thrombomodulin (TM) differs from the before-mentioned natural anticoagulants, as it not only directly inhibits a procoagulant (thrombin), but actually redirects the substrate specificity of thrombin towards the activation of the natural anticoagulant protein C (PC).

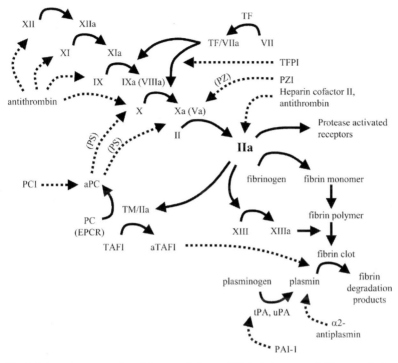

Fig. 1 Schematic presentation of the coagulation and fibrinolytic system. *Solid arrows* depict activation; *stippled arrows* depict inhibition; protein cofactors are shown in *brackets*. For details see text

Activation of PC by the TM-thrombin complex is almost 100-fold enhanced in the presence of the endothelial membrane receptor for PC, endothelial cell protein C receptor (EPCR) (Taylor et al. 2001). In concert with protein S (PS), activated PC proteolytically cleaves coagulation cofactors Va and VIIIa, providing a feedback inhibition for thrombin generation. Impairment of the TM–PC pathway in humans is among the most frequent risk factors for venous thrombosis (Seligsohn and Lubetsky 2001). The single most frequent recognized genetic risk factor, the fV Leiden mutation (R506Q), renders activated fV resistant to limited proteolysis by activated PC (Bara et al. 1999), and impairs the fV-dependent anticoagulant cofactor activity (towards activated PC-dependent fVIIIa inactivation) (Thorelli et al. 1999).

Once generated, thrombin activates platelets and cleaves fibrinogen to fibrin, thus contributing to both primary and secondary hemostasis. Thrombin interacts with protease-activated receptors (PARs) and integrin receptors (e.g., glycoprotein Ibα) expressed on platelets, resulting in secretion of α granules and dense body contents and ultimately aggregation of platelets. The thrombin-sensitive PARs on human platelets are PAR1 and PAR4, while on mouse platelets PAR3 and PAR4 are responsive to thrombin.

Thrombin cleaves the Aα- and Bβ-chains of fibrinogen, thus exposing polymerization sites and inducing the aggregation of polymeric fibrin strands. Covalent crosslinks between fibrin molecules, mediated by the transglutaminase fXIIIa, enhances the tensile strength of the clot and its resistance to plasmin degradation. Fibrin interacts with the glycoprotein $\alpha_{IIb}\beta_3$ of activated platelets through its C-terminus of the γ-chain, thus promoting platelet aggregation and the formation of a hemostatic platelet–fibrin clot.

Vascular integrity requires both clot formation, to prevent excessive blood loss, and clot lysis, to maintain vascular patency and thus tissue perfusion. Fibrin can be proteolytically degraded by the plasminogen-derived protease plasmin. Two physiological plasminogen activators have been identified: tissue-type plasminogen activator (tPA) and urokinase-type plasminogen activator (uPA). The activity of tPA increases markedly by the interaction with fibrin, while single-chain uPA acquires proteolytic activity when cleaved by plasmin or kallikrein into the two-chain form. tPA has a specific affinity for fibrin, resulting in clot-restricted plasminogen activation, while uPA is targeted to cell surfaces through interaction with a specific, high-affinity, GPI-anchored plasma membrane receptor (uPAR). Thus, tPA has been considered the predominant initiator of fibrinolysis, while pericellular proteolysis was attributed primarily to uPA-dependent mechanisms. The activation of plasminogen to plasmin by either tPA:fibrin or two-chain uPA is enhanced by binding of plasminogen to carboxyterminal lysine residues of fibrin. The carboxypeptidase thrombin activatable fibrinolysis inhibitor (TAFI), which is activated by the TM-thrombin complex, removes carboxyterminal lysine residues from fibrin, thus inhibiting the degradation of fibrin by plasmin. Plasmin has other substrates besides fibrin, including common extracellular matrix (ECM) glycoproteins, can activate matrix metalloproteases, and liberate latent growth factors (e.g., TGF-β, bFGF). In addition, angiostatin, a noncatalytic fragment of plasmin, has anti-angiogenic properties.

Plasminogen activation is mainly controlled by the serpin plasminogen activator inhibitor-1 (Pai-1), which forms an inactive 1:1 protease–inhibitor complex. The physiological role of the plasminogen activator inhibitor-2, which is mostly retained intracellularly, is still uncertain. Plasmin itself is rapidly inhibited by α_2-antiplasmin, which circulates in plasma at a high concentration (1 μmol/l). α_2-Antiplasmin is synthesized in the liver and released into the circulation, while Pai-1 is produced by several cell types, including endothelial cells and platelets.

Almost all regulators of the hemostatic and fibrinolytic pathways have been inactivated via gene-targeting in mice (Table 1). In some cases, mice with targeted mutations or transgenic mice expressing regulators of hemostasis or fibrinolysis—or functional domains thereof—have been generated. New insights into the hemostatic and fibrinolytic system have been obtained through these studies, and the availability of these mice provides useful tools for future in vivo studies.

Table 1 List of mutations in murine hemostatic and fibrinolytic proteins

Category	Gene mutation	Embryonic lethal?	Murine phenotype	Human deficiency	Relevant references
Promoting thrombin formation	TF$^{-/-}$	Yes (E8.5–10.5)	Lack of vascular integrity, hemorrhage into yolk sac cavity	Neither partial nor complete deficiency recorded	PNAS 93:6258 (1996); Nature 383:73 (1996); Blood 88:1583 (1996)
	FVII$^{-/-}$	No/Yes (before E12.5)	If carried by a FVII wildtype mother: postnatal lethality secondary to hemorrhage (within 24 h) If carried by a mother expressing low FVII levels: vascular defects and embryonic lethality	Variable bleeding, thrombosis reported rarely	Nature 390:290 (1997)
	FX$^{-/-}$	Partial (E11.5–12.5)	No vascular defects, death caused by hemorrhage in embryos and neonates, no survival beyond 20 days after birth	Variable bleeding	Thromb Haemost 83:185 (2000)
	FV$^{-/-}$	Partial (E9.5–10.5)	Vascular defects, death caused by hemorrhage in neonates, limited survival beyond 2 h after birth	Deficiencies <1% extremely rare Mild bleeding, complete deficiency not recorded	Nature 384:66 (1996)
	FII$^{-/-}$	Partial (E9.5–11.5)	Inconsistent reports of embryonic bleeding and vascular abnormalities, death caused by hemorrhage in neonates, no survival beyond several days after birth	Severe bleeding, complete deficiency not recorded	PNAS 95:7597 (1998); PNAS 95:7603 (1998)
	FIX$^{-/-}$	No	Hemorrhagic swelling of feet, death from internal hemorrhage	Hemophilia B; severe bleeding, spontaneous joint bleeds	Blood 90:3962 (1997); Blood 92:168 (1998)
	FVIII$^{-/-}$	No	Prolonged hemorrhage only after challenge (e.g., partial tail amputation)	Hemophilia A; severe bleeding, spontaneous joint bleeds	Nat Genet 10:119 (1995)

Table 1 (continued)

Category	Gene mutation	Embryonic lethal?	Murine phenotype	Human deficiency	Relevant references
Promoting thrombin formation	FXI⁻/⁻	No	Tendency for increased bleeding time, prolonged APTT	Mild bleeding	Blood Coagul Fibrinolysis 8:134 (1997)
Clot formation	Fbg⁻/⁻	No	Neonatal hemorrhage, females cannot support pregnancy	Severe bleeding associated with complete deficiency	Genes Dev 9:2020 (1995); Am J Pathol 157:703 (2000)
	γΔ5 Fbg	No	Impaired platelet aggregation, increased bleeding time	Not recorded	EMBO J 15:5760 (1996)
	Elevated Fbg	No	No increase in mortality, no gross or histological abnormalities	Correlated with various pathologies, thrombosis	Thromb Haemost 86:511 (2001)
	NF-E2⁻/⁻	No	Absolute thrombocytopenia, hemorrhage in neonates, less than 10% survive to adulthood	Not recorded	Cell 81:695 (1995)
	vWF⁻/⁻	No	Prolonged APTT, neonatal hemorrhage	Type III vWD; severe bleeding, reduced FVIII levels	PNAS 95:9524 (1998)
	TFPI⁻/⁻	Yes (E9.5–11.5)	GI bleeding, reduced FVIII levels Liver fibrin deposition, rarely intravascular thrombosis	May be associated with thrombosis, complete deficiency not recorded	Blood 90:944 (1997)
	PCI	No	Impaired spermatogenesis, resulting in infertility	Not recorded	JCI 106:1531 (2000)

Table 1 (continued)

Category	Gene mutation	Embryonic lethal?	Murine phenotype	Human deficiency	Relevant references
Curtailing clot formation	TM$^{-/-}$	Yes (E9.5)	Overall growth retardation and rapid resorption	Thrombosis, complete deficiency not recorded	PNAS 92:850 (1995)
	TM$^{Pro/Pro}$	No	Fibrin deposition in lungs, heart, spleen, and liver; phenotype exacerbated upon thrombogenic challenge	Not recorded	JCI 101:1983 (1998)
	PC$^{-/-}$	No	Signs of DIC as early as E12.5, no survival beyond 24 h after birth	DIC as neonates	JCI 102:1481 (1998)
	EPCR$^{-/-}$	Yes (E9.5–10.5)	Overall growth retardation and embryonic death	Not recorded	Thromb Haemost Suppl (2001)
	FV Leiden	No	APC resistance, fibrin deposition	Thrombosis	Blood 96:4222 (2000)
	ATIII$^{-/-}$	Yes (E15.5–16.5)	Subcutaneous and intracranial hemorrhage, thrombotic damage to embryonic heart and liver, DIC	Thrombosis, complete deficiency not recorded	JCI 106:873 (2000)
	HC$^{-/-}$	No	No overt phenotype	Thrombosis, typically in association with additional risk factors	JCI 109:213 (2002)
	PZ$^{-/-}$	No	No overt phenotype	Maybe associated with thrombosis, complete deficiency not recorded	PNAS 97:6734 (2000)

Table 1 (continued)

Category	Gene mutation	Embryonic lethal?	Murine phenotype	Human deficiency	Relevant references
Pro-fibrinolytic	Plasminogen	No	Spontaneous thrombosis, rectal prolapse, conjunctivitis, reduced bodyweight, impaired survival	Ligneous conjunctivitis in patients with hypoplasminogenemia, complete deficiency not recorded	Genes Dev 9:794 (1995)
	tPA	No	Increased tissue-fibrin deposition, normal life expectancy, reduced fertility	Deficiencies associated with thrombosis; complete deficiency not recorded	Nature 368:419 (1994)
	uPA	No	Spontaneous fibrin deposition, rectal prolapse, non-healing ulceration of the eyelids, reduced fertility	Not recorded	Nature 368:418 (1994)
Anti-fibrinolytic	α_2-Antiplasmin	No	No overt phenotype	Hemorrhagic complications	Blood 93:2274 (1999)
	Pai-1	No	No overt phenotype	Hemorrhagic complications	JCI 92:2756 (1993)
	TAFI	No	No overt phenotype	Acquired deficiencies (liver disease) without apparent phenotype; inherited deficiencies not recorded	JCI 109:101 (2002)

APC, activated protein C; APTT, activated partial thromboplastin time; DIC, disseminated intravascular coagulopathy; E, embryonic day; GI, gastrointestinal.

2
Intrauterine and Perinatal Defects in Mice with Disrupted Hemostasis

2.1
Yolk Sac Defects

2.1.1
Procoagulant Defects

Mice lacking TF, fVII, fV, or prothrombin fail to establish a functional yolk sac vasculature, resulting in embryonic lethality during midgestation [around day 10.5 *post coitum* (p.c.)] (Bugge et al. 1996a; Carmeliet et al. 1996; Cui et al. 1996; Toomey et al. 1996; Rosen et al. 1997; Sun et al. 1998; Xue et al. 1998) (see Fig. 2 for an overview). The penetrance of this midgestational phenotype depends on the genetic background. For example, on a mixed 129/SvJ-C57BL/6 background development of some TF-null embryos proceeds normally until birth, when these embryos nevertheless succumb to the perinatal hemostatic challenge (Toomey et al. 1997). The TF-dependent midgestational lethality persists independent of the cytoplasmic domain of TF, but requires binding of fVII/VIIa to TF and/or proteolytic activity of the TF/fVIIa complex, indicating that the developmental function of TF is related to its known interaction with fVII (Parry and Mackman 2000; Melis et al. 2001). The lethal yolk sac defect in fVII-deficient embryos is only apparent when these embryos are carried by females with minimal fVII levels, but not if the mother expresses wildtype fVII (Rosen et al. 1997; Chan et al. 2001a), suggesting that embryonic coagulation factor deficiency can be at least partially mitigated by trans-placental transfer of maternal coagulation factors. Thus, fVII levels in fVII-deficient embryos (carried by fVII expressing females) are below the detection limit (<0.05%), demonstrating that very low levels of coagulation factor can be sufficient for normal development. The latter observation is consistent with normal embryogenesis in mice with less than 1% of wildtype tissue factor activity (Parry et al. 1998), severely impaired TM-dependent PC activation (Weiler-Guettler et al. 1998), or minimal EPCR expression (Rosen et al. 2001). Low levels of maternally derived fX might prevent defects in the yolk sac vasculature of fX-deficient mice (Dewerchin et al. 2000). Of note, expression of an fV transgene, resulting in low fV levels in adult mice (<3%), does not prevent the lethal yolk sac hemorrhage affecting approximately half of fV knockout embryos (Yang et al. 2000). However, the liver-specific albumin promoter used for the fV transgene expression might have failed to mediate fV expression in non-hepatic tissue sites (e.g., yolk sac) or at sufficient levels during early midgestation. The observation that minimal coagulation regulator activity can maintain the hemostatic balance is consistent with the clinical experience that therapeutic substitution of coagulation factors at low levels (~1%) in coagulation factor-deficient individuals is adequate to prevent complications (High 2001).

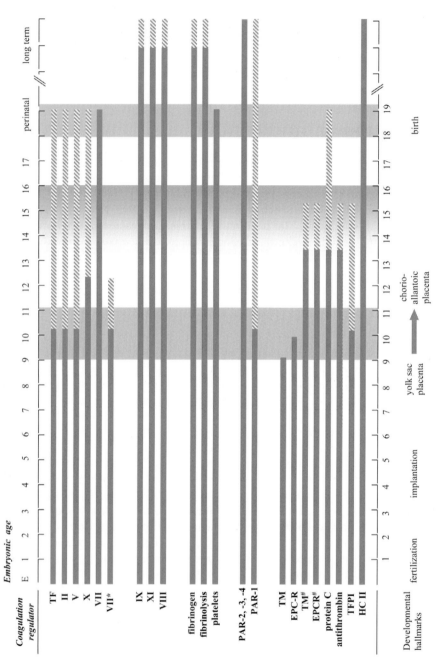

Fig. 2 Embryonic phenotypes in mice with genetically altered hemostasis. Three "risk windows" are apparent: (1) E9–E11, when the chorioallantoic placenta and the embryonic circulation are established; (2) E13–E16; (3) perinatal. *Solid bars* indicate normal development and survival; *striped bars* indicate partial survival and/or pathological phenotype. *VII**, fVII$^{-/-}$ embryos carried by mice with low fVII expression; *TM$^{\#}$* and *EPCR$^{\#}$*, embryos with tissue-restricted expression of TM and EPCR, respectively, in the placenta

2.1.2
Anticoagulants Defects

A subset of embryos lacking TFPI succumbs to lethal midgestational yolk sac hemorrhage closely resembling the phenotype observed in mice lacking TF (Huang et al. 1997). This lethal intrauterine yolk sac defect does not occur in mice with a compound TFPI and fVII deficiency (Chan et al. 1999), demonstrating that fVII and TFPI interact during development, most likely in a fashion related to their known hemostatic functions. This notion is supported by the recently reported survival of TFPI-null mice beyond 1 year of age in the absence of fibrinogen (Degen 2001). These preliminary reports did not clarify, however, whether fibrinogen deficiency corrected the early yolk sac defect, the consumptive coagulopathy at later stages (see below), or both defects. Future analyses of other double-knockout mice will yield further information about the exact nature of the TF, fVII, and TFPI interaction, the relevant substrates, and the mechanisms involved in yolk sac vascular development.

2.2
Placental Defects

2.2.1
Procoagulant Defects

A placental defect has been identified in mice expressing a human TF-minigene, resulting in low TF activity (less than 1% of wildtype TF-activity) (Erlich et al. 1999). Unlike completely TF-deficient mice (Bugge et al. 1996a; Carmeliet et al. 1996; Toomey et al. 1996), which die secondary to a yolk sac defect (see above), these mice survive into adulthood. Detailed analysis revealed placental hemorrhage within the labyrinthine layer of the placenta associated with a reduction of cellular contacts between trophoblast cells ("layer I" trophoblast cells) and reduced staining for cytokeratin. This defect predisposes pregnant mice to midgestational lethal hemorrhage only if both the embryo and the mother have low TF activity, indicating that maternal and embryonic coagulation regulators interact in the placenta.

In the absence of maternal, but not embryonic fibrinogen, hemorrhage at the placental implantation site occurs as early as embryonic day (E)6.0, and increases in severity until approximately E9.5, resulting in a separation of the placenta from the decidua at the giant trophoblast cell layer (Iwaki et al. 2002). Levels of laminin, fibronectin, and fXIII appear to be unaffected by the absence of maternal fibrinogen, indicating a critical role of fibrinogen itself for the development of the hemochorial placenta. The developmental delay of embryos derived from fibrinogen-null females presumably reflects the impaired placental function (Iwaki et al. 2002).

2.2.2
Anticoagulant Defects

The earliest developmental defects occur in TM- and EPCR-deficient mice (Healy et al. 1995; Gu et al. 2001). The absence of TM or EPCR results in embryonic lethality during early midgestation, before the establishment of a functional cardiovascular system in the embryo proper. Consistently, the primary defect in TM-null embryos occurs within placental tissue, and TM-expression restricted to the placenta (giant trophoblast and parietal endoderm cells) rescues TM-null embryos from early lethality (Isermann et al. 2001a). The developmental function of TM must be mediated through the EGF-like domains or the threonine-serine-rich domain, as targeted deletion of the cytoplasmic or lectin-like domain does not impair embryonic development (Conway et al. 1999, 2001). The developmental function of TM is at least in part related to its known anticoagulant role, as inhibition of the maternal coagulation system (via heparin or warfarin) or maternal fibrinogen deficiency prevents the rapid resorption of TM-null embryos. Interestingly, inhibition of the rapid resorption reveals a complete growth arrest of TM-null embryos at E8.5 (B. Isermann, H. Weiler, manuscript submitted). These findings establish that embryonic coagulation regulators interact with and control maternal hemostasis. However, the growth arrest of TM-null embryos is mediated by embryonic, but not maternal TF activity, and is independent of fibrin(ogen), implying a dual role of TM during development. The exact mechanism underlying the TM-null growth arrest, and whether TM and EPCR coordinately regulate embryonic development, is currently being investigated.

2.3
Defects of the Embryo Proper

2.3.1
Procoagulant Defects

Defects other than hemorrhage or thrombosis within the embryo proper have not been identified in mice lacking coagulation regulators. As mentioned, a proportion of embryos lacking TF (Bugge et al. 1996; Carmeliet et al. 1996; Toomey et al. 1996), fV (Cui et al. 1996), or prothrombin (Sun et al. 1998; Xue et al. 1998) survive until birth, when they succumb to hemorrhagic complications. Likewise, about one third of embryos lacking fX die during midgestation, but the remaining embryos survive until term and die during the postnatal period (Dewerchin et al. 2000). Lethal postnatal hemorrhage affects also 100% of fVII-deficient embryos that survive until term (Rosen et al. 1997). The partial rescue of some embryos with disrupted procoagulant pathways might reflect genetic heterogeneity, as demonstrated in TF-deficient mice (Toomey et al. 1997), or transfer of maternal coagulation factors, as demonstrated in fVII-deficient mice (Chan et al. 2001a). The latter provides a rationale for the lethal postnatal hemorrhage, when the birth-related trauma coincides with a sudden loss of maternally derived coagulation factors.

Deficiency of the fibrinogen $A\alpha$- or γ-chain, resulting in total fibrinogen deficiency, is compatible with murine embryonic development (Suh et al. 1995; Ploplis et al. 2000). However, depending on the genetic background, 10% (C57/6 J) to 30% (129/CF-1) of fibrinogen-deficient mice succumb to spontaneous postnatal hemorrhage (Suh et al. 1995). Thus, the consequences of fibrinogen deficiency are less severe than those seen in embryos lacking procoagulant coagulation regulators. The less severe phenotype in mice lacking fibrinogen has been attributed to compensatory platelet-dependent hemostasis in these mice. Like fibrinogen-deficient mice, embryos with a isolated platelet defect, secondary to impaired megakaryocyte maturation in the absence of the transcription factor NF-E2, develop normal until term, when the majority of embryos (90%) succumbs to a severe perinatal hemorrhage (Shivdasani et al. 1995). Perinatal hemorrhage in platelet-deficient embryos can be prevented by caesarian section, establishing birth-related trauma as the cause for the perinatal hemorrhage. Interesting, mice that lack fibrinogen and have functional impaired platelets [$Gq\alpha$ knockout mice (Offermanns et al. 1997)] develop normal until birth, when they again succumb to the severe perinatal hemostatic challenge (Degen 2001). These observations suggest that the two principal endpoints of the coagulation system, fibrinogen and platelets, are not required for normal embryonic development, and indicate that the endpoint of coagulation factor activation during midgestation might be unrelated to the formation of a platelet–fibrin clot.

A role for thrombin, independent of the formation of a platelet-fibrin clot, during development is supported by the vascular defects in embryos lacking the thrombin receptor PAR1 (Griffin et al. 2001). PAR1 is expressed in endothelial cells during development, and absence of PAR1 results in hemorrhage and cardiovascular failure during midgestation in a subset of embryos (Darrow et al. 1996; Griffin et al. 2001). Endothelial specific, tie-2-dependent expression of PAR1 prevents the hemorrhagic complications of PAR1 deficiency, identifying a role for endothelial PAR1 during development.

2.3.2
Anticoagulants Defects

TFPI-deficient embryos escaping the midgestational lethality succumb to a consumptive coagulopathy after day 11.5 p.c., which is associated with fibrin deposition in the liver and—rarely—intravascular thrombosis (Huang et al. 1997). A strikingly similar phenotype is apparent in embryos lacking the anticoagulant proteins antithrombin (Ishiguro et al. 2000) or PC (Jalbert et al. 1998), or in embryos with spatial-limited TM expression in the placenta (Isermann et al. 2001a). Conversely, mice lacking heparin cofactor II, a specific thrombin inhibitor, or PZ, a cofactor for fXa inhibition, do not develop spontaneous thrombosis pre- or postnatally (Yin et al. 2000; He et al. 2002). Antithrombin deficiency results in extensive fibrin(ogen) deposition in the myocardium and liver, but not the brain or lung. In the absence of PC or embryonic TM, fibrin deposition occurs as early as day 12.5 p.c., particularly in the brain and liver, ultimately resulting in a lethal consumptive hemorrhage. Consistent with the early intrauterine onset of the consumptive coagulopathy in PC-deficient embryos, caesarian section does not increase the survival of PC knockout mice, establishing that death occurs independent of the birth-related trauma (Jalbert et al. 1998). Inactivation of the fVII gene does not attenuate the phenotype of PC-deficient embryos, but rather aggravates the hemorrhagic complications (Chan et al. 2000). Conversely, mice with a compound fXI and PC deficiency are partially rescued from the consumptive perinatal lethality observed in mice with isolated PC deficiency (Chan et al. 2001a). These observations confirm that PC-dependent coagulation inhibition predominantly affects the amplification pathway of coagulation, and demonstrate the importance of fXI-dependent coagulation amplification during development.

3
Defects in Adult Mice with Disrupted Hemostasis or Fibrinolytic

3.1
Hemorrhagic Phenotypes

3.1.1
Procoagulant Defects

Mice lacking the coagulation factors VIII, IX, or XI are born at a slightly reduced frequency, indicating only minor fetal or perinatal wastage (Bi et al. 1995; Gailani et al. 1997; Lin et al. 1997; Kundu et al. 1998). Thus, contrary to the initiation pathway of coagulation, the amplification pathway appears to have little or no specific developmental function. Mice lacking fVIII or fIX have increased tail bleeding times. While spontaneous hemorrhage resulting in potentially lethal complications occurs in fIX-null mice (Bi et al. 1995, 1996; Lin et al. 1997), fVIII-Null mice lack signs of spontaneous hemorrhage and females carry pregnancy to birth without apparent problems. Therefore, the phenotype in fIX-deficient mice replicates the disease in humans (hemophilia B) more faithfully than the murine fVIII-null phenotype (hemophilia A).

FXI-null mice survive at expected frequency, and females carry pregnancies without apparent problems (Gailani et al. 1997). These mice have a markedly prolonged activated partial thromboplastin time (aPTT) but normal PT, as expected, and normal tail bleeding time, thus closely replicating the milder phenotype of humans with fXI deficiency when compared to patients with hemophilia A or B.

Absence of von Willebrand's factor (vWF) reduces fVIII levels (about 20% of wildtype levels), reflecting the increased proteolytic inactivation of fVIII in the absence of vWF. Mice lacking vWF have a hemorrhagic diathesis resulting in spontaneous hemorrhage in about 10% of newborn mice and a prolonged tail bleeding time (Denis et al. 1998). Compound vWF and fibrinogen deficiency, resulting in a loss of two important platelet ligands, increases the postnatal lethality of mice (to about 23%), but the remaining mice survive into adulthood (Ni et al. 2000).

Gene targeting has been employed to determine in vivo the role of the 5 carboxyterminal amino acids of the fibrinogen γ-chain for the interaction with integrin $\alpha_{IIb}\beta_3$, which can bind fibrinogen when "activated," resulting in enhanced platelet aggregation and clot retraction. Mice homozygous for a mutated fibrinogen γ-chain, lacking 5 carboxyterminal AS, have normal thrombin time, fibrin crosslinking, and clot retraction, but prolonged tail bleeding time and occasionally fatal neonatal hemorrhage (Holmback et al. 1996). In vitro analyses revealed a failure of platelets to aggregate and reduced binding of mutant fibrinogen to immobilized $\alpha_{IIb}\beta_3$ (Holmback et al. 1996). These in vivo structure–function analyses revealed that the carboxyterminal end of the fibrinogen γ-chain is critical for hemostasis, but not necessary for clot retraction.

3.1.2
Fibrinolytic Defects

Impairment of antifibrinolytic mechanisms by disrupting the genes for either plasminogen activator inhibitor-1 (Pai-1) or α_2-antiplasmin results in a hyperfibrinolytic state, as determined by enhanced in vivo lysis of ^{125}I-labled clots and reduced thrombus formation following lipopolysaccharide (LPS) challenge (Carmeliet et al. 1993a; Lijnen et al. 1999). However, unlike human Pai-1- or α_2-antiplasmin deficiencies, which result in hemorrhagic complications (Miles et al. 1982; Fay et al. 1997), these mice lack an apparent impairment of the hemostatic response, even after amputation of the tail tip. Transgenic liver-specific expression of uPA results in lethal abdominal and gastrointestinal hemorrhage in about 50% of newborns (Heckel et al. 1990). The hemorrhagic diathesis is associated with markedly reduced fibrinogen plasma levels despite normal mRNA levels. Normal platelet counts in these newborns argue against a consumptive coagulopathy as the underlying cause. The exact mechanism of the hypofibrinogenemia and the importance of increased fibrinolysis in these mice remain to be established. Targeting of the plasminogen activator inhibitor-2 (Pai-2) gene and subsequent generation of Pai-1 and Pai-2 double-knockout mice failed to uncover an overlap in function between these two related proteins (Dougherty et al. 1999). Pai-2-deficient mice exhibit normal development, survival, and fertility, normal response to bacterial challenge or endotoxin infusion, normal recruitment of monocytes into the peritoneum, and normal epidermal wound healing.

3.2
Thrombotic Phenotypes

3.2.1
Anticoagulant Defects

Mice carrying a targeted point mutation (R504Q) corresponding to the human fV Leiden mutation are viable, display a decreased APC resistance ratio associated with increased organ-specific fibrin deposition (in lung, heart, spleen, kidney, and brain, but not in the liver), and develop occasionally spontaneous phenotypic thrombosis, thus replicating closely the phenotype of humans carrying the fV Leiden mutation (Cui et al. 2000). The thrombin-generating potential is higher on a mixed 129Sv-C57BL/6 J than on a pure C57BL/6 J background, resulting in perinatal lethal disseminated intravascular coagulation activation in about one quarter of embryos. The prothrombotic diathesis of fV Leiden mice (129Sv-C57BL/6 J background) is further aggravated when mice lack in addition protein Z (PZ), resulting in increased intrauterine fibrin deposition (including the liver) associated with obvious signs of hemorrhage in about 90% of embryos, indicating a consumptive coagulopathy already in utero (Yin et al. 2000). Mice with a compound defect of fV and PZ exemplify the well-documented clinical experience, that the combination of prothrombotic traits significantly increases the risk for thrombosis. In addition, these in vivo experiments provided the first in vivo evidence for anticoagulant properties of PZ, demonstrating the value of studies combining mutant mice strains with mild or absent phenotypes.

Disruption of the murine TM gene constitutes an alternative approach to generate mice with a disrupted TM—PC pathway and has led to the identification of a vital developmental role of placental TM (see above). To circumvent the lethality associated with complete embryonic TM deficiency, several mice with partially impaired TM function have been generated. TM-null chimeric mice, displaying up to 40% chimerism based on the presence of embryonic stem (ES) cell-derived glycerol phosphate isoenzyme (Healy et al. 1998), and mice with a targeted point mutation in the TM gene (E404P), abolishing the cofactor activity of TM towards the thrombin-dependent PC activation (Weiler-Guettler et al. 1998), survive without an apparent phenotype into adulthood. Spontaneous fibrin deposition, however, is increased in both mouse models, and is further increased when mice are challenged (e.g., LPS or hypoxia). Interestingly, deposition of crosslinked fibrin co-localizes with TM-null regions in larger vessels of TM-null chimeric mice, emphasizing the role of local blood coagulation activation and subsequent fibrin deposition (Healy et al. 1998). The latter finding implies that spatially impairment of endothelial anticoagulant function, e.g., following invasive manipulations or at the site of arteriosclerotic lesions, is a strong risk factor for local thrombosis.

Endothelial TM deficiency has been achieved by tissue-specific inactivation of the TM gene (LoxP sequences flanking the endogenous TM gene, and tie-2 dependent Cre expression) (Isermann et al. 2001b). Mice with endothelial TM deficiency (TM^{Lox} mice) are born at a reduced frequency (about 60% of the expected numbers), but live-born TM^{Lox} mice appear undistinguishable compared to littermates during the neonatal period. Subsequently, TM^{Lox} mice develop spontaneous intravascular thrombosis, resulting in necrosis of extremities, skin, and internal organs. Anticoagulation with warfarin (coumadin) completely prevents the onset of spontaneous thrombosis in TM^{Lox} mice, implying that the consequences of endothelial TM deficiency are indeed caused by increased coagulation activation. Conversely, the importance of impaired TAFI activation in TM^{Lox} mice is likely of minor significance, considering the normal phenotype of TAFI-null mice even when challenged (arterial and venous thrombosis model, thrombin, LPS, writhing response) (Nagashima et al. 2002).

If left untreated TM^{Lox} mice develop a consumptive coagulopathy, thus replicating—although at a later age—the consequences of PC deficiency (Isermann et al. 2001b). The postnatal consumptive coagulopathy seen in PC-deficient mice is in part corrected on a fXI-deficient background (Chan et al. 2001a). The partial survival of PC-deficient mice lacking fXI demonstrates in vivo the importance of fXI-dependent, thrombin-mediated feedback amplification within the coagulation system. Conversely, inactivation of fVII has no beneficial effect on the perinatal consumptive coagulopathy of PC-deficient mice (Chan et al. 2000). These observations are consistent with the persistence of thrombosis in TM-deficient mice with minimal TF expression (B. Isermann, H. Weiler, manuscript submitted). Taken together, these results underline the importance of the TM–PC pathway in controlling the thrombin-dependent feedback amplification of coagulation, and demonstrate the thrombin generation potential despite genetic impairment of TF/VIIa-dependent coagulation initiation. Furthermore, these results confirm the pivotal role of fXI-dependent feedback amplification during coagulation activation.

A mild prothrombotic phenotype is observed in heterozygous antithrombin-deficient mice, resulting in spontaneous fibrin deposition in the kidney (glomeruli, peritubular capillaries), liver sinusoids, and small vessels of the myocardium in comparison to wildtype mice (Yanada et al. 2002). Fibrin depositions in heterozygous antithrombin mice are further increased in animals challenged with LPS or physical stress.

3.2.2
Fibrinolytic Defects

Isolated deficiency of either tPA or uPA does not impair embryogenesis, fertility, or normal lifespan, thus arguing against a crucial role of either plasminogen activator alone in development, reproduction, thrombosis, thrombolysis, or macrophage function (Carmeliet et al. 1994). Despite a reduced ex vivo thrombolytic potential and increased myocardial fibrin deposition (Christie et al. 1999) tPA mice appear healthy throughout life. Conversely, uPA-deficient mice, despite normal ex vivo thrombolytic potential, develop occasionally spontaneous fibrin deposition, non-infections rectal prolapse, and non-healing ulceration of the eyelids. If challenged (footpad injection of endotoxin), the frequency of intravascular thrombi is increased in both knockout mice when compared to wild-type mice. Postnatal growth and fertility are impaired in mice with a combined deficiency of tPA and uPA, but embryogenesis proceeds normally despite the absence of both plasminogen activators (Carmeliet et al. 1994). Fibrin deposition is markedly increased in tPA:uPA double-knockout mice (affected organs: liver, intestines, gonad, and lung) in comparison to singly deficient tPA or uPA mice. Furthermore, mice with tPA:uPA deficiency develop frequently rectal prolapse and occasionally non-healing skin ulcerations, and 17% become runted, cachectic, and dyspneic, resulting in premature death. These double-knockout studies demonstrated that the function of tPA and uPA are at least in part redundant and that uPA conveys an endogenous fibrinolytic potential.

Interestingly, tPA:uPA-deficient mice do not display spontaneous thrombosis and subsequent necrosis of extremities, which occurs in mice expressing a (human) Pai-1 transgene (Erickson et al. 1990). Conversely, Pai-1 transgenic mice survive the initial thrombotic challenge and—unlike tPA:uPA knockout mice— have a normal life expectancy. These discrepancies might reflect difference in the function of tPA/uPA and/or species- and age-dependent differences in the function and expression of the Pai-1 transgene.

Mice lacking uPAR have a surprisingly mild phenotype and display normal thrombolytic activity (despite impaired plasminogen activation in vitro) and ECM degradation in vivo (Dewerchin et al. 1996). In contrast to the severe and widespread fibrin deposition in tPA:uPA double-knockout mice, fibrin deposition is restricted to the liver sinusoids in mice lacking tPA and uPAR. This finding demonstrates that the function of uPA is at least in part independent of uPAR and that uPAR is not strictly needed for the fibrinolytic effect of uPA.

Plasminogen deficiency predisposes mice to spontaneous thrombosis, resulting in reduced bodyweight and reduced survival and rectal prolapse (Bugge et al. 1995; Ploplis et al. 1995), the latter reminiscence of those seen in mice with isolated uPA and compound tPA:uPA deficiency. Fibrin depositions in adult plasminogen-null mice are detected histologically in liver, and occasionally in lung and intestine, the latter associated with gastric ulcer. The similar phenotypes of tPA:uPA and plasminogen-deficient mice imply that tPA and uPA are the only physiologically relevant plasminogen activators. The chronic pseudo-membranous conductivities observed in plasminogen-deficient mice, characterized by acellular, fibrin-rich material and aberrant disrupted epithelium (Drew et al. 1998), is reminiscent of ligneous conjunctivitis seen in humans with plasminogen deficiency (Schuster et al. 2001).

The widespread occurrence of spontaneous thrombosis and the absence of other spontaneous phenotypes in mice with a compound plasminogen activator deficiency or plasminogen deficiency, and the absence of fibrin deposition and associated complications (such as thrombosis, wasting, reduced life expectancy, and impaired wound healing) in mice lacking both plasminogen and fibrinogen support the notion that the primary role of the plasminogen system is fibrinolysis (Bugge et al. 1996b). However, as discussed below, detailed analyses of these mice revealed some milder phenotypes, and the applications of various disease models identified functions of the plasminogen system independent of fibrinolysis.

3.3
Arterial Thrombosis, Arteriosclerosis, and Vascular Remodeling

3.3.1
Anticoagulant Defects

Considering the impact of arteriosclerotic disease for individual health and the associated socioeconomic burden, it is not surprising that much effort has been dedicated to improve our understanding of how the coagulation and fibrinolytic systems modulate arteriosclerotic disease. Disruption of natural anticoagulant mechanisms are primarily considered a risk factor for venous thrombosis (Lane and Grant 2000), and their role for arterial disease is less well defined. However, clinical studies suggest that natural anticoagulant mechanisms modify arterial disease (Salomaa et al. 1999)—a notion now backed by in vivo experiments employing genetically modified mice. Mice with impaired PC activation (TM^{Pro} mice), heparin cofactor II knockout mice, or heterozygous TFPI (TFPI$^{+/-}$) mice with compounding apoE deficiency lack spontaneous thrombosis or arteriosclerosis, but these mice display a significantly shortened occlusion time of the common carotid artery following experimental endothelial cell damage (Weiler et al. 2001; Westrick et al. 2001; He et al. 2002), demonstrating a role for these natural anticoagulants in platelet-rich thrombosis. Reduction of TFPI (TFPI heterozygous mice) promotes the spontaneous development of arteriosclerotic lesions, determined in the carotid and iliac arteries, in apoE-deficient mice (Westrick et al. 2001). Atherosclerosis in heterozygous TFPI, apoE-null mice coincides with increased plaque-associated TF activity. Taken together, these results indicate that endogenous anticoagulant mechanisms modulate acute arterial thrombosis, and development of atherosclerotic lesions.

Increased thrombin activation in prothrombotic mice might promote arteriosclerosis through the formation of platelet–fibrin clots, or—alternatively—through PAR1-dependent cellular effects. Indeed, vascular remodeling is impaired in PAR1-deficient mice, as the total diameter of injured blood vessels remains constant despite increased media thickness, resulting in a reduced vessel lumen (Cheung et al. 1999). These changes have to be independent of thrombin-mediated (and PAR-dependent) platelet activation as mouse platelets lack PAR1.

Platelets contribute largely, however, to acute arterial thrombosis. The interaction between (activated) platelets and the injured vessel wall are mostly mediated by binding of platelets to either fibrin (via $\alpha_{IIb}\beta_3$) or vWF (via glycoprotein Ib). Consistently, the absence of either platelet ligand impairs the formation of platelet-rich thrombi in injured arterioles, but vascular occlusion ultimately occurs (Ni et al. 2000). Surprisingly, vascular occlusion also occurs, albeit delayed, in the absence of both platelet ligands (fibrinogen and wWF double-knockout mice), indicating that in the absence of these ligands platelets interact with other substrates. It remains to be established to which extent these—currently unidentified—substrates contribute to arterioscleroses in humans.

3.3.2
Fibrinolytic Defects

The role of the fibrinolytic system for arterial thrombosis has been addressed in a number of in vivo studies, providing new insights, but also raising questions as some results appear contradictory. In principle, two different model systems have been applied to evaluate the role of the fibrinolytic system for acute arterial occlusion and arteriosclerosis: (1) acute arterial damage and (2) genetic models for spontaneous arteriosclerotic lesions.

Acute Arterial Injury. Following endothelial cell damage the formation of a predominately platelet-rich thrombi, defined as time to occlusion, appears to be unaffected by uPA or tPA levels, but prolonged in mice lacking Pai-1 or α_2-antiplasmin (Matsuno et al. 1999; Kawasaki et al. 2000). During acute arterial occlusion, Pai-1 is mostly derived from the injured endothelium, and not from platelets (Kawasaki et al. 2000). In addition, Pai-1 appears to modulate the persistence of thrombi at the site of endothelial cell damage, as the frequency and size of arterial thrombosis is about twice as high after 24 h in wildtype mice as compared to Pai-1-null mice (Farrehi et al. 1998). The redundant activities of uPA and tPA provide a rationale for the failure of isolated uPA or tPA deficiency to modify experimental acute arterial thrombosis. Conversely, spontaneous myocardial fibrin deposition is mediated by endogenous tPA levels, while endogenous uPA deficiency has only a minor effect (Christie et al. 1999). The severity of the spontaneous fibrin deposition and associated myocardial dysfunction in the absence of tPA can be aggravated by a superimposed TM (TM^{Pro}) or uPA deficiency. A critical role of tPA and its Pai-1-modulated activity for arterial fibrinolysis is supported by studies employing reperfusion models, in which tPA-dependent fibrinolysis is enhanced in the absence of Pai-1 (Zhu et al. 1999). These results imply that high Pai-1 levels can mediate thrombolysis resistance in humans.

Unlike early arterial thrombosis, plasminogen activators mediate mural thrombosis after initiation of vascular wall remodeling (e.g., after 2 or 3 weeks of vascular damage). Mural thrombosis is more pronounced in mice lacking uPA or plasminogen, and to a lesser degree in tPA-null mice, as compared to wildtype mice, indicating a predominant role of uPA during vascular wound healing (Carmeliet et al. 1997a). Likewise, arterial wound healing, characterized by the migration of smooth muscle cells into the injured vessel wall, and subsequent neointima formation is reduced in the absence of uPA and plasminogen, while the absence of Pai-1 accelerates the neointima formation (more neointima 1 week, but not 3 weeks after vascular wall injury) (Carmeliet et al. 1997a,b,c).

Neointima formation following acute arterial injury is modulated by uPA, plasminogen, and Pai-1 through regulation of smooth muscle cell migration, and not proliferation (Carmeliet et al. 1997b). Accumulation of neointima cells and migration of smooth muscle cells is independent of tPA or uPAR levels (Carmeliet et al. 1997c, 1998; Lijnen et al. 1998). Consistently, activity of tPA, as determined by zymography, does not change following acute arterial damage, while uPA activity increases (Lijnen et al. 1998). Interestingly, re-endothelization is not affected by genetic alterations of the plasminogen system following acute vascular injury, independent of the mode of vascular injury (Carmeliet et al. 1997a,b,c).

Increased uPA activity is associated with increased matrix metalloproteinase (MMP)-9 activity during vascular remodeling in the presence, but not in the absence of plasminogen, identifying MMP-9 and potentially other matrix metalloproteases as alternative endpoints of the fibrinolytic system (Lijnen et al. 1998). These results are supported by studies evaluating cardiac rupture following myocardial infarction in mice with defective plasminogen system or lacking MMPs (Heymans et al. 1999; Creemers et al. 2000). Deficiency of uPA, plasminogen, or MMP-9, or treatment with Pai-1 or TIMP-1, an MMP inhibitor, prevents early post myocardial failure (within 3 days) secondary to cardiac rupture. However, in the absence of uPA or plasminogen, granulation or fibrous tissue fails to replace necrotic cardiomyocytes, resulting in late cardiac failure due to depressed contractility, arrhythmias, and ischemia (after 14 days). Transient treatment with Pai-1 or tissue inhibitor of metalloprotease (TIMP)-1 protects mice from early cardiac rupture without impairing the formation of scar tissue (Heymans et al. 1999). A similar role of the fibrinolytic system has been suggested for late-graft arterial disease (after 15–45 days), as the absence of plasminogen attenuates fragmentation of elastic laminae, media necrosis, adventitial remodeling, and reduces macrophage infiltration (Moons et al. 1998).

Both fibrinogen-dependent and -independent roles of plasmin for vascular remodeling have been identified using a different model (arterial cuff placement) (Drew et al. 2000). In this model, compensatory vascular remodeling is impaired in the absence of plasminogen, but can be restored by superimposed fibrinogen deficiency, demonstrating that plasmin-mediated fibrinolysis, potentially within the adventitia, can be an important determinant for vascular remodeling. Conversely, medial atrophy of challenged blood vessels is enhanced in plasminogen-null mice independent of fibrinogen (Drew et al. 2000). While the relevant plasmin substrate preventing medial atrophy has not been identified, these results are consistent with a failure to clear and repopulate necrotic tissue, e.g., as a consequence of reduced ECM degradation. Unlike models using direct vascular injury (e.g., electric or chemical injury) neointima formation, migration of inflammatory and smooth muscle cells, and elastic membrane breakdown were independent of plasminogen levels in the vascular cuff model.

Spontaneous Arteriosclerotic Lesions. A role of the plasminogen system independent of fibrin is supported by the unaltered presence of arteriosclerotic lesions in apoE-null mice, both in the presence of absence of fibrinogen (Xiao et al. 1998). However, these results obtained in a murine model do not exclude a role of fibrin for the development of arteriosclerotic lesions in humans. Unlike humans, mice lack apo(a), a component of Lp(a), which has high sequence homology with plasminogen. Apo(a) might competitively inhibit binding of plasminogen to fibrin, thus contributing to atherosclerosis. Indeed, transgenic expression of apo(a) in mice induces fatty streak-like aortic lesions in the presence of a high-fat diet (Lou et al. 1998). These lesions coincide with decreased levels of plasmin and TGF-β and increased smooth muscle cell activation. The absence of fibrinogen largely reduces these lesions (by 81%) (Lou et al. 1998). Thus, fibrin/ogen promotes the development of arteriosclerotic lesions in the presence of apo(a). Fibrin has been identified as a risk factor for arteriosclerosis and myocardial infarction in humans (Thompson et al. 1995), and the above in vivo studies exemplify that results obtained in mice have to be interpreted critically considering clinical experience and species-specific differences.

Evaluations of arteriosclerotic lesions in hyperlipidemic mice with altered Pai-1 activity have yielded conflicting results. Spontaneous arteriosclerotic lesions (after 30 weeks) of the proximal aorta in ApoE or low-density lipoprotein cholesterol receptor (LDLR)-deficient mice appear to be independent of Pai-1 activity (Pai-1-null, Pai-1 wildtype, and transgenic—overexpressing—Pai-1 mice), while Pai-1 deficiency reduces plaque growth in the carotid bifurcation (Eitzman 2000; Sjoland 2000). The protective effect of Pai-1 deficiency is consistent with the accelerated formation of intimal lesions in apoE mice lacking plasminogen (Xiao et al. 1997). These studies suggest that plasmin attenuates the development of arteriosclerotic lesions, potentially by removing fibrin. Other studies, evaluating the role of the fibrinolytic system in apoE-deficient mice come to a different conclusion. Atherosclerotic plaques in the abdominal and thoracic aorta of apoE knockout mice (on a normal chow or a cholesterol-rich diet) were more advanced in the absence of Pai-1 (promoting plasminogen activation) after 25 weeks, but not after 5 or 10 weeks (Luttun et al. 2002). Pai-1 deficiency was associated with an increased number of macrophages, more matrix components, higher activity of MMPs, and higher levels of TGF-β. Consistently, uPA deficiency (impairing plasminogen activation) attenuated media destruction and aneurysm formation in apoE-deficient mice (Carmeliet et al. 1997d). The latter studies imply that increased plasmin activity promotes tissue remodeling with long-term detrimental effects on arteriosclerotic lesions. The differences in the above studies might reflect heterogeneous genetic backgrounds, variations in the model or the food used, or in the time and procedure of analyses, or vascular bed-specific differences. At any rate, it appears that the role of the plasminogen system in arteriosclerosis is complex, with both detrimental and beneficial effects.

The different results obtained from distinct models of acute vascular injury imply that the implications from these animal studies have to be cautiously compared with the corresponding clinical settings, if conclusions for clinical practice are to be made.

3.4
Stroke

A role of the fibrinolytic system in the central nervous system unrelated to fibrin/ogen has been demonstrated in mice, triggering a re-evaluation of plasminogen activators, especially tPA, for the treatment of thrombotic strokes. Both plasminogen and tPA are expressed by neurons, while tPA is in addition expressed in microglial and upregulated in the cerebellum during normal neuronal stimulation and changes in plasticity (Wu et al. 2000). Late long-term potentiation in the hippocampus (in Schaffer collaterals and the mossy fiber pathway) is reduced in tPA-null mice even in the absence of a challenge (Huang et al. 1996). In tPA- or plasminogen-null mice, but not in uPA- or fibrinogen-null mice, neuronal death is attenuated following excitotoxin (kainic acid)-induced cerebral damage (Tsirka et al. 1995, 1997; Chen and Strickland 1997; Tsirka 1997). Laminin and DSD-1-PG/phosphocan (a proteoglycan) have been identified as substrates for the tPA–plasmin extracellular proteolytic system in the hippocampus, which are related to tPA–plasmin-dependent neuronal cell death and tissue reorganization (Chen and Strickland 1997; Wu et al. 2000). In addition, tPA appears to have plasminogen-independent function in the hippocampus, as the absence of tPA, but not of plasminogen, attenuates microglial activation and mossy fiber pathfinding and outgrowth following excitotoxin challenge (Tsirka 1997; Wu et al. 2000).

In addition to these fibrin/ogen independent effects of the tPA–plasmin proteolytic system during cerebral damage and subsequent repair, the plasminogen system can reduce the ischemia-induced cerebrovascular thrombosis. Transient impairment of cerebral blood flow, followed by reperfusion results in an increased fibrin deposition, infarct volume, and reduced cerebral blood flow in tPA-null mice as compared to wildtype mice (Tabrizi et al. 1999). However, using models of persistent focal cerebral ischemia, the beneficial effects of endogenous tPA activity were not only abrogated, but increased tPA activity actually increased the infarct size, indicating that tPA is a double-edged sword for the treatment of persistent cerebral ischemia (Nagai et al. 1999). Conversely, enhancing endogenous plasmin-activity by depleting α_2-antiplasmin appears to have beneficial effects even in models of persistent focal ischemia, suggesting that the direct modulation of plasmin activity might be a better therapeutic approach for ischemic stroke, superior to tPA treatment (Nagai et al. 2001).

Mechanical injury of peripheral nerves (the sciatic nerve) revealed a fibrinogen-dependent role of the plasminogen system during peripheral neuronal cell damage and repair. tPA is induced in Schwann cells (myelinating cells surrounding the axon of peripheral nerves) following mechanical injury, suggesting a role of tPA in peripheral nerve injury. Demyelination is increased in tPA and plasminogen-deficient mice, indicating that tPA-mediated plasmin generation attenuates peripheral nerve damage in the crush model (Akassoglou et al. 2000). The consequences of plasminogen deficiency are corrected by superimposed fibrinogen deficiency, demonstrating that the tPA/plasminogen system protects the peripheral nerve through fibrinolysis (Akassoglou et al. 2000).

3.5
Wound Healing and Tissue Remodeling

3.5.1
Skin Wounds

Early observation describing impaired wound healing in fibrinogen-deficient mice indicated already that fibrinogen is important, but not strictly required for wound healing (Suh et al. 1995). These observations were confirmed using skin wound models, which demonstrated similar healing times in mice expressing or lacking fibrinogen, but marked histological alterations (Drew et al. 2001a). Granulation tissue and neovascularization appear indistinguishable between fibrinogen wildtype and knockout mice. However, granulation tissue is less stable at the early stages (e.g., after 24 h), and subsequently keratinocytes do not follow the typical re-epithelialization pattern (orientation of keratinocytes towards the center of the wound field), but appear rather disorganized, often projecting away from the wound field. These changes result in poor tensile strength of the resulting scar, a phenotype aggravated in sutured wounds.

Re-epithelialization of incisional skin wounds is even more impaired in mice lacking plasminogen as compared to fibrinogen-deficient mice, delaying wound healing on average by 3 weeks (Romer et al. 1996), while wound healing in Pai-1-deficient mice is accelerated (Chan et al. 2001b). Angiogenesis and formation of granulation tissue are unremarkable in plasminogen-deficient mice. Rather, delayed wound healing in the absence of plasminogen appears to be the consequence of increased fibrin and fibronectin deposition at the wound edge, compromising the migration of keratinocytes (Bugge et al. 1996b; Romer et al. 1996). The wound healing defect of plasminogen-deficient mice is corrected by superimposed fibrinogen deficiency, demonstrating that the relevant plasmin substrate during skin wound healing is fibrin (Bugge et al. 1996b).

3.5.2
Liver Injury

In contrast to the fibrin-dependent role of plasmin during healing of skin wounds, plasmin has a fibrin-independent function for the restoration of liver tissue following liver damage. In wildtype mice, normal liver architecture is restored as early as 7 days following carbon tetrachloride-induced liver damage, while the liver of plasminogen-deficient mice maintains a diffuse, pale appearance with persistent damage to centrilobular hepatocytes (Bezerra et al. 1999). Despite predominant fibrin and fibronectin deposition, which suggests that fibrin hampers tissue repair akin to its role in skin wound healing, superimposed fibrinogen deficiency does not restore the impaired tissue remodeling observed in plasminogen-deficient livers. Impaired proteolysis combined with increased matrix production, probably as a result of persistent activation of hepatic stellate cells, results in an enlargement of injured plasminogen-null livers (Ng et al. 2001; Pohl et al. 2001). Absence of tPA has only a mild effect, while uPA or—to a greater extent—combined tPA and uPA deficiency severely impairs liver repair (Bezerra et al. 2001). Both plasminogen activators are upregulated during liver repair, which is consistent with the notion that both tPA and uPA contribute to plasminogen activation in this setting. Following partial hepatectomy, regeneration of liver tissue is similarly impaired in the absence of uPA, while the absence of uPAR has no effect (Roselli et al. 1998). Furthermore, activity of MMP-9 is not altered in injured plasminogen-null livers. These results suggest that the plasminogen system acts independent of fibrin, uPAR, and—unlike in some extra-hepatic tissues (Lijnen et al. 1998; Heymans et al. 1999)—MMP-9 during liver remodeling.

3.5.3
Pulmonary Fibrosis

The fibrinolytic system modulates bleomycin-induced pulmonary fibrosis in a fashion similar to its role in liver remodeling, with the important distinction, that not only the absence of uPAR, but also uPA is without effect. Thus, tissue remodeling and lung hydroxyproline content as a measure for collagen deposition are increased in mice lacking plasminogen or tPA (Swaisgood et al. 2000), or in mice overexpressing Pai-1 (Eitzman et al. 1996a), while collagen deposition is reduced in mice heterozygous or completely deficient of Pai-1 (Eitzman et al. 1996a). Fibrin deposition is a predominant feature of bleomycin-injured lungs (Eitzman et al. 1996a), but is not required for bleomycin-induced pulmonary fibrosis, as the genetic absence of fibrinogen does not prevent the disease onset (Hattori et al. 2000; Ploplis et al. 2000). Furthermore, the increased fibrinolytic potential in injured lungs of Pai-1-null mice (resulting in less fibrin deposition and more fibrin degradation products) does not affect the disease progression (Hattori et al. 2000). Accumulation of inflammatory cells, vascular permeability, and fibronectin deposition is comparable between Pai-1-wildtype and -null mice (Hattori et al. 2000), suggesting that Pai-1 deficiency protects against bleomycin-induced lung fibrosis independent of these disease markers.

   Interestingly, hypoxia-induced lung injury, triggering an increase of arterial smooth muscle cells, resulting in increased media thickness, and a rarefaction of nonmuscularized vessels appears to be mediated by uPA-dependent plasminogen activation and—to some extent—engagement of uPAR (Levi et al. 2001a). These observations strongly suggest that the type of tissue injury determines in part the biological response of the fibrinolytic system. In addition, the biological response of the fibrinolytic system appears to differ in a tissue-specific manner, as illustrated by the profibrotic effect following myocardial ischemia (Heymans et al. 1999) and the antifibrotic effect following bleomycin-induced lung injury (Eitzman et al. 1996a). The variable effects of the fibrinolytic system might be determined by the amount of necrotic tissue, the composition of ECM, and the expression pattern and regulation of hemostatic, fibrinolytic, and other proteolytic regulators. This organ specificity of the fibrinolytic system resembles the tissue specificity of the hemostatic system.

3.6
Inflammation and Infection

3.6.1
Systemic Inflammation

The pro-inflammatory effects of thrombin and other activated coagulation factors as well as the pro-coagulant consequences of inflammation are well established and imply a close interaction between blood coagulation and inflammation (Esmon 2001). The advent of mice with disrupted coagulation and fibrinolytic systems provided the tools for the in vivo analyses of the interaction between these two systems. Mice with impaired PC activation secondary to a point mutation in the TM gene (TM^{Pro}, E404P) display an altered cytokine response and impaired survival when challenged with sublethal or lethal doses, respectively, of LPS (Weiler et al. 2001). Cytokine levels are not different in unchallenged animals, even in the complete absence of PC (Chan et al. 2001a) or endovascular TM (Isermann et al. 2001b), indicating that the TM–PC pathway has no major effect on baseline cytokine production, but modifies the cytokine response during acute inflammation. LPS injection also increases fibrin deposition in kidney glomeruli, the myocardium, and the brain in mice with heterozygous antithrombin deficiency, but cytokine levels were not determined in these experiments (Yanada et al. 2002). Fibrin deposition was also increased in various organs of LPS-challenged TM^{Pro} mice, including the kidney and the lung, but not in the brain (Weiler et al. 2001). These findings are congruent with the concept of vascular bed-specific coagulation regulation.

Fibrin deposition following LPS challenge is likewise altered in mice with a disrupted fibrinolytic system. Deficiency of either tPA or uPA increases the thrombotic burden (Carmeliet et al. 1994), while the absence of α_2-antiplamsin (Lijnen et al. 1999) or Pai-1 (Carmeliet et al. 1993b) reduces fibrin deposition in LPS-challenged animals. The effect of the fibrinolytic system on cytokine production was not determined in these studies.

3.6.2
Glomerulonephritis

Experimentally induced glomerulonephritis in mice is associated with fibrin deposition in glomerular capillaries. Genetic elimination of fibrinogen attenuates, but does not prevent, damage to glomeruli (Drew et al. 2001b). Extracellular mesangial matrix, necrotizing changes, and microthrombi are less frequent in the absence of fibrinogen, establishing that fibrin contributes to the renal damage (Drew et al. 2001b). Consistently, genetic tPA or plasminogen deficiency exacerbates experimental glomerulonephritis (Kitching et al. 1997). Interestingly, uPA deficiency, but not uPAR deficiency, reduces macrophage infiltration into damaged glomeruli without affecting the disease progression, indicating a minor uPAR-independent role of uPA (Kitching et al. 1997). The notion that macrophage recruitment is at least in part regulated by uPA during inflammatory response is supported by the finding that plasminogen enhances recruitment of monocytes and—to a lesser extent—of lymphocytes, but not of neutrophils, during thioglycollate-induced peritonitis (Ploplis et al. 1998). Glomerular accumulation of periodic acid–Schiff (PAS)-positive material, reflecting cell debris, plasma proteins, and IgG deposits as well as fibrin, is reduced by only one third in the absence of fibrinogen, consistent with fibrinogen-independent effects (Kitching et al. 1997). Indeed, deficiency of PAR1 reduces crescent formation, inflammatory cell infiltration, and serum creatinine levels in murine experimental glomerulonephritis (Cunningham et al. 2000), supporting the notion that activation of the hemostatic system aggravates glomerular damage through thrombin-mediated cellular activation and fibrin formation.

3.6.3
Arthritis

Intraarticular fibrin(ogen) deposition correlates with the severity of experimental arthritis in mice, suggesting that synovial fibrin depositions exacerbate joint inflammation and destruction (Busso et al. 1998). Impairment of the endogenous fibrinolytic response in mice lacking tPA, uPA, or plasminogen results in increased intraarticular fibrin(ogen) deposition associated with increased synovial thickness, bone erosion, and macrophage number (Busso et al. 1998; Yang et al. 2001). Of note, cartilage proteoglycan depletion did not differ between wildtype mice and mice with an impaired fibrinolytic system (Busso et al. 1998), indicating that proteases other than plasmin mediate cartilage erosion. Ancrod-induced defibrinogenation attenuates joint inflammation in uPA-null, but not in wildtype mice, indicating that the impaired fibrin removal in uPA-null mice is causative for the enhanced joint inflammation (Busso et al. 1998). Whether the consequences of genetic tPA deficiency could also be attenuated by fibrinogen deficiency has not been determined so far. Crosses with fibrinogen-deficient mice will help to determine whether the lingering inflammatory response following ancrod treatment of uPA-null mice reflects the residual fibrin deposition, or a fibrin-independent role of the fibrinolytic system during arthritis.

3.6.4
Infection

Neutrophil recruitment following pulmonary pseudomonas aeruginosa infection is impaired in uPAR-, but not uPA-deficient mice, implying a role of uPAR independent of uPA (Gyetko et al. 2000). As antibodies to CD11b/CD18 (Mac-1) reduce neutrophil recruitment to levels seen in uPAR knockout mice, the authors concluded that uPAR and CD11b/CD18 interact during neutrophil recruitment into pseudomonas aeruginosa-infected lungs—a finding consistent with previous in vitro results. However, in mice with a pulmonary *Cryptococcus neoformans* infection, recruitment of inflammatory (CD45$^+$) cells is modulated by uPA, as the number of CD11b/CD18$^+$ cells in infected lungs is reduced in the absence of uPA at early stages (3 weeks), but increased at later stages (Gyetko et al. 1996; Gyetko et al. 2002). *C. neoformans* ingested by monocytes persist in uPA-deficient mice, which ultimately fail to control the disease, resulting in dissemination and death of most uPA-null mice. The failure to clear the infection in the absence of uPA reflects (1) a quantitative defect in cell recruitment, and (2) a qualitative defect in cytokine production, characterized by a deficient T1-cytokine response (reduced IFN-γ and IL-12, increase IL-5 levels). Cytokine levels in healthy uPA-null mice do not differ from healthy wildtype controls, excluding differences in cytokine production in the absence of a stimulus. As the effect of fibrinogen deficiency has not been determined in this disease model, proinflammatory effects of fibrin or fibrin-split products can currently not be excluded.

As demonstrated in mice infected with the spirochete *Borrelia burgdorferi*, pathogens use the host's fibrinolytic system to their advantage. *B. burgdorferi* uses host-derived plasminogen activators and plasminogen to spread from the midgut of the vector (the tick *Ixodes scapularis*) and for the subsequent dissemination in the host (Coleman et al. 1997; Gebbia et al. 1999). Dissemination within the vector and the host are prevented or attenuated, respectively, in the absence of host-derived plasminogen.

3.7
Tumor Biology

Reports suggesting a role of the initiator of blood coagulation, TF, in tumor angiogenesis and tumor growth could not be replicated using teratomas and teratocarcinoma derived from TF-expressing and TF-deficient ES-cells (employing both RW4 and E14 ES cells) (Toomey et al. 1997). It will be interesting to explore other tumor models employing mice with altered TF activity or expressing TF mutants to explore the role of TF for tumor-associated angiogenesis in mice and/or tumor cells with an altered TF-gene.

Studies in fibrinogen-deficient mice evaluating the tumor progression of Lewis lung carcinoma and of B16-BL6 melanoma cells injected intravenously demonstrated that host fibrinogen enhances the establishment of metastatic foci, but does not affect tumor growth or tumor stroma formation (Palumbo et al. 2000). These studies support the notion that fibrin-mediated adherence of tumor cells to target organs enhances hematogenous metastasis. Interestingly, thrombin inhibition by the specific and potent inhibitor hirudin diminishes hematogenous metastasis of tumor cells in the presence and absence of fibrinogen, suggesting that thrombin has a prometastatic effect independent of fibrinogen

(Palumbo et al. 2000). In the same tumor model, plasminogen-mediated fibrinolysis appears to be without an effect on hematogenous metastasis after 17–21 days of tumor growth (Palumbo et al. 2000). At least Lewis lung carcinoma cells do not express plasminogen (Bugge et al. 1997), excluding that tumor-derived plasminogen might compensate for the absence of host-derived plasminogen.

Employing different tumor models, which evaluated either Lewis lung carcinoma cells implanted into the subcutis (Bugge et al. 1997) or spontaneous middle T antigen-induced mammary cancer (Bugge et al. 1998), the appearance rate of primary tumors was indistinguishable between plasminogen-expressing and -deficient mice. Nevertheless, in plasminogen-null mice subcutaneously implanted Lewis lung carcinomas appeared smaller, less hemorrhagic, and displayed less skin ulcerations at earlier stages (5–10 days) (Bugge et al. 1997). In the latter study, dissemination of tumor cells into lymph nodes (lymphatic metastasis) and re-growth of tumors following dissection was reduced in the absence of plasminogen (to about 1/6 of wildtype levels). Likewise, the metastatic burden of middle T antigen-induced mammary cancers was significantly smaller in plasminogen-deficient mice, based on the number of lung metastasis, which spread generally hematogenously.

Clinical studies suggested that Pai-1 expression by the tumor itself is associated with an invasive phenotype and a worse prognosis. Studies that investigated the role of host-derived Pai-1 for tumor growth using mice demonstrated that Pai-1 deficiency impairs tumor vascularization and subsequently impairs tumor growth and/or tumor invasion (Bajou et al. 1998, 2001; Gutierrez et al. 2000), while other studies suggested that tumor growth is independent of (Eitzman et al. 1996b) or even attenuated by (Soff et al. 1995) host-derived Pai-1 levels. The apparent inconsistent effects of endogenous host-derived Pai-1 levels on tumor growth might reflect specific properties of the tumor cell line (e.g., differential expression of plasminogen activators/inhibitors) or the tumor model employed (tissue site, mode of inoculation). Alternatively, the observed differences could reflect a dose-dependent effect of Pai-1 on tumor vascularization and subsequent growth (McMahon et al. 2001). The latter study suggests that both the absence of Pai-1 or high levels of active Pai-1 inhibit tumor angiogenesis, while slightly elevated Pai-1 levels increase angiogenesis, in part by regulating the interaction of the uPA/uPAR complex with integrins (e.g., $\alpha_v\beta_3$, $\alpha_v\beta_5$).

These results suggest a role of plasminogen and Pai-1 in modulating local tumor growth and tumor spread. Depending on the tumor model, primary tumor invasion and associated angiogenesis as well as lymphatic or hematogenous metastasis can be modulated by the plasminogen system, probably reflecting different biological properties of the tumor and/or the diseased tissue.

3.8
Reproduction

Studies with genetically modified mice have identified a role for some regulators of coagulation and hemostasis during reproduction unrelated to the embryonic lethality secondary to a developmental failure of the embryo proper or the placenta. TM, PC, and the serpin PC inhibitor are all expressed in the testis. While the embryonic lethality prevented the evaluation of TM's and PC's role in the male reproductive system, mice lacking the PC inhibitor are viable (Uhrin et al. 2000). Spermatogenesis in male mice lacking the PC inhibitor is impaired, resulting in immature and malformed sperms, increased cell death, and subsequent infertility. This phenotype is associated with a disruption of the Sertoli cell barrier, implying increased proteolytic activity in the testis of PC inhibitor-deficient mice.

Mice with compound tPA and uPA deficiency or plasminogen-null mice have markedly reduced fertility (Carmeliet et al. 1994; Ploplis et al. 1995; Lund et al. 2000). However, the reduced fertility might reflect the overall impaired health in these mice, rather than a specific defect in the absence of active plasmin. This notion is supported by the apparently normal estrus cycle and the normal ovulation of mice lacking plasminogen (Ny et al. 1999; Lund et al. 2000). Impaired ovulation of borderline significance is only apparent in plasminogen-deficient mice when "challenged" by injection of gonadotropin (Ny et al. 1999).

Expression of uPA in the mammary gland during development and post lactation suggests a role of the fibrinolytic system during lactation. Indeed, in plasminogen-deficient mice the lactational competence is severely impaired in primiparous mice and—to an even greater extent—in subsequent pregnancies (Lund et al. 2000). The lactational insufficiency is associated with smaller secretory alveolar volumes, accumulation of collagen and fibrotic stroma (in the absence of detectable fibrin deposition), and accumulation of basement membrane protein fragments. ECM breakdown is delayed during alveolar regression, which might result in the associated decrease in cell death. Whether these pathological changes in the mammary gland can be corrected by superimposed fibrinogen deficiency has not been determined, but appears unlikely considering the absence of increased fibrin deposition in the mammary glands of plasminogen-deficient mice.

These results establish that the coagulation and fibrinolytic system impair reproduction not only by predisposing to thrombosis, hemorrhage, or through increased coagulation activation in the placenta, but also by disrupting other biological functions relevant for reproduction through mechanisms which—based on currently available data—appear to be unrelated to thrombosis and fibrinolysis

3.9
Age-Dependent Expression of Coagulation Regulators

The generation of transgenic animals with defined promoter elements and mu-tated promoter sites leads to the identification of age-regulatory elements. Two age-regulatory elements have been identified to date (Kurachi et al. 1999; Zhang et al. 2002). An age-related stability element (ASE) is present in the 5′-region of human fIX and PC promoters. In both cases, the ASE is required and sufficient to mediated age-stable expression of the respective coagulation regulator. Of note, the ASE in the human fIX promoter, but not of the human PC promoter, is derived from a retrotransposed LINE-1 sequence, indicating an evolutionary distinct origin of both ASEs. The ASE consists of a 32-bp fragment, approxi-mately 790 bp from the transcription start signal, and contains a sequence ele-ment (GAGGAAG), which matches the consensus motif of polyomavirus en-hancer activator-3 (PEA-3, a member of the Ets family of transcription factors). This sequence element appears to be functionally relevant based on in vitro binding assays. An age-related increase element (AIE) is present in the 3′-region of the human fIX gene, but not of the human PC gene, consistent with an in-crease of fIX levels, but constant PC levels, with age. The age-dependent regula-tory elements seem to function independent of the gene, as the age-dependent expression pattern is maintained after substitution of the ASEs, and as introduc-tion of the ASI in the human PC gene (which normally lacks an ASI) results in an—unphysiological—increase of PC expression with age.

Using a similar approach (expression of transgenes with defined promoter el-ements) the age-dependent phenotype of hemophilia Leyden B could be ex-plained at a molecular level (Boland et al. 1995). Individuals with hemophilia B Leyden have a prepubescent hemorrhagic phenotype secondary to reduced fIX levels. However, after puberty fIX activity gradually increases with age, ulti-mately reaching about 60% of adult levels. Several mutations of the fIX gene, within less than 200 bp of the transcription start signal, have been identified in these patients. Introduction of one of these mutation (at position −13) into the promoter of a human fIX transgene resulted in an age-dependent increased of human fIX in 2-month-old transgenic mice, and thus at a time when mice reach sexual maturity. These results suggest that several age-regulatory elements mod-ulate the expression of coagulation regulators, as the mutation resulting in he-mophilia B Leyden lies outside the ASE described above. The identification of these age-regulatory elements provides the opportunity to design mice with age-dependent phenotypes, which might—maybe in combination with Cre-Lox-mediated in vivo recombination—allow us to circumvent neonatal phenotypes in mice, which would otherwise prevent in vivo studies.

4
Conclusion

Blood coagulation takes place in an environment of non-anticoagulated blood, in the presence of blood cells and vascular wall components, under flow conditions and in a constantly changing milieu, such as local hypoxia and acidosis. In vitro or ex vivo models can hardly recapitulate the complexity of in vivo blood coagulation. Gene-targeting and transgenic technology provide in vivo models to study these complex interactions, and have improved—and in some instances changed—our understanding of hemostasis. The possibility to generate mice with designed alterations of the genome raised expectations for animal models replicating spontaneous vascular disease in humans. The latter has proved difficult, but has finally been achieved (Cui et al. 2000; Chan et al. 2001a; Isermann et al. 2001b). Analyses of mice with disrupted homeostasis demonstrated their usefulness for the study of disease in humans, but also their limitations secondary to species-specific limitations. Nevertheless, accessibility of the mouse genome to experimental alteration will, without doubt, increase the proportion of animal studies employing mice in the field of coagulation and fibrinolysis, which in the past was below 4% (Levi et al. 2001b).

References

Akassoglou K, Kombrinck KW, Degen JL, Strickland S (2000) Tissue plasminogen activator-mediated fibrinolysis protects against axonal degeneration and demyelination after sciatic nerve injury. *J Cell Biol* 149: 1157–1166

Bajou K, Masson V, Gerard RD, Schmitt PM, Albert V, Praus M, Lund LR, Frandsen TL, Brunner N, Dano K, Fusenig NE, Weidle U, Carmeliet G, Loskutoff D, Collen D, Carmeliet P, Foidart JM, Noel A (2001) The plasminogen activator inhibitor PAI-1 controls in vivo tumor vascularization by interaction with proteases, not vitronectin. Implications for antiangiogenic strategies. *J Cell Biol* 152: 777–784

Bajou K, Noel A, Gerard RD, Masson V, Brunner N, Holst-Hansen C, Skobe M, Fusenig NE, Carmeliet P, Collen D, Foidart JM (1998) Absence of host plasminogen activator inhibitor 1 prevents cancer invasion and vascularization. *Nat Med* 4: 923–928

Bara L, Planes A, Samama MM (1999) Occurrence of thrombosis and haemorrhage, relationship with anti-Xa, anti-IIa activities, and D-dimer plasma levels in patients receiving a low molecular weight heparin, enoxaparin or tinzaparin, to prevent deep vein thrombosis after hip surgery. *Br J Haematol* 104: 230–240

Bezerra JA, Bugge TH, Melin-Aldana H, Sabla G, Kombrinck KW, Witte DP, Degen JL (1999) Plasminogen deficiency leads to impaired remodeling after a toxic injury to the liver. *Proc Natl Acad Sci USA* 96: 15143–15148

Bezerra JA, Currier AR, Melin-Aldana H, Sabla G, Bugge TH, Kombrinck KW, Degen JL (2001) Plasminogen activators direct reorganization of the liver lobule after acute injury. *Am J Pathol* 158: 921–929

Bi L, Lawler AM, Antonarakis SE, High KA, Gearhart JD, Kazazian HH, Jr. (1995) Targeted disruption of the mouse factor VIII gene produces a model of haemophilia A (letter). *Nat Genet* 10: 119–121

Bi L, Sarkar R, Naas T, Lawler AM, Pain J, Shumaker SL, Bedian V, Kazazian HH, Jr. (1996) Further characterization of factor VIII-deficient mice created by gene targeting: RNA and protein studies. *Blood* 88: 3446–3450

Boland EJ, Liu YC, Walter CA, Herbert DC, Weaker FJ, Odom MW, Jagadeeswaran P (1995) Age-specific regulation of clotting factor IX gene expression in normal and transgenic mice. *Blood* 86: 2198–2205

Bugge TH, Flick MJ, Daugherty CC, Degen JL (1995) Plasminogen deficiency causes severe thrombosis but is compatible with development and reproduction. *Genes Dev* 9: 794–807

Bugge TH, Kombrinck KW, Flick MJ, Daugherty CC, Danton MJ, Degen JL (1996b) Loss of fibrinogen rescues mice from the pleiotropic effects of plasminogen deficiency. *Cell* 87: 709–719

Bugge TH, Kombrinck KW, Xiao Q, Holmback K, Daugherty CC, Witte DP, Degen JL (1997) Growth and dissemination of Lewis lung carcinoma in plasminogen-deficient mice. *Blood* 90: 4522–4531

Bugge TH, Lund LR, Kombrinck KK, Nielsen BS, Holmback K, Drew AF, Flick MJ, Witte DP, Dano K, Degen JL (1998) Reduced metastasis of Polyoma virus middle T antigen-induced mammary cancer in plasminogen-deficient mice. *Oncogene* 16: 3097–3104

Bugge TH, Xiao Q, Kombrinck KW, Flick MJ, Holmback K, Danton MJ, Colbert MC, Witte DP, Fujikawa K, Davie EW, Degen JL (1996a) Fatal embryonic bleeding events in mice lacking tissue factor, the cell- associated initiator of blood coagulation. *Proc Natl Acad Sci USA* 93: 6258–6263

Busso N, Peclat V, Van Ness K, Kolodzieszczyk E, Degen J, Bugge T, So A (1998) Exacerbation of antigen-induced arthritis in urokinase-deficient mice. *J Clin Invest* 102: 41–50

Carmeliet P, Kieckens L, Schoonjans L, Ream B, van Nuffelen A, Prendergast G, Cole M, Bronson R, Collen D, Mulligan RC (1993b) Plasminogen activator inhibitor-1 gene-deficient mice. I. Generation by homologous recombination and characterization. *J Clin Invest* 92: 2746–2755

Carmeliet P, Mackman N, Moons L, Luther T, Gressens P, Van V, I, Demunck H, Kasper M, Breier G, Evrard P, Muller M, Risau W, Edgington T, Collen D (1996) Role of tissue factor in embryonic blood vessel development. *Nature* 383: 73–75

Carmeliet P, Moons L, Dewerchin M, Rosenberg S, Herbert JM, Lupu F, Collen D (1998) Receptor-independent role of urokinase-type plasminogen activator in pericellular plasmin and matrix metalloproteinase proteolysis during vascular wound healing in mice. *J Cell Biol* 140: 233–245

Carmeliet P, Moons L, Herbert JM, Crawley J, Lupu F, Lijnen R, Collen D (1997c) Urokinase but not tissue plasminogen activator mediates arterial neointima formation in mice. *Circ Res* 81: 829–839

Carmeliet P, Moons L, Lijnen R, Baes M, Lemaitre V, Tipping P, Drew A, Eeckhout Y, Shapiro S, Lupu F, Collen D (1997d) Urokinase-generated plasmin activates matrix metalloproteinases during aneurysm formation. *Nat Genet* 17: 439–444

Carmeliet P, Moons L, Lijnen R, Janssens S, Lupu F, Collen D, Gerard RD (1997b) Inhibitory role of plasminogen activator inhibitor-1 in arterial wound healing and neointima formation: a gene targeting and gene transfer study in mice. *Circulation* 96: 3180–3191

Carmeliet P, Moons L, Ploplis V, Plow E, Collen D (1997a) Impaired arterial neointima formation in mice with disruption of the plasminogen gene. *J Clin Invest* 99: 200–208

Carmeliet P, Schoonjans L, Kieckens L, Ream B, Degen J, Bronson R, De Vos R, van den Oord JJ, Collen D, Mulligan RC (1994) Physiological consequences of loss of plasminogen activator gene function in mice. *Nature* 368: 419–424

Carmeliet P, Stassen JM, Schoonjans L, Ream B, van den Oord JJ, De Mol M, Mulligan RC, Collen D (1993a) Plasminogen activator inhibitor-1 gene-deficient mice. II. Effects on hemostasis, thrombosis, and thrombolysis. *J Clin Invest* 92: 2756–2760

Chan JC, Carmeliet P, Moons L, Rosen ED, Huang ZF, Broze GJ, Jr., Collen D, Castellino FJ (1999) Factor VII deficiency rescues the intrauterine lethality in mice associated with a tissue factor pathway inhibitor deficit. *J Clin Invest* 103: 475–482

Chan JC, Cornelissen I, Collen D, Ploplis VA, Castellino FJ (2000) Combined factor VII/ protein C deficiency results in intrauterine coagulopathy in mice. *J Clin Invest* 105: 897–903

Chan JC, Duszczyszyn DA, Castellino FJ, Ploplis VA (2001b) Accelerated skin wound healing in plasminogen activator inhibitor-1- deficient mice. *Am J Pathol* 159: 1681–1688

Chan JC, Ganopolsky JG, Cornelissen I, Suckow MA, Sandoval-Cooper MJ, Brown EC, Noria F, Gailani D, Rosen ED, Ploplis VA, Castellino FJ (2001a) The characterization of mice with a targeted combined deficiency of protein c and factor XI. *Am J Pathol* 158: 469–479

Chen ZL, Strickland S (1997) Neuronal death in the hippocampus is promoted by plasmin-catalyzed degradation of laminin. *Cell* 91: 917–925

Cheung WM, D'Andrea MR, Andrade-Gordon P, Damiano BP (1999) Altered vascular injury responses in mice deficient in protease- activated receptor-1. *Arterioscler Thromb Vasc Biol* 19: 3014–3024

Christie PD, Edelberg JM, Picard MH, Foulkes AS, Mamuya W, Weiler-Guettler H, Rubin RH, Gilbert P, Rosenberg RD (1999) A murine model of myocardial microvascular thrombosis. *J Clin Invest* 104: 533–539

Coleman JL, Gebbia JA, Piesman J, Degen JL, Bugge TH, Benach JL (1997) Plasminogen is required for efficient dissemination of B. burgdorferi in ticks and for enhancement of spirochetemia in mice. *Cell* 89: 1111–1119

Conway EM, Pollefeyt S, Cornelissen J, DeBaere I, Steiner-Mosonyi M, Weitz JI, Weiler-Guettler H, Carmeliet P, Collen D (1999) Structure-function analyses of thrombomodulin by gene-targeting in mice: the cytoplasmic domain is not required for normal fetal development. *Blood* 93: 3442–3450

Creemers E, Cleutjens J, Smits J, Heymans S, Moons L, Collen D, Daemen M, Carmeliet P (2000) Disruption of the plasminogen gene in mice abolishes wound healing after myocardial infarction. *Am J Pathol* 156: 1865–1873

Cui J, Eitzman DT, Westrick RJ, Christie PD, Xu ZJ, Yang AY, Purkayastha AA, Yang TL, Metz AL, Gallagher KP, Tyson JA, Rosenberg RD, Ginsburg D (2000) Spontaneous thrombosis in mice carrying the factor V Leiden mutation. *Blood* 96: 4222–4226

Cui J, O'Shea KS, Purkayastha A, Saunders TL, Ginsburg D (1996) Fatal haemorrhage and incomplete block to embryogenesis in mice lacking coagulation factor V. *Nature* 384: 66–68

Cunningham MA, Rondeau E, Chen X, Coughlin SR, Holdsworth SR, Tipping PG (2000) Protease-activated receptor 1 mediates thrombin-dependent, cell-mediated renal inflammation in crescentic glomerulonephritis. *J Exp Med* 191: 455–462

Darrow AL, Fung-Leung WP, Ye RD, Santulli RJ, Cheung WM, Derian CK, Burns CL, Damiano BP, Zhou L, Keenan CM, Peterson PA, Andrade-Gordon P (1996) Biological consequences of thrombin receptor deficiency in mice. *Thromb Haemost* 76: 860–866

Degen JL (2001) Genetic interactions between the coagulation and fibrinolytic systems. *Thromb Haemost* 86: 130–137

Denis C, Methia N, Frenette PS, Rayburn H, Ullman-Cullere M, Hynes RO, Wagner DD (1998) A mouse model of severe von Willebrand disease: defects in hemostasis and thrombosis. *Proc Natl Acad Sci USA* 95: 9524–9529

Dewerchin M, Liang Z, Moons L, Carmeliet P, Castellino FJ, Collen D, Rosen ED (2000) Blood coagulation factor X deficiency causes partial embryonic lethality and fatal neonatal bleeding in mice. *Thromb Haemost* 83: 185–190

Dewerchin M, Nuffelen AV, Wallays G, Bouche A, Moons L, Carmeliet P, Mulligan RC, Collen D (1996) Generation and characterization of urokinase receptor-deficient mice. *J Clin Invest* 97: 870–878

Dougherty KM, Pearson JM, Yang AY, Westrick RJ, Baker MS, Ginsburg D (1999) The plasminogen activator inhibitor-2 gene is not required for normal murine development or survival. *Proc Natl Acad Sci USA* 96: 686–691

Drew AF, Kaufman AH, Kombrinck KW, Danton MJ, Daugherty CC, Degen JL, Bugge TH (1998) Ligneous conjunctivitis in plasminogen-deficient mice. *Blood* 91: 1616–1624

Drew AF, Liu H, Davidson JM, Daugherty CC, Degen JL (2001a) Wound-healing defects in mice lacking fibrinogen. *Blood* 97: 3691–3698

Drew AF, Tucker HL, Kombrinck KW, Simon DI, Bugge TH, Degen JL (2000) Plasminogen is a critical determinant of vascular remodeling in mice. *Circ Res* 87: 133–139

Drew AF, Tucker HL, Liu H, Witte DP, Degen JL, Tipping PG (2001b) Crescentic glomerulonephritis is diminished in fibrinogen-deficient mice. *Am J Physiol Renal Physiol* 281: F1157-F1163

Eitzman DT, Krauss JC, Shen T, Cui J, Ginsburg (1996b) Lack of plasminogen activator inhibitor-1 effect in a transgenic mouse model of metastatic melanoma. *Blood* 87: 4718–4722

Eitzman DT, McCoy RD, Zheng X, Fay WP, Shen T, Ginsburg D, Simon RH (1996a) Bleomycin-induced pulmonary fibrosis in transgenic mice that either lack or overexpress the murine plasminogen activator inhibitor-1 gene. *J Clin Invest* 97: 232–237

Erickson LA, Fici GJ, Lund JE, Boyle TP, Polites HG, Marotti KR (1990) Development of venous occlusions in mice transgenic for the plasminogen activator inhibitor-1 gene. *Nature* 346: 74–76

Erlich J, Parry GC, Fearns C, Muller M, Carmeliet P, Luther T, Mackman N (1999) Tissue factor is required for uterine hemostasis and maintenance of the placental labyrinth during gestation. *Proc Natl Acad Sci USA* 96: 8138–8143

Esmon CT (2001) Role of coagulation inhibitors in inflammation. *Thromb Haemost* 86: 51–56

Farrehi PM, Ozaki CK, Carmeliet P, Fay WP (1998) Regulation of arterial thrombolysis by plasminogen activator inhibitor- 1 in mice. *Circulation* 97: 1002–1008

Fay WP, Parker AC, Condrey LR, Shapiro AD (1997) Human plasminogen activator inhibitor-1 (PAI-1) deficiency: characterization of a large kindred with a null mutation in the PAI-1 gene. *Blood* 90: 204–208

Gailani D, Lasky NM, Broze GJ, Jr. (1997) A murine model of factor XI deficiency. *Blood Coagul Fibrinolysis* 8: 134–144

Gebbia JA, Monco JC, Degen JL, Bugge TH, Benach JL (1999) The plasminogen activation system enhances brain and heart invasion in murine relapsing fever borreliosis. *J Clin Invest* 103: 81–87

Griffin CT, Srinivasan Y, Zheng YW, Huang W, Coughlin SR (2001) A role for thrombin receptor signaling in endothelial cells during embryonic development. *Science* 293: 1666–1670

Gu JM, Ferrell G, She M, Esmon CT (2001) Generation and Characterization of the Endothelial Protein C receptor deficient mice . *Thromb Haemost* Suppl 2001:

Gutierrez LS, Schulman A, Brito-Robinson T, Noria F, Ploplis VA, Castellino FJ (2000) Tumor development is retarded in mice lacking the gene for urokinase- type plasminogen activator or its inhibitor, plasminogen activator inhibitor-1. *Cancer Res* 60: 5839–5847

Gyetko MR, Chen GH, McDonald RA, Goodman R, Huffnagle GB, Wilkinson CC, Fuller JA, Toews GB (1996) Urokinase is required for the pulmonary inflammatory response to Cryptococcus neoformans. A murine transgenic model. *J Clin Invest* 97: 1818–1826

Gyetko MR, Sud S, Chen GH, Fuller JA, Chensue SW, Toews GB (2002) Urokinase-type plasminogen activator is required for the generation of a type 1 immune response to pulmonary Cryptococcus neoformans infection. *J Immunol* 168: 801–809

Gyetko MR, Sud S, Kendall T, Fuller JA, Newstead MW, Standiford TJ (2000) Urokinase receptor-deficient mice have impaired neutrophil recruitment in response to pulmonary Pseudomonas aeruginosa infection. *J Immunol* 165: 1513–1519

Hattori N, Degen JL, Sisson TH, Liu H, Moore BB, Pandrangi RG, Simon RH, Drew AF (2000) Bleomycin-induced pulmonary fibrosis in fibrinogen-null mice. *J Clin Invest* 106: 1341–1350

He L, Vicente CP, Westrick RJ, Eitzman DT, Tollefsen DM (2002) Heparin cofactor II inhibits arterial thrombosis after endothelial injury. *J Clin Invest* 109: 213–219

Healy AM, Hancock WW, Christie PD, Rayburn HB, Rosenberg RD (1998) Intravascular coagulation activation in a murine model of thrombomodulin deficiency: effects of lesion size, age, and hypoxia on fibrin deposition. *Blood* 92: 4188–4197

Healy AM, Rayburn HB, Rosenberg RD, Weiler H (1995) Absence of the blood-clotting regulator thrombomodulin causes embryonic lethality in mice before development of a functional cardiovascular system. *Proc Natl Acad Sci USA* 92: 850–854

Heckel JL, Sandgren EP, Degen JL, Palmiter RD, Brinster RL (1990) Neonatal bleeding in transgenic mice expressing urokinase-type plasminogen activator. *Cell* 62: 447–456

Heymans S, Luttun A, Nuyens D, Theilmeier G, Creemers E, Moons L, Dyspersin GD, Cleutjens JP, Shipley M, Angellilo A, Levi M, Nube O, Baker A, Keshet E, Lupu F, Herbert JM, Smits JF, Shapiro SD, Baes M, Borgers M, Collen D, Daemen MJ, Carmeliet P (1999) Inhibition of plasminogen activators or matrix metalloproteinases prevents cardiac rupture but impairs therapeutic angiogenesis and causes cardiac failure. *Nat Med* 5: 1135–1142

High KA (2001) Gene transfer as an approach to treating hemophilia. *Circ Res* 88: 137–144

Holmback K, Danton MJ, Suh TT, Daugherty CC, Degen JL (1996) Impaired platelet aggregation and sustained bleeding in mice lacking the fibrinogen motif bound by integrin alpha IIb beta 3. *EMBO J* 15: 5760–5771

Huang YY, Bach ME, Lipp HP, Zhuo M, Wolfer DP, Hawkins RD, Schoonjans L, Kandel ER, Godfraind JM, Mulligan R, Collen D, Carmeliet P (1996) Mice lacking the gene encoding tissue-type plasminogen activator show a selective interference with late-phase long-term potentiation in both Schaffer collateral and mossy fiber pathways. *Proc Natl Acad Sci USA* 93: 8699–8704

Huang ZF, Higuchi D, Lasky N, Broze GJ, Jr. (1997) Tissue factor pathway inhibitor gene disruption produces intrauterine lethality in mice. *Blood* 90: 944–951

Isermann B, Hendrickson SB, Hutley K, Wing M, Weiler H (2001a) Tissue-restricted expression of thrombomodulin in the placenta rescues thrombomodulin-deficient mice from early lethality and reveals a secondary developmental block. *Development* 128: 827–838

Isermann B, Hendrickson SB, Zogg M, Wing M, Cummiskey M, Kisanuki YY, Yanagisawa M, Weiler H (2001b) Endothelium-specific loss of murine thrombomodulin disrupts the protein C anticoagulant pathway and causes juvenile-onset thrombosis. *J Clin Invest* 108: 537–546

Ishiguro K, Kojima T, Kadomatsu K, Nakayama Y, Takagi A, Suzuki M, Takeda N, Ito M, Yamamoto K, Matsushita T, Kusugami K, Muramatsu T, Saito H (2000) Complete antithrombin deficiency in mice results in embryonic lethality. *J Clin Invest* 106: 873–878

Iwaki T, Sandoval-Cooper MJ, Paiva M, Kobayashi T, Ploplis VA, Castellino FJ (2002) Fibrinogen stabilizes placental-maternal attachment during embryonic development in the mouse. *Am J Pathol* 160: 1021–1034

Jalbert LR, Rosen ED, Moons L, Chan JC, Carmeliet P, Collen D, Castellino FJ (1998) Inactivation of the gene for anticoagulant protein C causes lethal perinatal consumptive coagulopathy in mice. *J Clin Invest* 102: 1481–1488

Kawasaki T, Dewerchin M, Lijnen HR, Vermylen J, Hoylaerts MF (2000) Vascular release of plasminogen activator inhibitor-1 impairs fibrinolysis during acute arterial thrombosis in mice. *Blood* 96: 153–160

Kitching AR, Holdsworth SR, Ploplis VA, Plow EF, Collen D, Carmeliet P, Tipping PG (1997) Plasminogen and plasminogen activators protect against renal injury in crescentic glomerulonephritis. *J Exp Med* 185: 963–968

Kundu RK, Sangiorgi F, Wu LY, Kurachi K, Anderson WF, Maxson R, Gordon EM (1998) Targeted inactivation of the coagulation factor IX gene causes hemophilia B in mice. *Blood* 92: 168–174

Kurachi S, Deyashiki Y, Takeshita J, Kurachi K (1999) Genetic mechanisms of age regulation of human blood coagulation factor IX. *Science* 285: 739–743

Lane DA, Grant PJ (2000) Role of hemostatic gene polymorphisms in venous and arterial thrombotic disease. *Blood* 95: 1517–1532

Levi M, Dorffle-Melly J, Johnson GJ, Drouet L, Badimon L (2001b) Usefulness and limitations of animal models of venous thrombosis. *Thromb Haemost* 86: 1331–1333

Levi M, Moons L, Bouche A, Shapiro SD, Collen D, Carmeliet P (2001a) Deficiency of urokinase-type plasminogen activator-mediated plasmin generation impairs vascular remodeling during hypoxia-induced pulmonary hypertension in mice. *Circulation* 103: 2014–2020

Lijnen HR, Okada K, Matsuo O, Collen D, Dewerchin M (1999) Alpha2-antiplasmin gene deficiency in mice is associated with enhanced fibrinolytic potential without overt bleeding. *Blood* 93: 2274–2281

Lijnen HR, Van Hoef B, Lupu F, Moons L, Carmeliet P, Collen D (1998) Function of the plasminogen/plasmin and matrix metalloproteinase systems after vascular injury in mice with targeted inactivation of fibrinolytic system genes. *Arterioscler Thromb Vasc Biol* 18: 1035–1045

Lin HF, Maeda N, Smithies O, Straight DL, Stafford DW (1997) A coagulation factor IX-deficient mouse model for human hemophilia B. *Blood* 90: 3962–3966

Lou XJ, Boonmark NW, Horrigan FT, Degen JL, Lawn RM (1998) Fibrinogen deficiency reduces vascular accumulation of apolipoprotein(a) and development of atherosclerosis in apolipoprotein(a) transgenic mice. *Proc Natl Acad Sci USA* 95: 12591–12595

Lund LR, Bjorn SF, Sternlicht MD, Nielsen BS, Solberg H, Usher PA, Osterby R, Christensen IJ, Stephens RW, Bugge TH, Dano K, Werb Z (2000) Lactational competence and involution of the mouse mammary gland require plasminogen. *Development* 127: 4481–4492

Luttun A, Lupu F, Storkebaum E, Hoylaerts MF, Moons L, Crawley J, Bono F, Poole AR, Tipping P, Herbert JM, Collen D, Carmeliet P (2002) Lack of plasminogen activator inhibitor-1 promotes growth and abnormal matrix remodeling of advanced atherosclerotic plaques in apolipoprotein E-deficient mice. *Arterioscler Thromb Vasc Biol* 22: 499–505

Matsuno H, Kozawa O, Niwa M, Ueshima S, Matsuo O, Collen D, Uematsu T (1999) Differential role of components of the fibrinolytic system in the formation and removal of thrombus induced by endothelial injury. *Thromb Haemost* 81: 601–604

McMahon GA, Petitclerc E, Stefansson S, Smith E, Wong MK, Westrick RJ, Ginsburg D, Brooks PC, Lawrence DA (2001) Plasminogen activator inhibitor-1 regulates tumor growth and angiogenesis. *J Biol Chem* 276: 33964–33968

Melis E, Moons L, De Mol M, Herbert JM, Mackman N, Collen D, Carmeliet P, Dewerchin M (2001) Targeted deletion of the cytosolic domain of tissue factor in mice does not affect development. *Biochem Biophys Res Commun* 286: 580–586

Miles LA, Plow EF, Donnelly KJ, Hougie C, Griffin JH (1982) A bleeding disorder due to deficiency of alpha 2-antiplasmin. *Blood* 59: 1246–1251

Moons L, Shi C, Ploplis V, Plow E, Haber E, Collen D, Carmeliet P (1998) Reduced transplant arteriosclerosis in plasminogen-deficient mice. *J Clin Invest* 102: 1788–1797

Nagai N, De Mol M, Lijnen HR, Carmeliet P, Collen D (1999) Role of plasminogen system components in focal cerebral ischemic infarction: a gene targeting and gene transfer study in mice. *Circulation* 99: 2440–2444

Nagai N, Yamamoto S, Tsuboi T, Ihara H, Urano T, Takada Y, Terakawa S, Takada A (2001) Tissue-type plasminogen activator is involved in the process of neuronal death induced by oxygen-glucose deprivation in culture. *J Cereb Blood Flow Metab* 21: 631–634

Nagashima M, Yin ZF, Zhao L, White K, Zhu Y, Lasky N, Halks-Miller M, Broze GJ, Jr., Fay WP, Morser J (2002) Thrombin-activatable fibrinolysis inhibitor (TAFI) deficiency is compatible with murine life. *J Clin Invest* 109: 101–110

Ng VL, Sabla GE, Melin-Aldana H, Kelley-Loughnane N, Degen JL, Bezerra JA (2001) Plasminogen deficiency results in poor clearance of non-fibrin matrix and persistent activation of hepatic stellate cells after an acute injury. *J Hepatol* 35: 781–789

Ni H, Denis CV, Subbarao S, Degen JL, Sato TN, Hynes RO, Wagner DD (2000) Persistence of platelet thrombus formation in arterioles of mice lacking both von Willebrand factor and fibrinogen. *J Clin Invest* 106: 385–392

Ny A, Leonardsson G, Hagglund AC, Hagglof P, Ploplis VA, Carmeliet P, Ny T (1999) Ovulation in plasminogen-deficient mice. *Endocrinology* 140: 5030–5035

Offermanns S, Toombs CF, Hu YH, Simon MI (1997) Defective platelet activation in G alpha(q)-deficient mice. *Nature* 389: 183–186

Palumbo JS, Kombrinck KW, Drew AF, Grimes TS, Kiser JH, Degen JL, Bugge TH (2000) Fibrinogen is an important determinant of the metastatic potential of circulating tumor cells. *Blood* 96: 3302–3309

Parry GC, Erlich JH, Carmeliet P, Luther T, Mackman N (1998) Low levels of tissue factor are compatible with development and hemostasis in mice. *J Clin Invest* 101: 560–569

Parry GC, Mackman N (2000) Mouse embryogenesis requires the tissue factor extracellular domain but not the cytoplasmic domain. *J Clin Invest* 105: 1547–1554

Ploplis VA, Carmeliet P, Vazirzadeh S, Van V, I, Moons L, Plow EF, Collen D (1995) Effects of disruption of the plasminogen gene on thrombosis, growth, and health in mice. *Circulation* 92: 2585–2593

Ploplis VA, French EL, Carmeliet P, Collen D, Plow EF (1998) Plasminogen deficiency differentially affects recruitment of inflammatory cell populations in mice. *Blood* 91: 2005–2009

Ploplis VA, Wilberding J, McLennan L, Liang Z, Cornelissen I, DeFord ME, Rosen ED, Castellino FJ (2000) A total fibrinogen deficiency is compatible with the development of pulmonary fibrosis in mice. *Am J Pathol* 157: 703–708

Pohl JF, Melin-Aldana H, Sabla G, Degen JL, Bezerra JA (2001) Plasminogen deficiency leads to impaired lobular reorganization and matrix accumulation after chronic liver injury. *Am J Pathol* 159: 2179–2186

Romer J, Bugge TH, Pyke C, Lund LR, Flick MJ, Degen JL, Dano K (1996) Impaired wound healing in mice with a disrupted plasminogen gene. *Nat Med* 2: 287–292

Roselli HT, Su M, Washington K, Kerins DM, Vaughan DE, Russell WE (1998) Liver regeneration is transiently impaired in urokinase-deficient mice. *Am J Physiol* 275: G1472-G1479

Rosen ED, Chan JC, Idusogie E, Clotman F, Vlasuk G, Luther T, Jalbert LR, Albrecht S, Zhong L, Lissens A, Schoonjans L, Moons L, Collen D, Castellino FJ, Carmeliet P (1997) Mice lacking factor VII develop normally but suffer fatal perinatal bleeding. *Nature* 390: 290–294

Rosen ED, Zhong L, Cornelissen I, Martin A, Castellino FJ (2001) Coagulation Factor VII is Required for Embryoinc Development in Mice. *Blood Supplement* ASH, 2001:

Salomaa V, Matei C, Aleksic N, Sansores-Garcia L, Folsom AR, Juneja H, Chambless LE, Wu KK (1999) Soluble thrombomodulin as a predictor of incident coronary heart disease and symptomless carotid artery atherosclerosis in the Atherosclerosis Risk in Communities (ARIC) Study: a case-cohort study. *Lancet* 353: 1729–1734

Schuster V, Zeitler P, Seregard S, Ozcelik U, Anadol D, Luchtman-Jones L, Meire F, Mingers AM, Schambeck C, Kreth HW (2001) Homozygous and compound-hetero-zygous type I plasminogen deficiency is a common cause of ligneous conjunctivitis. *Thromb Haemost* 85: 1004–1010

Seligsohn U, Lubetsky A (2001) Genetic susceptibility to venous thrombosis. *N Engl J Med* 344: 1222–1231

Shivdasani RA, Rosenblatt MF, Zucker-Franklin D, Jackson CW, Hunt P, Saris CJ, Orkin SH (1995) Transcription factor NF-E2 is required for platelet formation independent of the actions of thrombopoietin/MGDF in megakaryocyte development. *Cell* 81: 695–704

Soff GA, Sanderowitz J, Gately S, Verrusio E, Weiss I, Brem S, Kwaan HC (1995) Expression of plasminogen activator inhibitor type 1 by human prostate carcinoma cells inhibits primary tumor growth, tumor-associated angiogenesis, and metastasis to lung and liver in an athymic mouse model. *J Clin Invest* 96: 2593–2600

Suh TT, Holmback K, Jensen NJ, Daugherty CC, Small K, Simon DI, Potter S, Degen JL (1995) Resolution of spontaneous bleeding events but failure of pregnancy in fibrino-gen-deficient mice. *Genes Dev* 9: 2020–2033

Sun WY, Witte DP, Degen JL, Colbert MC, Burkart MC, Holmback K, Xiao Q, Bugge TH, Degen SJ (1998) Prothrombin deficiency results in embryonic and neonatal lethality in mice. *Proc Natl Acad Sci USA* 95: 7597–7602

Swaisgood CM, French EL, Noga C, Simon RH, Ploplis VA (2000) The development of ble-omycin-induced pulmonary fibrosis in mice deficient for components of the fibrino-lytic system . *Am J Pathol* 157: 177–187

Tabrizi P, Wang L, Seeds N, McComb JG, Yamada S, Griffin JH, Carmeliet P, Weiss MH, Zlokovic BV (1999) Tissue plasminogen activator (tPA) deficiency exacerbates cere-brovascular fibrin deposition and brain injury in a murine stroke model: studies in tPA-deficient mice and wild-type mice on a matched genetic background. *Arterioscler Thromb Vasc Biol* 19 : 2801–2806

Taylor FB, Jr., Peer GT, Lockhart MS, Ferrell G, Esmon CT (2001) Endothelial cell protein C receptor plays an important role in protein C activation in vivo. *Blood* 97: 1685–1688

Thompson SG, Kienast J, Pyke SD, Haverkate F, van de Loo JC (1995) Hemostatic factors and the risk of myocardial infarction or sudden death in patients with angina pec-toris. European Concerted Action on Thrombosis and Disabilities Angina Pectoris Study Group. *N Engl J Med* 332: 635–641

Thorelli E, Kaufman RJ, Dahlback B (1999) Cleavage of factor V at Arg 506 by activated protein C and the expression of anticoagulant activity of factor V. *Blood* 93: 2552–2558

Toomey JR, Kratzer KE, Lasky NM, Broze GJ, Jr. (1997) Effect of tissue factor deficiency on mouse and tumor development. *Proc Natl Acad Sci USA* 94: 6922–6926

Toomey JR, Kratzer KE, Lasky NM, Stanton JJ, Broze GJ, Jr. (1996) Targeted disruption of the murine tissue factor gene results in embryonic lethality. *Blood* 88: 1583–1587

Tsirka SE (1997) Clinical implications of the involvement of tPA in neuronal cell death. *J Mol Med* 75: 341–347

Tsirka SE, Gualandris A, Amaral DG, Strickland S (1995) Excitotoxin-induced neuronal degeneration and seizure are mediated by tissue plasminogen activator. *Nature* 377: 340–344

Tsirka SE, Rogove AD, Bugge TH, Degen JL, Strickland S (1997) An extracellular proteo-lytic cascade promotes neuronal degeneration in the mouse hippocampus. *J Neurosci* 17: 543–552

Uhrin P, Dewerchin M, Hilpert M, Chrenek P, Schofer C, Zechmeister-Machhart M, Kronke G, Vales A, Carmeliet P, Binder BR, Geiger M (2000) Disruption of the pro-tein C inhibitor gene results in impaired spermatogenesis and male infertility. *J Clin Invest* 106: 1531–1539

Weiler-Guettler H, Christie PD, Beeler DL, Healy AM, Hancock WW, Rayburn H, Edelberg JM, Rosenberg RD (1998) A targeted point mutation in thrombomodulin generates viable mice with a prethrombotic state. *J Clin Invest* 101: 1983–1991

Weiler H, Lindner V, Kerlin B, Isermann BH, Hendrickson SB, Cooley BC, Meh DA, Mosesson MW, Shworak NW, Post MJ, Conway EM, Ulfman LH, von Andrian UH, Weitz JI (2001) Characterization of a mouse model for thrombomodulin deficiency. *Arterioscler Thromb Vasc Biol* 21: 1531–1537

Westrick RJ, Bodary PF, Xu Z, Shen YC, Broze GJ, Eitzman DT (2001) Deficiency of tissue factor pathway inhibitor promotes atherosclerosis and thrombosis in mice. *Circulation* 103: 3044–3046

Wu YP, Siao CJ, Lu W, Sung TC, Frohman MA, Milev P, Bugge TH, Degen JL, Levine JM, Margolis RU, Tsirka SE (2000) The tissue plasminogen activator (tPA)/plasmin extracellular proteolytic system regulates seizure-induced hippocampal mossy fiber outgrowth through a proteoglycan substrate. *J Cell Biol* 148: 1295–1304

Xiao Q, Danton MJ, Witte DP, Kowala MC, Valentine MT, Bugge TH, Degen JL (1997) Plasminogen deficiency accelerates vessel wall disease in mice predisposed to atherosclerosis. *Proc Natl Acad Sci USA* 94: 10335–10340

Xiao Q, Danton MJ, Witte DP, Kowala MC, Valentine MT, Degen JL (1998) Fibrinogen deficiency is compatible with the development of atherosclerosis in mice. *J Clin Invest* 101: 1184–1194

Xue J, Wu Q, Westfield LA, Tuley EA, Lu D, Zhang Q, Shim K, Zheng X, Sadler JE (1998) Incomplete embryonic lethality and fatal neonatal hemorrhage caused by prothrombin deficiency in mice. *Proc Natl Acad Sci USA* 95: 7603–7607

Yanada M, Kojima T, Ishiguro K, Nakayama Y, Yamamoto K, Matsushita T, Kadomatsu K, Nishimura M, Muramatsu T, Saito H (2002) Impact of antithrombin deficiency in thrombogenesis: lipopolysaccharide and stress-induced thrombus formation in heterozygous antithrombin- deficient mice. *Blood* 99: 2455–2458

Yang TL, Cui J, Taylor JM, Yang A, Gruber SB, Ginsburg D (2000) Rescue of fatal neonatal hemorrhage in factor V deficient mice by low level transgene expression. *Thromb Haemost* 83: 70–77

Yang YH, Carmeliet P, Hamilton JA (2001) Tissue-type plasminogen activator deficiency exacerbates arthritis. *J Immunol* 167: 1047–1052

Yin ZF, Huang ZF, Cui J, Fiehler R, Lasky N, Ginsburg D, Broze GJ, Jr. (2000) Prothrombotic phenotype of protein Z deficiency. *Proc Natl Acad Sci USA* 97: 6734–6738

Zhang K, Kurachi S, Kurachi K (2002) Genetic mechanisms of age regulation of protein C and blood coagulation. *J Biol Chem* 277: 4532–4540

Zhu Y, Carmeliet P, Fay WP (1999) Plasminogen activator inhibitor-1 is a major determinant of arterial thrombolysis resistance. *Circulation* 99: 3050–3055

Transgenic Animals in Primary Hemostasis and Thrombosis

C. Gachet · B. Hechler · C. Léon · J.-P. Cazenave · F. Lanza

INSERM U. 311, Etablissement Français du Sang-Alsace, 10, rue Spielmann,
BP N° 36, 67065 Strasbourg Cedex, France
e-mail:christian.gachet@efs-alsace.fr

Abstract Blood platelet activation at the contact of an injured vessel wall results in adhesion, shape change, aggregation and secretion, which are all tightly regulated biological processes to fulfill the main physiological function of platelets: the arrest of bleeding or primary hemostasis. The same mechanisms of activation are triggered when platelets encounter an atherosclerotic plaque rupturing or following mechanical or infectious injury of the vessel wall, resulting in arterial thrombosis or disseminated intravascular thrombosis. Knowledge of the molecular biology of hemostasis has increased considerably during the last few decades due to the accurate observation of defective hemostasis in patients exhibiting selective abnormalities in platelet surface glycoproteins involved in adhesive functions, defects of plasma adhesive proteins, or defects affecting the complex network of receptors and their transduction machinery. The era of gene targeting and transgenesis in living animals has largely confirmed previous knowledge about the molecular aspects of platelet functions. New insights have also emerged with the perspective of identifying as-yet-unexpected targets for antiplatelet drugs. Blood platelets of transgenic mice have been studied not only to explore hemostasis and thrombosis but also for purposes of general biochemistry and molecular biology. This accounts for the broad range of targeted genes resulting in platelet dysfunction, not all being relevant to pharmacological objectives in terms of antiplatelet drug research. However, these transgenic mice have greatly improved our general understanding of platelet physiology and represent useful models for preclinical pharmacology and basic science.

Keywords Platelets · Hemostasis · Arterial thrombosis · Antithrombotic drugs · G protein-coupled receptors · Thrombin · Integrins · Signaling · Vascular wall

1
Introduction

The major role of blood platelets is to stop bleeding occurring upon lesion of small vessels, a physiological function termed primary hemostasis. Platelet activation on contact with an injured vessel wall results in adhesion, shape change, aggregation and secretion, all of which are tightly regulated biological processes. The same mechanisms of activation are triggered when platelets encounter a rupturing atherosclerotic plaque or any other mechanical or infectious injury of the vessel wall. Antiplatelet drugs are therefore of critical importance for the prevention and treatment of acute arterial thrombosis. In addition, platelets are involved in many pathophysiological processes including inflammation, atherosclerosis, angiogenesis, and dissemination of metastases. Our knowledge of the molecular biology of hemostasis has increased considerably during the last few decades, and it is noteworthy that this progress has been mainly due to the fine observation of hemostatic deficiencies in patients presenting selective molecular defects of membrane glycoproteins involved in the adhesive functions of platelets, defects of adhesive plasma proteins, or defects in the complex network of receptors and their transduction machinery. Animal strains including mice, rats, dogs, cows, and pigs with naturally mutated genes have also provided information on specific aspects of primary hemostasis and are still employed in experimental models of thrombosis and hemorrhage. Since platelets are easy to sample, they have moreover often been used in biochemical and molecular biology studies. The new era of gene targeting and transgenesis in living animals has thus mainly confirmed previous knowledge concerning the molecular aspects of platelet functions. However, new insights have also emerged with the perspective of identifying as-yet-unexpected targets for antiplatelet drugs.

1.1
Molecular Mechanisms of Platelet Function and Related Bleeding Diatheses

The first step of platelet activation in flowing blood following vessel wall injury is attachment of the cells to the exposed subendothelial matrix proteins, of which collagens are the most thrombogenic (Fig. 1). This occurs through tethering of the platelet glycoprotein (GP) GPIbα to von Willebrand factor (vWF) bound to collagen on the matrix (adhesion step). GPIbα is a subunit of the multimolecular GPIb-V-IX complex. Molecular defects of subunits of this complex are responsible for a rare but severe bleeding diathesis known as Bernard-Soulier syndrome (BSS) (originally termed hemorrhagic dystrophic thrombocytopenia), where platelet adhesion is strongly impaired due to a lack of GPIb-V-IX expression at the plasma membrane (Bernard et al. 1975; Nurden and Caen 1975; de la Salle et al. 1995; Lopez et al. 1998; Rivera et al. 2000). The adherent platelets undergo shape change and spread on the surface through activation of integrins such as the $\alpha_2\beta_1$ collagen receptor and the $\alpha_{IIb}\beta_3$ fibrinogen/vWF receptor. The latter is also involved in the final common step of platelet activation, namely platelet-to-platelet aggregation through binding of soluble fibrinogen. Defects in the molecular structure of this integrin or its absence result in another severe thrombopathy, Glanzmann's thrombasthenia (GT), where platelets are unable to aggregate in response to any agonist. Cells from GT patients helped to discover the role of this canonical integrin specific to platelets (Nurden and

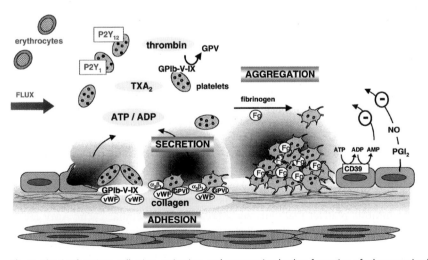

Fig. 1 Platelet functions: adhesion, activation, and aggregation lead to formation of a hemostatic plug

Caen 1974; Parise 1999; Savage et al. 2001). Multiple and complex transduction pathways then lead to platelet secretion and recruitment of circulating platelets, thus enabling thrombus growth and formation of the so-called hemostatic plug (aggregation step). Key steps here are platelet activation through the GPVI collagen receptor which induces signaling through the γ-chain of the Fc receptor and tyrosine phosphorylation (Clemetson and Clemetson 2001), reorganization of the cytoskeleton, secretion of the granule contents and subsequent activation of G protein-coupled receptors (GPCR) including the adenosine diphosphate (ADP) receptors $P2Y_1$ and $P2Y_{12}$ (Gachet 2001) and the $5\text{-HT}_{(2A)}$ serotonin receptor, release of thromboxane A_2 (TXA_2), and activation of thromboxane prostanoid (TP) receptors. Thrombin, the strongest platelet agonist and the central enzyme of the blood coagulation cascade, is formed as a result of tissue factor (TF) exposure and activates platelets directly through members of the protease activated receptor (PAR) family (Coughlin 1999b).

Dysfunction of most of these activation steps has been observed in rare patients suffering from mild to severe hereditary bleeding disorders. Patients have been described with impaired aggregation in response to collagen, which was attributed to defects in integrin $\alpha_2\beta_1$ (Nieuwenhuis et al. 1987; Kehrel et al. 1988) or in GPVI (Sugiyama et al. 1986; Moroi et al. 1989). In both cases, mild bleeding could be observed, but as collagen has multiple receptors on the platelet membrane, a deficiency in only one of them will not necessarily result in a profound diathesis. Patients with selective defects in one of the most important GPCR, the $P2Y_{12}$ receptor, have also been reported (Cattaneo et al. 1992; Nurden et al. 1995; Gachet 2001). A lack of granule contents referred to as storage pool disease (SPD) exists, with some selectivity of the deficiency concerning the α-granules, which contain mainly adhesive proteins and growth factors such as platelet derived growth factor (PDGF) or vascular endothelial growth factor (VEGF), or the dense granules which store large amounts of ATP and ADP, serotonin, and calcium (Cattaneo 2002). These disorders are frequently discovered during routine examination of platelet functions, before surgery, for example. Finally, patients have been described with intracellular transduction protein defects involving phospholipase C (PLC) isoforms (Gabbeta et al. 1997). A number of platelet abnormalities have consequences for the platelet count and size, as in Wiskott-Aldrich syndrome (small platelets) or BSS syndrome (giant platelets). Inherited thrombocytopenias with a normal platelet volume also exist, like thrombocytopenia with absent radii (Van Geet et al. 2002). Although in a growing number of these diseases the genetic defect has been identified, in many inherited platelet abnormalities the underlying mechanisms still remain unknown.

The antithrombogenicity of the vessel wall is regulated by several mechanisms including notably the continuous release of prostacyclin (PGI_2), which strongly inhibits platelet reactivity by increasing intracellular cyclic AMP levels and promotes vasodilation through production of nitric oxide (NO). Another important mechanism involves the ATP diphosphohydrolase enzyme activity of the endothelial CD39 molecule (E-NTDPase-1) (Zimmermann 2000). This enzyme sequentially degrades ATP and other triphosphate nucleotides into ADP and AMP, thus preventing interaction of platelets with the healthy vessel wall. It has been shown that this enzyme activity is downregulated in various pathological states where the endothelium is stimulated, which increases platelet–vessel wall interactions and the subsequent risk of thrombosis (Robson et al. 1997; Marcus et al. 2001). Finally, there exist natural inhibitors of coagulation such as protein S and protein C, thrombomodulin, tissue factor pathway inhibitor (TFPI) or plasmin activator inhibitors (PAI1 and PAI2), and congenital mutations leading to deficiencies with an increased risk of thrombosis have been reported (Plow et al. 1999).

1.2
Molecular Targets of Antiplatelet Drugs

The important antiplatelet drugs routinely used in humans to prevent and treat primary or secondary ischemic disease are at present limited to aspirin, which inhibits cyclooxygenase and hence the production of TXA_2, the thienopyridine compounds ticlopidine and clopidogrel, which irreversibly inhibit ADP-induced platelet aggregation by generating an active metabolite which binds covalently to the $P2Y_{12}$ receptor and inhibitors of integrin $\alpha_{IIb}\beta_3$ such as the chimeric human/murine monoclonal antibody fragment abciximab (ReoPro), a cyclic heptapeptide based on the KGD sequence eptifibatide (Integrilin), a peptidomimetic based on the RGD recognition sequence tirofiban (Aggrastat) (Coller 2001) or other inhibitors of fibrinogen binding. Numerous clinical trials have demonstrated the efficacy but also the undesirable effects of these different compounds. In addition to these widely used drugs, various molecules are undergoing preclinical and clinical trials including direct antithrombins like hirudin, direct antagonists of the ADP or TP receptors, and prostaglandins like iloprost which inhibit platelet functions by increasing intracellular levels of cyclic AMP. Considering the overall results for treatment of ischemic diseases, there is still a place and need for new drugs interfering with platelet activation. Transgenic animal models will undoubtedly not only generate a mine of information concerning the general physiology of hemostasis but also help in discovering new targets for efficient therapeutic strategies.

2
Transgenic Models

2.1
Adhesion Receptors

Integrin $\alpha_{IIb}\beta_3$ (GPIIb-IIIa) and the GPIb-V-IX complex are the two most important adhesive receptors (Table 1) in platelet physiology. The well-characterized bleeding syndromes of Glanzmann's thrombasthenia and Bernard-Soulier disease result from absence or anomaly of respectively GPIIb-IIIa or GPIb-V-IX

Table 1 Major phenotype of mice deficient in adhesion receptors

Disrupted gene	Ligand/ receptor	Phenotype of knockout mice	Reference(s)
β_3 Integrin	Fibrinogen, vWF ($\alpha_{IIb}\beta_3$), vitronectin ($\alpha_v\beta_3$)	Glanzmann's phenotype: prolonged bleeding time, defective aggregation to all agonists, reduced thrombosis	Hodivala-Dilke et al. 1999
β_1 Integrin	Collagen ($\alpha_2\beta_1$), fibronectin ($\alpha_5\beta_1$), laminin ($\alpha_6\beta_1$)	Normal bleeding time, delayed response to collagen	Nieswandt et al. 2001a
α_{IIb} Integrin	Fibrinogen, vWF ($\alpha_{IIb}\beta_3$)	Glanzmann's phenotype: prolonged bleeding time, defective aggregation to all agonists	Tronik-Le Roux et al. 2000
α_2 Integrin	Collagen ($\alpha_2\beta_1$)	Normal bleeding time, delayed response to collagen	Holtkötter et al. 2002
GPVI	Collagen	Normal bleeding time, absence of aggregation to collagen	Kato 2003
GPIbα	vWF	Bernard-Soulier phenotype: prolonged bleeding time, low number/giant platelets	Ware et al. 2000
GPV	Thrombin, collagen	Normal bleeding time, normal platelets, delayed response to collagen, increased response to low doses thrombin, thrombus instability	Ramakrishnan et al. 1999; Moog et al. 2001
P-Selectin	PSGL-1	Prolonged bleeding time, increased hemorrhage in Schwartzman reaction, abnormal thrombus geometry	Subramaniam et al. 1996; Furie et al. 2001
PECAM-1	PECAM-1	Increased response to collagen, prolonged bleeding time of vascular origin	Jones et al. 2001; Patil et al. 2001
CD9	?	Normal bleeding time, normal platelets, normal aggregation	F. Lanza (unpublished)
CD40L	CD40, $\alpha_{IIb}\beta_3$	Defective thrombosis	André et al. 2002
Fibrinogen		Prolonged bleeding time, defective aggregation and clotting	Suh et al. 1995
vWF	GPIb-V-IX, $\alpha_{IIb}\beta_3$	vWD phenotype: prolonged bleeding time, spontaneous bleeding, defective thrombosis	Denis et al. 1998

(see Sect. 1) and these disorders have been reproduced recently in mice by genetic manipulation. Platelets also bare other adhesive receptors belonging to various gene families. In most cases the in vivo function is less well established and production of animals with inherited deficiencies of these receptors will provide tools to study their function and physiological relevance. Recent work has revealed responses in such mice which differ from those induced by blocking the receptors with monoclonal antibodies or other antagonists.

2.1.1
Integrins

β_3 *Integrins.* The role of integrin $\alpha_{IIb}\beta_3$ in platelet functions is well established but reproduction of the deficiency in mice will be useful to study its involvement in thrombosis and other platelet-related pathologies such as atherosclerosis (Massberg et al. 2002). β_3 Integrin-deficient mice have been generated which are viable and fertile and display all the cardinal features of Glanzmann's thrombasthenia, namely defective platelet aggregation and clot retraction, a prolonged bleeding time and cutaneous and gastrointestinal bleeding (Hodivala-Dilke et al. 1999). β_3-Null mice were variably protected from thrombosis depending on the method used to initiate thrombosis. Arterial thrombosis was diminished as shown by a lack of occlusion in a model of ferric chloride injury of the carotid artery. Disseminated microvascular thrombosis was reduced after injection of ADP but was less affected in response to a mixture of collagen and adrenaline and there was no resistance to tissue factor (Smyth et al. 2001a). The animals were not protected from developing intimal hyperplasia, unlike P selectin-deficient mice (Smyth et al. 2001b). Mice in which tyrosines were mutated in the cytoplasmic domain displayed impaired outside-in $\alpha_{IIb}\beta_3$ signaling, with defective in vitro aggregation and clot-retraction responses and a tendency to rebleed (Law et al. 1999).

α_{IIb} *Subunit.* Inactivation of the α_{IIb} chain by insertion of the thymidine kinase (tk) gene into the α_{IIb} locus reproduces the features of Glanzmann's thrombasthenia. This construct placing tk under the control of the α_{IIb} promoter has also been used to abolish megakaryopoiesis following ganciclovir treatment (Tronik-Le Roux et al. 2000; Tronik-Le Roux et al. 1995).

β_1 *Integrins.* The proposed function of integrin $\alpha_2\beta_1$ is to support platelet adhesion to subendothelial collagen fibers, thus facilitating subsequent interactions with the activating platelet receptor for collagen, GPVI. Contrary to the phenotype observed in α_2 integrin-deficient patients, cre/loxP-mediated loss of β_1 integrin in mouse platelets had no significant effect on the bleeding time, suggesting a minor role of the three platelet β_1 integrins, $\alpha_5\beta_1$, $\alpha_6\beta_1$, and, most surprisingly, $\alpha_2\beta_1$ (Nieuwenhuis et al. 1985; Nieswandt et al. 2001a). Aggregation of β_1-null platelets in response to native fibrillar collagen was delayed but not reduced. Ablation of the α_2 integrin gene provided another unexpected finding, as these mice developed normally and showed no obvious anatomical or histological defects. This strain also enabled confirmation of the subtle defects of collagen-induced platelet adhesion and aggregation observed in β_1 knockout mice (Holtkötter et al. 2002).

2.1.2
The GPIb-V-IX Complex

Studies of the Bernard-Soulier bleeding disorder, due to defects in the genes coding for the GPIb$\alpha\beta$ and GPIX subunits of the GPIb-V-IX complex, have shown that this receptor is required for normal hemostasis and vWF-dependent platelet adhesion and that the bleeding diathesis is accompanied by an additional macrothrombocytopenic defect (Lopez et al. 1998). Mice deficient in the GPIbα or GPV subunit have been produced (Kahn et al. 1999; Ramakrishnan et al. 1999; Ware et al. 2000), but the role of the GPV subunit remains poorly defined.

GPIbα. GPIbα-deficient mice reproduce the Bernard-Soulier phenotype with an increased bleeding time, giant platelets and a low platelet count (Ware et al. 2000). Moreover, study of their bone marrow has revealed defective megakaryocyte maturation with poorly developed demarcation membranes and abnormal proplatelet formation (Poujol et al. 2002). These defects could be prevented by expression of a human GPIbα subunit (Ware et al. 2000), while improvement of the macrothrombocytopenia has been observed in knockout mice expressing a chimeric IL4R/GPIbα intracellular domain (Kanaji et al. 2002). No ex vivo or in vivo functional studies have been reported to date.

GPV. GPV is a subunit of the GPIb-V-IX complex which is cleaved by thrombin, but its role in platelet adhesion or activation is not precisely known. In two separate mouse strains, GPV deficiency did not lead to a Bernard-Soulier phenotype and was accompanied by an increased platelet response to low concentrations of thrombin (Kahn et al. 1999; Ramakrishnan et al. 1999; Moog et al. 2001). This could mean that GPV acts as a negative modulator of thrombin activation or be the consequence of increased thrombin availability due to substrate withholding. An unanticipated role of GPV as a collagen receptor was revealed in these mice by the reduced adhesion and activation of their platelets in response to collagen (Moog et al. 2001). Results in an intravital arterial thrombosis model differed between mouse strains, one being less prone to thrombus formation and the other displaying more rapid formation of thrombi, which were however less stable and embolized (Moog et al. 2001; Ni et al. 2001). Possible variations in genetic background could be responsible for these discrepancies and hopefully will be resolved by backcrossing onto a pure background.

2.1.3
P-Selectin

P-selectin is present in endothelial cells and platelet granules and is exposed at the cell surface following activation. Production of P-selectin-deficient mice has shown that endothelial P-selectin mediates not only leukocyte but also platelet rolling on the vessel wall (Subramaniam et al. 1996). The function of platelet P-selectin is less clear. However, studies of lymphocyte homing to peripheral lymph nodes indicate that activated platelets might participate in leukocyte recruitment. Work with the P-selectin mutant mice has further suggested an anti-inflammatory aspect of platelet P-selectin in that binding of the receptor to leukocytes promoted the transcellular production of an anti-inflammatory mediator limiting the extent of acute glomerulonephritis (Hartwell and Wagner 1999). A possible mechanism whereby platelet P-selectin could play a role in thrombosis would be to participate in monocyte recruitment, which in turn would transfer tissue factor to platelets and generate a platelet clot. P-selectin-deficient mice exhibit a bleeding tendency and an abnormal thrombus geometry in an ex vivo model (Furie et al. 2001). Mice have also been produced which express P-selectin lacking the cytoplasmic domain and this deletion did not affect the sorting of P-selectin into platelet (alpha) granules, unlike in endothelial cells (Hartwell et al. 1998).

2.1.4
Other Receptors

PECAM.1. PECAM.1 is a member of the IgG superfamily found in platelets, endothelial cells, and leukocytes. The presence of an intracellular immunoreceptor tyrosine-based inhibitory motif (ITIM) would suggest its involvement in negative regulation of the GPVI/FcRγ chain response. PECAM.1-deficient mice displayed enhanced platelet responses to collagen ex vivo (Jones et al. 2001; Patil et al. 2001) but no apparent abnormalities of thrombus formation in a venous or arterial in vivo model (Vollmar et al. 2001). These mice also have a prolonged bleeding time which has been attributed to vascular defects.

CD9. CD9 is a member of the tetraspanin superfamily which is highly expressed on platelets but also in many other tissues. It associates with integrins and could modulate their functions. CD9-deficient mice displayed reduced fertility of maternal origin (Le Naour et al. 2000) but no signs of hemostatic defects and the platelets had a normal structure and responded to all agonists (F. Lanza, unpublished data). The deficiency has not yet been examined in thrombosis models.

CD40L. CD40L belongs to the tumor necrosis factor ligand family and plays a role in immune responses by binding to its receptor CD40. CD40L has been detected on the surface of activated platelets where it binds to $\alpha_{IIb}\beta_3$ through its KGD integrin-recognition sequence. Its absence affected the stability of arterial thrombi and delayed arterial occlusion in vivo (André et al. 2002).

CDCrel-1. CDCrel-1 is a member of the septin family thought to be involved in neurotransmitter release. Its gene is located a short distance upstream of the GPIbβ gene in both the human and mouse species and has been found to be co-transcribed as a result of non-consensus polyadenylation. Deletion of the CD-Crel-1 gene in mice had no effect on development or neurophysiology, while the platelets were normal in number and size but exhibited enhanced secretion in response to low concentrations of agonists (Dent et al. 2002).

2.1.5
Adhesive Proteins

Although adhesive proteins do not fall directly within the scope of this chapter, the von Willebrand factor (vWF) and fibrinogen molecules will be considered as they are intimately involved in platelet physiology. These proteins are key ligands for adhesion and aggregation and are stored in the platelet granules.

Fibrinogen. Fibrinogen is critical both as a building block for fibrin formation and as a ligand for integrin $\alpha_{IIb}\beta_3$. Disruption of the α-chain of fibrinogen led to a bleeding tendency and failure of blood clotting and platelet aggregation in vitro, but did not allow discrimination between the in vivo importance of the two functions (Suh et al. 1995). Fibrinogen-deficient mice crossed with ApoE-deficient mice were not protected from atherosclerotic lesions, which ranged in appearance from fatty streaks to fibrous plaques (Xiao et al. 1998). The importance of the fibrinogen–$\alpha_{IIb}\beta_3$ interaction was examined in mice by deleting the last five residues (QAGDV) from the fibrinogen γ-chain (Holmback et al. 1996). These mice displayed normal clotting but defective platelet aggregation and an increased bleeding time similarly as in the integrin β_3 knockout strain.

Von Willebrand Factor. Von Willebrand factor is a multimeric glycoprotein necessary for thrombus formation under conditions of high shear, and its deficiency causes the bleeding disorder known as von Willebrand disease (vWD) in humans. vWF-deficient mice reproduced the severe vWD type III phenotype with an absence of vWF in plasma and extracellular and platelet compartments. These mice have a bleeding tendency and show defective thrombus formation in an in vivo mesenteric artery model (Denis et al. 1998). In mice lacking both vWF and the LDL receptor and placed on an atherogenic diet, fewer fatty streaks and fibrous cap lesions were observed than in vWF-positive controls, the reduction of atherosclerosis being more pronounced in regions of disturbed flow such as the branch points of the renal and mesenteric arteries (Methia et al. 2001).

Combined Fibrinogen/vWF Deficiency. Close analysis of intravital thrombosis experiments showed that mouse strains lacking either fibrinogen or vWF were both able to form an arterial thrombus, albeit of different nature and with different kinetics (Ni et al. 2000). Platelet adhesion was delayed in vWF knockout mice but stable thrombi still formed, while in fibrinogen knockout mice abundant thrombi appeared at the vessel wall but detached easily causing downstream occlusion. Surprisingly, mice deficient in both vWF and fibrinogen successfully formed thrombi with characteristics of both mutations, leading to occlusion in the majority of vessels.

Table 2 Major phenotype of knockout mice in relation to hemostasis and thrombosis

Disrupted gene	Endogenous ligand	Phenotype of knockout mice	Reference(s)
PAR1	Thrombin	Normal bleeding time, normal aggregation to thrombin	Connolly et al. 1996
PAR3	Thrombin	Partial inhibition of thrombin-induced platelet aggregation and resistance to thrombosis	Ishihara et al. 1997; Weiss et al. 2002
PAR4	Thrombin	Markedly prolonged bleeding time, absence of aggregation to thrombin and resistance to thrombosis	Sambrano et al. 2001
TP receptor	TXA_2	Markedly prolonged bleeding time and resistance to thromboembolism	Thomas et al. 1998
EP3 receptor	PGE_2	Normal or slightly increased bleeding time, resistance to arachidonic acid-induced thrombosis	Fabre et al. 2001; Ma et al. 2001
$P2Y_1$	ADP	Moderate increase of bleeding time, and resistance to thromboembolism	Léon et al. 1999; Fabre et al. 1999; Léon et al. 2001
$P2Y_{12}$	ADP	Markedly prolonged bleeding time	Foster et al. 2001
$P2X_1$	ATP	Slightly prolonged bleeding time, decreased aggregation to collagen and resistance to thromboembolism	B. Hechler, unpublished
α_{2A} adrenergic receptor	Adrenaline	?	
$5-HT_{(2A)}$ receptor	Serotonin	?	
IP receptor	PGI_2-PGE_1	Normal bleeding time, increased sensitivity to FeCl3-induced thrombosis of mesenteric arterioles	Murata et al. 1997
DP receptor	PGI_2	?	
A2a receptor	Adenosine	Increased ADP-induced platelet aggregation	Ledent et al. 1997
CD39	ATP, ADP	Prolonged bleeding time; platelet $P2Y_1$ receptor desensitization, resistance to thromboembolism	Enjyoji et al. 1999

2.2
Activation Receptors

Platelets in flowing blood may be exposed to various soluble or insoluble ligands which stimulate or inhibit their reactivity. These molecules interact with platelets by binding to specific receptors on the cell surface, either glycoprotein receptors of the immunoglobulin superfamily, which all signal through the

γ-chain of the Fc receptor and tyrosine kinases, G protein-coupled receptors, or ion channel receptors (Table 2).

2.2.1
The GPVI Collagen Receptor

As mentioned in the introduction, GPVI plays a major part in the platelet activation induced by collagen. Its contribution to stable adhesion and thrombus formation has been revealed by targeted gene deletion (Kato et al. 2003). Interestingly, tail bleeding time measurements revealed no severe bleeding tendency. This phenotype could well resemble that observed in FcRγ-deficient platelets (Poole et al. 1997) or in mice treated with a monoclonal antibody (mAb) against GVI (Nieswandt et al. 2001b), which causes disappearance of GPVI from the cell surface. Platelets from these mice exhibit a selective defect of collagen-induced activation. Human platelets express the FcγRIIA receptor, which mediates their responses to immunoglobulins and may play a role in immune-mediated thrombocytopenia. Mice lack the genetic equivalent of this receptor and have been used to study its function following insertion of the human transgene (McKenzie et al. 1999). FcγRIIA-transgenic mice reproduced the platelet activation and immune clearance responses observed in humans, as did a cross strain between FcγRIIA-transgenic and FcRγ-deficient mice.

2.2.2
G Protein-Coupled Receptors

Thrombin Receptors. Thrombin is the main effector protease of the coagulation cascade which converts circulating fibrinogen into fibrin, the unit element of the fibrous matrix of blood clots. It is also involved in endothelial cell activation and in inflammation and is the most potent activator of platelets. Thrombin activates cells at least in part by cleaving protease-activated G protein-coupled receptors (PARs) (Coughlin 1999a). Four PARs have been identified among which PAR1, PAR3, and PAR4 are activated by thrombin and PAR2 by trypsin and tryptase but not by thrombin (Coughlin 1999a). Thrombin acts on human PAR1 and PAR4 by binding to and cleaving the amino-terminal exodomain of the receptor to unmask a new amino terminus. This new terminus then serves as a tethered peptide ligand, binding intramolecularly to the body of the receptor to effect transmembrane signaling.

Gene disruption in mice has provided important information on the thrombin receptors involved in platelet activation. Mice lacking PAR1 have a high rate of embryonic death. As almost 50% of the animals nevertheless survive past birth and grow to adulthood without major abnormalities, this would indicate a role of PAR1 in embryonic development (Connolly et al. 1996). Surprisingly, these mice displayed a normal bleeding time and responded normally to activation by human thrombin, suggesting little or no hemostatic importance of PAR1 in mouse platelets despite its role in human platelets (Connolly et al. 1996). This observation prompted a search for additional thrombin receptors and led to the identification of PAR3 (Ishihara et al. 1997). PAR3 is expressed in mouse mega-karyocytes and platelets but not in human platelets. Although mice deficient in PAR3 develop normally and do not suffer from spontaneous bleeding (Ishihara et al. 1997), their platelets respond abnormally to thrombin, requiring high concentrations to achieve even a suboptimal response (Nakanishi-Matsui et al. 2000). Studies in PAR3-deficient mice have revealed that PAR3 is necessary for activation of mouse platelets at low but not high concentrations of thrombin. These animals are protected against $FeCl_3$-induced thrombosis of mesenteric arterioles and thromboplastin-induced pulmonary embolism (Weiss et al. 2002), indicating a key role of this receptor in thrombosis in mice. Persistent thrombin signaling in PAR3-null mouse platelets could be attributed to PAR4 (Kahn et al. 1998), which is also expressed on human platelets. Mice deficient in PAR4 do not exhibit spontaneous bleeding but display a markedly prolonged bleeding time as measured by tail transection. The platelets are unresponsive to thrombin as shown by the absence of shape change, calcium mobilization, aggregation, and secretion even in the presence of high concentrations of agonist (Sambrano et al. 2001). In addition, mice lacking PAR4, like those lacking PAR3, are protected against $FeCl_3$-induced thrombosis of mesenteric arterioles (Sambrano et al. 2001).

Thus, in both man and mouse, platelets utilize two thrombin receptors: A high-affinity receptor (PAR1 in man, PAR3 in mouse) is necessary for responses to low concentrations of thrombin, while a "low-affinity" receptor (PAR4 in both species) mediates responses to higher concentrations. Thrombin moreover not only binds to PAR-type receptors. The $GPIb\alpha$ subunit contains a binding site for thrombin and is thought to participate in platelet activation by thrombin, as shown by a decreased response of the cells following antibody treatment or $GPIb\alpha$ cleavage or in Bernard-Soulier patients. No data have yet been published for $GPIb\alpha$-deficient mice. As mentioned earlier, GPV-deficient platelets exhibit an enhanced response to low concentrations of thrombin, but further studies are needed to clarify this effect (Ramakrishnan et al. 1999; Moog et al. 2001).

ADP Receptors. ADP is with thrombin and collagen one of the most important platelet agonists and was identified very early (Gaarder et al. 1961). Adenine nucleotides interact with P2 receptors, which are widely distributed in many different cells and regulate a broad range of physiological processes. The P2 family consists of two classes of membrane receptors, P2X ligand-gated cation channels and G protein-coupled P2Y receptors (Ralevic and Burnstock 1998). Three P2 receptor subtypes have been identified on blood platelets, namely $P2Y_1$, $P2Y_{12}$, and $P2X_1$, the two P2Y receptors being essential for aggregation in response to ADP. Coactivation of the $P2Y_1$ and $P2Y_{12}$ receptors is necessary for normal ADP-induced platelet aggregation since inhibition of either receptor is sufficient to prevent it (Gachet 2001).

P2Y₁ Receptor. The presence of the $P2Y_1$ receptor on platelets was initially suggested by pharmacological studies using selective $P2Y_1$ antagonists and by detection of $P2Y_1$ mRNA in both megakaryocytes and platelets (Leon et al. 1997; Hechler et al. 1998). However, since all effects mediated by ADP in platelets were not inhibited by $P2Y_1$ antagonists, the existence of another receptor for ADP was proposed. Definite proof of the existence of a second ADP receptor distinct from $P2Y_1$ and coupled to adenylyl cyclase inhibition was provided by the generation of $P2Y_1$ knockout mice (Fabre et al. 1999; Leon et al. 1999). These mice have no apparent abnormalities affecting their development, survival, or reproduction, and their platelets display normal numbers and morphology. In contrast, platelet shape change and aggregation in response to usual concentrations of ADP are completely abolished, whereas the ability of ADP to inhibit cyclic AMP formation is maintained (Leon et al. 1999). Use of this strain in experimental models showed that the $P2Y_1$ receptor plays an essential role in systemic thromboembolism and localized arterial thrombosis (Leon et al. 1999, 2001; Lenain et al. 2003). Conversely, transgenic mice overexpressing the $P2Y_1$ receptor specifically in the megakaryocyte/platelet lineage have been generated using the promoter of the tissue-specific platelet factor 4 gene (Hechler et al. 2003). This led to a phenotype of platelet hyperreactivity in vitro. Overexpression of the $P2Y_1$ receptor also enabled ADP to induce granule secretion, unlike in wild-type platelets, which suggests that the level of $P2Y_1$ expression is critical for this event and that the weak responses of normal platelets to ADP are due to a limited number of $P2Y_1$ receptors rather than to the specific transduction pathway. These transgenic mice further display a shortened bleeding time and an increased sensitivity to the in vivo platelet aggregation induced by infusion of a mixture of collagen and adrenaline (Hechler et al. 2003).

P2Y₁₂ Receptor. The $P2Y_{12}$ receptor has been cloned from human and rat platelet cDNA libraries using an expression cloning strategy in Xenopus oocytes designed to detect G_i-linked receptors through their coupling to co-transfected inward-rectifying K^+ channels (Hollopeter et al. 2001) and also by screening an orphan receptor library (Zhang et al. 2001). Its tissue distribution seems to be restricted to platelets and subregions of the brain (Hollopeter et al. 2001). The $P2Y_{12}$ receptor coupled to $G\alpha_{i2}$ is essential for full platelet aggregation in response to ADP or other aggregating agents. This receptor is the target of the antithrombotic drugs ticlopidine and clopidogrel (Gachet 2001). It plays a specific role in activation of the $\alpha_{IIb}\beta_3$ integrin by ADP and also mediates the stabilization of platelet aggregates through triggering of a PI3 K pathway downstream of G_i activation and potentiation of platelet secretion (Trumel et al. 1999; Gachet 2001). $P2Y_{12}$-deficient mice are viable and fertile and display no spontaneous bleeding or other overt abnormalities (Foster et al. 2001). However, they have a prolonged bleeding time as compared to wild-type and probably to $P2Y_1$-deficient mice, while platelet aggregation in response to ADP is inhibited although shape change is conserved. Finally, these mice are insensitive to clopidogrel treatment (Foster et al. 2001), confirming that the $P2Y_{12}$ receptor is the target of this drug.

Prostanoid Receptors. Prostaglandins (PGs) and thromboxanes are important modulators of platelet activation. On the basis of their sensitivity to the five naturally occurring prostanoids PGD_2, PGE_2, $PGF_{2\alpha}$, PGI_2, and TXA_2, prostanoid receptors have been classified into five types: DP, EP, FP, IP and TP. Among these, platelets express TP, EP_3 and EP_4, DP, and IP receptors. While TXA_2 or low concentrations of PGE_2 are proaggregatory, PGI_2, high concentrations of PGE_2, and PGD_2 are inhibitors of aggregation (for PGI_2 and PGD_2, see Sects. 2.3.1 and 2.3.2).

TXA_2 Receptor. TXA_2 is a labile metabolite produced from arachidonic acid in the cyclooxygenase pathway. It is a potent vasoconstrictor and a platelet aggregating agent and release of TXA_2 from activated platelets is an important factor in the propagation of platelet activation. A single gene encodes the human thromboxane-prostanoid (TP) receptor, of which two splice variants have been identified, α and β. Although mRNA for both isoforms has been found in human platelets, only the $TP\alpha$ receptor is detectably translated (Habib et al. 1999), whereas both isoforms are expressed on human endothelial and vascular smooth muscle cells (Narumiya and FitzGerald 2001). In mice, only the $TP\alpha$ isoform is expressed. TP-deficient mice survive in expected numbers and do not exhibit organ abnormalities but display a marked prolongation of the bleeding time (Thomas et al. 1998). Platelet aggregation in response to the TXA_2 analog U46619 is totally abolished in these mice and the aggregation response to collagen is delayed, whereas ADP-induced aggregation is similar to that observed in wild-type mice. Infusion of U46619 causes a transient increase in blood pressure followed by cardiovascular collapse in wild-type mice but has no hemodynamic effect in TP-deficient animals. Mice lacking the TP receptor are also resistant to arachidonic acid-induced shock (Thomas et al. 1998).

EP Receptors for PGE_2. Human platelets express EP_3 and EP_4 receptors for PGE_2. If PGE_2 alone does not induce platelet aggregation, it has a biphasic effect on the platelet response, potentiating aggregation at low concentrations and inhibiting it at higher concentrations. Studies in prostanoid receptor-deficient mice have confirmed that the proaggregatory action of PGE_2 is mediated by an EP_3 receptor inhibiting adenylyl cyclase, while high concentrations of PGE_2 act on the prostacyclin (IP) receptor to block platelet activation. Consistent with this schema, lack of the EP_3 receptor protects against the formation of intravascular clots in a model of venous inflammation (Fabre et al. 2001). Moreover, when mice are challenged intravenously with arachidonic acid, mortality and thrombus formation in the lungs are significantly reduced in EP_3-deficient animals. In one study (Fabre et al. 2001), EP_3-deficient mice exhibited a normal bleeding time, whereas in another this parameter was slightly increased (Ma et al. 2001). Although PGE_2 is not usually considered an important physiological regulator of platelet functions, in an inflammatory reaction sufficient PGE_2 may be generated locally to enhance the aggregation induced by platelet agonists and oppose the inhibitory action of prostacyclin (see Sect. 2.3.1).

5-HT$_{(2A)}$ Serotonin Receptor. Serotonin is produced by enterochromaffin cells and carried by specific transporters from the plasma into the cytoplasm and then the dense granules of platelets, where it is stored at a concentration of about 65 mM. Once released from the dense granules, serotonin can in turn activate platelets by interacting with the 5-HT$_{(2A)}$ receptor subtype. It is a weak aggregating agent but can exert mild synergism with other agonists such as thrombin, collagen, or ADP. Although mice lacking the 5-HT$_{(2A)}$ receptor have been generated recently (Fiorica-Howells et al. 2002), no investigation of the consequences of the deficiency for platelet functions has been reported to date.

α_{2A} Adrenergic Receptor. Among the adrenergic receptor subtypes, human and mouse platelets express the α_{2A} adrenergic receptor, while rat platelets bare equal numbers of α_{2A} and β_2 adrenergic receptors (Siess 1989). This explains why adrenaline potentiates aggregation in human platelets whereas it inhibits the reactivity of rat platelets. Adrenaline, by activating α_{2A} adrenergic receptors which are negatively coupled to adenylyl cyclase, does not induce platelet aggregation itself but potentiates the aggregation induced by ADP or low concentrations of other platelet activators (Lanza et al. 1988). Mice lacking the α_{2A} adrenergic receptor subtype are viable, fertile, and apparently normal (Altman et al. 1999). However, the impact of α_{2A} adrenergic deficiency on platelet functions has not yet been explored (Kable et al. 2000).

2.2.3
P2X₁ Receptor

In addition to the G protein-coupled $P2Y_1$ and $P2Y_{12}$ receptors, platelets also express the $P2X_1$ receptor, a ligand-gated cation channel responsible for the fast calcium entry induced by ATP (MacKenzie et al. 1996; Mahaut-Smith et al. 2000). The functional role of this receptor in hemostasis and thrombosis has long been difficult to assess on account of its rapid desensitization during preparation of platelets for in vitro studies and a lack of potent and selective antagonists. $P2X_1$-deficient mice have been shown to exhibit male infertility due to loss of vas deferens contraction, indicating that the $P2X_1$ receptor is essential for normal male reproductive function (Mulryan et al. 2000). The bleeding time is mildly prolonged in this strain as compared to the wild type. $P2X_1$-deficient platelets display a decreased response to low concentrations of collagen and reduced platelet accumulation on a collagen-coated surface under flow conditions corresponding to the wall shear rates in small arteries (1,500 s^{-1}). Finally, $P2X_1$-deficient mice are resistant to both systemic thromboembolism and localized laser-induced arterial thrombosis (Hechler et al. 2003). This is a striking example of a case where in vivo evaluation of the phenotype was determinant in unmasking the role of a receptor.

2.3
Inhibitory Receptors

2.3.1
IP Receptor for PGI$_2$

Prostacyclin (PGI$_2$) acts on platelets and blood vessels to inhibit platelet aggregation and cause vasodilatation. PGI$_2$ activates a $G\alpha_s$-coupled receptor (IP) to produce fast stimulation of adenylyl cyclase and hence rapidly suppress platelet activity. The IP receptor also binds PGE$_1$ (Ashby 1994). IP-deficient mice are viable, reproductive, and normotensive and have a normal bleeding time, but they display increased sensitivity in a model of FeCl$_3$-induced carotid artery thrombosis (Murata et al. 1997).

2.3.2
DP Receptor for PGD$_2$

PGD$_2$ inhibits platelet aggregation by activating DP receptors positively coupled to adenylyl cyclase. DP-deficient mice have been generated recently (Matsuoka et al. 2000), but the impact of the deficiency on platelet functions has not been investigated as yet.

2.3.3
A2a Receptor for Adenosine

Adenosine is produced extracellularly through degradation of released ATP and is also released from cells by facilitated diffusion. It acts on numerous cell types including various neuronal populations, platelets, neutrophils, and smooth muscle cells and mainly helps to protect cells and tissues under stress conditions such as ischemia. Adenosine mediates its effects through four receptor subtypes, the A1, A2a, A2b, and A3 receptors. Among these, platelets express the A2a subtype which mediates the inhibitory effect of adenosine on platelet aggregation by stimulating adenylyl cyclase through $G\alpha_s$ signaling (Olah and Stiles 1995). Although A2a-deficient mice are viable and breed normally, platelet aggregation in response to ADP was consistently higher in this strain compared to the wild type (Ledent et al. 1997).

2.4
CD39, ATP Diphosphohydrolase

One important thromboregulatory mechanism is the expression of E-NTDPase-1 or CD39 on the healthy inactivated endothelium. CD39 is a transmembrane

Table 3 Knockout mice of genes involved in the intracellular signaling pathway

Disrupted gene	Viability	Phenotype of knockout mice	Reference(s)
G_q	30%–40% perinatal mortality	Ataxia, motor discoordination, increased bleeding time and resistance to thromboembolism	Offermanns 2000
$G\alpha_{13}$	Embryonic mortality at E10	Impaired embryonic angiogenesis	Gu et al. 2002
$G\alpha_{12}$	Viable	No phenotype	Gu et al. 2002
G_z	Viable	Resistant to thromboembolism/increased bleeding time	Yang et al. 2000; Kelleher et al. 2001
G_{i2}	Viable	Impairment of ADP-induced platelet activation	Jantzen et al. 2001
G_s	Embryonic mortality at E10	?	Yu et al. 1998
Fyn	Viable	Reduced platelet responses to collagen-related peptide (CRP)	Quek et al. 2000
Lyn	Viable	Delayed platelet responses to collagen-related peptide	Quek et al. 2000
Syk	Mortality within 1 to 5 days	Studies in chimeric mice: loss of aggregation to collagen, normal bleeding time	Poole et al. 1997
LAT	Viable	Impaired platelet responses to CRP	Pasquet et al. 1999
SLP-76	17% perinatal mortality	Fetal hemorrhage, impaired collagen-induced platelet aggregation	Clements et al. 1999
PLCγ2	30% perinatal mortality	Fetal hemorrhage, smaller size, loss of collagen-induced platelet aggregation	Wang et al. 2000; Mangin et al. 2003
Btk	Viable	Reduced aggregation and secretion in response to collagen	Quek et al. 1998
SHP-1	Mortality within 2 weeks	Mev mice, having a mutation in SHP-1gene, display severe defect in hematopoiesis	Shultz et al. 1993
SHP-2	Embryonic mortality at E9.5	Suppression of hematopoietic development	Saxton et al. 1997
SHIP-1	Viable	Increase responsiveness to CRP	Pasquet et al. 2000
PI3-K p85α	Viable	Partial inhibition of collagen and CRP-induced aggregation	Watanabe 2003
PI3-Kγ	Viable	Impaired platelet responses to ADP, normal responses to collagen and thrombin	Hirsch et al. 2001
Gelsolin	Viable	Decreased platelet shape change	Witke et al. 1995
WASP	Viable	Decreased peripheral blood lymphocytes and platelets	Snapper et al. 1998
VASP	Viable	Hyperplasia of megakaryocytes; defects in cAMP/cGMP-mediated inhibition of aggregation	Hauser et al. 1999; Aszodi et al. 1999
cGMP-K1	Viable	Increase in platelet adhesion and aggregation following ischemia/reperfusion	Massberg et al. 1999
Talin	Embryonic mortality at E9	Failure of cell migration at gastrulation	Monkley et al. 2000
Vinculin	Embryonic mortality at E10	Defective embryonic development	Xu et al. 1998
4.1	Viable	Moderate hemolytic anemia	Shi et al. 1999
Profilin	2-Cell stage mortality	?	Witke et al. 2001
Moesin	Viable	No phenotype; normal platelet aggregation	Doi et al. 1999

protein originally identified on lymphoid cells, the extracellular part of which exhibits apyrase or ATP diphosphohydrolase (ATPDase) activity. This thromboregulatory potential of CD39 has been highlighted by disruption of the gene (Enjyoji et al. 1999). CD39-deficient mice do not exhibit specific abnormalities of development or reproductive capacity, although they paradoxically display a prolonged bleeding time with minimally perturbed coagulation parameters. Platelet interactions with the injured mesenteric vasculature were considerably reduced in these mice. In addition, aggregation of platelets in response to ADP, collagen, or low-dose thrombin was diminished. This platelet hypofunction was due to desensitization of the $P2Y_1$ receptor and normal responses could be restored by incubating the cells with soluble apyrase. Consistent with a deficient mechanism of vascular protection, fibrin deposits were found at numerous organ sites in CD39-deficient mice and transplanted cardiac grafts. Hence, CD39 plays a dual role in modulating hemostasis and thrombotic reactions.

2.5
Intracellular Signaling Pathways

2.5.1
The Platelet G Proteins

Among the several G protein α subunits described to date, platelets express G_s, G_q, $G_{12/13}$, G_z, G_{i2} and G_{i3} (Offermanns 2000). Whereas G_s mediates PGI_2/PGE_1-dependent platelet inhibition by stimulating adenylyl cyclase, the other G proteins are involved in platelet activation (Table 3). G_q activates phospholipase $C\beta$ to trigger release of intracellular calcium and activation of protein kinase C, $G_{12/13}$ is involved in events leading to platelet shape change and G_z is able to inhibit adenylyl cyclase. G_{i2} and G_{i3} can likewise mediate repression of cAMP formation, while the released $\beta\gamma$ subunits can activate phospholipase $C\beta$ or other signaling molecules like phosphoinositide 3-kinases (PI3 K) (Brass and Molino 1997; Offermanns 2000) (Fig. 2).

$G\alpha_q$. G_q-deficient platelets exhibit defective calcium mobilization in response to ADP, thrombin, or the TXA_2 mimetic U46619. As a result, platelets from G_q-deficient mice are unable to fully aggregate or secrete the contents of their granules when stimulated with ADP, thrombin, U46619, or a low concentration of collagen alone (Offermanns et al. 1997a), while co-stimulation of the G_{12}/G_{13} and G_i pathways induces integrin $\alpha_{IIb}\beta_3$ activation (Nieswandt et al. 2002). This defect of primary hemostasis leads to an increased bleeding time and to protection against the thromboembolism induced by injection of collagen and adrenaline (Offermanns et al. 1997a,b). Platelet shape change persists except in response to ADP in G_q-deficient mice, demonstrating the involvement of the G_{12}/G_{13} proteins in shape change (Klages et al. 1999). These studies in G_q-null mice have confirmed observations in human platelets concerning the coexistence of

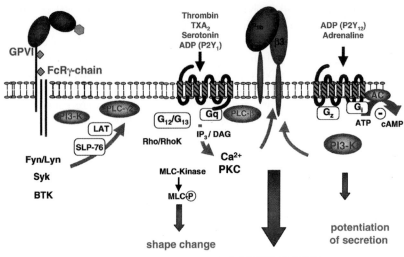

Fig. 2 Platelet signaling pathways. The FcRγ chain is tyrosine-phosphorylated by the kinases Lyn and Fyn, leading to recruitment of Syk kinase. Syk phosphorylates LAT, which leads to recruitment of PLCγ2 and SLP-76 to the cell membrane. LAT also associates with PI3 K, resulting in second messenger PI(3,4,5)P3 production and recruitment of Btk to the membrane, both of which contribute to PLCγ2 activation. Stimulation of GPCR results in activation of G proteins. Gα_q activates PLCβ, while G$\alpha_{i/z}$ activates PI3 kinase-dependent mechanisms and inhibits adenylyl cyclase, thus amplifying the platelet responses. Activation of PLCβ and PLCγ2 leads to second messenger IP3 and DAG production, which results in final events such as shape change, $\alpha_{IIb}\beta_3$ exposure, aggregation, and secretion. The G$_{12/13}$ proteins also participate in platelet shape change through a Rho/Rho kinase pathway

two independent pathways leading to platelet shape change, the calcium/cal-modulin and Rho/Rho kinase pathways (Bauer et al. 1999; Paul et al. 1999).

$G\alpha_{12/13}$. The ubiquitously expressed G_{12} and G_{13} proteins are members of the G_{12} subfamily. Several seven-transmembrane-domain receptors are coupled to G_{12} and/or G_{13}, including receptors for thrombin, TXA$_2$, LPA, and sphingosine-1 phosphate. Studies in Gα_q-deficient mice have shown that G_{12}/G_{13} activation, followed by Rho/Rho kinase signaling leading to phosphorylation of the myosin light chain, is involved in platelet shape change. Mice lacking G_{13} die at embryonic day 10 from impaired angiogenesis. In contrast, G_{12}-deficient mice are viable with no apparent abnormalities. However, intercrossing between G_{12} and G_{13} or G_q mutant mice suggests that G_{12} plays a role in mouse embryogenesis and functionally interacts with signaling pathways using both G_{13} and G_q (Gu et al. 2002).

$G\alpha_z$. G_z is mainly expressed in platelets and the brain. Platelets from G_z-deficient mice display abnormal responses only with regard to adrenaline-mediated inhibition of adenylyl cyclase and the potentiating effect of adrenaline on aggregation induced by other agonists. Consequently, these mice are resistant to the thromboembolism challenge triggered by injection of collagen and adrenaline (Yang et al. 2000).

$G\alpha_{i2}$. G_{i2} is the predominant platelet G alpha(i) subtype. ADP-dependent aggregation is reduced in G_{i2}-deficient mice, and their platelets also display a diminished response to low concentrations of thrombin due to impairment of platelet activation in response to secreted ADP (Jantzen et al. 2001).

$G\alpha_s$. G_s deficiency is embryonically lethal, leading to arrest of development before embryonic day 10.5 (Yu et al. 1998).

2.5.2
The FcRγ Chain-Initiated Pathway

The GPVI/FcRγ chain complex collagen receptor triggers platelet activation through a pathway resembling immune receptor signaling. The FcRγ chain of GPVI is phosphorylated on an ITAM (immunoreceptor tyrosine-based activation motif) by the Src kinases Lyn and Fyn, which leads to recruitment and activation of the non-Src tyrosine kinase Syk. Syk initiates a signaling cascade, resulting in activation of the central enzymes phosphatidylinositol 3-kinase (PI3 K) and PLCγ2. Several proteins are regulated downstream of Syk, including many adapters (LAT, Gads, and SLP-76) and the Tec family tyrosine kinase Brk (Watson et al. 2001) (Fig. 2). Knockout mice have been generated for most of the proteins involved in GPVI signaling and all strains display some impairment of collagen-induced platelet activation. These animals have been useful tools to help elucidate the GPVI-mediated signaling cascade and the more or less crucial roles of all the transduction proteins (Table 3).

Src Kinases. Fyn and Lyn are responsible for initial phosphorylation of the FcRγ chain ITAM (Ezumi et al. 1998). Lyn or Fyn deficiency results respectively in reduced or delayed phosphorylation, with nevertheless no dramatic impairment of collagen-induced platelet aggregation (Quek et al. 2000). Phosphorylation is further delayed in double-knockout mice, indicating the presence of another still-unknown protein kinase probably of the Src family (Quek et al. 2000). Fyn and Lyn are also activated by stimulation of G protein-coupled receptors, but a deficiency in these kinases does not impair the cytoskeletal changes underlying platelet shape change (Bauer et al. 2001).

Syk. Syk-deficient mice die perinatally or within 1–5 days of birth (Cheng et al. 1995; Turner et al. 1995). Hence the role of Syk in platelets has been studied in chimeric wild-type mice irradiated and repopulated with Syk-deficient hematopoietic cells. Syk deficiency leads to a complete loss of collagen-induced platelet aggregation, although the tail bleeding time is normal (Poole et al. 1997). The absence of Syk is associated with a lack of phosphorylation of LAT, SLP-76, and

PLCγ2, together with defective activation of integrin $\alpha_{IIb}\beta_3$ in response to ADP in the presence or absence of adrenaline (Law et al. 1999).

Adapter Proteins Regulating PLCγ2: LAT and SLP-76. Knockout mice deficient for expression of adapter proteins have been useful to determine the function of these proteins. In LAT-deficient platelets, tyrosine phosphorylation of SLP-76 is only weakly inhibited and a significant level of PLCγ2 phosphorylation persists (Pasquet et al. 1999). Mice lacking SLP-76 exhibit perinatal mortality probably due to fetal hemorrhage. If thrombin responsiveness is maintained, collagen-induced platelet aggregation and secretion is strongly impaired in these mice and is associated with a total loss of induction of PLCγ2 phosphorylation (Clements et al. 1999).

PLCγ2. Studies in PLCγ2-deficient mice have demonstrated a critical role of this phospholipase in collagen-induced aggregation and secretion. Although viable PLCγ2-deficient mice can be obtained, the absence of PLCγ2 leads to perinatal mortality and a smaller size of some animals, which most probably result from a bleeding disorder. Embryonic and adult mice display intraperitoneal and gastrointestinal hemorrhage (Wang et al. 2000). The ability of platelets to aggregate and release TXA_2 or ADP following collagen stimulation was severely affected in PLCγ2-deficient mice, although responses to thrombin, ADP, and U46619 were normal (Manging et al. 2003). This is consistent with the hypothesis that PLCγ2 is essential for signaling through collagen receptors, which require the FcRγ chain. Residual activation of PLCγ2-null platelets through a mechanism independent of GPVI but dependent on PI3 K and integrin $\alpha_{IIb}\beta_3$ was nevertheless observed at high collagen concentrations (Manging et al. 2003).

Tec Kinases. The Tec kinases Btk (Bruton tyrosine kinase) and Tec are expressed in platelets where they are phosphorylated during stimulation with collagen (Quek et al. 2000). Human platelets from patients with X-linked agammaglobulinemia (XLA), characterized by a primary immunodeficiency resulting from mutations in the Btk gene, exhibit reduced aggregation and secretion in response to collagen (Quek et al. 1998). This is accompanied by a partial decrease in PLCγ2 phosphorylation. In Xid mice (an X-linked immunodeficiency resulting from mutation of Btk), there is negligible reduction in PLCγ2 phosphorylation, which would suggest the involvement of Tec and/or another Src or Syk-related kinase (Pasquet et al. 2000). Mice deficient in both Btk and Tec will be useful to elucidate this point (Ellmeier et al. 2000).

2.5.3
Miscellaneous Pathways

SHP and SHIP Phosphatases. Receptors signaling through ITAM-dependent pathways can be regulated by transmembrane proteins containing ITIMs (immunoreceptor tyrosine-based inhibition motifs). After phosphorylation of the conserved tyrosine in the ITIM, tyrosine phosphatases containing an SH2 domain (SHP-1 and SHP-2) or inositol 5'-lipid phosphatases containing an SH2 domain (SHIP-1 and SHIP-2) are recruited to the plasma membrane. SHP-2 knockout mice are not viable and die by day 9.5 from suppression of hematopoietic development (Saxton et al. 1997). Mice lacking SHP-1 are called *motheaten* owing to their appearance and general state of ill-health and do not survive more than 2 weeks. Viable *motheaten* (mev) mice have a mutation in the SHP-1 gene which results in almost complete loss of catalytic activity. These mice survive several weeks although older animals are thrombocytopenic and their platelets display hypophosphorylation of Syk and Lyn in response to collagen-related peptide (CRP), accompanied by reduced P-selectin expression. Studies of resting *mev/mev* platelets have revealed a novel protein of 26 kDa, heavily tyrosine-phosphorylated, which remains to be identified (Pasquet et al. 2000). SHIP-1-deficient platelets show increased responsiveness to CRP in the presence of extracellular calcium. This finding has demonstrated a novel pathway of calcium entry, which is regulated through binding of PI(3,4,5)P3 to Btk and is independent of PLCγ2 (Pasquet et al. 2000). SHIP-2 has a broader distribution than SHIP-1 and is also expressed in hematopoietic tissues (Muraille et al. 1999) but no SHIP-2 knockout mice have been reported to date.

PI3 Kinases. Murine platelets express several forms of PI3 K: p85/p110α and β, and p110γ. Class IA PI3Ks are heterodimeric enzymes which regulate a large number of signal transduction pathways. The p85 regulatory subunit recruits the p110 catalytic subunit to the cell membrane, where p110 phosphorylates inositol lipids. PI3Kp85 null mice have been generated recently and exhibit a clear deficiency of collagen-induced platelet activation with impaired signalling of the GPVI/FcgammaR chain pathway. In contrast, platelet activation by soluble agonists such as ADP, thrombin or U46619 is not affected in these mice (Watanabe et al. 2003). PI3Kγ is a key downstream effector of G protein-coupled receptors. PI3Kγ-deficient platelets exhibit impaired aggregation in response to ADP, whereas responses to collagen and more surprisingly to thrombin are normal. The bleeding time is not affected, but the mice are resistant to the acute thromboembolism induced by injection of ADP (Hirsch et al. 2001).

2.5.4
Cytoskeletal Proteins and Platelet Signaling

One function of the cytoskeleton is to direct the contours of the membrane in resting platelets and the rapid shape changes of activated platelets resulting from phosphorylation or calpain-induced cleavage of cytoskeletal proteins. Mice deficient in several proteins of the membrane cytoskeleton have been generated but will not be discussed here as no platelet phenotype has yet been described. The cytoskeleton is also able to bind signaling molecules, thus confining them to specific cellular locations and playing a critical part in the integration of cellular activities. In particular, knockout mice for gelsolin, Wiskott-Aldrich syndrome protein (WASP), and vasodilator-stimulated phosphoprotein (VASP) have been useful to elucidate the important role of cytoskeletal proteins in platelet signaling (Table 3).

Gelsolin. Gelsolin is a 82-kDa actin-binding protein with potent actin filament severing activity in vitro. Gelsolin-null mice are viable and develop normally but their platelet shape change is impaired, which results in a prolonged bleeding time (Witke et al. 1995). On a CRP-coated surface, gelsolin expression is required for the extension of platelet lamellae but not for the formation of filopodia (Falet et al. 2000).

WASP. Wiskott-Aldrich syndrome (WAS) is a human X-linked immunodeficiency associated with a bleeding disorder, thrombocytopenia and small platelets. It arises from mutations in a gene encoding a cytoplasmic protein (WASP) implicated in regulating the actin cytoskeleton. WASP serves as an adapter protein which is recruited to submembrane sites containing actin. Here it activates CDC42 or Rac and in turn recruits signaling molecules, some of which are involved in actin polymerization. WASP-deficient mice have reduced numbers of peripheral blood lymphocytes and platelets and develop chronic colitis (Snapper et al. 1998). However, unlike in WASP-deficient patients, the decrease in platelet count is modest and is not associated with a reduced platelet size or bleeding diathesis.

VASP and cGMP Kinase I. Vasodilator-stimulated phosphoprotein (VASP) is associated with focal adhesions, cell–cell contacts, microfilaments and highly dynamic membrane regions, and is a substrate for cAMP- and cGMP-dependent protein kinases. VASP is expressed in most cell types and at particularly high levels in human platelets, where it is thought to be involved in actin filament formation and integrin $\alpha_{IIb}\beta_3$ inhibition. VASP-deficient mice exhibit hyperplasia of the megakaryocytes in bone marrow and spleen, although platelet numbers are normal (Hauser et al. 1999). These mice also display some defects of cAMP- and cGMP-mediated inhibition of platelet aggregation, suggesting that VASP is a negative modulator of platelet and integrin $\alpha_{IIb}\beta_3$ activation (Aszodi et al. 1999; Hauser et al. 1999). VASP is the only well-established substrate of cGMP kinase I and platelets from mice lacking cGMP kinase I display defective phosphorylation of VASP. This is associated with increased in vivo platelet adhesion and aggregation in a mouse model of ischemia/reperfusion of the intestinal microcirculation, with no compensatory effect of platelet cAMP kinase (Massberg et al. 1999).

2.6
Megakaryopoiesis

Platelets are fragmentation products of the cytoplasm of mature megakaryocytes generated in the bone marrow. Mature megakaryocytes develop from pro-

Table 4 Major phenotypes of mice deficient in megakaryopoiesis-related genes

Protein family	Disrupted gene	Phenotype	Reference(s)
Hormone	Thrombopoietin (TPO)	85% decrease in megakaryocyte and platelet number, modestly prolonged bleeding time	de Sauvage et al. 1996
Receptor	c-mpl	85% decrease in megakaryocyte and platelet number, modestly prolonged bleeding time	Gurney et al. 1994; Alexander et al. 1996
Transcription factor	GATA-1	Lethal	Fujiwara et al. 1996
	Megakaryocyte-targeted GATA-1	Thrombocytopenia, abnormal platelet ultrastructure, defective response to thrombin and ADP, prolonged bleeding time	Shivdasani et al. 1997
	p45 NF-E2	Complete absence of circulating platelets; mice die shortly after birth from extensive hemorrhage	Shivdasani et al. 1995
	Fli-1	Lethal	Hart et al. 2000

genitor cells through various processes including cellular proliferation, endomitosis, and differentiation and finally fragment to ensure platelet production (Table 4). All these events take place predominantly under the control of a hormone called thrombopoietin (TPO).

2.6.1
Thrombopoietin and c-Mpl Receptor

TPO is also known as Mpl ligand or megakaryocyte growth and differentiation factor (MGDF) and is the primary physiological regulator of megakaryocyte platelet production. It is synthesized in the liver and kidneys and its biological functions are mediated by specific binding to a cell surface receptor called c-Mpl, a member of the cytokine receptor superfamily present on platelets, megakaryocytes, and some CD34$^+$ progenitor cells. TPO-deficient mice (de Sauvage et al. 1996) and c-Mpl-deficient mice (Gurney et al. 1994; Alexander et al. 1996) present an almost identical phenotype. Consistent with the fact that TPO is the primary physiological regulator of platelet production in vivo, both knockout strains are severely thrombocytopenic, having only 5%–10% of the platelet numbers present in normal mice (Gurney et al. 1994; Alexander et al. 1996; de Sauvage et al. 1996). There is also an 85% reduction in megakaryocyte counts and a deficit of megakaryocyte progenitor cells (Alexander et al. 1996). Hence, TPO is critical for the maintenance of megakaryocyte numbers through its control of progenitor cell proliferation and maturation. The platelets produced in the absence of TPO signaling are morphologically normal and aggregate normally in response to various agonists. Despite the severely diminished platelet count, the knockout mice do not display spontaneous bleeding and their bleeding time is only mildly prolonged (Bunting et al. 1997). Therefore, although

TPO signaling is the major regulator of megakaryocytopoiesis, important TPO-independent mechanisms must exist in vivo which control residual platelet production in these mice. In addition, the TPO- and c-Mpl-deficient strains exhibit reduced numbers of progenitor cells in all hematopoietic lineages, indicating a central role of TPO signaling in hematopoietic stem cell regulation (Alexander 1999).

2.6.2
Transcription Factors

Megakaryocyte-restricted expression of genes is achieved through use of both lineage-restricted and more widely expressed transcriptional regulators. Particularly important for megakaryocyte differentiation and platelet production are three erythro-megakaryocytic transcriptional regulators, GATA-1, Fli-1, and NF-E2 (Kaluzhny et al. 2001; Shivdasani 2001).

GATA-1. GATA-1 is a specific erythro-megakaryocytic transcription factor and many of the genes selectively expressed in megakaryocytes such as the PF4 (Ravid et al. 1991), GPIIb (Uzan et al. 1991), GPIbα, or GPV genes (Lepage et al. 1999) contain active binding sites for GATA protein in their regulatory regions. Moreover, a naturally occurring mutation in the GATA-1 sequence located within the promoter element of GPIbβ has been described as one of the causes of macro thrombocytopenia (Freson et al. 2001), pointing to a major role of GATA-1 in thrombopoiesis. Since GATA-1 disruption is lethal in mice (Fujiwara et al. 1996), mice lacking GATA-1 selectively in megakaryocytes have been generated (Shivdasani et al. 1997). These mice present abnormally abundant and immature megakaryocytes accompanied by marked thrombocytopenia (Shivdasani et al. 1997). The platelets are enlarged, spherical, and ultrastructurally abnormal and display defective activation in response to thrombin or ADP and adrenaline (Vyas et al. 1999), while the bleeding time is prolonged compared to that of wild-type mice. Thus, GATA-1 function is not necessary for megakaryocytic lineage commitment but is critical for a proper balance between cell proliferation, death, and differentiation during megakaryopoiesis and for normal completion of the maturation process.

p45 NF-E2. p45 NF-E2 heterodimerizes with p18 to form the hematopoietic transcription factor NF-E2. A number of genes exclusively expressed in megakaryocytes such as the GPIIb, PF4, and GPIX genes contain binding sites for NF-E2, which would suggest that this transcription factor is involved in lineage development. This has now been confirmed by a study of NF-E2-deficient mice (Shivdasani et al. 1995). These mice display impaired megakaryopoiesis with a complete absence of circulating platelets and consequently a high mortality of the homozygous animals through hemorrhage (Shivdasani et al. 1995). Megakaryocytes are present in the spleen and bone marrow of the mutant mice, but the majority of these cells appear larger than control megakaryocytes and display severely impaired cytoplasmic maturation. NF-E2 is therefore not required for lineage commitment and megakaryopoiesis proceeds normally in the early phases. However, this transcription factor is necessary in the late stages of differentiation for proper final maturation and release of circulating platelets.

Ets Family. Although a number of transcription factors belonging to the Ets family including Ets-1, Fli-1 and PU.1 are expressed in megakaryocytes, to date only Fli-1 appears to play an important role in megakaryopoiesis. Fli-1-deficient mouse fetuses die at mid-gestation, principally as a result of aberrations of vascular development (Hart et al. 2000), while megakaryocytes derived from fetal liver and cultured in vitro display severely impaired cytoplasmic maturation. In contrast, PU.1-deficient mice failed to reveal defects of megakaryopoiesis or platelet production (Scott et al. 1994). Ets-1 is involved in positive regulation of the PF4 gene (Minami et al. 1998) and in activation of the Mpl receptor gene by TPO in megakaryocytes.

3
Concluding Remarks

The blood platelets of transgenic mice have been studied not only to explore hemostasis and thrombosis but also for purposes of general biochemistry and molecular biology. This explains why such a broad range of targeted genes lead to platelet dysfunction and not all are relevant for pharmacological objectives in terms of antiplatelet drug research. Most of the critical observations relating to hemostasis and thrombosis have confirmed previous knowledge of the roles of specific receptors or transduction proteins. However, these transgenic mice have greatly improved our general understanding of platelet physiology and represent convenient models for preclinical pharmacology and basic science. Future perspectives include the oncoming technology of tissue-restricted and/or inducible gene deletion, which will of course avoid the problems of lethality and those of compensatory mechanisms which can mask gene functions. Finally, tissue-targeted knock-in will further extend the transgenic strategies.

Acknowledgements. The authors would like to thank J.N. Mulvihill for reviewing the English of this chapter and EFS-Alsace, INSERM, ARMESA, and Fondation de France for continuous support.

References

Alexander WS (1999) Thrombopoietin and the c-Mpl receptor: insights from gene targeting. Int J Biochem Cell Biol 31:1027–1035
Alexander WS, Roberts AW, Nicola NA, Li R, Metcalf D (1996) Deficiencies in progenitor cells of multiple hematopoietic lineages and defective megakaryocytopoiesis in mice lacking the thrombopoietic receptor c-Mpl. Blood 87:2162–2170

Altman JD, Trendelenburg AU, MacMillan L, Bernstein D, Limbird L, Starke K, Kobilka BK, Hein L (1999) Abnormal regulation of the sympathetic nervous system in alpha2A- adrenergic receptor knockout mice. Mol Pharmacol 56:154–161

André P, Prasad KS, Denis CV, He M, Papalia JM, Hynes RO, Phillips DR, Wagner DD (2002) CD40L stabilizes arterial thrombi by a beta3 integrin–dependent mechanism. Nat Med 8:247–252

Ashby B (1994) Interactions among prostaglandin receptors. Receptor 4:31–42

Aszodi A, Pfeifer A, Ahmad M, Glauner M, Zhou XH, Ny L, Andersson KE, Kehrel B, Offermanns S, Fassler R (1999) The vasodilator-stimulated phosphoprotein (VASP) is involved in cGMP- and cAMP-mediated inhibition of agonist-induced platelet aggregation, but is dispensable for smooth muscle function. Embo J 18:37–48

Bauer M, Maschberger P, Quek L, Briddon SJ, Dash D, Weiss M, Watson SP, Siess W (2001) Genetic and pharmacological analyses of involvement of Src-family, Syk and Btk tyrosine kinases in platelet shape change. Src-kinases mediate integrin alphaIIb beta3 inside-out signalling during shape change. Thromb Haemost 85:331–340

Bauer M, Retzer M, Wilde JI, Maschberger P, Essler M, Aepfelbacher M, Watson SP, Siess W (1999) Dichotomous regulation of myosin phosphorylation and shape change by Rho-kinase and calcium in intact human platelets. Blood 94:1665–1672

Bernard J, Caen J, Nurden A, Tobelem G, Jeanneau C (1975) [Platelet membrane glycoprotein defect, molecular basis for the abnormal adhesion of platelets to the subendothelium in thrombocytic hemorrhagic dystrophy]. C R Acad Sci Hebd Seances Acad Sci D 280:2517–2520

Brass LF, Molino M (1997) Protease-activated G protein-coupled receptors on human platelets and endothelial cells. Thromb Haemost 78:234–241

Bunting S, Widmer R, Lipari T, Rangell L, Steinmetz H, Carver-Moore K, Moore MW, Keller GA, de Sauvage FJ (1997) Normal platelets and megakaryocytes are produced in vivo in the absence of thrombopoietin. Blood 90:3423–3429

Cattaneo M (2002) Congenital disorders of platelet secretion. In: Gresele P (ed) Platelets in thrombotic and non-thrombotic disorders. Cambridge University Press, Cambridge, U.K., pp 655–673

Cattaneo M, Lecchi A, Randi AM, McGregor JL, Mannucci PM (1992) Identification of a new congenital defect of platelet function characterized by severe impairment of platelet responses to adenosine diphosphate. Blood 80:2787–2796

Cheng AM, Rowley B, Pao W, Hayday A, Bolen JB, Pawson T (1995) Syk tyrosine kinase required for mouse viability and B-cell development. Nature 378:303–306

Clements JL, Lee JR, Gross B, Yang B, Olson JD, Sandra A, Watson SP, Lentz SR, Koretzky GA (1999) Fetal hemorrhage and platelet dysfunction in SLP-76-deficient mice. J Clin Invest 103:19–25

Clemetson KJ, Clemetson JM (2001) Platelet collagen receptors. Thromb Haemost 86:189–197

Coller BS (2001) Anti-GPIIb/IIIa drugs: current strategies and future directions. Thromb Haemost 86:427–443

Connolly AJ, Ishihara H, Kahn ML, Farese RV, Jr., Coughlin SR (1996) Role of the thrombin receptor in development and evidence for a second receptor. Nature 381:516–519

Coughlin SR (1999a) How the protease thrombin talks to cells. Proc Natl Acad Sci U S A 96:11023–11027

Coughlin SR (1999b) Protease-activated receptors and platelet function. Thromb Haemost 82:353–356

de la Salle C, Lanza F, Cazenave JP (1995) Biochemical and molecular basis of Bernard-Soulier syndrome: a review. Nouv Rev Fr Hematol 37:215–222

de Sauvage FJ, Carver-Moore K, Luoh SM, Ryan A, Dowd M, Eaton DL, Moore MW (1996) Physiological regulation of early and late stages of megakaryocytopoiesis by thrombopoietin. J Exp Med 183:651–656

Denis C, Methia N, Frenette PS, Rayburn H, Ullman-Cullere M, Hynes RO, Wagner DD (1998) A mouse model of severe von Willebrand disease: defects in hemostasis and thrombosis. Proc Natl Acad Sci U S A 95:9524–9529

Dent J, Kato K, Peng XR, Martinez C, Cattaneo M, Poujol C, Nurden P, Nurden A, Trimble WS, Ware J (2002) A prototypic platelet septin and its participation in secretion. Proc Natl Acad Sci U S A 99:3064–3069

Doi Y, Itoh M, Yonemura S, Ishihara S, Takano H, Noda T, Tsukita S (1999) Normal development of mice and unimpaired cell adhesion/cell motility/actin-based cytoskeleton without compensatory up-regulation of ezrin or radixin in moesin gene knockout. J Biol Chem 274:2315–2321

Ellmeier W, Jung S, Sunshine MJ, Hatam F, Xu Y, Baltimore D, Mano H, Littman DR (2000) Severe B cell deficiency in mice lacking the tec kinase family members Tec and Btk. J Exp Med 192:1611–1624

Enjyoji K, Sevigny J, Lin Y, Frenette PS, Christie PD, Esch JS, 2nd, Imai M, Edelberg JM, Rayburn H, Lech M, Beeler DL, Csizmadia E, Wagner DD, Robson SC, Rosenberg RD (1999) Targeted disruption of cd39/ATP diphosphohydrolase results in disordered hemostasis and thromboregulation. Nat Med 5:1010–1017

Ezumi Y, Shindoh K, Tsuji M, Takayama H (1998) Physical and functional association of the Src family kinases Fyn and Lyn with the collagen receptor glycoprotein VI-Fc receptor gamma chain complex on human platelets. J Exp Med 188:267–276

Fabre JE, Nguyen M, Athirakul K, Coggins K, McNeish JD, Austin S, Parise LK, FitzGerald GA, Coffman TM, Koller BH (2001) Activation of the murine EP3 receptor for PGE2 inhibits cAMP production and promotes platelet aggregation. J Clin Invest 107:603–610

Fabre JE, Nguyen M, Latour A, Keifer JA, Audoly LP, Coffman TM, Koller BH (1999) Decreased platelet aggregation, increased bleeding time and resistance to thromboembolism in P2Y1-deficient mice. Nat Med 5:1199–1202

Falet H, Barkalow KL, Pivniouk VI, Barnes MJ, Geha RS, Hartwig JH (2000) Roles of SLP-76, phosphoinositide 3-kinase, and gelsolin in the platelet shape changes initiated by the collagen receptor GPVI/FcR gamma-chain complex. Blood 96:3786–3792

Fiorica-Howells E, Hen R, Gingrich J, Li Z, Gershon MD (2002) 5-HT(2A) receptors: location and functional analysis in intestines of wild-type and 5-HT(2A) knockout mice. Am J Physiol Gastrointest Liver Physiol 282: G877–893

Foster CJ, Prosser DM, Agans JM, Zhai Y, Smith MD, Lachowicz JE, Zhang FL, Gustafson E, Monsma FJ, Jr., Wiekowski MT, Abbondanzo SJ, Cook DN, Bayne ML, Lira SA, Chintala MS (2001) Molecular identification and characterization of the platelet ADP receptor targeted by thienopyridine antithrombotic drugs. J Clin Invest 107:1591–1598

Freson K, Devriendt K, Matthijs G, Van Hoof A, De Vos R, Thys C, Minner K, Hoylaerts MF, Vermylen J, Van Geet C (2001) Platelet characteristics in patients with X-linked macrothrombocytopenia because of a novel GATA1 mutation. Blood 98:85–92

Fujiwara Y, Browne CP, Cunniff K, Goff SC, Orkin SH (1996) Arrested development of embryonic red cell precursors in mouse embryos lacking transcription factor GATA-1. Proc Natl Acad Sci U S A 93:12355–12358

Furie B, Furie BC, Flaumenhaft R (2001) A journey with platelet P-selectin: the molecular basis of granule secretion, signalling and cell adhesion. Thromb Haemost 86:214–221

Gaarder A, Jonsen J, Laland S, Hellem A, Owren PA (1961) Adenosine diphosphate in red cells as a factor in the adhesiveness of human blood platelets. Nature 192:531–532

Gabbeta J, Yang X, Kowalska MA, Sun L, Dhanasekaran N, Rao AK (1997) Platelet signal transduction defect with Galpha subunit dysfunction and diminished Galphaq in a patient with abnormal platelet responses. Proc Natl Acad Sci U S A 94:8750–8755

Gachet C (2001) ADP receptors of platelets and their inhibition. Thromb Haemost 86:222–232

Gu JL, Muller S, Mancino V, Offermanns S, Simon MI (2002) Interaction of G alpha(12) with G alpha(13) and G alpha(q) signaling pathways. Proc Natl Acad Sci U S A 99:9352–9357

Gurney AL, Carver-Moore K, de Sauvage FJ, Moore MW (1994) Thrombocytopenia in c-mpl-deficient mice. Science 265:1445–1447

Habib A, FitzGerald GA, Maclouf J (1999) Phosphorylation of the thromboxane receptor alpha, the predominant isoform expressed in human platelets. J Biol Chem 274:2645–2651

Hart A, Melet F, Grossfeld P, Chien K, Jones C, Tunnacliffe A, Favier R, Bernstein A (2000) Fli-1 is required for murine vascular and megakaryocytic development and is hemizygously deleted in patients with thrombocytopenia. Immunity 13:167–177

Hartwell DW, Mayadas TN, Berger G, Frenette PS, Rayburn H, Hynes RO, Wagner DD (1998) Role of P-selectin cytoplasmic domain in granular targeting in vivo and in early inflammatory responses. J Cell Biol 143:1129–1141

Hartwell DW, Wagner DD (1999) New discoveries with mice mutant in endothelial and platelet selectins. Thromb Haemost 82:850–857

Hauser W, Knobeloch KP, Eigenthaler M, Gambaryan S, Krenn V, Geiger J, Glazova M, Rohde E, Horak I, Walter U, Zimmer M (1999) Megakaryocyte hyperplasia and enhanced agonist-induced platelet activation in vasodilator-stimulated phosphoprotein knockout mice. Proc Natl Acad Sci U S A 96:8120–8125

Hechler B, Leon C, Vial C, Vigne P, Frelin C, Cazenave JP, Gachet C (1998) The P2Y1 receptor is necessary for adenosine 5'-diphosphate-induced platelet aggregation. Blood 92:152–159

Hechler B, Lenain N, Marchese P, Vial C, Heim V, Freund M, Cazenave JP, Cattaneo M, Ruggeri ZM, Evans R, Gachet C (2003) A role of the fast ATP-gated P2X1 cation cannel in thrombosis of small arteries in vivo. J Exp Med (in press)

Hechler B, Zhang Y, Eckly A, Cazenave JP, Gachet C, Ravid K (2003) Lineage specific overexpression of the P2Y1 receptor induces platelet hyperreactivity in transgenic mice. JTH 1: 155–163

Hirsch E, Bosco O, Tropel P, Laffargue M, Calvez R, Altruda F, Wymann M, Montrucchio G (2001) Resistance to thromboembolism in PI3Kgamma-deficient mice. Faseb J 15:2019–2021

Hodivala-Dilke KM, McHugh KP, Tsakiris DA, Rayburn H, Crowley D, Ullman-Cullere M, Ross FP, Coller BS, Teitelbaum S, Hynes RO (1999) Beta3-integrin-deficient mice are a model for Glanzmann thrombasthenia showing placental defects and reduced survival. J Clin Invest 103:229–238

Hollopeter G, Jantzen HM, Vincent D, Li G, England L, Ramakrishnan V, Yang RB, Nurden P, Nurden A, Julius D, Conley PB (2001) Identification of the platelet ADP receptor targeted by antithrombotic drugs. Nature 409:202–207

Holmback K, Danton MJ, Suh TT, Daugherty CC, Degen JL (1996) Impaired platelet aggregation and sustained bleeding in mice lacking the fibrinogen motif bound by integrin alpha IIb beta 3. Embo J 15:5760–5771

Holtkötter O, Nieswandt B, Smyth N, Muller W, Hafner M, Schulte V, Krieg T, Eckes B (2002) Integrin alpha 2-deficient mice develop normally, are fertile, but display partially defective platelet interaction with collagen. J Biol Chem 277:10789–10794

Ishihara H, Connolly AJ, Zeng D, Kahn ML, Zheng YW, Timmons C, Tram T, Coughlin SR (1997) Protease-activated receptor 3 is a second thrombin receptor in humans. Nature 386:502–506

Jantzen HM, Milstone DS, Gousset L, Conley PB, Mortensen RM (2001) Impaired activation of murine platelets lacking G alpha(i2). J Clin Invest 108:477–483

Jones KL, Hughan SC, Dopheide SM, Farndale RW, Jackson SP, Jackson DE (2001) Platelet endothelial cell adhesion molecule-1 is a negative regulator of platelet-collagen interactions. Blood 98:1456–1463

Kable JW, Murrin LC, Bylund DB (2000) In vivo gene modification elucidates subtype-specific functions of alpha(2)-adrenergic receptors. J Pharmacol Exp Ther 293:1-7

Kahn ML, Diacovo TG, Bainton DF, Lanza F, Trejo J, Coughlin SR (1999) Glycoprotein V-deficient platelets have undiminished thrombin responsiveness and Do not exhibit a Bernard-Soulier phenotype. Blood 94:4112–4121

Kahn ML, Zheng YW, Huang W, Bigornia V, Zeng D, Moff S, Farese RV, Jr., Tam C, Coughlin SR (1998) A dual thrombin receptor system for platelet activation. Nature 394:690–694

Kaluzhny Y, Poncz M, Ravid K (2001) Transcription factors in lineage-specific gene expression during megakaryopoiesis. In: Ravid K, Licht J (eds) Transcription factors: Normal and malignant develpment of blood cells. Wiley-Liss, New-York, pp 31–49

Kanaji T, Russell S, Ware J (2002) Amelioration of the macrothrombocytopenia associated with the murine Bernard-Soulier syndrome. Blood 100:2102–2107

Kato K, Kanaji T, Russell S, Kunicki TJ, Furihata K, Kanaji S, Marchese P, Reininger A, Ruggeri ZM, Ware J (2003) The contribution of glycoprotein VI to stable adhesion and thrombus formation illustrated by targeted gene deletion. Blood (online ahead of publication)

Kehrel B, Balleisen L, Kokott R, Mesters R, Stenzinger W, Clemetson KJ, van de Loo J (1988) Deficiency of intact thrombospondin and membrane glycoprotein Ia in platelets with defective collagen-induced aggregation and spontaneous loss of disorder. Blood 71:1074–1078

Kelleher KL, Matthaei KI, Hendry IA (2001) Targeted disruption of the mouse Gz-alpha gene: a role for Gz in platelet function? Thromb Haemost 85:529–532

Klages B, Brandt U, Simon MI, Schultz G, Offermanns S (1999) Activation of G12/G13 results in shape change and Rho/Rho-kinase- mediated myosin light chain phosphorylation in mouse platelets. J Cell Biol 144:745–754

Lanza F, Beretz A, Stierle A, Hanau D, Kubina M, Cazenave JP (1988) Epinephrine potentiates human platelet activation but is not an aggregating agent. Am J Physiol 255: H1276–1288

Law DA, Nannizzi-Alaimo L, Ministri K, Hughes PE, Forsyth J, Turner M, Shattil SJ, Ginsberg MH, Tybulewicz VL, Phillips DR (1999) Genetic and pharmacological analyses of Syk function in alphaIIbbeta3 signaling in platelets. Blood 93:2645–2652

Le Naour F, Rubinstein E, Jasmin C, Prenant M, Boucheix C (2000) Severely reduced female fertility in CD9-deficient mice. Science 287:319–321

Ledent C, Vaugeois JM, Schiffmann SN, Pedrazzini T, El Yacoubi M, Vanderhaeghen JJ, Costentin J, Heath JK, Vassart G, Parmentier M (1997) Aggressiveness, hypoalgesia and high blood pressure in mice lacking the adenosine A2a receptor. Nature 388:674–678

Lenain N, Freund M, Léon C, Cazenave JP, Gachet C (2003) Inhibition of localized thrombosis in P2Y1-deficient mice and in rodents treated with MRS2179, a P2Y1 receptor antagonist. The Journal of Thrombosis and Haemostasis 1:1144–1149

Léon C, Freund M, Ravanat C, Baurand A, Cazenave JP, Gachet C (2001) Key role of the P2Y(1) receptor in tissue factor-induced thrombin- dependent acute thromboembolism: studies in P2Y(1)-knockout mice and mice treated with a P2Y(1) antagonist. Circulation 103:718–723

Léon C, Hechler B, Freund M, Eckly A, Vial C, Ohlmann P, Dierich A, LeMeur M, Cazenave JP, Gachet C (1999) Defective platelet aggregation and increased resistance to thrombosis in purinergic P2Y(1) receptor-null mice. J Clin Invest 104:1731–1737

Léon C, Hechler B, Vial C, Leray C, Cazenave JP, Gachet C (1997) The P2Y1 receptor is an ADP receptor antagonized by ATP and expressed in platelets and megakaryoblastic cells. FEBS Lett 403:26–30

Lepage A, Uzan G, Touche N, Morales M, Cazenave JP, Lanza F, de La Salle C (1999) Functional characterization of the human platelet glycoprotein V gene promoter: A specific marker of late megakaryocytic differentiation. Blood 94:3366–3380

Lopez JA, Andrews RK, Afshar-Kharghan V, Berndt MC (1998) Bernard-Soulier syndrome. Blood 91:4397–4418

Ma H, Hara A, Xiao CY, Okada Y, Takahata O, Nakaya K, Sugimoto Y, Ichikawa A, Narumiya S, Ushikubi F (2001) Increased bleeding tendency and decreased susceptibility to thromboembolism in mice lacking the prostaglandin E receptor subtype EP(3). Circulation 104:1176–1180

MacKenzie AB, Mahaut-Smith MP, Sage SO (1996) Activation of receptor-operated cation channels via P2X1 not P2T purinoceptors in human platelets. J Biol Chem 271:2879–2881

Mahaut-Smith MP, Ennion SJ, Rolf MG, Evans RJ (2000) ADP is not an agonist at P2X(1) receptors: evidence for separate receptors stimulated by ATP and ADP on human platelets. Br J Pharmacol 131:108–114

Mangin P, Nonne C, Eckly A, Ohlmann P, Freund M, Nieswandt B, Cazenave JP, Gachet C, Lanza F (2003) A PLCgamma2-independent platelet collagen aggregation requiring functional association of GPVI and integrin alpha2beta1. FEBS Letters 542:53–59

Marcus AJ, Broekman MJ, Drosopoulos JH, Pinsky DJ, Islam N, Maliszewsk CR (2001) Inhibition of platelet recruitment by endothelial cell CD39/ecto- ADPase: significance for occlusive vascular diseases. Ital Heart J 2:824–830

Massberg S, Brand K, Gruner S, Page S, Muller E, Muller I, Bergmeier W, Richter T, Lorenz M, Konrad I, Nieswandt B, Gawaz M (2002) A critical role of platelet adhesion in the initiation of atherosclerotic lesion formation. J Exp Med 196:887–896

Massberg S, Sausbier M, Klatt P, Bauer M, Pfeifer A, Siess W, Fassler R, Ruth P, Krombach F, Hofmann F (1999) Increased adhesion and aggregation of platelets lacking cyclic guanosine 3',5'-monophosphate kinase I. J Exp Med 189:1255–1264

Matsuoka T, Hirata M, Tanaka H, Takahashi Y, Murata T, Kabashima K, Sugimoto Y, Kobayashi T, Ushikubi F, Aze Y, Eguchi N, Urade Y, Yoshida N, Kimura K, Mizoguchi A, Honda Y, Nagai H, Narumiya S (2000) Prostaglandin D2 as a mediator of allergic asthma. Science 287:2013–2017

McKenzie SE, Taylor SM, Malladi P, Yuhan H, Cassel DL, Chien P, Schwartz E, Schreiber AD, Surrey S, Reilly MP (1999) The role of the human Fc receptor Fc gamma RIIA in the immune clearance of platelets: a transgenic mouse model. J Immunol 162:4311–4318

Methia N, Andre P, Denis CV, Economopoulos M, Wagner DD (2001) Localized reduction of atherosclerosis in von Willebrand factor- deficient mice. Blood 98:1424–1428

Minami T, Tachibana K, Imanishi T, Doi T (1998) Both Ets-1 and GATA-1 are essential for positive regulation of platelet factor 4 gene expression. Eur J Biochem 258:879–889

Monkley SJ, Zhou XH, Kinston SJ, Giblett SM, Hemmings L, Priddle H, Brown JE, Pritchard CA, Critchley DR, Fassler R (2000) Disruption of the talin gene arrests mouse development at the gastrulation stage. Dev Dyn 219:560–574

Moog S, Mangin P, Lenain N, Strassel C, Ravanat C, Schuhler S, Freund M, Santer M, Kahn M, Nieswandt B, Gachet C, Cazenave JP, Lanza F (2001) Platelet glycoprotein V binds to collagen and participates in platelet adhesion and aggregation. Blood 98:1038–1046

Moroi M, Jung SM, Okuma M, Shinmyozu K (1989) A patient with platelets deficient in glycoprotein VI that lack both collagen-induced aggregation and adhesion. J Clin Invest 84:1440–1445

Mulryan K, Gitterman DP, Lewis CJ, Vial C, Leckie BJ, Cobb AL, Brown JE, Conley EC, Buell G, Pritchard CA, Evans RJ (2000) Reduced vas deferens contraction and male infertility in mice lacking P2X1 receptors. Nature 403:86–89

Muraille E, Pesesse X, Kuntz C, Erneux C (1999) Distribution of the src-homology-2-domain-containing inositol 5- phosphatase SHIP-2 in both non-haemopoietic and haemopoietic cells and possible involvement of SHIP-2 in negative signalling of B-cells. Biochem J 342 Pt 3:697–705

Murata T, Ushikubi F, Matsuoka T, Hirata M, Yamasaki A, Sugimoto Y, Ichikawa A, Aze Y, Tanaka T, Yoshida N, Ueno A, Oh-ishi S, Narumiya S (1997) Altered pain perception and inflammatory response in mice lacking prostacyclin receptor. Nature 388:678–682

Nakanishi-Matsui M, Zheng YW, Sulciner DJ, Weiss EJ, Ludeman MJ, Coughlin SR (2000) PAR3 is a cofactor for PAR4 activation by thrombin. Nature 404:609–613

Narumiya S, FitzGerald GA (2001) Genetic and pharmacological analysis of prostanoid receptor function. J Clin Invest 108:25–30

Ni H, Denis CV, Subbarao S, Degen JL, Sato TN, Hynes RO, Wagner DD (2000) Persistence of platelet thrombus formation in arterioles of mice lacking both von Willebrand factor and fibrinogen. J Clin Invest 106:385–392

Ni H, Ramakrishnan V, Ruggeri ZM, Papalia JM, Phillips DR, Wagner DD (2001) Increased thrombogenesis and embolus formation in mice lacking glycoprotein V. Blood 98:368–373

Nieswandt B, Brakebusch C, Bergmeier W, Schulte V, Bouvard D, Mokhtari-Nejad R, Lindhout T, Heemskerk JW, Zirngibl H, Fassler R (2001a) Glycoprotein VI but not alpha2beta1 integrin is essential for platelet interaction with collagen. Embo J 20:2120–2130

Nieswandt B, Schulte V, Bergmeier W, Mokhtari-Nejad R, Rackebrandt K, Cazenave JP, Ohlmann P, Gachet C, Zirngibl H (2001b) Long-term antithrombotic protection by in vivo depletion of platelet glycoprotein VI in mice. J Exp Med 193:459–469

Nieswandt B, Schulte V, Zywietz A, Gratacap MP, Offermanns S (2002) Costimulation of Gi- and G12/G13-mediated Signaling Pathways Induces Integrin alpha IIbbeta 3 Activation in Platelets. J Biol Chem 277:39493–39498

Nieuwenhuis HK, Akkerman JW, Houdijk WP, Sixma JJ (1985) Human blood platelets showing no response to collagen fail to express surface glycoprotein Ia. Nature 318:470–472

Nieuwenhuis HK, Akkerman JW, Sixma JJ (1987) Patients with a prolonged bleeding time and normal aggregation tests may have storage pool deficiency: studies on one hundred six patients. Blood 70:620–623

Nurden AT, Caen JP (1974) An abnormal platelet glycoprotein pattern in three cases of Glanzmann's thrombasthenia. Br J Haematol 28:253–260

Nurden AT, Caen JP (1975) Specific roles for platelet surface glycoproteins in platelet function. Nature 255:720–722

Nurden P, Savi P, Heilmann E, Bihour C, Herbert JM, Maffrand JP, Nurden A (1995) An inherited bleeding disorder linked to a defective interaction between ADP and its receptor on platelets. Its influence on glycoprotein IIb-IIIa complex function. J Clin Invest 95:1612–1622

Offermanns S (2000) The role of heterotrimeric G proteins in platelet activation. Biol Chem 381:389–396

Offermanns S, Hashimoto K, Watanabe M, Sun W, Kurihara H, Thompson RF, Inoue Y, Kano M, Simon MI (1997a) Impaired motor coordination and persistent multiple climbing fiber innervation of cerebellar Purkinje cells in mice lacking Galphaq. Proc Natl Acad Sci U S A 94:14089–14094

Offermanns S, Toombs CF, Hu YH, Simon MI (1997b) Defective platelet activation in G alpha(q)-deficient mice. Nature 389:183–186

Olah ME, Stiles GL (1995) Adenosine receptor subtypes: characterization and therapeutic regulation. Annu Rev Pharmacol Toxicol 35:581–606

Parise LV (1999) Integrin alpha(IIb)beta(3) signaling in platelet adhesion and aggregation. Curr Opin Cell Biol 11:597–601

Pasquet JM, Gross B, Quek L, Asazuma N, Zhang W, Sommers CL, Schweighoffer E, Tybulewicz V, Judd B, Lee JR, Koretzky G, Love PE, Samelson LE, Watson SP (1999) LAT is required for tyrosine phosphorylation of phospholipase cgamma2 and platelet activation by the collagen receptor GPVI. Mol Cell Biol 19:8326–8334

Pasquet JM, Quek L, Stevens C, Bobe R, Huber M, Duronio V, Krystal G, Watson SP (2000) Phosphatidylinositol 3,4,5-trisphosphate regulates Ca(2+) entry via btk in platelets and megakaryocytes without increasing phospholipase C activity. Embo J 19:2793–2802

Patil S, Newman DK, Newman PJ (2001) Platelet endothelial cell adhesion molecule-1 serves as an inhibitory receptor that modulates platelet responses to collagen. Blood 97:1727–1732

Paul BZ, Daniel JL, Kunapuli SP (1999) Platelet shape change is mediated by both calcium-dependent and—independent signaling pathways. Role of p160 Rho-associated coiled-coil- containing protein kinase in platelet shape change. J Biol Chem 274:28293–28300

Plow EF, Ploplis VA, Busuttil S, Carmeliet P, Collen D (1999) A role of plasminogen in atherosclerosis and restenosis models in mice. Thromb Haemost 82 Suppl 1:4-7

Poole A, Gibbins JM, Turner M, van Vugt MJ, van de Winkel JG, Saito T, Tybulewicz VL, Watson SP (1997) The Fc receptor gamma-chain and the tyrosine kinase Syk are essential for activation of mouse platelets by collagen. Embo J 16:2333–2341

Poujol C, Ware J, Nieswandt B, Nurden AT, Nurden P (2002) Absence of GPIbalpha is responsible for aberrant membrane development during megakaryocyte maturation. Ultrastructural study using a transgenic model. Exp Hematol 30:352–360

Quek LS, Bolen J, Watson SP (1998) A role for Bruton's tyrosine kinase (Btk) in platelet activation by collagen. Curr Biol 8:1137–1140

Quek LS, Pasquet JM, Hers I, Cornall R, Knight G, Barnes M, Hibbs ML, Dunn AR, Lowell CA, Watson SP (2000) Fyn and Lyn phosphorylate the Fc receptor gamma chain downstream of glycoprotein VI in murine platelets, and Lyn regulates a novel feedback pathway. Blood 96:4246–4253

Ralevic V, Burnstock G (1998) Receptors for purines and pyrimidines. Pharmacol Rev 50:413–492

Ramakrishnan V, Reeves PS, DeGuzman F, Deshpande U, Ministri-Madrid K, DuBridge RB, Phillips DR (1999) Increased thrombin responsiveness in platelets from mice lacking glycoprotein V. Proc Natl Acad Sci U S A 96:13336–13341

Ravid K, Doi T, Beeler DL, Kuter DJ, Rosenberg RD (1991) Transcriptional regulation of the rat platelet factor 4 gene: interaction between an enhancer/silencer domain and the GATA site. Mol Cell Biol 11:6116–6127

Rivera J, Lozano ML, Corral J, Gonzalez-Conejero R, Martinez C, Vicente V (2000) Platelet GP Ib/IX/V complex: physiological role. J Physiol Biochem 56:355–365

Robson SC, Kaczmarek E, Siegel JB, Candinas D, Koziak K, Millan M, Hancock WW, Bach FH (1997) Loss of ATP diphosphohydrolase activity with endothelial cell activation. J Exp Med 185:153–163

Sambrano GR, Weiss EJ, Zheng YW, Huang W, Coughlin SR (2001) Role of thrombin signalling in platelets in haemostasis and thrombosis. Nature 413:74–78

Savage B, Cattaneo M, Ruggeri ZM (2001) Mechanisms of platelet aggregation. Curr Opin Hematol 8:270–276

Saxton TM, Henkemeyer M, Gasca S, Shen R, Rossi DJ, Shalaby F, Feng GS, Pawson T (1997) Abnormal mesoderm patterning in mouse embryos mutant for the SH2 tyrosine phosphatase Shp-2. Embo J 16:2352–2364

Scott EW, Simon MC, Anastasi J, Singh H (1994) Requirement of transcription factor PU.1 in the development of multiple hematopoietic lineages. Science 265:1573–1577

Shi ZT, Afzal V, Coller B, Patel D, Chasis JA, Parra M, Lee G, Paszty C, Stevens M, Walensky L, Peters LL, Mohandas N, Rubin E, Conboy JG (1999) Protein 4.1R-deficient mice are viable but have erythroid membrane skeleton abnormalities. J Clin Invest 103:331–340

Shivdasani RA (2001) Molecular and transcriptional regulation of megakaryocyte differentiation. Stem Cells 19:397–407

Shivdasani RA, Fujiwara Y, McDevitt MA, Orkin SH (1997) A lineage-selective knockout establishes the critical role of transcription factor GATA-1 in megakaryocyte growth and platelet development. Embo J 16:3965–3973

Shivdasani RA, Rosenblatt MF, Zucker-Franklin D, Jackson CW, Hunt P, Saris CJ, Orkin SH (1995) Transcription factor NF-E2 is required for platelet formation independent of the actions of thrombopoietin/MGDF in megakaryocyte development. Cell 81:695–704

Shultz LD, Schweitzer PA, Rajan TV, Yi T, Ihle JN, Matthews RJ, Thomas ML, Beier DR (1993) Mutations at the murine motheaten locus are within the hematopoietic cell protein-tyrosine phosphatase (Hcph) gene. Cell 73:1445–1454

Siess W (1989) Molecular mechanisms of platelet activation. Physiol Rev 69:58–178

Smyth SS, Reis ED, Vaananen H, Zhang W, Coller BS (2001a) Variable protection of beta 3-integrin–deficient mice from thrombosis initiated by different mechanisms. Blood 98:1055–1062

Smyth SS, Reis ED, Zhang W, Fallon JT, Gordon RE, Coller BS (2001b) Beta(3)-integrin-deficient mice but not P-selectin-deficient mice develop intimal hyperplasia after vascular injury: correlation with leukocyte recruitment to adherent platelets 1 hour after injury. Circulation 103:2501–2507

Snapper SB, Rosen FS, Mizoguchi E, Cohen P, Khan W, Liu CH, Hagemann TL, Kwan SP, Ferrini R, Davidson L, Bhan AK, Alt FW (1998) Wiskott-Aldrich syndrome protein-deficient mice reveal a role for WASP in T but not B cell activation. Immunity 9:81–91

Subramaniam M, Frenette PS, Saffaripour S, Johnson RC, Hynes RO, Wagner DD (1996) Defects in hemostasis in P-selectin-deficient mice. Blood 87:1238–1242

Sugiyama T, Okuma M, Ushikubi F, Kanaji K, Sensaki S, Uchino H, Hattori A, Ihzumi T (1986) [Studies on platelets in a patient with a novel hereditary platelet function disorder–impaired aggregation in response to A 23187 with normal response to arachidonic acid]. Rinsho Ketsueki 27:1834–1842

Suh TT, Holmback K, Jensen NJ, Daugherty CC, Small K, Simon DI, Potter S, Degen JL (1995) Resolution of spontaneous bleeding events but failure of pregnancy in fibrinogen-deficient mice. Genes Dev 9:2020–2033

Thomas DW, Mannon RB, Mannon PJ, Latour A, Oliver JA, Hoffman M, Smithies O, Koller BH, Coffman TM (1998) Coagulation defects and altered hemodynamic responses in mice lacking receptors for thromboxane A2. J Clin Invest 102:1994–2001

Tronik-Le Roux D, Roullot V, Poujol C, Kortulewski T, Nurden P, Marguerie G (2000) Thrombasthenic mice generated by replacement of the integrin alpha(IIb) gene: demonstration that transcriptional activation of this megakaryocytic locus precedes lineage commitment. Blood 96:1399–1408

Tronik-Le Roux D, Roullot V, Schweitzer A, Berthier R, Marguerie G (1995) Suppression of erythro-megakaryocytopoiesis and the induction of reversible thrombocytopenia in mice transgenic for the thymidine kinase gene targeted by the platelet glycoprotein alpha IIb promoter. J Exp Med 181:2141–2151

Trumel C, Payrastre B, Plantavid M, Hechler B, Viala C, Presek P, Martinson EA, Cazenave JP, Chap H, Gachet C (1999) A key role of adenosine diphosphate in the irreversible platelet aggregation induced by the PAR1-activating peptide through the late activation of phosphoinositide 3-kinase. Blood 94:4156–4165

Turner M, Mee PJ, Costello PS, Williams O, Price AA, Duddy LP, Furlong MT, Geahlen RL, Tybulewicz VL (1995) Perinatal lethality and blocked B-cell development in mice lacking the tyrosine kinase Syk. Nature 378:298–302

Uzan G, Prenant M, Prandini MH, Martin F, Marguerie G (1991) Tissue-specific expression of the platelet GPIIb gene. J Biol Chem 266:8932–8939

Van Geet C, Freson K, Devos R, Vermylen J (2002) Platelets in thrombotic and non-thrombotic disorders. In: Gresele P (ed) Platelets in thrombotic and non-thrombotic disorders. Cambridge University Press, Cambridge, U.K., pp 515–527

Vollmar B, Schmits R, Kunz D, Menger MD (2001) Lack of in vivo function of CD31 in vascular thrombosis. Thromb Haemost 85:160–164

Vyas P, Ault K, Jackson CW, Orkin SH, Shivdasani RA (1999) Consequences of GATA-1 deficiency in megakaryocytes and platelets. Blood 93:2867–2875

Wang D, Feng J, Wen R, Marine JC, Sangster MY, Parganas E, Hoffmeyer A, Jackson CW, Cleveland JL, Murray PJ, Ihle JN (2000) Phospholipase Cgamma2 is essential in the functions of B cell and several Fc receptors. Immunity 13:25–35

Ware J, Russell S, Ruggeri ZM (2000) Generation and rescue of a murine model of platelet dysfunction: the Bernard-Soulier syndrome. Proc Natl Acad Sci U S A 97:2803–2808

Watanabe N, Nakajima H, Suzuki H, Oda A, Matsubara Y, Moroi M, Terauchi Y, Kadowaki T, Suzuki H, Koyasu S, Ikeda Y, Handa M (2003) Functional phenotyp of phospho-inositide 3-kinase p85alpha null platelets characterized by an impaired response to GPVI stimulation. Blood (online ahead of publication)

Watson SP, Asazuma N, Atkinson B, Berlanga O, Best D, Bobe R, Jarvis G, Marshall S, Snell D, Stafford M, Tulasne D, Wilde J, Wonerow P, Frampton J (2001) The role of ITAM- and ITIM-coupled receptors in platelet activation by collagen. Thromb Haemost 86:276–288

Weiss EJ, Hamilton JR, Lease KE, Coughlin SR (2002) Protection against thrombosis in mice lacking PAR3. Blood 100:3240–3244

Witke W, Sharpe AH, Hartwig JH, Azuma T, Stossel TP, Kwiatkowski DJ (1995) Hemostatic, inflammatory, and fibroblast responses are blunted in mice lacking gelsolin. Cell 81:41–51

Witke W, Sutherland JD, Sharpe A, Arai M, Kwiatkowski DJ (2001) Profilin I is essential for cell survival and cell division in early mouse development. Proc Natl Acad Sci U S A 98:3832–3836

Xiao Q, Danton MJ, Witte DP, Kowala MC, Valentine MT, Degen JL (1998) Fibrinogen deficiency is compatible with the development of atherosclerosis in mice. J Clin Invest 101:1184–1194

Xu W, Baribault H, Adamson ED (1998) Vinculin knockout results in heart and brain defects during embryonic development. Development 125:327–337

Yang J, Wu J, Kowalska MA, Dalvi A, Prevost N, O'Brien PJ, Manning D, Poncz M, Lucki I, Blendy JA, Brass LF (2000) Loss of signaling through the G protein, Gz, results in abnormal platelet activation and altered responses to psychoactive drugs. Proc Natl Acad Sci U S A 97:9984–9989

Yu S, Yu D, Lee E, Eckhaus M, Lee R, Corria Z, Accili D, Westphal H, Weinstein LS (1998) Variable and tissue-specific hormone resistance in heterotrimeric Gs protein alpha-subunit (Gsalpha) knockout mice is due to tissue-specific imprinting of the gsalpha gene. Proc Natl Acad Sci U S A 95:8715–8720

Zhang FL, Luo L, Gustafson E, Lachowicz J, Smith M, Qiao X, Liu YH, Chen G, Pramanik B, Laz TM, Palmer K, Bayne M, Monsma FJ, Jr. (2001) ADP is the cognate ligand for the orphan G protein-coupled receptor SP1999. J Biol Chem 276:8608–8615

Zimmermann H (2000) Extracellular metabolism of ATP and other nucleotides. Naunyn Schmiedebergs Arch Pharmacol 362:299–309

Chemokine Receptors

G. Bernhardt · O. Pabst · H. Herbrand · R. Förster

Institute of Immunology, Hannover Medical School,
Feodor-Lynen-Str. 21, 30625 Hannover, Germany
-mail: Foerster.Reinhold@MH-Hannover.de

Abstract The past decade has witnessed a breakthrough in our understanding of one of the most puzzling phenomena of immunology: leukocyte homeostasis and homing. Being very similar in their underlying concepts, both processes rely on identical mechanisms, i.e. the induction and control of the migration of immune-competent cells via the chemokine/chemokine receptor system. According to their basic function, chemokines fall into one of two groups: inflammatory and homeostatic. The former are implicated in processes of inflammation whereas the latter contribute in large part to the maintenance of the lymphocyte pool. However, there is no absolute discrimination between these two branches as reflected by the intimate links between inflammatory and immunoregulatory pathways in order to perform proper immunological responses. Insights into the function of the chemokine network were brought about by studying mice deficient for distinct chemokine receptors. Such a strategy turned out to be indispensable when analysing an intricate balance as seen in lymphocyte homeostasis/migration, but it experienced some difficulties when targeting chemokine receptors of the inflammatory branch. This is due to the functional reliability-born-by-redundancy inherent in this system and may be cured by the analysis of double-knockout animals. In addition, the mice deficient for diverse chemokine receptors provided the basis for model systems for the study of autoimmune diseases and transplant rejection. These aspects as well as the aforementioned regulation of lymphocyte homeostasis and migration will be discussed in this review.

Keywords Chemokine · Chemokine receptor · Lymphocyte migration · Autoimmune disease · Allograft tolerance · Knockout mouse · Disease model · Haematopoietic cell

1
Overview

The aim of this review is to describe the biological functions of chemokine receptors based on the data obtained from gene-targeted mice. We will first give a brief overview on chemokines and their receptors followed by a summary of the key information about each receptor as far as data derived from gene-targeted mice are concerned.

1.1
Chemokines and Their Receptors

Chemokines constitute a family of chemotaxis-inducing peptides composed of 70–130 amino acids. They are produced by a plethora of cells including epithelial cells, endothelial cells, other tissue cells and immune cells. Chemokines share four conserved cysteine residues forming two distinct disulphide bonds. CC and CXC chemokines are classified based on the position of the first two conserved cysteine residues which are either adjacent (CCL) or separated by a single amino acid (CXCL). Thus far, 28 members of the CC and 16 members of the CXC chemokine family have been identified. In addition to these chemokines, two chemokines have been identified possessing only two (instead of four) cysteines (XCL), whereas another chemokine is characterized by three amino acids between the first two cysteines (CX$_3$CL) (for reviews see: Baggiolini et al. 1997; Rollins 1997; Murphy et al. 2000). Sequence analysis revealed that chemokines encompass a short amino-terminal domain, a β-strand-based backbone, connecting loops between the second and the forth cysteine and a carboxy-terminal α-helix. Initially, chemokines were identified by their ability to attract inflammatory cells such as neutrophils, monocytes and eosinophils to places of inflammation and infection. Secretion of CXCL8 and a variety of other chemokines are induced by microbial toxins and inflammatory cytokines. Consequently, these chemokines are referred to as inflammatory chemokines.

In addition, some chemokines could be identified within secondary lymphoid organs, being constitutively expressed (rather than being induced during inflammatory processes). More recent work has demonstrated that these chemokines regulate homeostatic lymphocyte trafficking to and from lymphoid compartments. The chemokines CCL17-22, CCL25, CCL27, CCL28, CXCL12 and CXCL13 each participate in these processes (Cyster 1999) and are now generally addressed as homeostatic chemokines, whereas all others are regarded to represent inflammatory chemokines. Chemokines act on target cells via seven-transmembrane spanning receptors coupled to Pertussis toxin-sensitive G proteins. Eleven receptors for CC chemokines, six for CXC chemokines and one each binding CX3C and XC chemokines have been identified so far. As outlined in Table 1 most of the chemokine receptors bind more than one chemokine and several chemokines bind to more than one receptor, suggesting a high degree of redundancy and versatility. The redundancy is particularly apparent in the inflammatory branch of the chemokine system with different chemokines acting on the same receptor. In contrast, several one-ligand-to-one-receptor interactions exist in the homeostatic chemokine branch, and it is thus not surprising that gene targeting of these members in mice revealed fundamental functions of the homeostatic chemokines in lymphocyte trafficking and immune surveillance. Table 1 summarizes the chemokine receptors identified so far, their ligands, the receptor-expressing cell type, their allocation to the inflammatory or homeostatic branch of the chemokine system and the most important publications describing the phenotype of gene-targeted mice.

1.2
Chemokines and Leukocyte Migration

The capacity of immune cells to recirculate through almost all compartments of the body represents an essential feature of immune surveillance and requires the ability of these cells to leave and re-enter the vasculature continuously. Leukocyte migration has been intensely studied on high endothelium venules (HEV) of secondary lymphoid organs. These vessels are characterized by a single layer of cubic endothelial cells decorated with several chemokines and adhesion molecules facilitating lymphocyte entry to lymphoid organs. The binding of leukocytes to endothelial cells occurs as a complex process. Based on early experimental data, a multistep model of leukocyte adhesion and transendothe-

Table 1 Chemokine receptors and their ligands. Receptors are listed with regard to their homeostatic (H) or inflammatory (I) function

Receptor	H/I	Ligand(s)	Receptor-expressing cell type	Reference(s) describing gene knock-out
CCR1	I	CCL3, CCL5, CCL7, CCL8, CCL13, CCL14, CCL15, CCL23	Mo, iDC, T, Neu, Eo, mesangial cell, platelet	Gao et al. 1997; Gerard et al. 1997
CCR2	I	CCL2, CCL7, CCL8, CCL13	Mo, iDC, Ba, T, Nk, endothelium, fibroblast	Boring et al. 1997; Kurihara et al. 1997; Kuziel et al. 1997
CCR3	I	CCL5, CCL7, CCL8, CCL11,CCL13, CCL14, CCL15, CCL24, CCL26	Eo, Ba, Th2, iDC, platelet	Humbles et al. 2002; Ma et al. 2002
CCR4	H	CCL17, CCL22	iDC, Ba, Th2, platelet	Chvatchko et al. 2000; Reiss et al. 2001
CCR5	i	CCL3, CCL4, CCL5, CCL8, CCL11, CCL13, CCL14	Th1, iDC, mDC, Mo, Nk, thymocyte	Zhou et al. 1998; Nansen et al. 2000; Tran et al. 2000
CCR6	H	CCL20	iDC, B, T, LC	Cook et al. 2000; Lukacs et al. 2001; Varona et al. 2001
CCR7	H	CCL19, CCL21	Naïve T cell, central memory T cell, B, mDC	Förster et al. 1999; Reif et al. 2002
CCR8	I	CCL1, CCL16	Mo, B, T, thymocyte	Chensue et al. 2001
CCR9	H	CCL25	T, thymocyte	Wurbel et al. 2001; Uehara et al. 2002
CCR10	H	CCL27, CCL28	T, melanocyte, endothelial cell, fibroblast, LC	n.d.
CCR11*	H	CCL19, CCL21, CCL25	Astrocyte	n.d.
CXCR1	I	CXCL5, CXCL6, CXCL8	Neu, Mo, astrocyte, endothelium	n.d.
CXCR2	I	CXCL1, CXCL2, CXCL3, CXCL5, CXCL7, CXCL8	Neu, Mo, astrocyte, endothelium	Cacalano et al. 1994; Godaly et al. 2000;
CXCR3	I	CXCL9, CXCL10, CXCL11	Th1, B, mesangial cell	Del Rio et al. 2001; Tateda et al. 2001
CXCR4	H	CXCL12	Mo, iDC, mDC, Neu, T, B, platelet astrocyte	Hancock et al. 2000; Ma et al. 1998; Tachibana et al. 1998; Zou et al. 1998
CXCR5	H	CXCL13	B, astrocyte, follicular Th	Förster et al. 1999; Ansel et al. 2000; Reif et al. 2002
CXCR6	I	CXCL16	Th1	n.d.
CX3CR1	I	XCL1, XCL2	T	Haskell et al. 2001
XCR1	I	CX3L1	Astrocyte, NK, T	n.d.

B, B cell; Ba, basophil; Eo, eosinophil; iDC, immature dendritic cell; LC, Langerhans cell; mDC, mature dendritic cell; Mo, monocyte; n.d., not determined; Neu, neutrophil; Nk, natural killer cell; T, T cell; Th, T helper cell.   * See footnote in text under the heading "CCR11".

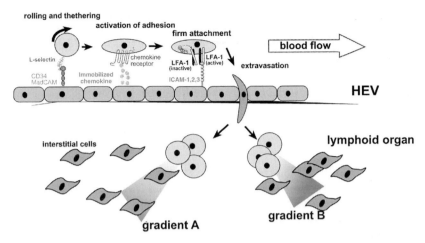

Fig. 1 Proposed model of lymphocyte extravasation. Selectin receptors bind carbohydrate counter-structures expressed on leukocytes permitting low-affinity interactions and rolling of the endothelial cells. Chemokines immobilized to the luminal side of the endothelium bind to and activate chemokine receptors, which transmit signals most likely initiating a conformational change and activation of integrins. Activated integrins now bind with high affinity to adhesion molecules expressed on the endothelium (such as ICAM-1) resulting in extravasation. Once lymphocytes have entered the lymphoid organ, they follow a hierarchy of chemokine gradients which guide them into functional microanatomical compartments. (Modified model initially proposed by Butcher 1991; Lawrence et al. 1991; Springer 1994)

lial migration was proposed shortly after the first chemokine receptors had been identified (Butcher 1991; Lawrence et al. 1991; Springer 1994). In an initial step, leukocytes tether to and roll along the endothelium of the vessel wall by the interaction of selectins with their counter receptors. In the particular case of lymphocytes entering lymphoid organs through HEV, this binding is facilitated between lymphocyte-expressed L-selectin and endothelial CD34 or MAdCAM (Fig. 1). Firm binding subsequently involves another set of adhesion molecules, lymphocytic integrins (such as LFA-1) and intracellular adhesion molecules (ICAMs). However, such firm binding will not occur unless the lymphocyte-borne integrins are converted into a binding-competent conformational stage. The signal required to initiate this event is provided by active G proteins released by chemokine receptors which in turn were induced by binding to their respective chemokines. Therefore, only the presence of chemokines trapped at the luminal surface of the endothelial cells, is capable of triggering the extravasation program of lymphoid cells consisting not only of tight lymphocyte/endothelial interaction but also providing the stimuli for the extensive cell reshaping occurring during transmigration. Once the cells have entered a lymphoid organ, they become exposed to new chemokine gradients, which are responsible for the segregation of B and T cells into their characteristic compartments, i.e. the lymphoid follicles and the T cell zones (Fig. 1). Although less intensively studied, it is believed that similar mechanisms regulate leukocyte extravasation during inflammatory processes. However, in contrast to the situation described for HEV, most of the chemokines and adhesion molecules have to be induced on the endothelium by inflammatory stimuli.

2
The Biological Consequences of Chemokine Receptor Deficiency

2.1
Introductory Remarks

A plethora of literature exists describing the expression of chemokine receptors on cell types or tissues. In part the presented data are conflicting. Care should be taken in two respects. Was the corresponding receptor detectable as protein using a specific antibody or was the evidence based on RNA data? In the case of the latter, it should be rated less reliable. Second, differences may also relate to expression profiles varying between species. Here we concentrate on conclusions drawn from mouse data and to a lesser extent from human data. A similar scenario holds true for the question regarding whether a distinct chemokine is indeed a ligand for a receptor. Mere binding studies, even if correlated signalling events were evidenced in heterologous expression systems, may not translate to the correct in vivo situation. Therefore, it is difficult to reconcile some contradictory data, and everybody who is interested in a particular receptor/ligand interaction must critically evaluate the literature. Another source of confusion so far has been the baptizing of chemokines and their receptors, which followed no uniform guidelines. In this review, we will refer to the recent renaming published by the IUIS/WHO Nomenclature Committee (2001).

Before starting detailed descriptions of each particular receptor, it is necessary to briefly discuss the combined expression of several chemokine receptors on distinct cell types, which helped us to understand basic mechanisms of their regulation and trafficking. Chemokine receptor expression profiles became landmarks of cell subtype assignments, and newly emerging concepts such as the diversification of memory T cells imposed problems on well-established ideas like the T helper (Th)1/Th2-paradigm. Accumulating data demonstrate that blood phagocytes express a limited set of chemokine receptors, whereas T lymphocytes express a wide array of these receptors, depending on their developmental as well as their activation stage. Monocytes are distinguished by CCR1, CCR2 and CCR5 expression, eosinophils characteristically express CCR1 and CCR3, which are also found on basophils (in addition to CCR2). Immature dendritic cells competent to migrate into inflamed tissue express CCR1, CCR2 and CCR5. Upon maturation these receptors are replaced by CCR4 and CCR7, enabling the immigration into the draining lymph nodes.

We first will describe the chemokine receptors which are of importance for the efferent pathway, i.e. those directing expressing cells to sites of inflammations: CCR1, CCR2, CCR3, CCR4, CCR5, CCR8 and CXCR3 (Kaplan 2001). These are also called the inflammatory chemokine receptors in contrast to the homeostatic or afferent chemokine receptors listed below (Moser et al. 2001). The latter names were coined to emphasize the role of these receptors in maintenance and homing of immunocompetent cells. Since the functions of the chemokine receptors providing the basis for such a classification are not defined in all details, and some receptors fulfil tasks belonging in either category, such listings are subject to some arbitrary decisions. Consequently, this should be interpreted as a guideline rather than a fixed concept.

2.2
The Inflammatory Chemokine Receptors

For the study of receptor functions, the generation and characterization of knockout mice was indispensable and will therefore constitute the backbone of the information given here. However, inactivation of chemokine receptors of the inflammatory type in many instances showed no apparent phenotype. These observations suggested a widespread redundancy in this class of chemokine receptors that might be caused by the overlapping binding profiles of chemokines as well as receptors [no less than nine chemokines were reported to bind to CCR1 or CCR3 (Baggiolini 2001)]. Therefore, a distinct phenotype could frequently be made visible upon provocation only, by confronting the knockout mice with pathogenic or allergic challenges. Largely, such experimental setups were chosen to mirror certain autoimmune or allergic diseases. For this reason, animal models for these malfunctions will be of considerable interest here.

2.2.1
CCR1: Th1/Th2; Neutrophils

CCR1 belongs to those chemokine receptors with an apparent binding capacity for a variety of chemokines (see Table 1). CCR1 was found to be expressed on myeloid progenitor cells ($CD34^+$), a finding in line with the observation that mice deficient for CCR1 fail to mobilize these cells from bone marrow in response to lipopolysaccharide (LPS) (Gao et al. 1997). The steady-state level of myeloid progenitors in femur is normal but found to be decreased in spleen and blood. Despite receptor/ligand redundancy, mature neutrophils obtained from peripheral blood of knockout animals failed to chemotax towards CCL3. Therefore, knockout mice displayed an accelerated mortality upon *Aspergillus fumigatus* infections (Gao et al. 1997). This infection is controlled predominantly by neutrophils which block tissue invasion of the pathogen from blood yet cannot prevent inflammation once penetration occurred. Granuloma formation in the lung induced by *Schistosoma mansoni* infection is greatly reduced in knockout animals. Remarkably, the cells of these granulomas differ in neither type nor relative percentage between knockout and wild-type littermates (Gao et al. 1997), rendering it less likely that this phenotype is caused by the selective lack of a CCR1-mediated chemotactic function. Lung lymph-node cells deficient for CCR1, challenged with a *Schistosoma* antigen, produce more interferon (IFN)-γ

and less interleukin (IL)-4 compared to wild-type cells, strengthening earlier reports that type 1 cytokines like IFN-γ inhibit, while those of type 2 (IL-4) promote, granuloma formation. Gerard et al. (1997) tested their knockout mice in a model for human adult respiratory distress syndrome. In wild-type mice, infiltration/inflammation of the lung was brought about by leukocytes activated in the course of an acute pancreatitis. Inflammation of the lung is paralleled by increased tumour necrosis factor (TNF)-α levels in the bronchoalveolar lavage fluid (BAL). The CCR1 deficiency protected these animals from lung injury. At the same time, the TNF-α levels in the BALs of knockout mice remained unchanged, although the mutant mice also suffered from pancreatitis.

While being a poor agonist for murine CCR1, CCL5 strongly activates human CCR1 even though the binding affinities are comparable in both systems. On the other hand, CCL3 is a potent activator of both human and murine CCR1, for example in inducing Ca-influx, yet CCL3 does not chemoattract human neutrophils (in contrast to mouse neutrophils) which were reported to score negative for CCR1 expression (Su et al. 1996). Apparently, species differences are profound regarding CCR1 and its ligands. It was speculated that in mouse neutrophils CCR1 compensates for the lack of CXCR1, which is of primordial importance in recruiting human neutrophils. Therefore, animal models may be of only limited use when asking for potential pharmaceutical strategies affecting CCR1 function in human disease.

2.2.2
CCR2: Th1 Bias; Monocyte/Macrophage; Multiple Sclerosis; Rheumatoid Arthritis; Atherosclerosis

From the earlier studies it was known that CCL2, one of the CCR2 ligands, attracts monocytes, which suggested an assignment of this chemokine receptor in inflammation resulting in a Th1-dominated response. Three groups established in 1997 knockout mouse lines. Kuziel et al. tested rolling/adhesion of leukocytes to microvessels and found that the number of firmly adherent leukocytes to CCL2-treated venules was markedly reduced in knockout mice, whereas rolling was unaffected. Concomitantly the number of emigrated cells was also reduced (Kuziel et al. 1997). An i.p. injection of thioglycollate, mimicking in its outcome an acute peritonitis, usually results in an elevated level of peritoneal macrophages. In knockout animals this level was found to be decreased, indicating that CCR2 is an important determinant of macrophage infiltration into the peritoneal cavity. These observations were confirmed by Kurihara et al. (1997) and Boring et al. (1997). The latter group also studied the effect of injecting *Mycobacterium bovis* antigen, which provoked a lung inflammation/granuloma formation and initiated a typical Th1 cytokine profile. Wild-type but not knockout mice developed a monocytosis, and cells derived from the draining lymph nodes of knockout mice did not respond with an increased IFN-γ production upon exposure to *M. bovis* antigen (as seen in wild-type animals). In continuation of this work, evidence was presented that this phenomenon is caused by an impaired migration of monocytes/macrophages into the inflamed tissue and, later on, of the antigen-presenting cells (APCs) to the draining lymph nodes such that an appropriate T cell stimulation does not take place (Peters et al. 2000). A different picture emerged when CCR2-deficient mice were treated with dextran sodium sulphate causing a colitis (initiating a Th1-type response in wild-type animals). The intestinal mucosa of both wild-type and knockout mice contained equal densities of infiltrating macrophages (and CD4$^+$ T cells). As above, however, decreased IFN-γ levels but elevated amounts of IL-10 were monitored, giving rise to the speculation that in this scenario the immune response shifted partially from a Th1 to a more Th2 type. This shift may also be responsible for the less severe clinical course of colitis in the CCR2-deficient mice (Andres et al. 2000) by attenuating the inflammatory functions of the attracted macrophages. The CCR2-deficient mice were also used to study the role of this chemokine receptor in the migration/differentiation of Langerhans cells (Sato et al. 2000). Although the number of skin-resident Langerhans cells lacking CCR2 was indistinguishable from that observed in wild-type animals, their migration to draining lymph nodes was impaired (not observed for CCR5-deficient Langerhans cells). It is well known that an infection with *Leishmania major* provokes a Th1-like response in C57/BL6 but a Th2-dominated answer in BALB/C mice. Only the former strain is capable of clearing the infection by expanding IFN-γ- and IL-12-producing T cells. Substantially decreased numbers of CD8α^+ dendritic cells (DCs) were observed in the spleens of C57/BL6, CCR2-null mice. Upon infection with *L. major*, splenic CD8α^+-DCs failed to migrate to the T cell areas. Strikingly, CD8α^+-DCs are thought to direct contacting T cells towards a Th1 differentiation pathway. These findings may explain why C57/BL6 mice deficient for CCR2 (but not for CCR5) develop a Th2-biased response resembling the non-healing phenotype seen in BALB/C (Sato et al. 2000). This picture is complemented by the observation of (1) increased levels of CXCL13, the B cell attractant, in the lymph nodes of infected C57/BL6, CCR2-null mice, and (2) a prominent B cell proliferation in these lymph nodes. Moreover, a massive neutrophil infiltration into the site of inflammation occurred in infected C57/BL6, CCR2-null mice as well as BALB/C but not wild-type C57/BL6 animals.

2.2.3
CCR3: Th2 Bias; Eosinophil; Ulcerative Colitis

One of the many CCR3 ligands, CCL11, was reported to be of particular importance in regulating homing of eosinophils to tissues (Matthews et al. 1998). Accordingly, CCR3-deficient mice were found to possess reduced levels of eosinophils in the small intestine but heavily increased eosinophil numbers in the spleen (lung and thymus content remained unchanged) (Humbles et al. 2002). Mice were sensitized/immunized i.p. with OVA (ovalbumin) and subsequently challenged with an OVA-containing aerosol. In addition, an airway hyperresponsiveness can be elicited in the animals upon inhalation of methacholine, mimicking bronchoconstriction in allergic asthma. Although resembling asthma in its clinical manifestations, the entire setup does not represent an appropriate model for this human disease (Gerard et al. 2001) which is characterized by monocytes, eosinophils and mast cells infiltrating the inflamed lung tissue. When studying airway inflammation, it should also be kept in mind that in humans two arterial systems maintain the blood flow in the lung, with the pulmonary system supplying the parenchyma, and the bronchial circulation delivering blood to the airways (D'Ambrosio et al. 2001). The latter system does not exist in mice. CCR3 deficiency resulted in decreased levels of lung-infiltrating eosinophils compared to wild-type, although the blood eosinophil count is equally elevated in wild-type and knockout mice (Humbles et al. 2002), suggesting a defect in eosinophil recruitment to the lung. Eosinophils lacking CCR3 adhered and transmigrated through the lung vessels but could not enter the parenchyma, indicating that CCR3 is not required for extravasation but for further migration into the tissue. Surprisingly, knockout mice overreacted in the hyperresponsiveness assay in what might be explained by the dramatically increased number in infiltrating intraepithelial mast cells. In striking contrast, the same mice did not develop a methacholine-induced hyperreactivity at all when the OVA-sensitization step was performed epicutaneously (Ma et al. 2002), correlating with a barely increased mast cell colonization of the lung. Eosinophil recruitment into the lung following challenge was almost absent in this model. The epicutaneous sensitization route seemed to favour a Th2 helper profile (identical in knockout and wild-type) as evidenced by IL-4 and IL-5 production of challenged splenocytes, whereas peritoneal administration corresponded to a response characterized by more Th1-like features. Another interesting yet unexplained observation was made when analyzing the skin of CCR3-deficient mice, revealing that skin homing of eosinophils is absent in knockout animals in either case, untreated and antigen sensitized.

2.2.4
CCR4: Th2 Bias; T Memory Skin Homing

Despite that CCR4 has been known for a while, it has proved to be difficult to elucidate its function. In addition, reports describing the expression profile of CCR4 were remarkably contradictory. Expectedly, the splenocytes of CCR4-deficient mice did not chemotax towards CCL17 or CCL22 (Chvatchko et al. 2000). Unexpectedly, however, these cells did not react to CCL3 either, suggesting that CCL3 is a physiological ligand for CCR4 in this context. It remains to be determined why CCR1 and CCR5—being expressed on splenocytes and known to be functional CCL3 receptors—did not elicit chemotaxis (Chvatchko et al. 2000). Even though not in accordance with the given evidence, it should be considered whether CCR4-deficient splenocytes may have evolved secondary defects due to the knockout, thereby preventing migration and explaining these surprising findings. The CCR4-deficient mice were analysed following the ovalbumin sensitizing/challenging protocol described above (ovalbumin given intraperitoneally) but CCR4-specific effects could not be detected. In light of the current knowledge, the observation that the knockout mice were significantly protected against an LPS-induced endotoxic shock remains unexplained. In contrast to wild-type littermates, macrophages producing TNF-α and IL-1β mediating the shock syndrome were not retained in the peritoneal cavity (place of LPS administration) of knockout animals (Chvatchko et al. 2000). In another set of experiments, the CCR4-deficient mice were sensitized and challenged epicutaneously with 2,4-dinitrofluorobenzene (skin painting with 2,4-DNFB). Wild-type and knockout animals displayed no differences in their immunological responses. In particular, homing of Th2 cells to skin was equally efficient (Reiss et al. 2001). Since it was evident by then that CCR4 might be involved in the specific homing of skin memory T cells, this observation was puzzling. However, a concomitant antibody-mediated block of CCL27 prevented recruitment of CCR4-deficient T cells to the skin, suggesting that either receptor CCR4 or CCR10 (the CCL27 receptor) confers homing capacity to the T cells. A detailed analysis of human haematopoietic cells using newly generated antibodies confirmed the expression of CCR4 on skin-homing memory T cells (CLA$^+$, CD45RA$^-$) whereas those positive for the integrin $\alpha_4\beta_7$ distinguishing gut homing T memory cells, are virtually devoid of CCR4 (Andrew et al. 2001). Likewise, CCR4 was not found to be expressed on B cells, eosinophils, basophils or NK cells. In thymus, CD3$^+$CD4$^+$CD8$^-$CCR9$^+$ cells express CCR4. CCR4 downregulation may render them competent to exit the thymus as naïve CD45RA$^+$ peripheral blood cells (Andrew et al. 2001). An interesting finding relates to the observation that a T memory subpopulation in the blood co-expresses CXCR3, CCR5 (classical Th1 cell marker) and CCR4 (a typical Th2-associated marker), suggesting that the current model of Th1/Th2 generation may prove insufficient in explaining the existence of distinct in vivo T cell subsets.

2.2.5
CCR5: Th1 Bias; HIV Receptor

For some good reasons it would have been justified to describe CCR5 along with CCR2 in one subsection. The genes coding CCR2 and CCR5 reside in direct proximity on human chromosome three (mouse chromosome nine) and are highly related to each other in their sequence (Mackay 2001). Evolutionary diversification in function is, however, indicated by different ligand usage as well as by different susceptibilities of the corresponding knockout mice towards several immunological challenges. This is illustrated by the example of mice lacking either CCR2 or CCR5 in an infection with a mouse-adapted strain of influenza virus. Whereas CCR5-deficient mice displayed an enhanced mortality rate caused by an accelerated macrophage influx into the lung, the CCR2 knockout animals exerted increased survival rates compared to wild-type littermates due to an early block in pulmonary macrophage infiltration (Dawson et al. 2000).

Apparently the highest expression rates for CCR5 are found on peritoneal macrophages. Yet the CCR5-deficient mice exert no defect in macrophage recruitment following a thioglycollate-induced peritonitis or a glucan-induced granuloma formation in lung or liver (Zhou et al. 1998). CCR5 deficiency resulted in a slightly impaired capacity to clear an infection with *Listeria monocytogenes* but caused an enhanced humoral response to T cell-dependent antigenic challenges, suggesting a function of CCR5 in negatively regulating a T cell-dependent response (Zhou et al. 1998). Given the prominent role assigned to CCR5 by the mere fact that it is, along with CXCR3, a resident marker of Th1 cells and immature DCs, its lack results in surprisingly mild aberrations upon immunological provocations [see also experimental autoimmune encephalomyelitis (EAE), a model for multiple sclerosis (Tran et al. 2000) or lymphocytic choriomeningitis virus (LCMV) infection (Nansen et al. 2002)]. This may not be unexpected, however, considering the observation that humans deficient for CCR5 are perfectly healthy. Probably this naturally occurring genotype would have escaped detection if it had not correlated with an unexpected phenotype. A small but noticeable percentage of Caucasians are protected from infection by HIV because they harbour defective copies of the CCR5 gene in their genome (a 32-bp deletion) rendering the corresponding protein non-functional. Although not yet of satisfactory statistical relevance, a picture emerges indicating that heterozygous individuals benefit from carrying a defective allele by showing reduced risks of getting asthma, developing a less severe clinical course of rheumatoid arthritis, and developing a later onset of multiple sclerosis and AIDS. Yet these people may pay by being exposed to a higher risk for more severe forms of sarcoidosis and a worsened clinical course after onset of AIDS unless they are homozygous carriers for the mutated CCR5 gene in the latter case.

2.2.6
CCR8: Th2 Bias; Indirect Eosinophilic; Asthma

Similar to CCL3, CCL1 is an effective attractant for mouse but not for human neutrophils, suggesting that a functional diversification between mouse and human CCR8 took place during evolution. Data regarding CCR8 expression are scarce. In mouse thymus, CCR8 expression is first encountered at a CD4⁻CD8⁻ stage. Later, only those thymocytes committed to develop into CD4⁺CD8⁻ cells continue to express CCR8 (Kremer et al. 2001). In the periphery, CCR8 expression was observed on T cells of the Th2 type (Zingoni et al. 1998). Since CCL1 is also acting on monocytes and CCR8 mRNA was found to be expressed by these cells, CCR8/CCL1 may be of importance in monocyte function. This assumption could not be corroborated when analysing mice deficient for CCR8 (Chensue et al. 2001). The results rather suggested an involvement of this receptor in the establishment of a proper Th2 response which was characterized in different disease models by a partial defect in the recruitment of eosinophils (but not lymphocytes and macrophages) to the site of inflammation. This was puzzling since eosinophils themselves do not express CCR8. In an asthma model using cockroach antigen, which is a major cause of asthma in childhood, it was found that the diseased lungs of the knockout animals produced much less IL-4, IL-5 and IL-13 than those of their wild-type littermates. Since there is an already dramatically decreased blood level of eosinophils in the allergic knockout animals, it was assumed that there is an insufficient rate of eosinophil differentiation in the bone marrow due to the decreased level of the eosinophilopoietic cytokine IL-5. The latter finding remained unexplained, since abnormalities in gross lymphocyte recruitment were not detected (Chensue et al. 2001).

2.2.7
CXCR2: Neutrophils; Inflammation, Wound Healing

In contrast to humans with two interleukin-8 (CXCL8) receptors, CXCR1 and CXCR2, only one functional receptor is described in mouse to date that binds to human IL-8 as well as to the mouse chemokines macrophage inflammatory protein (MIP)-2 and KC (Cacalano et al. 1994; Lee et al. 1995). In inflammatory processes, CXCL8 is crucially involved in epithelial–neutrophil interactions, and anti-CXCL8 antibodies have been shown to block neutrophil migration across infected epithelial cell layers in in vitro transwell assays (Godaly et al. 1997). In line with this, administration of the CXCR2 ligand, CXCL1, increased rolling, adhesion and tissue recruitment of CXCR2-expressing neutrophils (Zhang et al. 2001). Interestingly analysis of CXCR2 gene-targeted mice not only revealed a diminished capacity to recruit neutrophils to inflammatory sites, but also identified an expansion of the B cell compartment (Cacalano et al. 1994). Infection of CXCR2-deficient mice revealed an increased susceptibility to uropathogenic strains of *Escherichia coli*. This defect was not due to a failure of neutrophil recruitment to the infected tissue but due to the inability of these cells to cross the epithelial barrier and kill the bacteria. Instead, neutrophils accumulated in large number under the epithelium and eventually filled the tissues surrounding the inflammatory focus (Godaly et al. 2000). Severe defects in correct targeting of neutrophils were also observed after infection of CXCR2-deficient mice with the parasite *Toxoplasma gondii* (Del Rio et al. 2001), in *Legionella pneumoniae*-induced lung infection (Tateda et al. 2001), and in experimental *Staphylococcus aureus*-induced brain abscesses (Kielian et al. 2001). Similarly, an antibody-mediated neutralization of CXCR2 results in increased mortality following *Pseudomonas aeruginosa*-induced pulmonary infection (Tsai et al. 2000) and the development of invasive pulmonary aspergillosis (Mehrad et al. 1999) due to defective neutrophil recruitment. During wound healing, CXCR2 and its ligand CXCL2 are expressed by keratinocytes and endothelial cells at areas where epithelization and neovascularization occur. CXCR2-deficient mice exhibit defective neutrophil recruitment and an altered pattern of monocyte recruitment, resulting in delayed wound healing and decreased neovascularization (Devalaraja et al. 2000). In vitro wounding experiments with cultures of keratinocytes also argue for a role of CXCR2 in epithelial surfacing of keratinocytes

2.2.8
CXCR3: Th1; Allograft Tolerance

CXCR3 is well recognized as a chemokine receptor implicated in the establishment of an immune response governed by Th1 cells. Accordingly, its expression was reported on infiltrating lymphocytes triggering in part the Th1-dominated disease syndromes such as multiple sclerosis, rheumatoid arthritis and atherosclerosis. CXCR3 is expressed widely on memory T cells homing to tissue without a noticeable tendency to mark a distinct subpopulation of these cells, as is observed in the case of CCR4 (skin homing) (Kunkel et al. 2002). CXCR3 is also expressed on a variety of cell types of non-haematopoietic origin (see Table 1). However, CXCR3 elimination did not cause an apparent phenotype in mice, yet its study is promising because it is the major player in transplant rejection, a process ruled by a Th1 immune response. Upon transplantation of an allograft, the host develops an acute rejection several days later. This stage is accompanied by an onset of CXCL10, CXCL11 and CXCL19 synthesis inside the grafted tissue, which causes massive infiltration of CXCR3-expressing Th1 cells, which initiates the destruction of the graft. Although other chemokine receptor deficiencies (CCR1, CCR2, CCR5 and CX3CR1) extended graft survival as well, the most pronounced effect was seen in the CXCR3 knockout mice (Hancock et al. 2000). Here, allograft survival extends from approximately 7 and up to 60 days. In synergy with low doses of cyclosporin A, a drug frequently used in transplant medicine for its useful effect of suppressing T cell function, permanent engraftment is achieved. Even long-term effects of chronic rejection were undetectable. Therefore, instead of broadly inactivating the immune system by application of drugs like cyclosporin A, antagonists specific for CXCR3 may represent promising therapeutical agents. Interestingly, the agonist/antagonist principle is exploited by nature itself. The ligands of CXCR3 function as CCR3 antagonists, thus reinforcing the onset of a Th1 response whilst suppressing a Th2 answer (Loetscher et al. 2001). The CCR3 ligand CCL11 in turn exerts antagonistic effects on CCR2 with the same net effect of amplifying the discrepancies between Th1 and Th2 (Baggiolini 2001). Apparently, many immunological challenges trigger a mixed-type answer at their onset with the propensity towards a Th1 or a Th2 phenotype seen only later. This concept may also help researchers to design strategies to force an autoimmune response in either direction, Th1 or Th2, depending on which one is coupled to a less harmful clinical manifestation. Or seen from a different perspective: A block of a chemokine receptor favouring a Th1 or Th2-like response may result in unwanted amplifications of answers of the other subtype. This scenario was already experienced in some instances when analysing the knockout animals (see above).

2.2.9
CX3CR1: Brain; Allograft Tolerance

CX$_3$CR1 is the receptor for fractalkine (CX$_3$CL1), a unique chemokine that combines properties of both chemoattractants and adhesion molecules. Structurally, CX$_3$CL1 is characterized by a CX$_3$C spacing of the cysteine motif and the chemokine region located on top of a mucin-like stalk. CX$_3$CL1has been shown to exist as a membrane-bound and a shorter, secreted protein (Bazan et al. 1997). Soluble CX$_3$CL1 has potent chemoattractant activity for CX$_3$CR1-expressing T cells and monocytes (Bazan et al. 1997), whereas the membrane-bound CX$_3$CL1 protein, which is induced on activated endothelial cells, promotes initial capture, firm adhesion and activation of circulating leukocytes (Bazan et al. 1997). CX3CR1 expression is upregulated by proinflammatory cytokines and LPS (Bazan et al. 1997), thus forming part of the inflammatory branch of chemokine receptors. Both receptor and ligand are mainly expressed in the CNS, CX$_3$CL1 in neurons, CX$_3$CR1 in astrocytes and microglia (Nishiyori et al. 1998), as well as in intestinal epithelial cells (Muehlhoefer et al. 2000). Within the CNS, CX$_3$CL1 was shown to induce microglial cell migration and activation (Harrison et al. 1998) and to inhibit Fas-mediated microglial cell death in vitro. Mice deficient for either CX3CR1 (Haskell et al. 2001) or its ligand, CX$_3$CL1 (Cook et al. 2001) do not exhibit any behavioural changes or gross histological abnormalities. Furthermore, they show normal responses to inflammatory stimuli. In detail, CX3CR1-deficient mice exhibit similar injury and proteinuria in induced glomerulonephritis and similar levels of disease in induced autoimmune encephalomyelitis as observed in the wild-type controls. CX3CR1 deficiency revealed a role for this receptor in cardiac allograft rejection. Similar to mice deficient for other chemokine receptors of the inflammatory branch (CCR1, CCR2, CCR5 and CXCR3) immunosuppressed CX3CR1$^{-/-}$ mice show a significantly increased graft survival time from 7 to approximately 29 days following heterotopic cardiac transplantation. This phenotype is in accordance with the observation that CX$_3$CL1 expression is upregulated in inflamed rejected cardiac allografts (Robinson et al. 2000).

2.3
The Homeostatic Chemokine Receptors

As outlined above, mice deficient for inflammatory chemokine receptors frequently showed a distinct phenotype only after immunologic challenges such as exposure to defined allergic or infectious agents, which is most likely due to versatility as well as to some degree of redundancy within the inflammatory part of the chemokine network. In contrast, chemokines that are constitutively expressed in lymphoid organs hardly show any promiscuity with regard to receptor binding, and most of the homeostatic chemokine receptors do not bind more than one or two chemokines. This constitutive expression of chemokines and the low degree of anticipated redundancy seem to explain that mice deficient for homeostatic chemokine receptors showed a disturbed homeostasis of immune cells within the different compartments of the immune system already in its naïve, unchallenged stage.

2.3.1
CCR6: Lung, Intestine; Allergic Infection, Positioning of Dendritic Cells

CCR6 is one of the few chemokine receptors that has only one known ligand, CCL20 (Hieshima et al. 1997; Hromas et al. 1997; Rossi et al. 1997). CCL20 has been identified in tonsillar epithelial crypts (Dieu et al. 1998a), the intestinal epithelium (Tanaka et al. 1999) and the epithelium of the subendothelial dome (SED) of Peyer's patches (Cook et al. 2000). Expression of CCR6 was shown on B cells and memory T cells (Liao et al. 1999) as well as on immature in vitro differentiated DCs (Greaves et al. 1997; Power et al. 1997). This particular expression pattern of CCR6 and its ligand suggested a role in lymphocyte and dendritic cell trafficking, especially in the mucosa-associated immune system.

This anticipated function of CCR6 could be confirmed by gene targeting. CCR6-deficient mice show defects in lymphocyte homing to the intestinal mucosa as evidenced by small Peyer's patches, and increased numbers of intraepithelial lymphocyte (IEL) and lamina propria lymphocyte (LPL) subpopulations. Furthermore, these mice show a defect in the positioning of CD11b$^+$CD11c$^+$ DC to the SED of PP. CCR6-deficient mice show an impaired humoral response to orally administered antigens and rotavirus, whereas they react normally to systemically applied antigen (Cook et al. 2000; Varona et al. 2001). These findings demonstrate that CCR6 is a mucosa-specific regulator of humoral immunity and lymphocyte homeostasis in the small intestine. In addition, in a cockroach antigen model for allergic pulmonary inflammation, CCR6-deficient mice had reduced airway resistance, fewer eosinophils located around the airways, reduced levels of IL-5 in the lung and lower levels of IgE in the serum (Lukacs et al. 2001), suggesting a pivotal role of CCR6 in allergic pulmonary inflammation.

2.3.2
CCR7: Homing of Naïve T Cells and B Cells, Mobilization of Dendritic Cells

CCR7—together with CXCR5, CXCR3, CCR5 and further chemokine receptors—has been identified as a marker that allows the differentiation of functionally diverse subsets of effector and memory T cells. CCR7 is found on T cells, B cells, thymocytes and mature dendritic cells (Schweickart et al. 1994; Burgstahler et al. 1995; Dieu et al. 1998b; Sallusto et al. 1998; Sozzani et al. 1998; Yanagihara et al. 1998). On T cells, CCR7 is highly expressed on the majority of naïve T cells and on a subpopulation of memory T cells, now known as "central memory T cells" (Sallusto et al. 1999). Since the ligands for CCR7, ELC/CCL19 and SLC/CCL21 are both expressed on HEV (in addition to other cells) (Tangemann et al. 1998; Breitfeld et al. 2000), it was likely that the interaction of CCR7 with its ligands is required for effective trans-endothelial migration of CCR7-positive lymphocytes into secondary lymphoid organs. Lymph nodes of CCR7-deficient mice harbour few naïve T cells and DC. In contrast, the T cell population is strongly expanded in the blood, the bone marrow and the splenic red pulp. B cells seem to be chronically activated in these mice and upon activation, Langerhans cells of the skin fail to be mobilized and do not migrate to the draining lymph nodes. Based on these migration defects, it is not surprising that CCR7-deficient mice show delayed antibody response and lack contact sensitivity and delayed-type hypersensitivity reactions. Adoptive transfer experiments to wild-type recipients revealed that the entering of CCR7-deficient B cells and T cells into lymph nodes and Peyer's patches, and of T cells into the splenic periarteriolar lymphoid sheath is profoundly affected. Interestingly, CCR7-deficient B cells rapidly leave the outer T zone of the peri-arteriolar lymphoid sheath (PALS) after adoptive transfer into wild-type recipients, demonstrating that expression of CCR7 allows B cells to stay in close contact with T cells to effectively facilitate T–B cell interactions. Taken together, the disorganized architecture of lymphoid organs, disturbed microarchitecture of secondary lymphoid organs, originated by the ineffective entry and maintenance of lymphocytes and DC, likely explains the observed deficiency of CCR7-deficient mice to rapidly mount an adaptive immune response (Förster et al. 1999). Studies on CCR7-deficient or CXCR5-deficient B cells elucidated the mechanism that controls B cell recirculation from the B cell follicle to the adjacent T-zone during their survey for antigen. The positioning of B cells to the B cell follicle is mediated by the interaction of CXCR5 on B cells with the ligand CXCL13 expressed by stroma cells of the follicle (see also the chapter on CXCR5). However, once B cells get activated by antigen through the B cell receptor they quickly upregulate surface expression of CCR7, which makes them more responsive towards the chemokines CCL19 and CCL21, both of which are strongly expressed within the T cell area. Interestingly, over-expression of CXCR5 on antigen-activated cells is sufficient to counteract the antigen-induced B cell migration to the T cell area (Reif et al. 2002). After being activated by T cells within the outer T cell area, B cells migrate back to the B cell follicle and under certain circumstances start to initiate the germinal centre reaction. Taken together, these findings define the molecular mechanisms of antigen-induced B cell migration, and demonstrate that the positioning of single cells in vivo is controlled by adjacent chemokine gradients.

2.3.3
CCR9: Thymus; Intestine; Homeostasis of IEL

The only know receptor for the thymus-expressed chemokine (TECK/CCL25) is CCR9. CCL25 is predominantly expressed in thymic epithelial cells starting during fetal development and in the small intestine of mouse and human. CCR9 on the other hand is expressed on the majority of double-positive $CD4^+$ $CD8^+$ immature thymocytes and is rapidly downregulated on transitional single-positive and mature thymocytes (Uehara et al. 2002b). Based on this expression profile, CCR9 has been implicated in recruiting T progenitor cells to the thymus and in intestine-specific homing of circulating CCR9-positive lymphocytes that coexpress the intestinal homing receptor $\alpha_4\beta_7$. Indeed, small intestinal lymphocytes as well as thymocytes show a chemotactic response to CCL25, and this migration can be hampered by addition of anti CCR9 antibody (Kunkel et al. 2000; Papadakis et al. 2000; Wurbel et al. 2001).

Surprisingly, loss of CCR9 causes only mild defects, although chemotaxis of CCR9 mutant cells to CCL25 is abolished, suggesting that CCR9 is indeed the sole receptor for CCL25. In CCR9-deficient thymi, the appearance of double-positive cells is delayed by 1 day compared to wild-type animals. However, this difference is lost by embryonic day 18.5. In adult mice, no differences could be found in numbers or in the expression of relevant cell surface markers between wild-type and CCR9-deficient thymocytes (Wurbel et al. 2001). In the bone marrow, loss of CCR9 results in a threefold reduction of pre-pro-B-cells. However comparable to the situation in fetal thymi, homeostatic adjustments seem to occur during later stages of development. In the periphery, loss of CCR9 results in a threefold increase in the number of TCR$\gamma\delta^+$, while the absolute number of TCR$\gamma\delta^+$ intraepithelial lymphocytes (IEL) in the small intestine is reduced to 20% when compared to wild-type (Wurbel et al. 2001; Uehara et al. 2002a). Thus, it is tempting to speculate that this redistribution might be due to an impaired ability of CCR9-deficient TCR$\gamma\delta^+$ cells to migrate into the small intestine.

2.3.4
CXCR4: Organ Development, B Cell Precursors; HIV Receptor

CXCR4 is the chemokine receptor for stromal-derived factor 1 (SDF-1; CXCL12). It is broadly expressed in the CNS and the immune system, by CD34$^+$ haematopoietic progenitors, B cell precursors, mature B and T lymphocytes, monocytes and neutrophils (Förster et al. 1998; Ohtani et al. 1998; Aiuti et al. 1999; Schabath et al. 1999). Both CXCR4- and CXCL12-deficient mice display the same phenotype: they die perinatally and have defects in neuron migration, organ vascularization and haematopoiesis (Nagasawa et al. 1996; Ma et al. 1998; Tachibana et al. 1998; Zou et al. 1998), suggesting a high receptor-ligand selectivity, with CXCR4 being the only physiological receptor for CXCL12 and vice versa. In mutant embryos, B lymphopoiesis and myelopoiesis are heavily impaired. The number of B cell progenitors is severely reduced in fetal liver and bone marrow. Myelopoiesis is quantitatively decreased in fetal liver and virtually absent in bone marrow (Nagasawa et al. 1996; Ma et al. 1998; Tachibana et al. 1998; Zou et al. 1998). By examination of fetal blood in CXCR4$^{-/-}$ mice and reconstitution experiments of lethally irradiated mice with CXCR4-deficient fetal liver cells, it could be shown that these haematopoietic defects are due insufficient retainment of B cell and myeloid precursors in the haematopoietic compartments, fetal liver and bone marrow, for proper maturation (Ma et al. 1999). In contrast, despite otherwise high-level expression of CXCR4 in immature CD4CD8 double-positive thymocytes in wild-type animals, T lymphopoiesis seems unaffected in CXCR4 knockout. At E17.5, double-positive thymocytes are generated in normal cellularity and can differentiate in vitro to mature single-positive cells (Ma et al. 1998). Due to perinatal death of CXCR4 mutants, further steps of T cell development were analysed by transferring E17.5 mutant thymuses to T cell receptor α-deficient recipients. These transplants were shown to result in normal T cell maturation and differentiation. (Zou et al. 1998).

In addition to their roles in haematopoiesis, CXCR4 and its ligand are also required for proper vascularization of the gastrointestinal tract: mice lacking CXCR4 or CXCL12 have defective formation of the large vessels supplying the gastrointestinal tract (Tachibana et al. 1998). Within the central nervous system, both genes, CXCR4 and CXCL12, are required for neuron migration within the cerebellum. The microarchitecture of the cerebellum is highly distorted and proliferative granule cells from the most peripheral cell layer invade the Purkinje cell layer (Zou et al. 1998).

2.3.5
CXCR5: Development of Two Lymphoid Organs; B Cell Migration

The chemokine receptor CXCR5 has been identified in an subtractive hybridization approach in order to identify gene products involved in the pathogenesis of Burkitt's lymphoma and has been originally termed Burkitt's lymphoma receptor (BLR)-1 (Dobner et al. 1992). Anti-CXCR5 monoclonal antibodies, the first ever produced anti-chemokine receptor antibodies, identified mature B cells and a subpopulation of $CD4^+$ T cells (but not any inflammatory cells, such as granulocytes or monocytes) to express this receptor (Förster et al. 1994). This distinct expression rendered CXCR5 a prime candidate for controlling B cell migration into lymphoid follicles. This early hypothesis could be confirmed by gene targeting. CXCR5 deficiency severely affects the development of Peyer's patches and some skin-draining lymph nodes (Förster et al. 1996). In addition, the formation of follicles in the spleen of CXCR5-deficient mice was found to be disturbed. By means of in vivo repopulation experiments, it could be shown that B cells isolated from these mice fail to migrate into the splenic B cell follicles of wild-type recipients, thus explaining the lack of organized GC within B cell follicles. Similarly, CXCR5-deficient B cells were unable to repopulate all B cell follicles in Peyer's patches and those follicles in lymph nodes which contain follicular dendritic cells. These results identified CXCR5 as the first chemokine receptor to be involved in the regulation of B cell migration and localization of these cells within specific anatomic compartments (Förster et al. 1996). Although CXCR5-deficient mice develop only small germinal centres dislocated to the T cell area, it was recently shown that B cell within these structures nevertheless undergo somatic mutation and affinity maturation as has been observed in wild-type mice (Voigt et al. 2000). Interestingly, when comparing mice deficient for CXCR5 with mice deficient for its ligand, BLC/CXCL13, a very similar phenotype between both strains of mice including the absence of various peripheral lymph nodes was found. These studies also revealed a positive-feedback loop of chemokines on lymphotoxin (LT) expression as exposure to CXCL13 induces B cells to up regulate membrane-bound $LT\alpha_1\beta_2$, a cytokine known to induce follicular dendritic cell (FDC) development and the expression of CXCL13 (Ansel et al. 2000). The identical phenotypes of CXCL13 and CXCR5 strongly supports the idea that CXCL13 mainly acts through CXCR5 and that CXCR5 binds no other chemokine than CXCL13. However, it became obvious recently that B1 cells need CXCL13 expression to populate the peritoneal cavity, a process that is independent of CXCR5. These data suggest that CXCL13 binds to an additional chemokine receptor on B1 cells.

2.4
Chemokine Receptors Not Studied So Far by Gene-Targeting

Although the function of most chemokine receptors has been elucidated by gene targeting in mice, there are still some examples for which no knockout has been described so far.

2.4.1
CCR10: T Memory Cells; Skin Homing

CCR10 is the former orphan receptor GPR2 (Marchese et al. 1994). Two ligands have been identified binding to this receptor: CCL27 (also known as CTACK or ESkine) and CCL28 (Homey et al. 2000; Wang et al. 2000). Both chemokines are expressed in the skin, attract skin homing memory T cells and regulate inflammatory skin processes (Reiss et al. 2001; Homey et al. 2002). Furthermore, CCR10 expressed on tumour cells is implicated in metastasis formation in situ (Muller et al. 2001).

2.4.2
CCR11

Expression of CCR11[1] has been described in various organs including lymph node and spleen. Regarding ligand specificity, CCR11 binds with high affinity to CCL19, CCL21 and CCL25 and with lower affinity to CXCL13. Thus, CCR11 represents one of the very few examples binding both CCL and CXCL chemokines (Gosling et al. 2000).

---

[1] Note added in proof: Since there is no signalling response ascribed for the receptor addressed as CCR11 in this manuscript, this molecule does not qualify for a chemokine receptor designation. The term CCR11 is no longer used to describe this chemokine-binding protein.

2.4.3
CXCR6: Th1; HIV receptor

CXCR6 (also known as Bonzo, STRL33, or TYMSTR) is the sole receptor for CXCL16 (Gosling et al. 2000) and has been initially described as a coreceptor for HIV-1 and SIV (Deng et al. 1997). Expression of CXCR6 has been identified on subsets of CD4, CD8 and natural killer T cells (Gosling et al. 2000) and seems to be characteristic for a subset of Th1 cells. CXCR6-expressing cells show tissue-homing potential, particularly to inflamed tissues (Kim et al. 2001).

2.4.4
XCR1

XCR1, formerly known as GPR5, is the only receptor known for the chemokines XCL1 (lymphotactin, ATAC) and XCL2. The receptor is expressed on T cells, but little is known about its biological function (Yoshida et al. 1998).

2.4.5
CXCR1

So far a murine homologue of human CXCR1 has not been identified.

3
Concluding Remarks

Herakleitos' revelation that nobody can enter the same river for a second time (fifth century B.C.) became a key feature of modern life science. Preserving their shape and function, the body's organs are, for the most part, under constant reconstruction. This process is particularly intricate in the case of the immune system, since the cells of no other organ need to adjust to such diverse microenvironments inside the body whilst constantly checking for self and non-self and reacting accordingly. This multi-task may translate into: what to become, when to divide, where to go, what to perform and similar questions to be answered by those who want to seek insight into the function of the immune network. Exactly such answers were provided when examining the function of chemokine receptors and their ligands, thereby explaining why this area of research has been the focus of so much interest for quite a while now. In this review, we confined ourselves to the description of immunological defects exerted by mice deficient for chemokine receptors to emphasize that many insights depended on applying this technology (to a comparable extent as they already did in developmental biology). Therefore, it is conceivable to assume that this concept will continue to provide information, especially when analysing mice deficient for more than one chemokine/receptor. This may be of primordial importance to those studying the inflammatory chemokine receptors. In the homeostatic branch for example, the identification of subsets of T cells and DCs helped us to recognize an immune net that is gaining in complexity but also elegance. It will be interesting to see whether a similar scenario holds true for cells of the inflammatory path such as basophils or eosinophils.

References

(2001) Chemokine/chemokine receptor nomenclature. J Leukoc Biol 70(3): 465–466

Aiuti A, Tavian M, Cipponi A, Ficara F, Zappone E, Hoxie J, Peault B, Bordignon C (1999) Expression of CXCR4, the receptor for stromal cell-derived factor-1 on fetal and adult human lympho-hematopoietic progenitors. Eur J Immunol 29(6): 1823–1831

Andres PG, Beck PL, Mizoguchi E, Mizoguchi A, Bhan AK, Dawson T, Kuziel WA, Maeda N, MacDermott RP, Podolsky DK, Reinecker HC (2000) Mice with a selective deletion of the CC chemokine receptors 5 or 2 are protected from dextran sodium sulfate-mediated colitis: lack of CC chemokine receptor 5 expression results in a NK1.1$^+$ lymphocyte-associated Th2-type immune response in the intestine. J Immunol 164(12): 6303–6312

Andrew DP, Ruffing N, Kim CH, Miao W, Heath H, Li Y, Murphy K, Campbell JJ, Butcher EC, Wu L (2001) C-C chemokine receptor 4 expression defines a major subset of circulating nonintestinal memory T cells of both Th1 and Th2 potential. J Immunol 166(1): 103–111

Ansel KM, Ngo VN, Hyman PL, Luther SA, Forster R, Sedgwick JD, Browning JL, Lipp M, Cyster JG (2000) A chemokine-driven positive feedback loop organizes lymphoid follicles. Nature 406(6793): 309–314

Baggiolini M (2001) Chemokines in pathology and medicine. J Intern Med 250(2): 91–104

Baggiolini M, Dewald B, Moser B (1997) Human chemokines: an update. Annu. Rev. Immunol. 15:675–705

Bazan JF, Bacon KB, Hardiman G, Wang W, Soo K, Rossi D, Greaves DR, Zlotnik A, Schall TJ (1997) A new class of membrane-bound chemokine with a CX3C motif. Nature 385(6617): 640–644

Boring L, Gosling J, Chensue SW, Kunkel SL, Farese RV, Jr., Broxmeyer HE, Charo IF (1997) Impaired monocyte migration and reduced type 1 (Th1) cytokine responses in C-C chemokine receptor 2 knockout mice. J Clin Invest 100(10): 2552–2561

Breitfeld D, Ohl L, Kremmer E, Ellwart J, Sallusto F, Lipp M, Forster R (2000) Follicular B helper T cells express CXC chemokine receptor 5, localize to. J. Exp. Med. 192(11): 1545–1552.

Burgstahler R, Kempkes B, Steube K, Lipp M (1995) Expression of the chemokine receptor BLR2/EBI-1 is specifically transactivated by Epstein Barr virus nuclear antigen 2. Biochem. Biophys. Res. Com. 215(2): 737–743

Butcher EC (1991) Leukocyte-endothelial cell recognition: three (or more) steps to specificity and diversity. Cell 67(6): 1033–1036

Cacalano G, Lee J, Kikly K, Ryan AM, Pitts-Meek S, Hultgren B, Wood WI, Moore MW (1994) Neutrophil and B cell expansion in mice that lack the murine IL-8 receptor homolog. Science 265(5172): 682–684

Chensue SW, Lukacs NW, Yang TY, Shang X, Frait KA, Kunkel SL, Kung T, Wiekowski MT, Hedrick JA, Cook DN, Zingoni A, Narula SK, Zlotnik A, Barrat FJ, O'Garra A, Napolitano M, Lira SA (2001) Aberrant in vivo T helper type 2 cell response and impaired eosinophil recruitment in CC chemokine receptor 8 knockout mice. J Exp Med 193(5): 573–584

Chvatchko Y, Hoogewerf AJ, Meyer A, Alouani S, Juillard P, Buser R, Conquet F, Proudfoot AE, Wells TN, Power CA (2000) A key role for CC chemokine receptor 4 in lipopolysaccharide-induced endotoxic shock. J Exp Med 191(10): 1755–1764

Cook DN, Prosser DM, Forster R, Zhang J, Kuklin NA, Abbondanzo SJ, Niu XD, Chen SC, Manfra DJ, Wiekowski MT, Sullivan LM, Smith SR, Greenberg HB, Narula SK, Lipp M, Lira SA (2000) CCR6 mediates dendritic cell localization, lymphocyte homeostasis, and immune responses in mucosal tissue. Immunity 12(5): 495–503

Cook DN, Chen SC, Sullivan LM, Manfra DJ, Wiekowski MT, Prosser DM, Vassileva G, Lira SA (2001) Generation and analysis of mice lacking the chemokine fractalkine. Mol Cell Biol 21: 3159–3165

Cyster JG (1999) Chemokines and cell migration in secondary lymphoid organs. Science 286(5447): 2098–2102

D'Ambrosio D, Mariani M, Panina-Bordignon P, Sinigaglia F (2001) Chemokines and their receptors guiding T lymphocyte recruitment in lung inflammation. Am J Respir Crit Care Med 164(7): 1266–1275

Dawson TC, Beck MA, Kuziel WA, Henderson F, Maeda N (2000) Contrasting effects of CCR5 and CCR2 deficiency in the pulmonary inflammatory response to influenza A virus. Am J Pathol 156(6): 1951–1959

Del Rio L, Bennouna S, Salinas J, Denkers EY (2001) CXCR2 deficiency confers impaired neutrophil recruitment and increased susceptibility during Toxoplasma gondii infection. J Immunol 167(11): 6503–6509

Deng HK, Unutmaz D, KewalRamani VN, Littman DR (1997) Expression cloning of new receptors used by simian and human immunodeficiency viruses. Nature 388(6639): 296–300

Devalaraja RM, Nanney LB, Du J, Qian Q, Yu Y, Devalaraja MN, Richmond A (2000) Delayed wound healing in CXCR2 knockout mice. J Invest Dermatol 115(2): 234–244

Dieu MC, Vanbervliet B, Vicari A, Bridon JM, Oldham E, Ait-Yahia S, Briere F, Zlotnik A, Lebecque S, Caux C (1998a) Selective recruitment of immature and mature dendritic cells by distinct chemokines expressed in different anatomic sites. J Exp Med 188(2): 373–386

Dieu MC, Vanbervliet B, Vicari A, Bridon JM, Oldham E, Ait-Yahia S, Briere F, Zlotnik A, Lebecque S, Caux C (1998b) Selective recruitment of immature and mature dendritic cells by distinct chemokines expressed in different anatomic sites. J. Exp. Med. 188(2): 373–386

Dobner T, Wolf I, Emrich T, Lipp M (1992) Differentiation-specific expression of a novel G protein-coupled receptor from Burkitt's lymphoma. Eur. J. Immunol. 22(11): 2795–2799

Förster R, Emrich T, Kremmer E, Lipp M (1994) Expression of the G-protein-coupled receptor BLR1 defines mature recirculating B cells and a subset of T memory helper cells. Blood 84(3): 830–840

Förster R, Kremmer E, Schubel A, Breitfeld D, Kleinschmidt A, C. N, Bernhardt G, Lipp M (1998) Intracellular and surface expression of the HIV-1 co-receptor CXCR4/fusin on various leukocyte subsets: rapid internalization and recycling upon activation. J. Immunol. 160:1522–1531

Förster R, Mattis EA, Kremmer E, Wolf E, Brem G, Lipp M (1996) A putative chemokine receptor, BLR1, directs B cell migration to defined lymphoid organs and specific anatomic compartments of the spleen. Cell 87:1037–1047

Förster R, Schubel A, Breitfeld D, Kremmer E, Renner-Müller I, Wolf E, Lipp M (1999) CCR7 coordinates the primary immune response by establishing functional microenvironments in secondary lymphoid organs. Cell 99:23–33

Gao JL, Wynn TA, Chang Y, Lee EJ, Broxmeyer HE, Cooper S, Tiffany HL, Westphal H, Kwon-Chung J, Murphy PM (1997) Impaired host defense, hematopoiesis, granulomatous inflammation and type 1-type 2 cytokine balance in mice lacking CC chemokine receptor 1. J Exp Med 185(11): 1959–1968

Gerard C, Frossard JL, Bhatia M, Saluja A, Gerard NP, Lu B, Steer M (1997) Targeted disruption of the beta-chemokine receptor CCR1 protects against pancreatitis-associated lung injury. J Clin Invest 100(8): 2022–2027

Gerard C, Rollins BJ (2001) Chemokines and disease. Nat Immunol 2(2): 108–115

Godaly G, Hang L, Frendeus B, Svanborg C (2000) Transepithelial neutrophil migration is CXCR1 dependent in vitro and is defective in IL-8 receptor knockout mice. J Immunol 165(9): 5287–5294

Godaly G, Proudfoot AE, Offord RE, Svanborg C, Agace WW (1997) Role of epithelial interleukin-8 (IL-8) and neutrophil IL-8 receptor A in Escherichia coli-induced transuroepithelial neutrophil migration. Infect Immun 65(8): 3451–3456

Gosling J, Dairaghi DJ, Wang Y, Hanley M, Talbot D, Miao Z, Schall TJ (2000) Cutting edge: identification of a novel chemokine receptor that binds dendritic cell- and T cell-active chemokines including ELC, SLC, and TECK. J Immunol 164(6): 2851–2856

Greaves DR, Wang W, Dairaghi DJ, Dieu MC, Saint-Vis B, Franz-Bacon K, Rossi D, Caux C, McClanahan T, Gordon S, Zlotnik A, Schall TJ (1997) CCR6, a CC chemokine receptor that interacts with macrophage inflammatory protein 3alpha and is highly expressed in human dendritic cells. J Exp Med 186(6): 837–844

Hancock WW, Lu B, Gao W, Csizmadia V, Faia K, King JA, Smiley ST, Ling M, Gerard NP, Gerard C (2000) Requirement of the chemokine receptor CXCR3 for acute allograft rejection. J Exp Med 192(10): 1515–1520

Harrison JK, Jiang Y, Chen S, Xia Y, Maciejewski D, McNamara RK, Streit WJ, Salafranca MN, Adhikari S, Thompson DA, Botti P, Bacon KB, Feng L (1998) Role for neuronally derived fractalkine in mediating interactions between neurons and CX3CR1-expressing microglia. Proc Natl Acad Sci U S A 95(18): 10896–10901

Haskell CA, Hancock WW, Salant DJ, Gao W, Csizmadia V, Peters W, Faia K, Fituri O, Rottman JB, Charo IF (2001) Targeted deletion of CX(3)CR1 reveals a role for fractalkine in cardiac allograft rejection. J Clin Invest 108(5): 679–688

Hieshima K, Imai T, Opdenakker G, Van Damme J, Kusuda J, Tei H, Sakaki Y, Takatsuki K, Miura R, Yoshie O, Nomiyama H (1997) Molecular cloning of a novel human CC chemokine liver and activation-regulated chemokine (LARC) expressed in liver. Chemotactic activity for lymphocytes and gene localization on chromosome 2. J Biol Chem 272(9): 5846–5853

Homey B, Alenius H, Muller A, Soto H, Bowman EP, Yuan W, McEvoy L, Lauerma AI, Assmann T, Bunemann E, Lehto M, Wolff H, Yen D, Marxhausen H, To W, Sedgwick J, Ruzicka T, Lehmann P, Zlotnik A (2002) CCL27-CCR10 interactions regulate T cell-mediated skin inflammation. Nat Med 8(2): 157–165

Homey B, Wang W, Soto H, Buchanan ME, Wiesenborn A, Catron D, Muller A, McClanahan TK, Dieu-Nosjean MC, Orozco R, Ruzicka T, Lehmann P, Oldham E, Zlotnik A (2000) Cutting edge: the orphan chemokine receptor G protein-coupled receptor-2 (GPR-2, CCR10) binds the skin-associated chemokine CCL27 (CTACK/ALP/ILC). J Immunol 164(7): 3465–3470

Hromas R, Gray PW, Chantry D, Godiska R, Krathwohl M, Fife K, Bell GI, Takeda J, Aronica S, Gordon M, Cooper S, Broxmeyer HE, Klemsz MJ (1997) Cloning and characterization of exodus, a novel beta-chemokine. Blood 89(9): 3315–3322

Humbles AA, Lu B, Friend DS, Okinaga S, Lora J, Al-Garawi A, Martin TR, Gerard NP, Gerard C (2002) The murine CCR3 receptor regulates both the role of eosinophils and mast cells in allergen-induced airway inflammation and hyperresponsiveness. Proc Natl Acad Sci U S A 99(3): 1479–1484

Kaplan AP (2001) Chemokines, chemokine receptors and allergy. Int Arch Allergy Immunol 124(4): 423–431

Kielian T, Barry B, Hickey WF (2001) CXC chemokine receptor-2 ligands are required for neutrophil-mediated host defense in experimental brain abscesses. J Immunol 166(7): 4634–4643

Kim CH, Kunkel EJ, Boisvert J, Johnston B, Campbell JJ, Genovese MC, Greenberg HB, Butcher EC (2001) Bonzo/CXCR6 expression defines type 1-polarized T-cell subsets with extralymphoid tissue homing potential. J Clin Invest 107(5): 595–601

Kremer L, Carramolino L, Goya I, Zaballos A, Gutierrez J, Moreno-Ortiz MdC, Martinez AC, Marquez G (2001) The transient expression of C-C chemokine receptor 8 in thymus identifies a thymocyte subset committed to become CD4+ single-positive T cells. J Immunol 166(1): 218–225

Kunkel EJ, Boisvert J, Murphy K, Vierra MA, Genovese MC, Wardlaw AJ, Greenberg HB, Hodge MR, Wu L, Butcher EC, Campbell JJ (2002) Expression of the Chemokine Receptors CCR4, CCR5, and CXCR3 by Human Tissue-Infiltrating Lymphocytes. Am J Pathol 160(1): 347–355

Kunkel EJ, Campbell JJ, Haraldsen G, Pan J, Boisvert J, Roberts AI, Ebert EC, Vierra MA, Goodman SB, Genovese MC, Wardlaw AJ, Greenberg HB, Parker CM, Butcher EC, Andrew DP, Agace WW (2000) Lymphocyte CC chemokine receptor 9 and epithelial thymus-expressed chemokine (TECK) expression distinguish the small intestinal immune compartment: Epithelial expression of tissue-specific chemokines as an organizing principle in regional immunity. J Exp Med 192(5): 761–768

Kurihara T, Warr G, Loy J, Bravo R (1997) Defects in macrophage recruitment and host defense in mice lacking the CCR2 chemokine receptor. J Exp Med 186(10): 1757–1762

Kuziel WA, Morgan SJ, Dawson TC, Griffin S, Smithies O, Ley K, Maeda N (1997) Severe reduction in leukocyte adhesion and monocyte extravasation in mice deficient in CC chemokine receptor 2. Proc Natl Acad Sci U S A 94(22): 12053–12058

Lawrence MB, Springer TA (1991) Leukocytes roll on a selectin at physiologic flow rates: distinction from and prerequisite for adhesion through integrins. Cell 65(5): 859–873

Lee J, Cacalano G, Camerato T, Toy K, Moore MW, Wood WI (1995) Chemokine binding and activities mediated by the mouse IL-8 receptor. J Immunol 155(4): 2158–2164

Liao F, Rabin RL, Smith CS, Sharma G, Nutman TB, Farber JM (1999) CC-chemokine receptor 6 is expressed on diverse memory subsets of T cells and determines responsiveness to macrophage inflammatory protein 3 alpha. J Immunol 162(1): 186–194

Loetscher P, Pellegrino A, Gong JH, Mattioli I, Loetscher M, Bardi G, Baggiolini M, Clark-Lewis I (2001) The ligands of CXC chemokine receptor 3, I-TAC, Mig, and IP10, are natural antagonists for CCR3. J Biol Chem 276(5): 2986–2991

Lukacs NW, Prosser DM, Wiekowski M, Lira SA, Cook DN (2001) Requirement for the chemokine receptor CCR6 in allergic pulmonary inflammation. J Exp Med 194(4): 551–555

Ma Q, Jones D, Borghesani PR, Segal RA, Nagasawa T, Kishimoto T, Bronson RT, Springer TA (1998) Impaired B-lymphopoiesis, myelopoiesis, and derailed cerebellar neuron migration in CXCR4- and SDF-1-deficient mice. Proc Natl Acad Sci U S A 95(16): 9448–9453

Ma Q, Jones D, Springer TA (1999) The chemokine receptor CXCR4 is required for the retention of B lineage and granulocytic precursors within the bone marrow microenvironment. Immunity 10(4): 463–471

Ma W, Bryce PJ, Humbles AA, Laouini D, Yalcindag A, Alenius H, Friend DS, Oettgen HC, Gerard C, Geha RS (2002) CCR3 is essential for skin eosinophilia and airway hyperresponsiveness in a murine model of allergic skin inflammation. J Clin Invest 109(5): 621–628

Mackay CR (2001) Chemokines: immunology's high impact factors. Nat Immunol 2(2): 95–101

Marchese A, Docherty JM, Nguyen T, Heiber M, Cheng R, Heng HH, Tsui LC, Shi X, George SR, O'Dowd BF (1994) Cloning of human genes encoding novel G protein-coupled receptors. Genomics 23(3): 609–618

Matthews AN, Friend DS, Zimmermann N, Sarafi MN, Luster AD, Pearlman E, Wert SE, Rothenberg ME (1998) Eotaxin is required for the baseline level of tissue eosinophils. Proc Natl Acad Sci U S A 95(11): 6273–6278

Mehrad B, Strieter RM, Moore TA, Tsai WC, Lira SA, Standiford TJ (1999) CXC chemokine receptor-2 ligands are necessary components of neutrophil-mediated host defense in invasive pulmonary aspergillosis. J Immunol 163(11): 6086–6094

Moser B, Loetscher P (2001) Lymphocyte traffic control by chemokines. Nat Immunol 2(2): 123–128

Muehlhoefer A, Saubermann LJ, Gu X, Luedtke-Heckenkamp K, Xavier R, Blumberg RS, Podolsky DK, MacDermott RP, Reinecker HC (2000) Fractalkine is an epithelial and endothelial cell-derived chemoattractant for intraepithelial lymphocytes in the small intestinal mucosa. J Immunol 164: 3368–3376

Muller A, Homey B, Soto H, Ge N, Catron D, Buchanan ME, McClanahan T, Murphy E, Yuan W, Wagner SN, Barrera JL, Mohar A, Verastegui E, Zlotnik A (2001) Involvement of chemokine receptors in breast cancer metastasis. Nature 410(6824): 50–56

Murphy PM, Baggiolini M, Charo IF, Hebert CA, Horuk R, Matsushima K, Miller LH, Oppenheim JJ, Power CA (2000) International union of pharmacology. XXII. Nomenclature for chemokine receptors. Pharmacol Rev 52(1): 145–176

Nagasawa T, Hirota S, Tachibana K, Takakura N, Nishikawa S, Kitamura Y, Yoshida N, Kikutani H, Kishimoto T (1996) Defects of B-cell lymphopoiesis and bone-marrow myelopoiesis in mice lacking the CXC chemokine PBSF/SDF-1. Nature 382(6592): 635–638

Nansen A, Marker O, Bartholdy C, Thomsen AR (2000) CCR2+ and CCR5+ CD8+ T cells increase during viral infection and migrate to sites of infection. Eur J Immunol 30(7): 1797–1806

Nansen A, Christensen JP, Andreasen SS, Bartholdy C, Christensen JE, Thomsen AR (2002) The role of CC chemokine receptor 5 in antiviral immunity. Blood 99(4): 1237–1245

Nishiyori A, Minami M, Ohtani Y, Takami S, Yamamoto J, Kawaguchi N, Kume T, Akaike A, Satoh M (1998) Localization of fractalkine and CX3CR1 mRNAs in rat brain: does fractalkine play a role in signaling from neuron to microglia? FEBS Lett 429(2): 167–172

Ohtani Y, Minami M, Kawaguchi N, Nishiyori A, Yamamoto J, Takami S, Satoh M (1998) Expression of stromal cell-derived factor-1 and CXCR4 chemokine receptor mRNAs in cultured rat glial and neuronal cells. Neurosci Lett 249(2–3): 163–166

Papadakis KA, Prehn J, Nelson V, Cheng L, Binder SW, Ponath PD, Andrew DP, Targan SR (2000) The role of thymus-expressed chemokine and its receptor CCR9 on lymphocytes in the regional specialization of the mucosal immune system. J Immunol 165(9): 5069–5076

Peters W, Dupuis M, Charo IF (2000) A mechanism for the impaired IFN-gamma production in C-C chemokine receptor 2 (CCR2) knockout mice: role of CCR2 in linking the innate and adaptive immune responses. J Immunol 165(12): 7072–7077

Power CA, Church DJ, Meyer A, Alouani S, Proudfoot AE, Clark-Lewis I, Sozzani S, Mantovani A, Wells TN (1997) Cloning and characterization of a specific receptor for the novel CC chemokine MIP-3alpha from lung dendritic cells. J Exp Med 186(6): 825–835

Reif K, Ekland EH, Ohl L, Nakano H, Lipp M, Forster R, Cyster JG (2002) Balanced responsiveness to chemoattractants from adjacent zones determines B-cell position. Nature 416(6876): 94–99

Reiss Y, Proudfoot AE, Power CA, Campbell JJ, Butcher EC (2001) CC chemokine receptor (CCR)4 and the CCR10 ligand cutaneous T cell-attracting chemokine (CTACK) in lymphocyte trafficking to inflamed skin. J Exp Med 194(10): 1541–1547

Robinson LA, Nataraj C, Thomas DW, Howell DN, Griffiths R, Bautch V, Patel DD, Feng L, Coffman TM (2000) A role for fractalkine and its receptor (CX3CR1) in cardiac allograft rejection. J Immunol 165(11): 6067–6072

Rollins BJ (1997) Chemokines. Blood 90(3): 909–928

Rossi DL, Vicari AP, Franz-Bacon K, McClanahan TK, Zlotnik A (1997) Identification through bioinformatics of two new macrophage proinflammatory human chemokines: MIP-3alpha and MIP-3beta. J Immunol 158(3): 1033–1036

Sallusto F, Lenig D, Forster R, Lipp M, Lanzavecchia A (1999) Two subsets of memory T lymphocytes with distinct homing potentials and effector functions. Nature 401(6754): 708–712

Sallusto F, Schaerli P, Loetscher P, Schaniel C, Lenig D, Mackay CR, Qin S, Lanzavecchia A (1998) Rapid and coordinated switch in chemokine receptor expression during dendritic cell maturation. Eur. J. Immunol. 28(9): 2760–2769

Sato N, Ahuja SK, Quinones M, Kostecki V, Reddick RL, Melby PC, Kuziel WA, Ahuja SS (2000) CC chemokine receptor (CCR)2 is required for langerhans cell migration and localization of T helper cell type 1 (Th1)-inducing dendritic cells. Absence of CCR2 shifts the Leishmania major-resistant phenotype to a susceptible state dominated by Th2 cytokines, B cell outgrowth, and sustained neutrophilic inflammation. J Exp Med 192(2): 205–218

Schabath R, Muller G, Schubel A, Kremmer E, Lipp M, Forster R (1999) The murine chemokine receptor CXCR4 is tightly regulated during T cell development and activation. J. Leukoc. Biol. 66(6): 996–1004

Schweickart VL, Raport CJ, Godiska R, Byers MG, Eddy RJ, Shows TB, Gray PW (1994) Cloning of human and mouse EBI1, a lymphoid-specific G-protein-coupled receptor encoded on human chromosome 17q12-q21.2. Genomics 23(3): 643–650

Sozzani S, Allavena P, G DA, Luini W, Bianchi G, Kataura M, Imai T, Yoshie O, Bonecchi R, Mantovani A (1998) Differential regulation of chemokine receptors during dendritic cell maturation: a model for their trafficking properties. J. Immunol. 161(3): 1083–1086

Springer TA (1994) Traffic signals for lymphocyte recirculation and leukocyte emigration: the multistep paradigm. Cell 76(2): 301–314

Su SB, Mukaida N, Wang J, Nomura H, Matsushima K (1996) Preparation of specific polyclonal antibodies to a C-C chemokine receptor, CCR1, and determination of CCR1 expression on various types of leukocytes. J Leukoc Biol 60(5): 658–666

Tachibana K, Hirota S, Iizasa H, Yoshida H, Kawabata K, Kataoka Y, Kitamura Y, Matsushima K, Yoshida N, Nishikawa S, Kishimoto T, Nagasawa T (1998) The chemokine receptor CXCR4 is essential for vascularization of the gastrointestinal tract. Nature 393(6685): 591–594

Tanaka Y, Imai T, Baba M, Ishikawa I, Uehira M, Nomiyama H, Yoshie O (1999) Selective expression of liver and activation-regulated chemokine (LARC) in intestinal epithelium in mice and humans. Eur J Immunol 29(2): 633–642

Tangemann K, Gunn MD, Giblin P, Rosen SD (1998) A high endothelial cell-derived chemokine induces rapid, efficient, and subset-selective arrest of rolling T lymphocytes on a reconstituted endothelial substrate. J Immunol 161(11): 6330–6337

Tateda K, Moore TA, Newstead MW, Tsai WC, Zeng X, Deng JC, Chen G, Reddy R, Yamaguchi K, Standiford TJ (2001) Chemokine-dependent neutrophil recruitment in a murine model of Legionella pneumonia: potential role of neutrophils as immunoregulatory cells. Infect Immun 69(4): 2017–2024

Tran EH, Kuziel WA, Owens T (2000) Induction of experimental autoimmune encephalomyelitis in C57BL/6 mice deficient in either the chemokine macrophage inflammatory protein-1alpha or its CCR5 receptor. Eur J Immunol 30(5): 1410–1415

Tsai WC, Strieter RM, Mehrad B, Newstead MW, Zeng X, Standiford TJ (2000) CXC chemokine receptor CXCR2 is essential for protective innate host response in murine Pseudomonas aeruginosa pneumonia. Infect Immun 68(7): 4289–4296

Uehara S, Grinberg A, Farber JM, Love PE (2002a) A role for CCR9 in T lymphocyte development and migration. J Immunol 168(6): 2811–2819

Uehara S, Song K, Farber JM, Love PE (2002b) Characterization of CCR9 expression and CCL25/thymus-expressed chemokine responsiveness during T cell development:

CD3(high)CD69+ thymocytes and gammadeltaTCR+ thymocytes preferentially respond to CCL25. J Immunol 168(1): 134–142

Varona R, Villares R, Carramolino L, Goya I, Zaballos A, Gutierrez J, Torres M, Martinez AC, Marquez G (2001) CCR6-deficient mice have impaired leukocyte homeostasis and altered contact hypersensitivity and delayed-type hypersensitivity responses. J Clin Invest 107(6): R37–45

Voigt I, Camacho SA, de Boer BA, Lipp M, Forster R, Berek C (2000) CXCR5-deficient mice develop functional germinal centers in the splenic T. Eur.J. Immunol. 30(2): 560–567.

Wang W, Soto H, Oldham ER, Buchanan ME, Homey B, Catron D, Jenkins N, Copeland NG, Gilbert DJ, Nguyen N, Abrams J, Kershenovich D, Smith K, McClanahan T, Vicari AP, Zlotnik A (2000) Identification of a novel chemokine (CCL28), which binds CCR10 (GPR2). J Biol Chem 275(29): 22313–22323

Wurbel MA, Malissen M, Guy-Grand D, Meffre E, Nussenzweig MC, Richelme M, Carrier A, Malissen B (2001) Mice lacking the CCR9 CC-chemokine receptor show a mild impairment of early T- and B-cell development and a reduction in T-cell receptor gammadelta(+) gut intraepithelial lymphocytes. Blood 98(9): 2626–2632

Yanagihara S, Komura E, Nagafune J, Watarai H, Yamaguchi Y (1998) EBI1/CCR7 is a new member of dendritic cell chemokine receptor that is up-regulated upon maturation. J. Immunol. 161(6): 3096–3102

Yoshida T, Imai T, Kakizaki M, Nishimura M, Takagi S, Yoshie O (1998) Identification of single C motif-1/lymphotactin receptor XCR1. J Biol Chem 273(26): 16551–16554

Zhang XW, Liu Q, Wang Y, Thorlacius H (2001) CXC chemokines, MIP-2 and KC, induce P-selectin-dependent neutrophil rolling and extravascular migration in vivo. Br J Pharmacol 133(3): 413–421

Zhou Y, Kurihara T, Ryseck RP, Yang Y, Ryan C, Loy J, Warr G, Bravo R (1998) Impaired macrophage function and enhanced T cell-dependent immune response in mice lacking CCR5, the mouse homologue of the major HIV-1 coreceptor. J Immunol 160(8): 4018–4025

Zingoni A, Soto H, Hedrick JA, Stoppacciaro A, Storlazzi CT, Sinigaglia F, D'Ambrosio D, O'Garra A, Robinson D, Rocchi M, Santoni A, Zlotnik A, Napolitano M (1998) The chemokine receptor CCR8 is preferentially expressed in Th2 but not Th1 cells. J Immunol 161(2): 547–551

Zou YR, Kottmann AH, Kuroda M, Taniuchi I, Littman DR (1998) Function of the chemokine receptor CXCR4 in haematopoiesis and in cerebellar development. Nature 393(6685): 595–599

Part 6
Endocrinology

Steroid Receptors

E. F. Greiner[1, 2] · T. Wintermantel[2] · G. Schütz[2]

[1] Life Science Technology, Evotec OAI AG, Schnackenburgallee 114,
22525 Hamburg, Germany
e-mail:erich.greiner@evotecoai.com
[2] Division Molecular Biology of the Cell I, German Cancer Research Center,
Im Neuenheimer Feld 280, 69120 Heidelberg, Germany

Abstract Steroids are lipophilic hormones and regulate multiple functions in development, physiology, and reproduction by binding to their cognate receptors. Steroid receptors are intracellular proteins that transduce biological signals into direct transcriptional responses. Because of both the lipophilic nature of the steroid signal and the immediacy of the signal transmission, steroid receptors make ideal drug targets. Sex steroid receptors (estrogen receptor, progesterone receptor, androgen receptor) have shown to be dispensable for mammalian development and survival. The fact that estrogen, progesterone, and androgen receptor knockout mice survive until adulthood has made these mouse models versatile tools for pharmacological studies in vivo. Corticosteroid receptors (glucocorticoid and mineralocorticoid receptor) have been shown to be essential for survival by early lethality of the respective knockout mouse models. Conditional gene targeting strategies for generating, restricting, and refining mutations in mice facilitate analysis of glucocorticoid and mineralocorticoid receptor functions in later development and adult physiology. For instance, allelic series of glucocorticoid receptor mutants with a wide range of cell-specific and function-selective defects allow dissecting glucocorticoid receptor functions in mice. For steroid pharmacology, these mouse models provide an unprecedented resource to understand drug action and drug target functions in vivo.

Keywords Steroid receptors · Androgen · Estrogen · Glucocorticoid · Mineralocorticoid · Progesterone · Mutation · Germline · Conditional · Allelic series

1
Steroids and Steroid Receptors

Steroids are lipophilic hormones. Because they diffuse from their synthesis site and permeate to their target, steroids are ideal regulators for integrating multiple signals throughout the organism. Steroid hormone-based therapeutics including glucocorticoids, mineralocorticoids, and sex steroids have been discovered to be important drugs with a range of diverse medical applications including treatment of cancer, cardiovascular disease, skin disorders, bone and joint disorders, inflammation, asthma therapy and contraception. In 2002, steroid-based therapeutics constituted about 20% of all prescription drugs and generated more than US $20 billion in sales.

Steroid receptors are intracellular proteins and act as signal-dependent transcription factors. By binding to small lipophilic ligands they transduce biological signals into direct transcriptional responses (Laudet and Gronemeyer 2001). Because steroid receptors are ideal drug targets, but limited in numbers, in-depth molecular understanding of specific receptor functions in vivo is the ultimate prerequisite for developing novel and better therapeutics.

1.1
Modular Structure and Function of Steroid Receptors

Molecular cloning and structure/function analyses revealed that steroid receptors are structurally related and display a common modular organization with several functional domains. This includes a variable amino-terminal (A/B) domain with an autonomous activation function AF-1 important for transactivation of transcription; a well conserved DNA-binding (C) domain, crucial for recognition of specific DNA-responsive elements and protein–protein interactions; and a complex carboxy-terminal end (D/E/F domains), including signals for nuclear localization, a ligand-binding domain (LBD), important for hormone binding and protein–protein interactions, and a ligand-dependent activation function AF-2 (Laudet and Gronemeyer 2001).

Although the structure of some independently expressed single domains of a few of these receptors have been solved, no holoreceptor structure or structure of any two domains together is yet available. Thus, the three-dimensional structure of the DNA-binding domains (DBDs) of the glucocorticoid and the estrogen receptors, and of the LBDs of estrogen, glucocorticoid, and progesterone receptors has been solved. The structural studies available provide a basis for understanding some of the topological details of the interaction of the receptor complexes with DNA-responsive elements, agonists, antagonists, coactivators, and corepressors. Therefore, receptor protein structures can guide the design of function-selective mutations (Brzozowski et al. 1997; Bledsoe et al. 2002; Bredenberg and Nilsson 2002; Shiau et al. 2002).

1.1.1
Amino-Terminal (A/B) Domain

The aminoterminal A/B domains with up to 550 amino acids in length harbor autonomous activation functions (AF-1) in steroid receptors. These regions are subject to alternative splicing and differential promoter usage. Phosphorylation and other posttranslational events are reported to modify the A/B domain and impinge on both, the transactivation potential of the autonomous activation function AF-1 and the intramolecular interaction with the ligand-dependent activation function AF-2 (Laudet and Gronemeyer 2001).

1.1.2
DNA Binding Domain (C) and Steroid Hormone Receptor Response Elements

Steroid receptors recognize bipartite palindromic target sequences (hormone-responsive elements, HREs) composed of six base pair half-sites. There are two canonical types of half-sites, which differ only in their central two base pairs (Laudet and Gronemeyer 2001).

Crystal and nuclear magnetic resonance (NMR)-derived structures of the steroid receptor DBDs include nine conserved cysteine residues, which have been shown to coordinate two zinc ions. Zinc has been shown to be required for the structural integrity and DNA-binding ability of the steroid receptor DBD (Freedman et al. 1988). The family of steroid/nuclear receptors, with their related DNA-binding sites, has specific determinants for DNA sequence recognition. A segment close to the aminoterminal zinc ion, the so-called P-box, has been shown to be responsible for target specificity of glucocorticoid and estrogen receptors by recognizing the actual core of the HREs. Protein–protein interactions facilitate dimeric DNA binding and a segment responsible for these interactions has been identified close to the C-terminal zinc-binding site, the so-called D-box, a loop region for dimerization with significant flexibility. The DNA-induced dimer fixes the separation of the subunits' recognition surfaces so that the spacing between the half-sites becomes a critical feature of the target sequence's identity (Luisi et al. 1991).

1.1.3
Ligand Binding

Steroid-induced changes in receptor protein conformation constitute a logical means of translating the variations in steroid structures into the observed array of whole-cell biological activities. Ligands for steroid receptors are small hydrophobic molecules. Structural studies have shown that hydrophobicity plays an important role not only in the physiological diffusion (and, consequently, signal transmission) processes, but also in the mechanism of receptor binding and function. The LBD of steroid hormone receptors is a 12 α-helical structure with a hydrophobic core, and the steroid ligand is deeply immersed in that core. Ligand binding is a key step in the mechanism of action of hormones, since it induces conformational modifications which modulate AF-2 and enable interactions with coactivators. X-ray crystallographic analyses of apo- and ligand-bound receptors have led to a "mousetrap" model, in which the ligand-binding pocket is accessible in the apo-receptor, and closes upon ligand binding. Helix 12 of the LBD folds back toward the core of the protein and snaps over the opening of the pocket, leading to a more compact structure and a novel interaction surface. This relocation creates a new structure on the surface of the LBD, providing a binding site for coactivators (Laudet and Gronemeyer 2001).

Various ligand-binding domain crystal structures of the estrogen receptor α revealed at the atomic level how natural or synthetic agonists and antagonists can promote recruitment of co-activator and co-repressor proteins (Brzozowski et al. 1997; Shang and Brown 2002; Shiau et al. 2002). Interestingly, it was recently shown that nucleotide polymorphisms located in steroid receptor LBDs could alter or even reverse the response of the receptors to small molecule ligands (Geller et al. 2000; Robin-Jagerschmidt et al. 2000; Matias et al. 2002).

1.2
Molecular Mechanisms of Transcriptional Regulation

Steroid hormone receptors constitute a broad platform for integration of multiple signals for transcriptional regulation. Orchestrated DNA–protein, protein–protein interactions, chromatin and histone modification are regulated precisely in time and space as exemplified for the estrogen receptor (Shang et al. 2000; Shang and Brown 2002).

Full transcriptional activation by steroid hormone receptors requires functional synergy between two transcriptional activation domains (AF) located in the amino (AF-1) and carboxyl (AF-2) terminal regions. Cell- and promoter-specific transcription activation by steroid receptors has been shown to be dependent on the differential action of the N- and C-terminal transcription activation functions AF-1 and AF-2, respectively (Lees et al. 1989; Jacq et al. 1994; Metzger et al. 1995; Parker 1998).

1.3
Non-genomic Steroid Effects

Several rapid actions of steroid ligands have been described which do not require transcriptional activation (Rae et al. 1998; Hinz and Hirschelmann 2000; Simoncini et al. 2000; Harvey et al. 2002). These effects do not require nuclear or transcriptional events to occur, are independent from modulating gene expression, and for this reason are defined as "non-genomic" (n.b., non-genomic effects of steroid hormones should not be mistaken for non-DNA binding-dependent signaling of steroid hormone receptors). Non-genomic effects are characterized by a rapid response (seconds/minute) and insensitivity to inhibitors of gene transcription and protein synthesis. There is a growing body of evidence that at least some of these effects are mediated by the respective steroid hormone receptor localized to the cytoplasm or cell membrane. On the other hand, binding sites other than and unrelated to the classical receptors have been described, e.g., ion channel subunits for estrogen, that also could mediate some of the rapid effects of steroids (Dick et al. 2001). Mouse models deficient for steroid receptor genes are invaluable tools to define and dissect receptor-mediated, non-genomic actions of steroids.

1.4
Gene Structure

The modular structure of the steroid hormone receptor protein is paralleled by the genomic structure of the locus encoding it: In most steroid hormone receptor genes, the translation start codon ATG resides on the second transcribed exon, which also encodes for AF-1. The DNA binding domain is encoded by the following two exons, one coding for one Zn-finger structure. The remaining exons code for the hinge- and ligand-binding domain.

This genomic organization has important consequences for gene-targeting experiments. In early knockout approaches (Lubahn et al. 1993; Cole et al. 1995) the first coding exon was targeted, destroying the ATG, but leaving intact all coding sequences for the DBD and the LBD. Physiological splice variants omitting this exon [as described for the estrogen receptor (Kos et al. 2002a,b)] will not be knocked out by this gene targeting strategy. For the glucocorticoid receptor knockout initially published, it has been shown that this gene targeting approach does not result in a complete inactivation, as some mice homozygous for this allele survive. If the glucocorticoid receptor gene is inactivated by removal of exon 3, thereby destroying the genomic information for the DBD and the open reading frame of possible splice variants, the allele is lethal with 100% penetrance (Tronche et al. 1998). Recent evidence suggests also that some activity of the estrogen receptor α (ERα) is retained in the classical ER knockout (ERKO) (Pendaries et al. 2002).

1.5
Steroid Hormone Receptor Genetics

Steroid hormones regulate body functions to which a multitude of organs and cell types contributes. Steroids are lipophilic hormones, which diffuse from their source and permeate to their targets. To this end, steroid hormones and their receptors are always embedded in regulatory circuits.

Mouse models could open avenues to innovative therapeutic strategies for human diseases, specific medical applications and drug development at various stages. First, mouse models could serve for pharmacological studies. Second, mouse models could guide the discovery and development process of function-selective and tissue-specific drugs based on in-depth understanding of drug targets in vivo.

Sex steroid receptors (estrogen receptor, progesterone receptor, androgen receptor) have shown to be dispensable for mammalian development and survival. The fact that estrogen, progesterone, and androgen receptor knockout mice survive until adulthood has made these animal models versatile tools for pharmacological investigations in vivo. For instance, using the knockout mouse models for estrogen receptors α and β, it has been possible to experimentally isolate the biological effects of estradiol that are dependent upon the presence of estrogen receptor α, as opposed to those in which estrogen receptor β is an essential mediator or as opposed to receptor-independent actions of estradiol. The key role for sex steroids as regulators of reproduction is underlined by the infertility of most of these models. Care has to be taken in the interpretation of these infertility phenotypes, as both organ function on a cellular level and neuroendocrine regulation of reproductive organs are severely affected by receptor deletions. Furthermore, in both the estrogen receptor α and the progesterone receptor knockout models, all female reproductive and accessory sex organs show striking phenotypic aberrations, which at least in part are interdependent. The primary cellular target of steroid hormone receptor action has yet to be determined in these cases.

The receptors for adrenal steroids (glucocorticoid and mineralocorticoid receptor) have been shown to be essential for survival by the lethality of the respective knockout models. Knocking out these genes results in early lethal phenotypes, reflecting the non-redundant role of the genes, and precludes an analysis of its function in later development.

Both null-mutations of corticosteroid and sex steroid receptors perturb neuroendocrine and/or endocrine feed-back loops. Conventional knockout models, although powerful, do not allow for the generating of spatially and temporally restricted and function-selective mutations. It is therefore highly desirable to develop mouse mutants which have more refined mutations in the gene of interest, thus limiting the effect of the mutation to a specific organ or a specific cell type, but which allow the dissection of cell-autonomous, cell-non-autonomous, or systemic effects in the whole animal. The advances in mouse molecular genetics have allowed enormous progress in the analysis of the function of steroid receptors (Gu et al. 1994; Tronche et al. 1998; Reichardt et al. 1999). By exploiting the Cre/loxP recombination system, it has become possible to generate cell- and organ-specific mutations as well as function-selective alterations (Gu et al. 1994). The generation of somatic mutations will not only bypass the lethality of mutant mice, but will also allow to analyze functions of the GR in a particular cell or tissue and to estimate to which extent this function contributes to the physiology of the organism. Furthermore, it might be of great interest to selectively alter a particular function, for example crippling the activating functions of the receptor, but retaining its inhibitory activity as achieved for the glucocorticoid receptor.

2
Estrogen Receptor α (NR3A1) and β (NR3A2)

Estrogenic responses are now known to be mediated by two forms of estrogen receptors (ER), ERα and ERβ, encoded by two genes. They can function both as homodimers or heterodimers. Homodimers have been recently shown to exhibit distinct transcriptional responses to estradiol, antiestrogens, and coactivators, suggesting that the ER complexes are not functionally equivalent. The existence of a second estrogen receptor gene and the dimerization of ERα and β add greater levels of complexity to transcription activation in response to estrogens.

2.1
αERKO: Germline Deletion of the Estrogen Receptor α Gene

Differences have been observed between the original αERKO^{neo}, consisting in the introduction of a neomycin cassette in exon 2 (Lubahn et al. 1993), and a recently generated null allele, in which exon 3 of the ERα has been removed (αERKO$^{\Delta 3}$) (Dupont et al. 2000). In the following, both knockout models are referred to as αERKO, but will be distinguished when differences between αERKO^{neo} and αERKO$^{\Delta 3}$ have been reported, i.e., in smooth muscle and the cardiovascular system.

In some studies, residual ERα activity was observed in αERKO^{neo} mice. These data also imply that in previously published experiments using the αERKO^{neo} mice, some of the conclusions drawn on whether or not ERα regulates specific functions may be premature (Pendaries et al. 2002).

The effect of loss of ERα on the reproductive system, however, was found to be identical in both knockout models. αERKO females are infertile.

2.1.1
Reproductive Phenotypes of ERKO Models

Estrogen has many roles in reproduction, ERs are found in the highest levels in female tissues critical to reproduction, including the ovaries, uterus, cervix, mammary glands, and pituitary gland. The generation of the αERKO mice has further illustrated its roles and mechanisms. Interestingly, both sexes of the αERKO mice are infertile. In the male αERKO mice, infertility is due to deficits at several points in the reproductive process, including severe reduction in sperm count and lack of sperm function, as well as abnormal sexual behavior. The seminiferous tubules of the αERKO testes show progressive dilation that is accompanied by degeneration of the epithelium (Korach et al. 1996; Couse and Korach 1999).

2.1.2
Ovarian Dysfunction and Neuroendocrinology in the ERKO Mouse

The hallmark phenotype of the αERKO female is the enlarged hemorrhagic cystic ovary, although the prepubertal αERKO ovary looks similar to its wildtype littermate. This phenotype begins to develop progressively as the animal matures and is apparently due to a lack of estradiol feedback inhibition in the pituitary, which results in chronically elevated luteinizing hormone (LH) and subsequent hyperstimulation of the ovary. This indicates that ERα is responsible for mediating the LH feedback inhibition in the hypothalamic–pituitary axis. The constant LH stimulation in the αERKO mice results in an abnormal endocrine environment in the αERKO female, with elevated estradiol and testosterone, and chronic preovulatory basal progesterone levels (Couse and Korach 1999).

The central role of neuroendocrine regulation in the development of the αERKO ovarian phenotype has been shown by a partial rescue of αERKO females using a gonadotropin-releasing hormone (GnRH) antagonist that suppresses LH signaling. Under this treatment, cysts and hemorrhages do not develop (Couse et al. 1999).

2.1.3
Uterine Phenotype: Evidence for Cross-talk with Growth Factor Signaling Pathways

Normally, the female rodent reproductive tract grows and matures in response to cycling ovarian hormones, including estradiol. The growth and maturation of the epithelial portion and the preparation of the stromal layer in the uterus is thought to be important for successful implantation and pregnancy to occur. The infertility of the female αERKO mouse is due in part to the insensitivity of the uterus to the mitogenic and differentiative actions of estrogen.

The uterus in the αERKO knockout female is formed normally, as all cell types and layers (endometrium, stroma, myometrium) are present at birth. However, in the αERKO mouse, the uterus remains immature and hypoplastic. Estrogen treatment leads to hyperemia and increased water imbibition, followed by DNA synthesis and cell proliferation in wildtype mice. In the αERKO mouse, the uterus is resistant to these growth-promoting effects of estrogens (Couse and Korach 1999).

In these uterine growth processes, paracrine growth factors have long been known to play an important role. Transgenic and knockout models have revealed an intriguing cross-talk between the protein kinase signaling pathways triggered by peptide hormones and steroid receptors (Kato et al. 1995). The cross-talk mechanism has been described for the ERα and the epidermal growth factor (EGF)-signaling pathway. The αERKO mouse reveals that estrogen-like effects of EGF require the ERα in vivo. Induction of DNA synthesis and the target gene, progesterone receptor, however, were abolished in αERKO mice, confirming that the estrogen-like effects of EGF in the mouse uterus do require the ER. Biochemical studies indicate that the EGF receptor is present and the pathway is functional in the αERKO mouse, as EGF induced c-fos, an EGF-responsive gene (Curtis et al. 1996). In addition, studies of transgenic reporter mice carrying an estrogen response element (ERE)-dependent luciferase gene demonstrated that IGF1 can activate ER-dependent transcription in vivo (Klotz et al. 2002)

2.1.4
Mammary Gland: Systemic and Local Control of Growth

Estrogen and progesterone, in concert with pituitary factors, regulate mammary gland growth and development in virgin, pregnant lactating female mice. Furthermore, estrogen exposure is an important risk factor for breast cancer. A role for ERα is illustrated by the lack of pubertal growth of the epithelial ductal rudiment in the αERKO female despite elevated circulating serum estradiol levels. This striking lack of any development has been shown to result from a combination of systemic and local defects in the αERKO^{neo} knockout mouse (Bocchinfuso et al. 2000). Breast-specific estrogen receptor α knockout models will address this open issue (Wintermantel et al. 2002).

2.1.5
Cardiovascular Tissue: Is the Original αERKO a Hypomorph Allele?

A role for estrogen in the cardiovascular system has also been implied by clinical observations correlating hormonal status with cardiovascular disease risk factors. Additionally, ER has been detected in the vasculature. In the αERKO^{neo} male heart, an increased number of calcium channels and an associated delay in cardiac depolarization have been observed (Couse and Korach 1999). In the αERKO^{neo} vasculature, lower basal nitric oxide activity is detected and, interestingly, the ability of estrogen to play a protective role in a vascular injury model is not lost in the αERKO^{neo} mice (Iafrati et al. 1997). It should not, from these data, be concluded that there is no function for ERα in mediating these estrogen effects: In ovariectomized ERα wildtype mice, estradiol increases both uterine weight and basal production of endothelial nitric oxide (NO). Both of these effects are abolished in αERKO$^{\Delta 3}$ mice. In contrast, both of these effects of estradiol are partially (uterine weight) or totally (endothelial NO production) preserved in αERKO^{neo}. The presence of two ERα mRNA splice variants in uterus and aorta from αERKO^{neo} mice probably explains the persistence of the estradiol effects in αERKO^{neo} mice (Pendaries et al. 2002). Therefore, some of the conclusions drawn from observations in the vascular system of αERKO^{neo} mice may be subject to reevaluation.

2.1.6
Bone Tissue

Clinical as well as experimental data imply a role for estrogen as well as other endocrine factors in maintaining bone mass. For example, menopause or castration increases the rate of osteoporosis progression in women. The ERKO model is a very useful tool for elucidating the mechanism of estrogen effects in bone and whether these effects are mediated, directly or indirectly, through ERs. ERα is present at very low levels in bone cells. In the αERKO female, the bone is normal in terms of density, but it is significantly shorter and smaller in diameter in both sexes of the αERKO mice. This indicates the possibility of a role for estrogen in bone lengthening. αERKO mice have IGF-1 levels 30% lower than normal mice, which might account for the shorter bone. The altered hormonal environment (elevated estradiol and testosterone) as well as the increased body weight of the αERKO mouse should also be considered when interpreting this phenotype. The αERKO males do show a decrease in bone mineral density, a phenotype that is similar to one clinical case of estrogen insensitivity in a man (Korach et al. 1996; Couse and Korach 1999).

2.2
βERKO and DERKO: Germline Mutation of the Estrogen Receptor β Gene and Compound Knockouts of Both Estrogen Receptors Genes

ERβ cloned in 1996 is highly homologous to the "classical" ERα. ERβ binds estrogens with an affinity similar to that of ERα, and activates expression of reporter genes containing estrogen response elements in an estrogen-dependent manner (Kuiper et al. 1996). ERβ seems only to regulate a subset of estrogen effects in the organism. The functions of estrogen receptors in mouse ovary and genital tracts were investigated by generating null mutants for ERα(αERKO), ERβ (βERKO), and both ERs (DERKO). Although the expression pattern of ERβ suggested a role for this molecule in reproductive physiology, both male and female mice deficient in ERβ (βERKOs) are fertile, and females have normal mammary gland development. βERKO females display impaired fertility/subfertility, but a key role in mediating estrogen effects on the reproductive system could not be attributed to ERβ (Krege et al. 1998).

2.2.1
Reproductive Phenotype of βERKO and DERKO Mutant Mice

The βERKO ovaries produce normal serum levels of estradiol and testosterone, and the circulating serum gonadotropin levels are also normal. However, the βERKO ovaries function suboptimally, with numerous unruptured follicles following superovulation appearing. Attempts to superovulate the βERKO female have resulted in some ovulation, but the number of oocytes released is reduced compared with wildtype females. A role for ERβ in ovulation is thus indicated, but the mechanism is still not defined (Krege et al. 1998). Interestingly, although both ERα and ERβ are detected in the ovary, their localization differs with ERβ in the granulosa cells and ER α in the theca and interstitial cells of the ovary. The differential expression of these receptors makes compensatory activity of one receptor in the absence of the other unlikely (Korach 2000).

In the female reproductive system, DERKO mice display similar phenotypic alterations compared to αERKO, thereby confirming the essential role of ERα. However, partial transdifferentiation of female ovarian follicles into male tubuli could only be observed in DERKO, but neither in αERKO nor βERKO mice (Couse et al. 1999).

2.2.2
Cardiovascular Tissue

Estradiol has been recognized to exert several vasculoprotective effects in several species. With the use of αERKO, βERKO, and DERKO mice, it has been possible to define the roles of the respective receptors in mediating estrogen effects on the vessel wall: Basal NO production was increased and the sensitivity to acetylcholine decreased in ERβ knockout mice in response to estradiol. In αERKO (αERKO$^{\Delta3}$) mice this effect was abolished. Thus, ERα, but not ERβ, mediates the beneficial effect of estradiol on basal NO production (Darblade et al. 2002). Upon ovariectomy, estradiol accelerated reendothelialization in wildtype and female βERKO mice, whereas this effect was abolished in female αERKO (αERKO$^{\Delta3}$) mice. This study demonstrates that ERα but not ERβ mediates the beneficial effect of estradiol on reendothelialization and potentially the prevention of atherosclerosis (Brouchet et al. 2001). In contrast, an essential role for ERβ in mediating estrogen's effects on vascular smooth muscle cells has been suggested by Zhu et al. (2002). Vascular smooth muscle cells and blood vessels from βERKO mice exhibit multiple functional abnormalities. In wildtype mouse blood vessels, estrogen attenuates vasoconstriction by an ERβ-mediated increase in inducible NO synthase expression. In blood vessels from βERKO mice, estrogen augments vasoconstriction. Vascular smooth muscle cells isolated from βERKO mice show multiple abnormalities of ion channel function. βERKO mice develop sustained systolic and diastolic hypertension as they age. According to this report, estrogens modulate the regulation of vascular function and blood pressure by βER.

2.2.3
Bone Tissue

Evaluation of the bones of the βERKO mouse shows no apparent difference from the wild type (unpublished data), indicating the lack of a major role for ERβ in bone physiology. αERKO and DERKO, but not βERKO, demonstrated decreased longitudinal as well as radial skeletal growth associated with decreased serum levels of IGF-1. ERα, but not ERβ, mediates important effects of estrogen in the skeleton of male mice during growth and maturation (Vidal et al. 2000).

2.3
ERα^{floxed}: Conditional Somatic Mutations of the Estrogen Receptor α Gene

Conditional alleles for ERα have been generated in two independent groups and will be exploited for studying tissue-specific functions of ERα (Dupont et al. 2000; Wintermantel et al. 2002).

2.4
Function-Selective Mutations of the Estrogen Receptor α

In the classical signaling pathway, the ER binds directly to EREs to regulate gene transcription. In addition to this classical pathway of estrogen action, the ER can also alter gene transcription by a mechanism that does not require direct ER binding to an ERE. Instead, protein–protein interactions between the ER and other transcription factors, such as Sp1, Jun, or nuclear factor (NF)-κB, lead to changes in target gene transcription including low-density lipoprotein receptor, lipoprotein lipase, collagenase, IGF-1, and interleukin (IL)-6. ER action through the activator protein (AP)-1 response element involves interactions with other promoter-bound proteins instead of, or in addition to, direct binding to DNA. Interactions with coactivators were required for both pathways. ER-mediated transcriptional activation or repression is dependent on the ligand and the nature of the response element in the target gene (Jakacka et al. 2001; Shang and Brown 2002). Many of the nonclassical pathway target genes are paradoxically stimulated by ER antagonists, raising the possibility that selective estrogen receptor modulators may act as agonists through the nonclassical pathway (Paech et al. 1997).

An estrogen receptor knock-in mouse model was generated by introducing a mutation (E207A/G208A) into the P box of the first zinc finger of the DBD-encoded by exon 3 to selectively eliminate classical ER signaling through EREs, while preserving the nonclassical ER pathway. The E207A/G208A mutant is inactive in the classical pathway. In the nonclassical pathway, the ER ligands exhibit effects that are the opposite of those seen in the classical pathway: E2 represses transcription, and ICI 182,780 activates transcription on an AP-1 reporter gene. Heterozygous females are infertile due to anovulation and the occurrence of endometrial hyperplasia, but the mutation should not confer a dominant-negative effect. The presence of such a strong phenotype in the heterozygous state confirms the role of nonclassical ER signaling in vivo and suggests that these features may be caused by dysregulation of classical and nonclassical signaling (Jakacka et al. 2002).

2.5
Estradiol-Responsive Reporter Mice

In addition to their well-known control of reproductive functions, estrogens modulate important physiological processes. The identification of compounds with tissue-selective activity could lead to new drugs mimicking the beneficial effects of estrogen on the prevention of osteoporosis and cardiovascular or neurodegenerative diseases, while avoiding its detrimental proliferative effects. ER reporter mice provide systems to measure estrogenic activity in different target tissues and to study ER-mediated estrogen pharmacology in vivo. Two different reporter mouse models have been established: ERE-TK β-galactosidase (ERIN) mice with an estrogen-responsive promoter (three copies of the vitellogenin ERE with a minimal thymidine kinase promoter) linked to the reporter gene beta-galactosidase (Nagel et al. 2001) and ERE luciferase mice with a luciferase reporter gene driven by a dimerized ERE, a minimal promoter, and flanking insulator sequences (Ciana et al. 2001; Ciana et al. 2002). They could assist in in vivo identification of new selective estrogen receptor modulators (SERMs) in defining the cellular and molecular mechanisms that determine agonist and antagonist activity, but clearly cannot reflect the combinatorial nature and the complexity of the naturally occurring ER-dependent promoters (Shang et al. 2000; Shang and Brown 2002).

3
Glucocorticoid Receptor (NR3C1)

Glucocorticoids are synthesized in the adrenal cortex and regulate multiple organ functions including carbohydrate and lipid metabolism, the stress response, and control of innate and acquired immunity, and modulation of behavior. Glucocorticoids induce the synthesis of gluconeogenic enzymes in liver, thereby increasing glucose synthesis and blood glucose levels. Glucocorticoids promote maturation of the lung and differentiation of erythroid progenitors. Glucocorticoids exert potent anti-inflammatory and immunosuppressive effects. Glucocorticoids can induce apoptosis of thymocytes. Glucocorticoid production in the adrenal gland is tightly controlled by a feedback mechanism involving the hypothalamus and the pituitary gland, the hypothalamic–pituitary–adrenal (HPA) axis. Repression of corticotropin-releasing hormone (CRH) and adrenocorticotropic hormone (ACTH) at the level of both transcription and secretion results from increased glucocorticoid levels. Glucocorticoids are released in response to stress, a protective mechanism that prepares the organism to react to threatening stimuli. They activate the HPA axis, which coordinates behavioral and physiological responses. Chronic dysregulation of the HPA axis leads to pathological consequences including depression- and anxiety-related disorders.

The glucocorticoid receptor (GR) mediates the effects of glucocorticoids by positively or negatively modulating gene transcription. Transcription regulation by the GR is achieved by both DNA binding-dependent and independent mechanisms (Beato et al. 1995). Binding to so-called negative GREs (nGRE) which have been found in several genes that are negatively regulated by glucocorticoids has also been described (Drouin et al. 1993).

3.1
GRKO: Germline Deletion of the Glucocorticoid Receptor Gene

Two GR-inactivating mutations have been generated: a hypomorphic allele which resulted from insertion of a neomycin resistance cassette right after the ATG start codon of the receptor coding sequence (Cole et al. 1995) and a null allele which has been generated by excision of exon 3 (Tronche et al. 1998). In the former case, alternative splicing leads to a truncated mRNA and the synthesis of a shortened protein. Deletion of exon 3 results in a complete ablation of the GR, shows complete penetrance, and a more severe phenotype in comparison to mice with hypomorphic GR alleles. Mice without functional GR die shortly after birth and suffer from atelectasis of the lungs, thereby demonstrating an essential function of the receptor in survival. Perinatal induction of gluconeogenic enzymes in the liver is impaired. Regulation of the glucocorticoid synthesis via the HPA axis is perturbed, leading to increased plasma levels of corticosterone and ACTH. Activation of the HPA axis results in extensive hypertrophy and hyperplasia of the cortical zones of the adrenal and induction of genes involved in steroidogenesis (Cole et al. 1995). Thymocytes derived from GRKO mice are resistant to glucocorticoid-dependent apoptosis. Under hypoxic stress conditions, the rapid expansion of GRKO erythroid progenitors is impaired (Bauer et al. 1999).

3.2
GR^{dim}: Dimeric DNA Binding-Deficient Mutation of the Glucocorticoid Receptor

Dimerization-defective GR mutant mice were generated to study DNA binding-independent mechanisms of glucocorticoid receptor action in vivo. By exploiting the Cre-loxP technology, a knock-in mouse model (GR^{dim}) carrying the point mutation A458T in the D-loop of the GR was established (Reichardt et al. 1998). The mutation selectively abolishes homodimeric DNA binding of the receptor and thereby impairs binding of GR to DNA, while regulation of gene activity by protein–protein interaction remains intact. Positive and negative transcriptional activation responses resulting from DNA binding-independent mechanism of the glucocorticoid receptor could be defined. GR^{dim} are viable, indicating that DNA binding of the receptor is not required to guarantee survival of the animals. DNA binding is not required for prevention of the atelectatic lung phenotype. Important anti-inflammatory activities of the receptor are maintained in this animal model. Inhibition of cytokine synthesis following treatment with lipopolysaccharide (LPS) of thymocytes and macrophages derived from GR^{dim} could be achieved by glucocorticoids. Glucocorticoids repress the pro-inflammatory activity of NF-κB even when the receptor is impaired for DNA binding (Reichardt et al. 2001). Systemic and local inflammatory responses could be repressed by glucocorticoids in GR^{dim}. GR^{dim} mice represent a very useful model to determine the contribution of protein–protein interactions between GR and other transcription factors in anti-inflammatory responses in vivo. Many of the side effects of glucocorticoids like osteoporosis and steroid-induced diabetes are mediated by DNA binding-dependent activities of the receptor. Selective glucocorticoid receptor modulators preventing receptor dimerization and DNA binding can be expected to reduce osteoporotic and/or diabetogenic side effects, but to display full anti-inflammatory potential.

GR^{dim} mice also represent a tool to study control mechanisms in the HPA axis with respect to the steroid synthesis feedback loop. In the hypothalamus, CRH levels do not differ in wildtype mice from GR^{dim}, arguing for GR-mediated control of CRH synthesis at the level of protein–protein interaction. Expression of the ACTH precursor gene pro-opiomelanocortin (POMC) is elevated by almost an order of magnitude demonstrating loss of negative control of POMC transcription in GR^{dim} mice (Reichardt et al. 1998).

3.3
GR^{floxed}: Conditional Somatic Mutations of the Glucocorticoid Receptor Gene

Since mice without a functional GR are not viable and die shortly after birth, cell-/tissue-specific mutations have been developed to analyze organ-/cell-specific functions of GR. To analyze the functions of GR in various cells/tissues, exon 3 of the receptor gene was flanked by two loxP sites using homologous recombination in embryonic stem cells (Tronche et al. 1998). Expression of Cre recombinase directs the specific mutation to the desired cells or tissues. The penetrance of the somatic mutation depends on the expression pattern of the recombinase. Yeast and bacterial artificial chromosomes have been employed to guarantee the desired expression selectivity and to minimize mosaic expression.

3.3.1
Corticosteroid Receptor Function in Brain

Deletion of GR in neuronal precursor cells and consequently in the entire nervous system was achieved by expressing the Cre recombinase under the control of the nestin promoter (GR^{NesCre}) (Tronche et al. 1999). Lack of the GR in the nervous system is not lethal, but profoundly alters the HPA axis equilibrium. GR^{NesCre} mice allow the discrimination between receptor functions in the hypothalamus and the anterior lobe of the pituitary, since the nestin promoter does not lead to expression of the Cre recombinase in this part of the pituitary. GR^{NesCre} mice lack the central glucocorticoid feedback in the nucleus paraventricularis of the hypothalamus, thereby releasing the inhibition of CRH production. In consequence, POMC mRNA and ACTH immunoreactivity increased in corticotroph cells of GR^{NesCre} mice. GR-mediated repression of POMC gene activity in the pituitary is not sufficient to counterbalance the increased levels of CRH caused by the hypothalamic GR ablation.

Inactivation of the GR in the nervous system reduces anxiety-related behavior. GR^{NesCre} mice are less anxious in the elevated zero maze and the dark-light box, two tasks which are exploiting the behavioral conflict between exploring and avoiding an aversive compartment. The reduced anxiety-related responses reveal an important role of GR signaling in emotional behavior (Tronche et al. 1999).

Detailed characterization of mice carrying highly defined mutations in the nervous system will provide a better understanding of the role of these receptors in the development of psychiatric diseases such as depression and anxiety disorders. Primary action of antidepressants could be the stimulation of corticosteroid receptor gene expression that renders the HPA system more susceptible to feedback inhibition by cortisol. Brain-specific GR knockout mouse models open up new insight into antidepressant drug action and suggest a line of approach to the development of new drugs by focusing on this action.

Brain functions leading to drug addiction are modulated by the glucocorticoid signaling system (Sillaber et al. 2002). In this context, the observation of loss of sensitization after cocaine treatment in brain-specific GRKO mice is extremely stimulating (F. Tronche, unpublished). An important role for GR in control of circadian timing was recently established, since glucocorticoids are able to phase shift peripheral oscillators in animals (Balsalobre et al. 2000).

3.3.2
Corticosteroid Receptor Function in Liver:
The Glucocorticoid Receptor's Important Function in Postnatal Body Growth

Hepatocyte-specific deletion of the GR ($GR^{AlfpCre}$) was achieved by employing gene regulatory sequences of the albumin gene for controlling the expression of the Cre recombinase in liver (Kellendonk et al. 2000). Mice with a hepatocyte-specific GR mutation displayed a severe growth deficit after 4 weeks. Alterations in serum glucocorticoid and growth hormone levels could not be detected; the growth deficit seems to reside in hepatic growth hormone receptor signaling. Growth hormone can affect growth through stimulation of IGF-1 by activating the transcription factor signal transducer and activator of transcription 5 (STAT5) (Chow et al. 1996; Metcalf et al. 2000). mRNA levels of IGF-1 and other growth hormone-regulated genes in the liver were drastically reduced in $GR^{AlfpCre}$ mice. Glucocorticoid receptor function in hepatocytes is crucial for body growth. Liver-specific deletion of the GR does not result in altered phosphorylation or expression levels of STAT5α and β, the transducers of growth hormone receptor signaling in liver. Mice with the dimerization-defective mutation are of normal size; the expression of IGF-1 and other growth hormone-regulated genes is unaltered. GR^{dim} mice compared to $GR^{AlfpCre}$ mice provide strong evidence that the growth-promoting activity of the receptor does not require binding to a glucocorticoid-responsive element. GR rather functions as a coactivator for STAT5-mediated transcription in vivo, along the same lines as suggested for GR and STAT5 in prolactin receptor signaling in cell culture (Stocklin et al. 1996).

Comparison of liver-specific mutations and function-selective mutations of the glucocorticoid receptor with wildtype mice demonstrates the potential and power of allelic series for understanding drug target functions in vivo.

3.4
YGR: Yeast Artificial Chromosome Transgenic Mice Overexpressing the Glucocorticoid Receptor

Transgenic GR-overexpressing mice (YGR) were generated by adding copies of the GR gene embedded in a 290-kb yeast artificial chromosome. Increased gene dosage of the GR alters the basal regulation of the HPA axis, resulting in reduced expression of both CRH and ACTH and a fourfold reduction in the level of circulating glucocorticoids. Primary thymocytes isolated from YGR mice show an enhanced sensitivity to glucocorticoid-induced apoptosis. When challenged by restraint stress, overexpression of the glucocorticoid receptor leads to a weaker response. Upon LPS-induced endotoxic shock, YGR mice display an increased resistance to the endotoxin. Hence, tight regulation of glucocorticoid receptor expression is important for the control of physiological and pathological processes including the susceptibility to inflammatory diseases or stress (Reichardt et al. 2000).

3.5
Allelic Series of the Glucocorticoid Receptor Gene

3.5.1
Studying Glucocorticoid Receptor-Mediated Anti-inflammatory Activities In Vivo

Cell-specific inactivation in thymocytes, monocytes/macrophages, dendritic cells, mast cells, and eosinophiles and other cellular compartments of the immune system leads to understanding the action and function of the glucocorticoid receptor in inflammation, in innate and acquired immunity. Both mice lacking the receptor in monocytes/macrophages and overexpressing the glucocorticoid receptor reveal an important role for the receptor in the immune response (Reichardt et al. 2000). Mice without a functional receptor in macrophages die within 36 h when challenged by LPS treatment, whereas wildtype mice survived this challenge. In contrast, YGR mice with two additional copies of the receptor showed enhanced resistance to this endotoxic shock paradigm and reduced inflammatory responses.

3.5.2
Dissecting Molecular Mechanisms of Glucocorticoid Receptor Functions In Vivo

Artificial chromosome transgenesis and Cre/loxP technology were instrumental to generate a series of alleles for the glucocorticoid receptor in mouse and to perform a comprehensive molecular genetic analysis of glucocorticoid receptor functions in vivo. Besides tissue-specific functions of the GR, four different modes of selective GR actions could be defined. The receptor is able to activate gene transcription by binding as a dimer to a glucocorticoid response element in the control region of a regulated gene. The receptor inhibits expression of genes such as the POMC gene and the prolactin gene in the anterior pituitary by binding to so-called negative GREs in the control regions of these genes. Elevated levels of the mRNAs encoding these proteins in mice with the dimerization-defective and thus DNA binding-deficient GR support this hypothesis. GR can modulate target gene activity by DNA binding-independent mechanism. Transcriptional activity of the STAT5 proteins can be enhanced by GR acting as a coactivator in vivo. GR can also inhibit the activity of AP-1- and NF-κB-dependent transcription in vivo, thereby acting as a corepressor.

In general, comparative analyses of allelic series for drug targets are invaluable tools to guide the development of novel function-selective and organ-specific therapeutics with reduced side effects.

3.6
Transgenic Mice Expressing Glucocorticoid Receptor Antisense RNA

Transgenic mice with impaired glucocorticoid receptor (GR) function were produced by partially knocking down GR gene expression with antisense RNA. When treated with increasing doses of dexamethasone, these mice require a tenfold higher dexamethasone dose to induce full suppression of plasma ACTH and corticosterone than normal mice, although the transgenic mice showed basal plasma ACTH and corticosterone levels similar to those of the normal control animals. Exposure to a defective GR, through development, programs major changes in endogenous neuroendocrine and immune mechanisms. These transgenic mice could serve as a model to study the negative feedback disturbance of the HPA system in affective or autoimmune disorders (Marchetti et al. 1994; Stec et al. 1994; Barden 1994; Barden 1999; Marchetti et al. 2001). Through expression of GR antisense RNA in brain, transgenic mice with a hyperactive hypothalamic–pituitary–adrenocortical (HPA) system have been generated. This model supports the hypothesis that disturbed corticosteroid receptor regulation could lead to increased activity of the HPA system (Barden 1996; Barden et al. 1997)

4
Mineralocorticoid Receptor (NR3C2)

Mineralocorticoids control genes involved in transepithelial sodium transport and thereby regulate sodium and potassium homeostasis and water balance. Aldosterone, the main circulating mineralocorticoid, has a major role in blood-pressure volume regulation in normal subjects, and is thought to be involved in the pathogenesis of hypertension and target-organ damage.

Mineralocorticoids activate selectively the mineralocorticoid receptor (MR, NR3C2), and glucocorticoids are able to activate both receptors—the mineralocorticoid and the glucocorticoid receptor (NR3C1) (Funder et al. 1988; Pearce and Funder 1988). In tissues expressing both receptors, e.g., the brain, glucocorticoids can affect gene expression by signaling through either receptor. Mineralocorticoid-responsive cells such as the principal cells of the collecting duct in kidney express the enzyme 11-beta-hydroxysteroid dehydrogenase 2. Conversion of cortisol to cortisone constitutes a prereceptor control mechanism, protecting the mineralocorticoid receptor from binding glucocorticoids and ensuring mineralocorticoid-specific effects.

4.1
MRKO: Germline Deletion of the Mineralocorticoid Receptor Gene

MR-deficient mice (MRKO) generated by gene targeting undergo a normal prenatal development. During the first week of life, MRKO mice developed symptoms of pseudohypoaldosteronism. At day 8, MRKO mice showed hyperkalemia, hyponatremia, and a strong increase in renin, angiotensin II, and aldosterone plasma concentrations. MRKO mice die mainly at day 9/10 after birth. Weight loss precedes death of homozygous mutant mice and is correlated with an increase in the hematocrit. Plasma levels of renin and aldosterone are elevated. MRKO mice are not able to compensate renal Na^+-loss and water uptake and die 8.5 days after birth because of impaired Na^+-reabsorption that results in severe Na^+ and water loss. Amiloride-sensitive Na^+-reabsorption is reduced in these mice but the abundance of transcripts encoding the Epithelial Sodium Channel (ENaC) and Na^+/K^+-ATPase is unchanged in knockout mice. Control of Na^+ reabsorption is not achieved by transcriptional regulation of ENaC and Na^+/K^+-ATPase but by the transcriptional control of yet unidentified genes (Berger et al. 1996, 1998). Components of the renin–angiotensin–aldosterone system (RAAS) that regulates blood pressure via aldosterone are upregulated in MRKO, presenting a condition of extreme sodium depletion that is never observed in wildtype animals. Renin was the most stimulated component in kidneys and adrenal glands of MRKO mice. Angiotensinogen and AT-I in the liver were also increased, but the other elements of the RAAS are not affected (Hubert et al. 1999).

MRKO mice can be rescued by timely and matched NaCl substitutions. This enables the animals to develop through a critical phase of life, after which they adapt their oral salt and water intake to match the elevated excretion rate; however, the renal salt-losing defect persists (Berger et al. 1998; Bleich et al. 1999).

4.2
MR^floxed: Conditional Somatic Mutations of the Mineralocorticoid Receptor Gene

Mice harboring conditional MR alleles have been generated. Experimental data on genetic dissection of corticosteroid signaling by glucocorticoid receptor and mineralocorticoid receptor in brain will be published in the near future.

4.3
Transgenic Mice Expressing Mineralocorticoid Receptor Antisense RNA

Cardiac failure is a common feature in the evolution of cardiac disease. Among the determinants of cardiac failure, the RAA-system has a central role, and antagonism of the MR has been proposed as a therapeutic strategy. An inducible and cardiac-specific transgenic mouse model was produced to address the role of the MR, not of aldosterone, on heart function. In a conditional knock-down model, an antisense mRNA directed against the MR, a transcription factor with unknown targets in cardiomyocytes was expressed in heart under tetracycline control. Within 2–3 months, mice developed severe heart failure and cardiac fibrosis in the absence of hypertension or chronic hyperaldosteronism. Moreover, cardiac failure and fibrosis were fully reversible when MR antisense mRNA expression was subsequently suppressed (Jaisser 2000; Beggah et al. 2002). This transgenic antisense model cannot be supported by data from rescued MR knockout mice. Cardiac-specific MR knockout mice should clarify this important pharmacological issue.

5
Progesterone Receptor (NR3C3)

Progesterone plays a central coordinating role in diverse reproductive events associated with establishment and maintenance of pregnancy. The progesterone receptor (PR) exists as two functionally distinct isoforms, PR-A and PR-B that arise from the same gene and function as progesterone activated transcription factors. PR-A and PR-B exhibit different transcription regulatory activities and elicit distinct, physiological responses to progesterone. Mouse models have been established for both selective (PRAKO, PRBKO) and compound (PRKO) ablation of PR isoforms (Conneely et al. 2001; Conneely and Jericevic 2002; Conneely et al. 2002). PR-A and PR-B knockout mice allow to discriminate distinct functions of the receptors in progesterone action in vivo. These mouse models could guide the identification of suitable targets for generation of tissue-selective progestins.

5.1
PRKO: Germline Deletion of the Progesterone Receptor

Male and female mice homozygous for the PR mutation (PRKO) developed normally to adulthood. The adult female PRKO displayed significant defects in all reproductive tissues. These included an inability to ovulate, uterine hyperplasia and inflammation, severely limited mammary gland development, and an inability to exhibit sexual behavior.

In PRAKO mice, the PR-B isoform functions in a tissue-specific manner to mediate a subset of the reproductive functions of PRs. Selective ablation of PR-A does not affect responses of the mammary gland or thymus to progesterone but results in severe abnormalities in ovarian and uterine function, leading to female infertility. PR-B could be demonstrated to modulate a subset of reproductive functions of progesterone by regulation of a subset of progesterone-responsive target genes in reproductive tissues. Ablation of PR-B does not affect ovarian, uterine, or thymic responses to progesterone but rather results in reduced mammary ductal morphogenesis. PR-A is both necessary and sufficient to elicit the progesterone-dependent reproductive responses necessary for female fertility, while PR-B is required to elicit normal proliferative responses of the mammary gland to progesterone (Mulac-Jericevic et al. 2000; Conneely et al. 2002).

The PRKO mice exhibit abnormal mammary gland development. The ductal growth accompanying puberty is not compromised in these mice, but lateral ductal branching and lobulo-alveolar growth characteristic of pregnancy do not occur. These animals do not exhibit estrous cycles and fail to become pregnant, so the full extent of the mammary gland defect cannot be studied. By transplanting PRKO breasts into wildtype mice, it was demonstrated that the primary target for progesterone is the mammary epithelium and that the mammary stroma is not required for the progesterone response (Brisken et al. 2000).

Recently, an interesting connection between the progesterone and the Wnt signaling pathways was observed (Robinson et al. 2000). The defect in the mammary gland development observed in PRKO animals can be overcome by ectopic expression of the proto-oncogene Wnt1. In addition, PR and Wnt4, another member of the Wnt family, are coexpressed in the luminal compartment of the ductal epithelium. In accordance with this coexpression, progesterone regulates Wnt4 expression in mammary epithelial cells. Wnt4 has an essential role in side-branching of the mammary ducts early in pregnancy. This new model suggests that progesterone induces Wnt4 production, which in turn induces the branching of mammary ducts during puberty and pregnancy (Brisken et al. 2000)

5.2
Transgenic Mice Overexpressing Progesterone Receptors

Mice with altered ratio of A and B forms of PR have been generated by transgenic overexpression of additional A or B form under the control of the mouse mammary tumor virus (MMTV) promoter. In PR-A transgenic mice, mammary glands exhibit increased ductal branching and hyperplasia (Shyamala et al. 1998). Transgenic mice carrying additional B form of PR also display abnormal mammary development, characterized by limited ductal elongation and branching (Shyamala et al. 2000). PR transgenic mice do not mimic the effects of isoform-selective PR ablation on mammary glands (Conneely et al. 2002). Regulated expression of both PR isoforms seems to be critical for appropriate cellular response to progesterone in mammary gland.

6
Androgen Receptor (NR3C4)

Male sex steroids testosterone and dihydrotestosterone bind and activate the androgen receptor (AR). 17β-Estradiol can also induce AR transactivation in the presence of selective coregulators in selective tissues. Initiation, maintenance, and reinitiation of spermatogenesis are androgen-dependent processes. Besides regulating male sex functions, androgen and AR also play important roles in female physiological processes, including folliculogenesis, bone metabolism, autoimmune diseases, maintenance of brain functions, and several female cancers, including breast, ovary, and endometrium.

For AR, the testicular feminization (Tfm) male mice and the patients with the androgen-insensitive syndrome are the natural models for the study of the loss of androgen function in males. Female models have been lacking, because localization of the AR gene on the X chromosome, which is critical for male fertility, impedes conventional gene targeting strategies. Female ARKO mice and tissue-specific ARKO mice were generated by a Cre-loxP strategy for conditional gene targeting The Cre-lox ARKO mouse provides a model to study androgen functions in the selective androgen target tissues in female or male mice. In addition, androgen actions mediated by AR could be dissociated from effects caused upon aromatase-mediated conversion of androgen to estradiol.

6.1
ARKO: Germline Deletion of the Androgen Receptor Gene

Two AR-null mutant (ARKO) mouse lines were generated from independent groups by means of a Cre-loxP system (Sato et al. 2002; Yeh et al. 2002; Sato et al. 2003). The male ARKO mice generated by Kato's laboratory exhibited typical features of Tfm disease in external reproductive organs with growth retardation. Growth curves of the male ARKO mice do not differ from that of their wildtype female littermates up to 10 weeks of age. Then a drastic increase in growth and development of obesity was observed. Clear increase in the wet weights of white adipose tissues, but not of brown adipose tissue, was found in the 30-week-old male ARKO mice. No significant alteration in serum lipid parameters and food intake could be detected. Thus, AR may serve as a negative regulator of adipose development in adult males.

Male ARKO mice produced by Yeh et al. (2002) have a female-like appearance and body weight. All male sexual organs including penis, vas deferens, epididymis, seminal vesicle, and prostate are hypoplastic or agenic. The scrotum is poorly developed and resembles the female labia major. Testes are small in size and cryptorchid similar to Tfm mice or humans with complete androgen-insensitive syndrome. No vaginal opening and no fallopian tubes or uterus can be found. Testes from ARKO mice are 80% smaller, less cellular, and thin in the tubules. No round spermatids, elongated spermatids, or mature spermatozoa could be detected in ARKO testis. Spermatogenesis is arrested at pachytene spermatocytes. Sertoli cells show fibrillary degeneration and Leydig cells are hypertrophic. Serum testosterone concentration in adult ARKO mice is lower than in wildtype mice.

ARKO male mice have a reduced body weight when compared to that of age-matched wildtype male mice, but it equals the body weight of age-matched wildtype female mice. Number and size of adipocytes differ between wildtype and ARKO mice. Besides these effects on adipogenesis, androgens have been reported to mediate site-specific adipose distribution and metabolism. Brown tissue is developed well and shows no obvious difference between wildtype and ARKO mice.

Bone volumes of ARKO male mice are reduced compared to wildtype littermates. Osteoclast numbers in the femoral metaphyses are higher in ARKO than in wildtype mice. In the absence of the AR, mice develop osteopenia although both mineral apposition and bone formation are increased in ARKO mice. Increased osteoclast numbers cause increased bone resorption and outbalance the increase in bone formation, thereby resulting in an osteopenic phenotype.

Female ARKO mice were fertile, the average number of the pups per litter from heterozygous and homologous ARKO females are reduced as compared to wildtype female mice. Compared to wildtype mice, ARKO mice show no major differences in breast morphology (Yeh et al. 2002).

6.2
AR^floxed: Conditional Somatic Mutations of the Androgen Receptor Gene

Floxed AR mice provide a base to generate tissue-specific ARKO in selective tissues such as bone, breast, skeletal muscle, prostate, and liver. Several laboratories are in the process of generating these tissue-specific ARKO mice to study the roles of AR in these tissues. These mouse models could support the development of tissue-specific androgens and anti-androgens.

6.3
Transgenic Mice Overexpressing the Androgen Receptor

Overexpression of AR in liver and brain of transgenic mice has been reported. Liver is an important target of androgens; mouse liver displays sexually dimorphic and temporally programmed expression of AR causing marked sex-dependent changes in androgen sensitivity. Liver-specific overexpression of AR under the control of the human phenylalanine hydroxylase (hPAH) gene promoter leads to perturbation of the expression of androgen-controlled steroidogenic enzymes. These transgenic mice produce a 30-fold higher level of the AR in the liver as compared to nontransgenic control animals. In the transgenic female, the hepatic expression of the dehydroepiandrosterone sulfotransferase was approximately fourfold lower than in normal females, a level comparable to that of normal males (Chatterjee et al. 1996)

The expansion of trinucleotide repeat sequences underlies a number of hereditary neurological disorders. X-linked spinal and bulbar muscular atrophy (SBMA) is caused by a CAG repeat expansion in the first exon of the androgen receptor (AR) gene encoding the AF-1 function. Disease-associated alleles (37–66 CAGs) change in length when transmitted from parents to offspring. Unlike the disease allele in humans, transgenic mice carrying human AR cDNAs with 45 and 66 CAG repeats do not display repeat instability and show no change in repeat length with transmission. Expression of the SBMA AR was found in transgenic mice, but at a lower level than normal endogenous expression. The lack of a physiological pattern of expression may explain why no phenotypic effects of the transgene were observed (Bingham et al. 1995). Trinucleotide repeat instability was modeled by generating transgenic mice with yeast artificial chromosomes (YACs) carrying AR CAG repeat expansions in their genomic context. Studies of independent lines of AR YAC transgenic mice with CAG 45 alleles reveal intergenerational instability. The 45 CAG repeat tracts are significantly more unstable with maternal transmission and as the transmitting mother ages. Of all the CAG/CTG repeat transgenic mice produced to date, the AR YAC CAG 45 mice are unstable with the smallest trinucleotide repeat mutations (La Spada et al. 1998).

7
Summary

Functional genomic technologies, including artificial chromosome-based transgenesis and conditional gene inactivation, allow us to generate mouse models harboring genes with loss-of-function mutations, gain-of-function mutations, temporal restricted mutations, tissue-specific mutations, and function-selective mutations. Such "allelic series" for drug targets in mouse models provide an unprecedented resource towards understanding drug targets, drug target functions, and therapeutic strategies, and they increase the probability of identifying the optimal target function for therapeutic intervention.

Mouse models provide opportunities for the identification of compounds that regulate steroid receptors in a tissue-specific and function-selective manner. These models will also support the identification of steroid receptor target genes. Mouse models will guide and help to evaluate distinct steroid receptor function for therapeutic intervention and conduct development of drugs specific for distinct functions of steroid receptors exemplified by allelic series for the

- *glucocorticoid receptor.* Function-selective and/or tissue-specific mutations of the glucocorticoid receptor dissect activating and inhibitory functions and in turn will guide the search for dissociated glucocorticoids (selective glucocorticoid response modulators) conferring a desired anti-inflammatory activity without diabetogenic, osteoporotic, or deleterious skin side effects.
- *estrogen receptors.* Tissue-specific and/or function-selective mutations of the estrogen receptors dissociate regulatory mechanisms exerted by estrogens and growth factors. Functional genomics of the estrogen receptor will direct the development of dissociated estrogens (selective estrogen response modulators SERMs) such as bone-specific estrogens that lack activity in reproductive tissue and breast, or cardiovascular protective estrogens without effects on the reproductive system and the breast. Specific efforts will help to understand and exploit the ligand-independent activity of the estrogen receptor.
- *progesterone receptors.* Selective mutations of progesterone receptor isoforms in mice could guide the generation of tissue-selective progestins.

References

Balsalobre, A., Brown, S. A., Marcacci, L., Tronche, F., Kellendonk, C., Reichardt, H. M., Schutz, G., and Schibler, U. (2000) Resetting of circadian time in peripheral tissues by glucocorticoid signaling. Science *289*, 2344–7

Barden, N. (1994) Corticosteroid receptor modulation in transgenic mice. Ann N Y Acad Sci *746*, 89–98; discussion 98–100, 131–3

Barden, N. (1996) Modulation of glucocorticoid receptor gene expression by antidepressant drugs. Pharmacopsychiatry *29*, 12–22

Barden, N. (1999) Regulation of corticosteroid receptor gene expression in depression and antidepressant action. J Psychiatry Neurosci *24*, 25–39

Barden, N., Stec, I. S., Montkowski, A., Holsboer, F., and Reul, J. M. (1997) Endocrine profile and neuroendocrine challenge tests in transgenic mice expressing antisense RNA against the glucocorticoid receptor. Neuroendocrinology *66*, 212–20

Bauer, A., Tronche, F., Wessely, O., Kellendonk, C., Reichardt, H. M., Steinlein, P., Schutz, G., and Beug, H. (1999) The glucocorticoid receptor is required for stress erythropoiesis. Genes Dev *13*, 2996–3002

Beato, M., Herrlich, P., and Schutz, G. (1995) Steroid hormone receptors: many actors in search of a plot. Cell *83*, 851–7

Beggah, A. T., Escoubet, B., Puttini, S., Cailmail, S., Delage, V., Ouvrard-Pascaud, A., Bocchi, B., Peuchmaur, M., Delcayre, C., Farman, N., and Jaisser, F. (2002) Reversible cardiac fibrosis and heart failure induced by conditional expression of an antisense mRNA of the mineralocorticoid receptor in cardiomyocytes. Proc Natl Acad Sci USA 7, 7

Berger, S., Bleich, M., Schmid, W., Cole, T. J., Peters, J., Watanabe, H., Kriz, W., Warth, R., Greger, R., and Schutz, G. (1998) Mineralocorticoid receptor knockout mice: pathophysiology of Na+ metabolism. Proc Natl Acad Sci USA 95, 9424–9

Berger, S., Cole, T. J., Schmid, W., and Schutz, G. (1996) Analysis of glucocorticoid and mineralocorticoid signalling by gene targeting. Endocr Res 22, 641–52

Bingham, P. M., Scott, M. O., Wang, S., McPhaul, M. J., Wilson, E. M., Garbern, J. Y., Merry, D. E., and Fischbeck, K. H. (1995) Stability of an expanded trinucleotide repeat in the androgen receptor gene in transgenic mice. Nat Genet 9, 191–6

Bledsoe, R. K., Montana, V. G., Stanley, T. B., Delves, C. J., Apolito, C. J., McKee, D. D., Consler, T. G., Parks, D. J., Stewart, E. L., Willson, T. M., Lambert, M. H., Moore, J. T., Pearce, K. H., and Xu, H. E. (2002) Crystal structure of the glucocorticoid receptor ligand binding domain reveals a novel mode of receptor dimerization and coactivator recognition. Cell 110, 93–105

Bleich, M., Warth, R., Schmidt-Hieber, M., Schulz-Baldes, A., Hasselblatt, P., Fisch, D., Berger, S., Kunzelmann, K., Kriz, W., Schutz, G., and Greger, R. (1999) Rescue of the mineralocorticoid receptor knock-out mouse. Pflugers Arch 438, 245–54. ny.com/link/service/journals/00424/bibs/438n3p245.html

Bocchinfuso, W. P., Lindzey, J. K., Hewitt, S. C., Clark, J. A., Myers, P. H., Cooper, R., and Korach, K. S. (2000) Induction of mammary gland development in estrogen receptor-alpha knockout mice. Endocrinology 141, 2982–94

Bredenberg, J., and Nilsson, L. (2002) Conformational states of the glucocorticoid receptor DNA-binding domain from molecular dynamics simulations. Proteins 49, 24–36

Brisken, C., Heineman, A., Chavarria, T., Elenbaas, B., Tan, J., Dey, S. K., McMahon, J. A., McMahon, A. P., and Weinberg, R. A. (2000) Essential function of Wnt-4 in mammary gland development downstream of progesterone signaling. Genes Dev 14, 650–4

Brouchet, L., Krust, A., Dupont, S., Chambon, P., Bayard, F., and Arnal, J. F. (2001) Estradiol accelerates reendothelialization in mouse carotid artery through estrogen receptor-alpha but not estrogen receptor-beta. Circulation 103, 423–8

Brzozowski, A. M., Pike, A. C., Dauter, Z., Hubbard, R. E., Bonn, T., Engstrom, O., Ohman, L., Greene, G. L., Gustafsson, J. A., and Carlquist, M. (1997) Molecular basis of agonism and antagonism in the oestrogen receptor. Nature 389, 753–8

Chatterjee, B., Song, C. S., Jung, M. H., Chen, S., Walter, C. A., Herbert, D. C., Weaker, F. J., Mancini, M. A., and Roy, A. K. (1996) Targeted overexpression of androgen receptor with a liver-specific promoter in transgenic mice. Proc Natl Acad Sci USA 93, 728–33

Chow, J. C., Ling, P. R., Qu, Z., Laviola, L., Ciccarone, A., Bistrian, B. R., and Smith, R. J. (1996) Growth hormone stimulates tyrosine phosphorylation of JAK2 and STAT5, but not insulin receptor substrate-1 or SHC proteins in liver and skeletal muscle of normal rats in vivo. Endocrinology 137, 2880–6

Ciana, P., Di Luccio, G., Belcredito, S., Pollio, G., Vegeto, E., Tatangelo, L., Tiveron, C., and Maggi, A. (2001) Engineering of a mouse for the in vivo profiling of estrogen receptor activity. Mol Endocrinol 15, 1104–13

Ciana, P., Raviscioni, M., Mussi, P., Vegeto, E., Que, I., Parker, M. G., Lowik, C., and Maggi, A. (2002) In vivo imaging of transcriptionally active estrogen receptors. Nat Med 16, 16

Cole, T. J., Blendy, J. A., Monaghan, A. P., Krieglstein, K., Schmid, W., Aguzzi, A., Fantuzzi, G., Hummler, E., Unsicker, K., and Schutz, G. (1995) Targeted disruption of the glucocorticoid receptor gene blocks adrenergic chromaffin cell development and severely retards lung maturation. Genes Dev 9, 1608–21

Conneely, O. M., and Jericevic, B. M. (2002) Progesterone regulation of reproductive function through functionally distinct progesterone receptor isoforms. Rev Endocr Metab Disord 3, 201–9

Conneely, O. M., Mulac-Jericevic, B., DeMayo, F., Lydon, J. P., and O'Malley, B. W. (2002) Reproductive functions of progesterone receptors. Recent Prog Horm Res 57, 339–55

Conneely, O. M., Mulac-Jericevic, B., Lydon, J. P., and De Mayo, F. J. (2001) Reproductive functions of the progesterone receptor isoforms: lessons from knock-out mice. Mol Cell Endocrinol 179, 97–103

Couse, J. F., Bunch, D. O., Lindzey, J., Schomberg, D. W., and Korach, K. S. (1999) Prevention of the polycystic ovarian phenotype and characterization of ovulatory capacity in the estrogen receptor-alpha knockout mouse. Endocrinology 140, 5855–65

Couse, J. F., Hewitt, S. C., Bunch, D. O., Sar, M., Walker, V. R., Davis, B. J., and Korach, K. S. (1999) Postnatal sex reversal of the ovaries in mice lacking estrogen receptors alpha and beta. Science 286, 2328–31

Couse, J. F., and Korach, K. S. (1999) Estrogen receptor null mice: what have we learned and where will they lead us? Endocr Rev 20, 358–417

Curtis, S. W., Washburn, T., Sewall, C., DiAugustine, R., Lindzey, J., Couse, J. F., and Korach, K. S. (1996) Physiological coupling of growth factor and steroid receptor signaling pathways: estrogen receptor knockout mice lack estrogen-like response to epidermal growth factor. Proc Natl Acad Sci USA 93, 12626–30

Darblade, B., Pendaries, C., Krust, A., Dupont, S., Fouque, M. J., Rami, J., Chambon, P., Bayard, F., and Arnal, J. F. (2002) Estradiol alters nitric oxide production in the mouse aorta through the alpha-, but not beta-, estrogen receptor. Circ Res 90, 413–9

Dick, G. M., Rossow, C. F., Smirnov, S., Horowitz, B., and Sanders, K. M. (2001) Tamoxifen activates smooth muscle BK channels through the regulatory beta 1 subunit. J Biol Chem 276, 34594–9

Drouin, J., Sun, Y. L., Chamberland, M., Gauthier, Y., De Lean, A., Nemer, M., and Schmidt, T. J. (1993) Novel glucocorticoid receptor complex with DNA element of the hormone- repressed POMC gene. Embo J 12, 145–56

Dupont, S., Krust, A., Gansmuller, A., Dierich, A., Chambon, P., and Mark, M. (2000) Effect of single and compound knockouts of estrogen receptors alpha (ERalpha) and beta (ERbeta) on mouse reproductive phenotypes. Development 127, 4277–91

Freedman, L. P., Luisi, B. F., Korszun, Z. R., Basavappa, R., Sigler, P. B., and Yamamoto, K. R. (1988) The function and structure of the metal coordination sites within the glucocorticoid receptor DNA binding domain. Nature 334, 543–6

Funder, J. W., Pearce, P. T., Smith, R., and Smith, A. I. (1988) Mineralocorticoid action: target tissue specificity is enzyme, not receptor, mediated. Science 242, 583–5

Geller, D. S., Farhi, A., Pinkerton, N., Fradley, M., Moritz, M., Spitzer, A., Meinke, G., Tsai, F. T., Sigler, P. B., and Lifton, R. P. (2000) Activating mineralocorticoid receptor mutation in hypertension exacerbated by pregnancy. Science 289, 119–23

Gu, H., Marth, J. D., Orban, P. C., Mossmann, H., and Rajewsky, K. (1994) Deletion of a DNA polymerase beta gene segment in T cells using cell type-specific gene targeting. Science 265, 103–6

Harvey, B. J., Doolan, C. M., Condliffe, S. B., Renard, C., Alzamora, R., and Urbach, V. (2002) Non-genomic convergent and divergent signalling of rapid responses to aldosterone and estradiol in mammalian colon. Steroids 67, 483–91

Hinz, B., and Hirschelmann, R. (2000) Rapid non-genomic feedback effects of glucocorticoids on CRF-induced ACTH secretion in rats. Pharm Res 17, 1273–7

Hubert, C., Gasc, J. M., Berger, S., Schutz, G., and Corvol, P. (1999) Effects of mineralocorticoid receptor gene disruption on the components of the renin-angiotensin system in 8-day-old mice. Mol Endocrinol 13, 297–306

Iafrati, M. D., Karas, R. H., Aronovitz, M., Kim, S., Sullivan, T. R., Jr., Lubahn, D. B., O'Donnell, T. F., Jr., Korach, K. S., and Mendelsohn, M. E. (1997) Estrogen inhibits the vascular injury response in estrogen receptor alpha-deficient mice. Nat Med 3, 545–8

Jacq, X., Brou, C., Lutz, Y., Davidson, I., Chambon, P., and Tora, L. (1994) Human TAFII30 is present in a distinct TFIID complex and is required for transcriptional activation by the estrogen receptor. Cell 79, 107–17

Jaisser, F. (2000) Inducible gene expression and gene modification in transgenic mice. J Am Soc Nephrol 11 Suppl 16, S95-S100

Jakacka, M., Ito, M., Martinson, F., Ishikawa, T., Lee, E. J., and Jameson, J. L. (2002) An estrogen receptor (ER)alpha deoxyribonucleic acid-binding domain knock-in mutation provides evidence for nonclassical ER pathway signaling in vivo. Mol Endocrinol 16, 2188–201

Jakacka, M., Ito, M., Weiss, J., Chien, P. Y., Gehm, B. D., and Jameson, J. L. (2001) Estrogen receptor binding to DNA is not required for its activity through the nonclassical AP1 pathway. J Biol Chem 276, 13615–21

Kato, S., Endoh, H., Masuhiro, Y., Kitamoto, T., Uchiyama, S., Sasaki, H., Masushige, S., Gotoh, Y., Nishida, E., Kawashima, H., and et al. (1995) Activation of the estrogen receptor through phosphorylation by mitogen- activated protein kinase. Science 270, 1491–4

Kellendonk, C., Opherk, C., Anlag, K., Schutz, G., and Tronche, F. (2000) Hepatocyte-specific expression of Cre recombinase. Genesis 26, 151–3

Klotz, D. M., Hewitt, S. C., Ciana, P., Raviscioni, M., Lindzey, J. K., Foley, J., Maggi, A., DiAugustine, R. P., and Korach, K. S. (2002) Requirement of estrogen receptor-alpha in IGF-1-induced uterine responses and in vivo evidence for IGF- 1/estrogen receptor cross-talk. J Biol Chem 277, 8531–7

Korach, K. S. (2000) Estrogen receptor knock-out mice: molecular and endocrine phenotypes. J Soc Gynecol Investig 7, S16–7

Korach, K. S., Couse, J. F., Curtis, S. W., Washburn, T. F., Lindzey, J., Kimbro, K. S., Eddy, E. M., Migliaccio, S., Snedeker, S. M., Lubahn, D. B., Schomberg, D. W., and Smith, E. P. (1996) Estrogen receptor gene disruption: molecular characterization and experimental and clinical phenotypes. Recent Prog Horm Res 51, 159–86

Kos, M., Denger, S., Reid, G., and Gannon, F. (2002a) Upstream open reading frames regulate the translation of the multiple mRNA variants of the estrogen receptor alpha. J Biol Chem 277, 37131–8

Kos, M., Denger, S., Reid, G., Korach, K. S., and Gannon, F. (2002b) Down but not out? A novel protein isoform of the estrogen receptor alpha is expressed in the estrogen receptor alpha knockout mouse. J Mol Endocrinol 29, 281–6

Krege, J. H., Hodgin, J. B., Couse, J. F., Enmark, E., Warner, M., Mahler, J. F., Sar, M., Korach, K. S., Gustafsson, J. A., and Smithies, O. (1998) Generation and reproductive phenotypes of mice lacking estrogen receptor beta. Proc Natl Acad Sci USA 95, 15677–82

Kuiper, G. G., Enmark, E., Pelto-Huikko, M., Nilsson, S., and Gustafsson, J. A. (1996) Cloning of a novel receptor expressed in rat prostate and ovary. Proc Natl Acad Sci USA 93, 5925–30

La Spada, A. R., Peterson, K. R., Meadows, S. A., McClain, M. E., Jeng, G., Chmelar, R. S., Haugen, H. A., Chen, K., Singer, M. J., Moore, D., Trask, B. J., Fischbeck, K. H., Clegg, C. H., and McKnight, G. S. (1998) Androgen receptor YAC transgenic mice carrying CAG 45 alleles show trinucleotide repeat instability. Hum Mol Genet 7, 959–67

Laudet, V., and Gronemeyer, H. (2001) The Nuclear Receptor FactsBook, 1st edition (November 2001) Edition: Academic Press)

Lees, J. A., Fawell, S. E., and Parker, M. G. (1989) Identification of two transactivation domains in the mouse oestrogen receptor. Nucleic Acids Res 17, 5477–88

Lubahn, D. B., Moyer, J. S., Golding, T. S., Couse, J. F., Korach, K. S., and Smithies, O. (1993) Alteration of reproductive function but not prenatal sexual development after insertional disruption of the mouse estrogen receptor gene. Proc Natl Acad Sci USA *90*, 11162–6

Luisi, B. F., Xu, W. X., Otwinowski, Z., Freedman, L. P., Yamamoto, K. R., and Sigler, P. B. (1991) Crystallographic analysis of the interaction of the glucocorticoid receptor with DNA. Nature *352*, 497–505

Marchetti, B., Morale, M. C., Testa, N., Tirolo, C., Caniglia, S., Amor, S., Dijkstra, C. D., and Barden, N. (2001) Stress, the immune system and vulnerability to degenerative disorders of the central nervous system in transgenic mice expressing glucocorticoid receptor antisense RNA. Brain Res Brain Res Rev *37*, 259–72

Marchetti, B., Peiffer, A., Morale, M. C., Batticane, N., Gallo, F., and Barden, N. (1994) Transgenic animals with impaired type II glucocorticoid receptor gene expression. A model to study aging of the neuroendocrine-immune system. Ann N Y Acad Sci *719*, 308–27

Matias, P. M., Carrondo, M. A., Coelho, R., Thomaz, M., Zhao, X. Y., Wegg, A., Crusius, K., Egner, U., and Donner, P. (2002) Structural basis for the glucocorticoid response in a mutant human androgen receptor (AR(ccr)) derived from an androgen-independent prostate cancer. J Med Chem *45*, 1439–46

Metcalf, D., Greenhalgh, C. J., Viney, E., Willson, T. A., Starr, R., Nicola, N. A., Hilton, D. J., and Alexander, W. S. (2000) Gigantism in mice lacking suppressor of cytokine signalling-2. Nature *405*, 1069–73

Metzger, D., Ali, S., Bornert, J. M., and Chambon, P. (1995) Characterization of the amino-terminal transcriptional activation function of the human estrogen receptor in animal and yeast cells. J Biol Chem *270*, 9535–42

Mulac-Jericevic, B., Mullinax, R. A., DeMayo, F. J., Lydon, J. P., and Conneely, O. M. (2000) Subgroup of reproductive functions of progesterone mediated by progesterone receptor-B isoform. Science *289*, 1751–4

Nagel, S. C., Hagelbarger, J. L., and McDonnell, D. P. (2001) Development of an ER action indicator mouse for the study of estrogens, selective ER modulators (SERMs), and Xenobiotics. Endocrinology *142*, 4721–8

Paech, K., Webb, P., Kuiper, G. G., Nilsson, S., Gustafsson, J., Kushner, P. J., and Scanlan, T. S. (1997) Differential ligand activation of estrogen receptors ERalpha and ERbeta at AP1 sites. Science *277*, 1508–10

Parker, M. G. (1998) Transcriptional activation by oestrogen receptors. Biochem Soc Symp *63*, 45–50

Pearce, P. T., and Funder, J. W. (1988) Steroid binding to cardiac type I receptors: in vivo studies. J Hypertens Suppl *6*, S131–3

Pendaries, C., Darblade, B., Rochaix, P., Krust, A., Chambon, P., Korach, K. S., Bayard, F., and Arnal, J. F. (2002) The AF-1 activation-function of ERalpha may be dispensable to mediate the effect of estradiol on endothelial NO production in mice. Proc Natl Acad Sci USA *99*, 2205–10

Rae, M. T., Menzies, G. S., McNeilly, A. S., Woad, K., Webb, R., and Bramley, T. A. (1998) Specific non-genomic, membrane-localized binding sites for progesterone in the bovine corpus luteum. Biol Reprod *58*, 1394–406

Reichardt, H. M., Kaestner, K. H., Tuckermann, J., Kretz, O., Wessely, O., Bock, R., Gass, P., Schmid, W., Herrlich, P., Angel, P., and Schutz, G. (1998) DNA binding of the glucocorticoid receptor is not essential for survival. Cell *93*, 531–41

Reichardt, H. M., Kellendonk, C., Tronche, F., and Schutz, G. (1999) The Cre/loxP system–a versatile tool to study glucocorticoid signalling in mice. Biochem Soc Trans *27*, 78–83

Reichardt, H. M., Tuckermann, J. P., Gottlicher, M., Vujic, M., Weih, F., Angel, P., Herrlich, P., and Schutz, G. (2001) Repression of inflammatory responses in the absence of DNA binding by the glucocorticoid receptor. Embo J *20*, 7168–73

Reichardt, H. M., Umland, T., Bauer, A., Kretz, O., and Schutz, G. (2000) Mice with an increased glucocorticoid receptor gene dosage show enhanced resistance to stress and endotoxic shock. Mol Cell Biol 20, 9009–17

Robin-Jagerschmidt, C., Wurtz, J. M., Guillot, B., Gofflo, D., Benhamou, B., Vergezac, A., Ossart, C., Moras, D., and Philibert, D. (2000) Residues in the ligand binding domain that confer progestin or glucocorticoid specificity and modulate the receptor transactivation capacity. Mol Endocrinol 14, 1028–37

Robinson, G. W., Hennighausen, L., and Johnson, P. F. (2000) Side-branching in the mammary gland: the progesterone-Wnt connection. Genes Dev 14, 889–94

Sato, T., Kawano, H., and Kato, S. (2002) Study of androgen action in bone by analysis of androgen-receptor deficient mice. J Bone Miner Metab 20, 326–30

Sato, T., Matsumoto, T., Yamada, T., Watanabe, T., Kawano, H., and Kato, S. (2003) Late onset of obesity in male androgen receptor-deficient (AR KO) mice. Biochem Biophys Res Commun 300, 167–71

Shang, Y., and Brown, M. (2002) Molecular determinants for the tissue specificity of SERMs. Science 295, 2465–8

Shang, Y., Hu, X., DiRenzo, J., Lazar, M. A., and Brown, M. (2000) Cofactor dynamics and sufficiency in estrogen receptor-regulated transcription. Cell 103, 843–52

Shiau, A. K., Barstad, D., Radek, J. T., Meyers, M. J., Nettles, K. W., Katzenellenbogen, B. S., Katzenellenbogen, J. A., Agard, D. A., and Greene, G. L. (2002) Structural characterization of a subtype-selective ligand reveals a novel mode of estrogen receptor antagonism. Nat Struct Biol 9, 359–64

Shyamala, G., Yang, X., Cardiff, R. D., and Dale, E. (2000) Impact of progesterone receptor on cell-fate decisions during mammary gland development. Proc Natl Acad Sci USA 97, 3044–9

Shyamala, G., Yang, X., Silberstein, G., Barcellos-Hoff, M. H., and Dale, E. (1998) Transgenic mice carrying an imbalance in the native ratio of A to B forms of progesterone receptor exhibit developmental abnormalities in mammary glands. Proc Natl Acad Sci USA 95, 696–701

Sillaber, I., Rammes, G., Zimmermann, S., Mahal, B., Zieglgansberger, W., Wurst, W., Holsboer, F., and Spanagel, R. (2002) Enhanced and delayed stress-induced alcohol drinking in mice lacking functional CRH1 receptors. Science 296, 931–3

Simoncini, T., Hafezi-Moghadam, A., Brazil, D. P., Ley, K., Chin, W. W., and Liao, J. K. (2000) Interaction of oestrogen receptor with the regulatory subunit of phosphatidyl-inositol-3-OH kinase. Nature 407, 538–41

Stec, I., Barden, N., Reul, J. M., and Holsboer, F. (1994) Dexamethasone nonsuppression in transgenic mice expressing antisense RNA to the glucocorticoid receptor. J Psychiatr Res 28, 1–5

Stocklin, E., Wissler, M., Gouilleux, F., and Groner, B. (1996) Functional interactions between Stat5 and the glucocorticoid receptor. Nature 383, 726–8

Tronche, F., Kellendonk, C., Kretz, O., Gass, P., Anlag, K., Orban, P. C., Bock, R., Klein, R., and Schutz, G. (1999) Disruption of the glucocorticoid receptor gene in the nervous system results in reduced anxiety. Nat Genet 23, 99–103. java/Propub/genetics/ng0999_99.fulltext java/Propub/genetics/ng0999_99.abstract

Tronche, F., Kellendonk, C., Reichardt, H. M., and Schutz, G. (1998) Genetic dissection of glucocorticoid receptor function in mice. Curr Opin Genet Dev 8, 532–8

Vidal, O., Lindberg, M. K., Hollberg, K., Baylink, D. J., Andersson, G., Lubahn, D. B., Mohan, S., Gustafsson, J. A., and Ohlsson, C. (2000) Estrogen receptor specificity in the regulation of skeletal growth and maturation in male mice. Proc Natl Acad Sci USA 97, 5474–9

Wintermantel, T. M., Mayer, A. K., Schutz, G., and Greiner, E. F. (2002) Targeting mammary epithelial cells using a bacterial artificial chromosome. Genesis 33, 125–30

Yeh, S., Tsai, M. Y., Xu, Q., Mu, X. M., Lardy, H., Huang, K. E., Lin, H., Yeh, S. D., Altuwairi, S., Zhou, X., Xing, L., Boyce, B. F., Hung, M. C., Zhang, S., Gan, L., and Chang, C.

(2002) Generation and characterization of androgen receptor knockout (ARKO) mice: an in vivo model for the study of androgen functions in selective tissues. Proc Natl Acad Sci USA 99, 13498–503

Zhu, Y., Bian, Z., Lu, P., Karas, R. H., Bao, L., Cox, D., Hodgin, J., Shaul, P. W., Thoren, P., Smithies, O., Gustafsson, J. A., and Mendelsohn, M. E. (2002) Abnormal vascular function and hypertension in mice deficient in estrogen receptor beta. Science 295, 505–8

Reproductive System

M. Poutanen · F.-P. Zhang · S. Rulli · S. Mäkelä · P. Sipilä · J. Toppari · I. Huhtaniemi

Department of Physiology, Institute of Biomedicine, University of Turku,
Kiinamyllynkatu 10, 20520 Turku, Finland
e-mail: matti.poutanen@utu.fi

Abstract Reproduction differs from other physiological functions in the sense that it is not essential for survival of an individual, only for that of the species. However, the prevalence of infertility is on the rise, and it seriously affects the quality of life of the couples affected. Since both contraception and infertility problems concern young, otherwise healthy individuals, the possibilities to do clinical research on human reproduction are limited. We therefore need novel experimental approaches, for which gene-modified animals provide excellent platforms. In the present chapter, we have summarized some of the key techniques typically used to analyze reproductive physiology and pathophysiology in gene-modified mouse models. The techniques involve, e.g., macroscopic anatomy and histology of the reproductive organs at various ages, assessment of reproductive capacity and behavior, analyses of hormones and their receptors in circulation, endocrine glands and target organs, and analyses of expression of specific gene transcription and translation products by various techniques. As the reproductive system is under dynamic change during life, the analyses should done with different age groups of animals, e.g., at fetal life, postnatally, during puberty, at young adult age, and with aging mice. The different periods of life, representing differentiation, development, maturation, and involution present with different functional characteristics and pathologies, and allow us to obtain a global view about the reproductive functions during an individual's life span.

Keywords Reproduction · Infertility · Gonad · Testis · Epididymis · Prostate · Ovary · Steroid hormone · Gonadotropin · Lipoprotein · Lipid metabolism · Atherosclerosis · Endocytosis · Lipase · Apoprotein · Cholesterol · Vascular wall

1
General Principles for Analyzing the Reproductive Tract Biology

A growing number of gene-modified (GM) animals, mainly mice, have been produced providing novel information about the genes playing important role in the reproductive tract biology, and several genes essential for gonadal differentiation and function have been identified or their roles have been confirmed using GM mice. In principle, any severe dysfunction in reproductive organs of both sexes does lead to subfertility or infertility. This is readily detected in the breeding colony of mice, by recording the litter sizes and time interval between births. However, a lot of novel information about the reproductive tract biology can also be obtained by analyzing in detail the reproductive tract of fertile mice.

The function of the reproductive system is regulated by a complex hormonal network, involving the hypothalamus–pituitary–gonadal axis. Dysfunction induced by a gene modification at any level of this regulatory cascade may result in altered function of the reproductive organs, or vice versa; dysfunction in the gonads resulting in altered hormone production affects the hypothalamic–pituitary level through altered feedback regulation. As the reproductive system is also tightly connected to the other endocrine regulatory systems, unbalanced secretion of reproductive hormones has frequently wider consequences, such as hyperstimulation of adrenocortical function, and unbalanced energy metabolism associated with obesity (Kero et al. 2000, 2003; Li et al. 2001; Rulli et al. 2002), for example. Hence, manipulation of the reproductive hormones often results in secondary effects caused by multiple hormonal disturbances. Analyzing the sequence of hormonal disturbances leading to the phenotypic features in the GM mouse models is therefore a demanding task.

The generation of knockout (KO) mice applies a universal gene-targeting technology, independent of the target tissues. However, the production of specific transgenic (TG) mouse models in the field of reproductive biology has been hindered by the lack of efficient cell-specific promoters directing the transgenes to different somatic cells present in gonads. Considering the limitations of the present chapter, it is impossible to introduce all the outstanding work carried out in the field of reproductive tract biology. Hence, we will focus on some basic methodological aspects and experimental approaches typically used to analyze reproductive tract phenotypes in GM mice, and several of the methods are introduced using examples of GM mice recently generated in our own laboratories. Methods used to analyze the reproductive physiology in mice involve hormone measurements, and morphological, histological, and physiological evaluation of the basic features of the reproductive tract biology. However, as in other organs systems, these methods do not necessary penetrate very deeply into the mechanisms causing the altered phenotypes. Therefore, analyzing gene expression profiles of known key genes in the reproductive tissues is important. Furthermore, also for a reproductive biologist, large-scale gene expression, and protein and metabolic profiling systems are becoming methods of choice, in order to screen for the signaling systems involved in the phenotypes obtained.

2
Fetal Development of the Reproductive Tract

The fetal development of both male and female reproductive organs shares significant similarities between mouse and human (for reviews see, e.g., Nef and Parada 2000; Hughes 2001). By following the morphology of the gonadal development, several of the genes essential for development of the bipotential gonads have been identified by KO mouse models. Mice presenting with gene disruption of, for example, the steroidogenic factor-1 (SF-1), Wilms tumor-associated gene (WT-1), transcription factors Lhx1 and Lhx9 all lack gonads (Kreidberg et al. 1993; Luo et al. 1994; Shawlot and Behringer 1995; Birk et al. 2000). Depending on the site of action, these mice also present some other dysfunctions: The SF-1 KO mice lack adrenals, in WT-1 KO mice the kidneys do not develop, and Lhx1 is also essential for the head development. The KO mouse models with total lack of gonads also show the power of simple macroscopic evaluation of the organogenesis as part of the phenotype analyses in GM mice. SF-1 has been shown to be involved in the regulation of gonadal and adrenal function and steroidogenesis at multiple levels also in adults. The lack of gonads in SF-1 KO mice hinders the use of this model for analyzing the role of SF-1 in adult gonads. To solve this problem, cell-specific deletion of SF-1 by the Cre/loxP technique has recently been developed (Zhao et al. 2001), and the studies showed that the lack of SF-1 function in pituitary gonadotropes reduces severely luteinizing hormone (LH) and follicle-stimulating hormone (FSH) secretion, consequently leading to gonadal dysfunction.

Once the gonads are formed, the expression of a transcription factor, SRY, is essential for initiating the male development. Many of the genetic factors and signaling networks involved in differentiation of the various gonadal cell types both in testis and ovaries are still unknown, but some of the genes involved have been recently discovered. One of the most interesting recent findings is the identification of the Wnt family of proteins as essential signals for normal ovarian development. According to the past dogma of mammalian sex development, no specific signal is needed for ovarian development. However, the mice deficient of the Wnt-4 signaling display masculinized ovaries, with the presence of testosterone-producing cells resembling testicular Leydig cells (Vainio et al. 1999).

The data thus show the apparent need of Wnt-4 for suppression of Leydig cell development in ovaries. Another signaling protein of the same family, Wnt-7a, is needed to complete the development of Müllerian ducts into certain structures of the internal female genital tract (Parr and McMahon 1998).

3
Analyzing the Male Phenotype

3.1
General Principles

As mentioned above, analyzing fertility by setting up a mating colony is a powerful way to measure reproductive functions. If the mating behavior is normal, we can conclude that a lack or lowered number of sperm in the uterus after mating or a dysfunction in the sperm function is the final cause for the reduced fertilization capacity in males. Mating behavior and sperm maturation are partially regulated by the same hormonal factors, and infertility could involve both of

Table 1 The tests suggested for preliminary analysis of the reproductive phenotype in GM mice

Female
1. Measure birth weight and record weight gain (growth curve)
2. Measure anogenital distance in newborns
3. Record age of vaginal opening and appearance of nipples
4. Analyze mating: record mating plugs, pregnancies, litter size, birth weights and sex ratio
5. Analyze success of lactation and survival of offspring (weight gain of pups during lactation)
6. Analyze estrus cycle and ovulation
7. Analyze the weight and macroscopic anatomy of reproductive organs
8. Analyze the histology of ovary, oviduct, uterus, vagina, mammary gland (also whole-mounts), pituitary gland
9. Analyze the hormonal levels in mice (testosterone, estradiol, progesterone, prolactin LH, FSH)
10. Analyze mRNA for a set of key genes for reproductive functions
11. Analyze possible secondary effects: adrenal function, obesity, insulin resistance
12. Use the data for generating the plan for more detailed analysis
Male
1. Measure birth weight and record weight gain (growth curve)
2. Measure anogenital distance in newborns
3. Analyze testicular descent/cryptorchidism
4. Analyze mating: calculate mating plugs, pregnancies, litter size and sex ratio
5. Analyze the weight and macroscopic anatomy of reproductive organs
6. Analyze the histology of testis, epididymis, vas deferens, seminal vesicles, urethro-prostatic block, pituitary gland
7. Analyze the hormonal levels in mice (testosterone, estradiol, progesterone, prolactin LH, FSH)
8. Analyze number of spermatozoa in epididymis, and uterus after mating
9. Analyze sperm number, structure, motility
10. Analyze mRNA for a set of key genes for reproductive functions
11. Analyze possible secondary effects: adrenal function, obesity, insulin resistance
12. Use the data for generating the plan for more detailed analysis

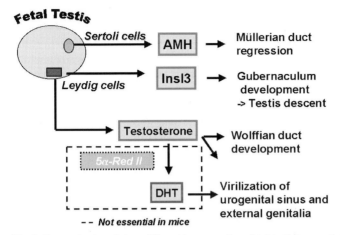

Fig. 1 The production of three different hormones from fetal testis is essential for the normal development of male reproductive tract: anti-Müllerian hormone (*AMH*) is responsible for the regression of the Müllerian duct in the males. Insulin-like factor 3 (*Insl3*) is essential for gubernaculum development, and hence, is needed, together with androgens, for the normal testicular descent. Testosterone is known to be essential for normal male sexual characteristics, including the normal development of the male external genitalia

these components. The typical measures involved in the basic phenotype analysis in the male reproductive tract are presented in Table 1.

3.2
Testicular Development and Function

Many of the key factors leading to differentiation of the two main testicular structures, the interstitial space with the Leydig cells and the seminiferous tubules with the Sertoli cells and developing germ cells, remain unknown. Once the fetal testes are present they produce three main hormones essential for full masculinization of the male during the fetal life (Fig. 1): testosterone (T), anti-Müllerian hormone (AMH; also termed Müllerian inhibiting substance, MIS) and insulin-like factor 3 (Insl3). The role of these hormones in male sex development has also been confirmed by GM mouse models. The lack of AMH expression results to the presence of Müllerian duct-derived structures (upper vagina, uterus, and Fallopian tubes) also in the male (Behringer et al. 1994; for review see Teixeira et al. 2001). The lack of functional androgen receptor in testicular feminized male mice (TFM) leads to male pseudohermaphroditism: genetic males with female external genitalia (Lyon and Hawkes 1970; He et al. 1991), and mice deficient in Insl3 are cryptorchid (Nef and Parada 1999; Zimmermann et al. 1999).

T is the main steroid produced by the Leydig cells, both in mice and humans, and in addition to the masculinization of the external genitalia, proper androgen action through high intratesticular T concentration is needed for the initiation and maintenance of normal spermatogenesis. The usefulness of serum T (Huh-taniemi et al. 1985) and LH (the main gonadotropin regulating T secretion) measurements in the male mouse is hindered by the high normal variation observed in their concentrations. However, in our laboratory we have successfully measured mouse serum gonadotropin concentrations (LH and FSH) by using a time-resolved fluoroimmunoassays developed for the corresponding rat gonadotropins (Haavisto et al. 1993; van Casteren et al. 2000). In addition, the measurement of intratesticular T concentration is a good measure to evaluate testicular androgen production in mice, and the variation is less than typically detected in the serum samples. Using these methods, we were able to show that, in contrast to that in human, LH receptor function is not essential for fetal T production in mouse. This was confirmed by identification of normally differentiated, but macroscopically hypoplastic, genitalia of the LH receptor knockout (LuRKO) mice (Lei et al. 2001; Zhang et al. 2001). Interestingly, recent findings also indicate that the conversion of T to DHT via 5α-reductase type II is not essential for the development of male urogenital region in mice (Mahendroo et al 2001), being opposite to that shown in human patients with 5α-reductase type II deficiencies.

Another marked difference between man and mouse in development of the male urogenital organs is the fact that the scrotal phase of testicular descent in the mice occurs postnatally, while in the human full testicular descent take place in the fetal life. However, the process of testicular descent seems to be mechanistically similar in both species. This process is divided in two distinguished phases: the trans-abdominal descent and inguino-scrotal descent. Development of the ligament mainly responsible for the testicular trans-abdominal descent, gubernaculum, can be histologically analyzed in fetal mice, e.g., at the embryonic day (E)17.5 (Zimmermann et al. 1999; Emmen et al 2000; Koskimies et al. 2003). In addition, scanning electron microscopy has been shown to be a powerful technique in analyzing the development of the ligament structures in fetal mice (Nef and Parada 1999; Zimmermann et al. 1999). Recently, a novel hormone involved in the development of gubernaculum, and hence, essential for the intra-abdominal descent of testes, was discovered by KO technology. The results showed that mice deficient in Insl3 were lacking normal gubernaculum structures, and were cryptorchid, with testes locating in the abdomen (Nef and Parada 1999; Zimmermann et al. 1999). Insl3 KO mice are present with normal androgen status, indicating that the cryptorchidism was not due to the lack of T (Nef and Parada 2000). The second phase of testicular descent, the inguino-scrotal phase, is clearly androgen dependent. Thus, mice lacking postnatal and pubertal androgen action (such as LuRKO males) lack normal scrotal development, and are cryptorchid with the testes localized in the abdomen (Lei et al. 2001; Zhang et al. 2001). As expected, the phenotype of LuRKO mice showed that LH receptor function is essential for the postnatal androgen production in mice, similar to that in human. In male mice, the endocrine puberty occurs at the age of around 45 days, and the seminal vesicle (SV) weight and size is a direct, and easily measured, biomarker for androgen production in adult male

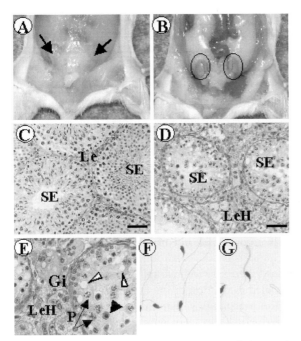

Fig. 2. A, B AROM+ mice are present with cryptorchid testes (*arrows*), located at the bottom of the abdominal cavity. **C** Testis histology in wild type adult mice. **D, E** Testis histology of AROM+ mice, showing Leydig cell hyperplasia (*LeH*) with disrupted spermatogenesis with degenerating germ cells within the seminiferous epithelium (*SE*). No germ cells beyond the stage of pachytene spermatocytes (*P*) were found, and numerous vacuoles (*arrowheads*) of different sizes are present. Also giant cells (*Gi*) are present in the interstitium, and cells with intensively stained nuclei and eosinophilic cytoplasm (*arrows*) are frequently present in the seminiferous epithelium of AROM+ mice. **F, G** Structure of the wildtype epididymal spermatozoa (*F*), and spermatozoa with angulated tail caused by an epididymal dysfunction in mice expressing SV-40 large T antigen in the epididymal epithelium

mice. Mice with large SVs are likely to have high T production, while hypoandrogenic mice have small SV size, such as seen in LuRKO males (Lei et al. 2001; Zhang et al. 2001). We have recently also produced hypo-androgenic/hyper-estrogenic male mice by expressing the human P450 aromatase in TG mice (AROM+). These mice present with rudimentary SV and are cryptorchid (Fig. 2A, B; Li et al. 2001). As fetal exposure to high concentrations of estrogens also causes cryptorchidism in rodents by downregulating Insl3 gene expression (Emmen et al. 2000; Nef et al. 2000), the lack of androgens and high exposure to estrogens and consequent lack of Insl3 may cause cryptorchidism in AROM+ mice.

Histological evaluation of the structure and number of Leydig cells in testicular interstitium belong to the basic testicular characterization in TG mice with subfertility or infertility. By histological evaluation, both Leydig cell hyperplasia and hypertrophy were detected, e.g., in the 4-month-old AROM+ males (Fig. 2D, F; Li et al. 2001). Unlike the fetal Leydig cells that are able to produce physiologically significant levels of androgens without gonadotropin stimulation, the adult-type Leydig cells are critically dependent on LH action. Therefore, it was not a surprise that the number of adult type of Leydig cells was highly reduced in LuRKO mice. This in turn resulted in lack of pubertal increase in T, and resulted in arrested spermatogenesis (Zhang et al. 2001). In the testis, the steroid biosynthetic pathway is present in Leydig cells, and together with the affected histology of the testis, the putative changes in the expression of steroid biosynthetic enzymes and their mRNAs are good indicators for altered Leydig cell function. In addition to the Leydig cells, the interstitial tissue contains also other cell types such as stromal cells and macrophages. The exact role of the latter in testicular function is not currently known, but they might well interact with Leydig cells in T production (Lukyanenko et al. 2001). An alteration in the relative proportion of the different cell types in the interstitium, e.g., the appearance of a large amount of multinucleated giant cells (Fig. 2E), as detected in the AROM+ mice (Li et al. 2001), is a good indicator of severely altered testicular function.

Compared with the above-described relatively simple structural analyses of the testicular interstitium, a detailed evaluation of the defects in spermatogenesis is a demanding task. Based on morphology of the seminiferous epithelium, spermatogenesis in mice can be divided into 12 recognizable stages, and all the stages have specific histological features for the germ cells of that stage, and several gene disruptions are associated with a disruption of proper germ cell maturation in the testis (Zirkin 1998; Plant and Marshall 2001). The weight of the testis, as such, is a good basic indicator of proper spermatogenesis and should be routinely analyzed as part of the phenotype characterization of the reproductive tract. Small testis could result from several reasons, such as a lack of germ cells, lack of Leydig cells, or a dysfunction in the developmental period leading to a reduced size of the seminiferous tubules. The development of germ cells in seminiferous tubules is regulated mainly via two hormones: pituitary FSH and T produced by the Leydig cells stimulated by LH. Hence, a direct or indirect affect on the production of these hormones leads to disruption of spermatogenesis. The LuRKO mouse model is a typical example with a cascade of events leading to reproductive dysfunction. In these mice, the lack of pubertal LH action leads into the lack of adult-type Leydig cells. This in turn results in the lack of pubertal androgens, which results in suppressed spermatid development, with sperms developing to steps 7–8 at the age of 2–3 months (Zhang et al. 2001).

Spermatogenesis is disrupted also in AROM+ mice, present with low T and elevated E2 concentration, and at the age of 4 months no germ cells beyond the pachytene spermatocytes could be identified (Fig. 2D, E). Furthermore, both of these mouse models are present with cryptorchidism, which as such also contributes to the germ cell development. Hence, it is evident that the final testicular dysfunction in several GM mouse models is a result of several factors. Reduced testicular size in adulthood, without apparent disruption of the histological picture, is a common finding with suppressed prepubertal secretion of gonadotropins, especially of FSH. This hormone is seminal for the prepubertal

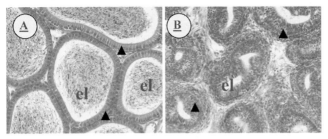

Fig. 3. A Histology of a normal mouse epididymal epithelium at the corpus region. **B** Histological appearance of dysplastic epididymal epithelium (*arrowheads*) in mouse expressing a transforming oncogene in the epididymis. *el*, epididymal lumen

proliferation of Sertoli cells. Testis total volume correlates closely to the total length of seminiferous tubules and thereby to total testicular size.

3.3
Epididymis

The spermatozoa produced in the testis are further maturing in the epididymis, where they gain their motility and fertilizing capacity. The epididymis develops from the Wolffian duct, and consists of enlarged head (caput), a central body (corpus), and an interior pointed tail (cauda), and the different epididymal regions are characterized by morphologically distinguishable epithelial cell types. Figure 3 represents a histological view of the corpus epididymidis of wild-type mice (A) and of mice with an oncogene-induced dysplasia (B). The well-segmented tubular structure of the epididymis plays an active role in sperm development, while the epididymal sperm maturation is dependent on the unique luminal environment, including specific proteins synthesized and secreted by the epididymal epithelium. During their transit through the epididymis, spermatozoa undergo biochemical remodeling of the acrosome, and the protein, glycoprotein, and lipid composition of their plasma membrane is altered. The most consistent morphological change is the migration of the cytoplasmic droplet from the neck region of the flagellum to the end of the midpiece. Also the sperm tails become disulfide-bond stabilized during their epididymal transit (for a review see Olson et al. 2002).

Only few TG models exist with a direct epididymal defect leading to disrupted sperm maturation. However, mice deficient of the c-ros tyrosine kinase receptor fail to undergo prepubertal differentiation of the proximal epididymal tubule, and therefore lack structurally the initial segment of caput epididymides (Sonnenberg-Rietmacher et al. 1996; Yeung et al. 1998). The data indicate an essential role for this orphan receptor in proper development of the epididymal segmentation. The defect in regionalized differentiation of epithelial cells in the epididymis results to various extents in flagellar angulation of the sperm, which can be readily analyzed in a squash preparation of caudal sperm (Fig. 2F, G; Yeung et al. 1999; Sipilä et al. 2002). We have recently developed an epididymal defect with angulated sperm in TG mice by specifically expressing the SV-40 T antigen in epididymis (Sipilä et al. 2002). These mice do have histologically distinguishable initial segment, but it is not functionally normal. The sperm with bent tails obtained both from the c-ros KO mice and T antigen-expressing TG mice are able to move, but are not able to fertilize the oocyte in vivo. This is likely to result from the failure of sperm to reach the oviduct during mating (Yeung et al. 2000). Kinematic parameters of mouse sperm can be monitored in vitro similarly to that carried out for humans by using computer-assisted sperm analyses (Yeung et al. 2000; Sipilä et al. 2002). Interestingly, in this type of analysis, sperm from c-ros KO mice showed rather normal motility (Yeung et al. 1999), but were still unable to pass the uterotubal junction (Yeung et al. 2000).

Furthermore, epididymal fluid can be collected from different epididymal regions, and several physiological parameters can be monitored in the fluid, such as pH and osmolality (Sipilä 2002). Also, the lack of ejaculation is to be considered a reason for infertility. Accordingly, recently a KO mouse model, deficient in $P2X_1$ receptor, was found to be infertile because a reduced contraction of the vas deferens (Mulryan et al. 2000). Estrogen receptor α-deficient mice, (αERKO mice) have been also shown to have an abnormal epididymal phenotype (for a review see Hess et al 2002), revealing the importance of functional ERα for normal epididymal function. However, infertility in these animals is most likely caused by an altered male sexual behavior and ejaculation (Ogawa et al. 1997).

3.4
Prostate and Seminal Vesicles

In rodents, the prostate consists of four paired lobes that are clearly distinguished from each other, and surrounded by a rich network of blood and lymph vessels, autonomic nerves, autonomic ganglia, and a loose capsule of connective and adipose tissue. The names of the prostatic lobes indicate their location around the prostatic urethra: ventral, lateral, dorsal, and anterior. Histologically, all lobes have their specific features, and differ from each other as regards the epithelial folding, epithelial cell staining properties, and thickness of the stromal layer. The collecting ducts from the dorsolateral and anterior lobes, seminal vesicles, and ejaculatory ducts all traverse the dorsolateral aspect of urethral wall, forming a complex aggregation of ducts of varied sizes and histological appearances. The distal end of vas deferens, prior entering the posterior urethral wall, is surrounded by a small gland, the ampullary gland. The urethral wall consists of a thick circular or C-shaped layer of striated muscle, called the rhabdosphincter, urethral mucosa, and between the mucosa and muscle, a thick layer of small spheroid periurethral glands.

Typically, there is considerable variation in the prostatic weights of individual mice of the same age and strain. The weight determined does not only represent the amount of tissue itself, but also the amount of secretory fluid in the glands. The organ weights correlate with body weight, and it is useful to use their rela-

Table 2 Examples of reproductive tract phenotypes in gene-modified mouse models

Gene modified	Representative phenotype	Reference(s)
Testis		
Transgenic		
Bcl-2	Accumulation of spermatogonia and spermatocytes and subsequent loss of germ cells	Furuchi et al., Development 1996 122:1703–9
Follistatin	Leydig cell hyperplasia, tubular degeneration	Guo et al., Mol Endocrinol 1998 12:96–106
DAX1	Male-to-female sex reversal	Swain et al., Nature 1998 391:761–7
MMTV-aromatase	Leydig cell tumorigenesis	Fowler et al., Am J Pathol 1999 156:347–53
Ubiquitin-c/aromatase (AROM+)	Cryptorchidism, Leydig cell hyperplasia	Li et al., Endocrinology 2001 142:2435–42
GDNF	Accumulation of undifferentiated spermatogonia	Meng et al., Science 2000 287:1489–93
Dhh	Loss of adult-type Leydig cells	Clark et al., Biol Reprod 2000 63:1825–38
Sox9	Female-to-male sex reversal in XX animals	Vidal et al., Nature Genet. 2001 28:216–7
Knockout		
Wt-1	Developmental arrest of kidneys and gonads	Kreidberg et al., Cell 1993 74:679–91
SF-1	Developmental arrest of adrenal glands and gonads	Luo et al., Cell 1994 77:481–90
LIM1	No formation of gonads and kidneys	Shawlot et al., Nature 1995 346:240–4
CREM	Early arrest in spermiogenesis	Nantel et al., Nature 1996 380:159–62
PDGF-A	Reduction of testis size, loss of Leydig cells, spermatogenic arrest	Boström et al., Cell 1996 85:863–73; Gnessi et al., J Cell Biol 149:1019–1025
EMX2	Developmental arrest of gonad and kidney	Miyamoto et al., Development 1997 124:1653–64
Bclw	Gradual loss of both Sertoli cells and germ cells apoptosis of Leydig cells	Print et al., PNAS 1998 95:12323–31; Ross et al., Nat Genet 1998 18:251–6; Russell et al., Biol. Reprod 2001 65:318–22
CYP19 (ArKO)	Initially fertile but developed progressive infertile spermatogenesis arrest in early stages Leydig cell hyperplasia and hypertrophy	Fisher et al., PNAS 1998 95:6965–70; Robertson et al., PNAS 1999 96:7986–91
LIMK2, gonad-specific	Degeneration of seminiferous tubules in adult mice Leydig cell hyperplasia and hypertrophy	Yu et al., Nature Genet. 1998 20:353–357
Insl-3	Cryptorchidism, disruption of gubernacular development	Zimmermann et al., Mol Endocrinol 1999 13:681–91; Nef and Parada, Nat Genet 1999 22:295–9

Table 2 (continued)

Gene modified	Representative phenotype	Reference(s)
GDNF heterozygous	Depletion of spermatogonia	Meng et al., Science 2000 287:1489–93
Lhx9	All mice were phenotypically female, no gonad formation	Birk et al., Nature 2000 403:909–913
Dmrt1	Hypoplastic testes, disorganized seminiferous tubules, missing germ cells, and degeneration of Leydig cells	Raymond et al., Genes & Dev 200014:2587–2595
TLF (TBP-like factor)	Late arrest in spermiogenesis	Martianov et al., Mol Cell 2001 7:509–15; Martianov et al., Development 2002 129:945–55
Trf2	Spermatogenesis arrest in elongated stage	Zhang et al., Science 2001 292,1153–5
FGF 9	Testicular hypoplasia or complete sex reversal	Colvin et al., Cell 2001 104:875–89
Atk1	Degeneration of spermatogenesis	Chen et al., Genes Dev. 2001 15:2203–8
LH receptor (LuRKO)	Spermatogenesis arrest at round spermatids, poorly differentiated Leydig cells	Zhang et al., Mol Endocrinol 200115:172–83; Lei et al., Mol Endocrinol 2001 15:184–200
Epididymis		
Transgenic		
MMTV/c-neu	Epithelial hypertrophy and hyperplasia	Muller et al., Cell 1988 54:105–15; Bouchard et al., Cell 1989 57:931–6; Lucchini et al., Cancer Letters 1992 64:203–9
MMTV/N-*ras* oncogene	Reduced motility of sperm, failure of spermatozoa to fertilize oocytes in vitro, male infertility	Mangues et al., Oncogene 1990 5:1491–7
MMTV/*int*-3 C3(1)/Polyomavirus middle T gene	Epithelial hyperplasia, pseudolumens, male infertility Focal hyperplasia, papillary proliferation of epididymal epithelium	Jhappan et al., Genes Dev 1992 6:345-; Tehranian et al., Am J Pathol 1996 149:1177–91
MMTV/c-erbB-2 L-type pyruvate-kinase/H-*ras*	Epithelial hyperplasia, male infertility Epithelial hyperplasia, inflammatory granulomas in the epididymal interstitium	Guy et al., J Biol Chem 1996 271:7673–8; Gilbert et al., Int J Cancer 1997 73:749–56
MMTV/d.n. RARα	Epithelial squamous metaplasia, reduced fertility, dense ductal fluid that blocked epididymal lumen	Costa et al., Biol Reprod 1997 56:985–90
MMTV/VEGF	Epithelial hyperplasia, pseudolumens, male infertility	Korpelainen et al., J Cell Biol 1998 143:1705–12

Table 2 (continued)

Gene modified	Representative phenotype	Reference(s)
MMTV/FGF-3	Enlarged epididymis	Chua et al., Oncogene 2002 21:1899–1908
GPX5/SV40 large T antigen	Reduction of spermatozoa in epididymis Severe dysplasia in all epididymal regions, hyperplasia, male infertility	Sipilä et al., Mol Endocrinol 2002 11:2603–17
Knockout		
hoxa-11 and *hoxd-11*	Homeotic transformation of vas deferens towards epididymis	Davis et al., Nature 1995 375:791–5
Apolipoprotein B	Male heterozygous mice have severely reduced fertility, sperm motility, count and survival time are reduced	Huang et al., Proc Natl Acad Sci USA 1996 93:10903–07
γ-Glutamyl transpeptidase	Hypoplastic epididymides	Lieberman et al., Proc Natl Acad Sci USA 1996 93:7923–26
c-ros	Failure to develop initial segment, male infertility	Sonnenberg-Riethmacher et al., Gene Develop 1996 10:1184
CSF-1	Lower density of macrophages in the caput and cauda epididymidis. Remaining macrophages failed to take up normal positions lining the epididymal tubules	Pollard et al., Biol Reprod 1997 56:1290–1300
β-Hexosaminidase A	Principal, narrow and halo cells increase in size and number of lysosomes in the initial segment and intermediate zone	Adamali et al., J Androl 1999 20:803–24
β-Hexosaminidase B	Principal, narrow and clear cells increase in size and number of lysosomes in all epididymal regions	Adamali et al., J Androl 1999 20:779–802
ERα (ERKO)	Disruption of fluid reabsorption in the efferent ducts, dilation of initial segment tubules, abnormality of apical narrow and clear cells in some epididymal regions	Hess et al., J Androl 2000 21:107–21
P2X₁	Reduced male fertility caused by reduced contraction of the vas deferens	Mulryan et al., Nature 2000 403:86–9

Table 2 (continued)

Gene modified	Representative phenotype	Reference(s)
Prostate		
Transgenic		
Transfection of *ras* in prostate reconstitution model system	Prostatic dysplasia and angiogenesis	Thompson et al., Cell 1989 56:917–30
Transfection of *myc* in prostate reconstitution model system	Prostatic hyperplasia	Thompson et al., Cell 1989 56:917–30
Co-transfection of *ras* and *myc*, prostate reconstitution model system	Prostatic carcinoma	Thompson et al., Cell 1989 56:917–30
MMTV/Int-2	Androgen-dependent benign prostatic epithelial hyperplasia	Muller et al., EMBO J 1990 9:907–13; Tutrone et al., J Urol 1993 149:633–639
Probasin/SV 40 T antigen	Metastatic prostate cancer	Greenberg et al., PNAS 1995 92:3439–43; Gingrich et al., Cancer Res 1996 56:4095–102
Mt-1/prolactin	Progressive prostatic hyperplasia	Wennbo et al., Endocrinology 1997 138:4410–15; Kindblom et al., Prostate 2002 53:24–33
MMTV-LTR/int-2+FGF-3	Normal prostate	Donjacour A et al., Differentiation 1998 62:227–37
	Hyperplasia in ampullary gland and seminal vesicles	
IGF-I in mouse prostate epithelium	Prostatic hyperplasia, atypical hyperplasia, well-differentiated small cell carcinoma	DiGiovanni et al., PNAS 2000 97:3455–60
Probasin/SV 40 T antigen	Androgen-dependent prostatic adenocarcinoma	Asamoto et al., Cancer Res 2001 61:4693–700
Probasin/AR	Increased proliferation of epithelium and PIN-lesions	Stanbrough et al., PNAS 2001 98:10823–628
Ubiquitin-c/aromatase (AROM+)	Inhibition of prostatic development and growth	Li et al., Endocrinology 2001 142:2435–42
Probasin/FGF-8b	Epithelial hyperplasia and PIN-lesions	Song et al., Cancer Res 2002 62:5096–105
G gamma/-T-15/SV 40 T antigen	Androgen-independent prostatic adenocarcinoma	Perez-Stable et al., Cancer Epidemiol Biomarkers Prev 2002 11:555–63
MMTV-HMMB/FGF-3	Epithelial hyperplasia and PIN-lesions	Chua et al., Oncogene 2002 21:1899–1908
	Cystic ampullary glands and vas deferens	
	Reduction of secretions in seminal vesicles	

Table 2 (continued)

Gene modified	Representative phenotype	Reference(s)
Knockout		
p53	Suppression of castration-induced apoptosis in ventral prostate	Colombel et al., Oncogene 1995 10:1269–74
Loss of p53 in *ras+myc*-initiated mouse prostate tissue	Metastatic prostatic carcinoma	Thompson et al., Oncogene 1995 10:869–79
mxi1	Increased number of prostatic glands, enlarged and hypercellular acini, epithelial dysplasia	Schreiber-Agus et al., Nature 1998 393:483–7
ERα (ERKO)	Enlarged prostate and seminal vesicles with normal histology	Couse and Korach, Endocr Rev 1999 20:358–417; Jarred et al., Tends Endocrinol Metab 2002 13:163–8
Nkx3.1	Defects in prostate development (ductal branching morphogenesis, prostatic secretion, epithelial hyperplasia and dysplasia)	Bhatia-Gaur et al., Genes Dev 1999 13:966–977
Rb-deficient prostate tissue grafted in adult nude mice	Testosterone+estradiol-induced atypical hyperplasia in prostatic epithelium, prostatic carcinoma in situ and adenocarcinoma	Wang et al., Cancer Res 2000 60:6008–17
CYP19 (ArKO)	Benign prostatic enlargement associated with elevated androgens and prolactin	McPherson et al., Endocrinology 2001 142:2458–67
ERβ (BERKO)	Prostatic epithelial hyperplasia and PIN-like lesions	Weihua et al., PNAS 2001 98:6330–5
LH receptor (LuRKO)	Undeveloped prostate	Zhang et al., Mol Endo 2001 15:172–183
Pten+/− xTRAMP mice	Promotion of prostate cancer progression	Kwabi-Addo et al., PNAS 2001 98:11563–68
Conditional disruption of *Nkx3.1*	PIN-lesions	Abdulkadir et al., Mol Cell Biol 2002 22:1495–1503
Nkx3.1−/− xPten+/−	Atypical hyperplasia in prostate epithelium and high-grade PIN-lesions	Kim et al., PNAS 2002 99:2884–89; Park et al., Am J Pathol 2002 161:727–35
Ovary		
Transgenic		
MIS	Postnatal ovarian degeneration	Behringer et al., Nature 1990 345:167–70.
Bcl-2	Decreased follicle apoptosis, enhanced folliculogenesis, germ cell tumors	Hsu et al., Endocrinology 1996 137:4837–43

Table 2 (continued)

Gene modified	Representative phenotype	Reference(s)
Follistatin	Defective folliculogenesis, infertile	Guo et al., Mol Endocrinol 1998 12:96–106
IGF-I	Polycystic ovaries	Dyck et al., Mol Reprod Dev 2001 59:178–185
Insl3	Descent of the ovaries	Adham et al., Mol Endocrinol 2002 16:244–252; Koskimies et al., Mol Cell Endocrinol 2003, in press
Knockout		
Inhibin α	Gonadal stromal tumors	Matzuk et al., Nature 1992 360:313–9
c-mos	Parthenogenetic development, germ cell tumor	Colledge et al., Nature 1994 370:65–8
Cyclin D2	Reduced granulosa cell proliferation, anovulatory, luteinized unruptured follicles	Sicinski et al., Nature 1996 384:470–4
GDF-9	Early block in folliculogenesis	Dong et al., Nature 1996 383:531–5 Carabatsos et al., Dev Biol 1998 204:373–84
	Impaired oogenesis	Lydon et al., Genes Dev 9:2266–78
Progesterone receptor	Inability to ovulate, reproductive defects	Ruggiu et al., Nature 1997 389:73–7
Dazl	Loss of germ cells and absence of gamete production	Ormandy et al., Genes Dev 1997 11:167–78
Prolactin receptor	Impaired luteal function, defective implantation	Dierich et al., Proc Natl Acad Sci USA 1998 95:13612–17; Abel et al., Endocrinology 2000 141:1795–803
FSH receptor	Ovulatory defects, disrupted folliculogenesis, infertility	
ERβ (BERKO)	Anovulatory, lack of corpora lutea, disrupted folliculogenesis	Fisher et al., Proc Natl Acad Sci USA 1998 95:6965–70
	Reduced ovarian efficiency	Krege et al., Proc Natl Acad Sci USA 1998 95:15677-82
ERα (ERKO)	Anovulatory, hemorrhagic and cystic ovaries, absent corpora lutea	Schomberg et al. Endocrinology 1999 140:2733–44
ERαβ	Morphological sex reversal of ovaries	Couse et al., Science 1999 286:2328–31
Nrip 1	Ovulatory dysfunction, luteinized unruptured follicles	White et al., Nature Med 2000 6:1368–74
Figα	Massive depletion of oocytes	Soyal et al., Development 2000 127:4645–54
LH receptor (LuRKO)	Underdeveloped external genitalia, altered folliculogenesis	Zhang et al., Mol Endocrinol 2001 15:172–83; Lei et al., Mol Endocrinol 2001 15:184–200
Growth hormone receptor	Reduced ovulation rate, reduced follicular growth	Bachelot et al., Endocrinology 2002 143:4104–12

Table 2 (continued)

Gene modified	Representative phenotype	Reference(s)
Hypothalamus/pituitary gland		
Transgenic		
GnRH	Correction of the hypogonadal *hpg* phenotype	Mason et al., Science 1986 234:1372–8
hGnRH/SV40 T antigen	Blockage of GnRH neuron migration, hypogonadism	Radovick et al., Proc Natl Acad Sci USA 1991 88:3402–6
Diphtheria toxin/α-subunit	Gonadotrope cells lost; hypogonadism	Kendall et al., Mol Endocrinol 1991 5:2025–36
α-Subunit/LHβ/CTP	Infertility, granulose cell tumors	Risma et al., Proc Natl Acad Sci USA 1995 92:1322–6
Inhibin-α/SV40 T antigen	Gonadal tumors, suppressed gonadotropins	Kananen et al. Mol Endocrinol 1996 10:1667–77
mMT-1/hFSH α:β	Infertility, hyperstimulated gonadal steroidogenesis in males, hemorrhagic and cystic ovaries in females	Kumar et al., Endocrinology 1998 139:3289–95
GH	Infertility/subfertility in both sexes	Bartke, Steroids 1999 64:598–604.
mMT-1/inhibin-α	Female subfertility	Cho et al., Endocrinology 2001 142:4994–5004
Ubiquitin/aromatase (AROM+)	Lactrotrope adenomas	Li et al., Endocrinology 2001 142:2435–42; Li et al., Endocrinology 2002 143:4074–83
Ubiquitin C/hCGβ	Mammary gland and pituitary tumors	Rulli et al., Endocrinology 2002 143:4084–95
Knockout		
Leptin	Hypogonadotropic hypogonadism	Swerdloff et al., Endocrinology 1976 98:1359–64
GnRH	Hypogonadotropic hypogonadism	Mason et al., Science 1986 234:1366–71
Pit 1	Anterior pit. hormone deficiency, hypogonadism	Li et al., Nature 1990 347:528–33
Common α-subunit	Infertility, hypogonadotropic hypogonadism, hypothyroidism	Kendall et al., Genes Dev 1995 9:2007–19
Egr1	Infertility, LH deficiency	Lee et al., Science 1996 273:1219–21
Leptin receptor	Hypogonadotropic hypogonadism	Chua et al., Science 1996 271:994–6
Prop 1	Anterior pit. hormone deficiencies, hypogonadism	Sornson et al., Nature 1996 384:327–33
FSHβ subunit	Female infertility, males fertile	Kumar et al., Nat Genet 1997 15:201–4
Prolactin	Female infertility	Horseman et al., EMBO J 1997 16:6926–35
TSHβ subunit	Hypothyroidism, female subfertility	Jiang et al., Reproduction 2001 122:695–700

tive organ weights instead of the absolute weights. Furthermore, the accessory sex glands continue to grow during the whole adult life, and the relative organ weights are usually higher in older animals. In order to obtain high-quality microscopic sections it may be advisable to dissect a larger organ block which contains the prostate, seminal vesicles, prostatic urethra, and urinary bladder, and special attention must be paid to the orientation of the tissue block when cutting the sections, in order to prepare comparable sections. By using serial sections and computer-aided morphometric analysis, it is possible to perform quantitative analysis of tissue composition (e.g., to determine the relative volumes of different tissue components), and reconstitute the three-dimensional image of the organ (for example, see Timms et al. 1994 and VomSaal et al. 1997). Several specific markers for prostatic structure and function are available, and can be used for further characterization of the phenotype. These include markers of different cell types, hormone responsiveness, differentiation, secretory activity, proliferative activity, and apoptosis.

Prostate development and growth is regulated by multiple hormonal factors, most notably androgens, estrogens, and prolactin. As expected, GM mice with altered hormone biosynthesis, and/or altered expression of hormone receptors, display a wide variety of changes in prostate growth or function (Wennbo et al. 1997; Couse and Korach 1999; Li et al. 2001; Mcpherson et al. 2001; Stanborough et al. 2001; Weihua et al. 2001; Zhang eta l. 2001; Jarred et al. 2002; summarized in Table 2). However, the presence of prostatic phenotype does not necessarily indicate that the genetic manipulation causes direct defects in prostatic cells. It is clear that any alteration in the hormone profile (e.g., gonadotropin, androgen, estrogen, prolactin) may induce pronounced changes in prostate, even though the gland itself would have the capacity to function normally.

Several GM mouse models with altered expression of growth factors, proto-oncogenes or tumor suppressor genes in the prostate, leading to the development of prostatic epithelial hyperplasia and premalignant prostatic intraepithelial neoplasia (PIN)-like lesions, have been characterized. These include overexpression of fibroblast growth factors 3 and 8 (Muller et al. 1990; Tutrone et al. 1993; Chua et al. 2002; Song et al. 2002), expression of *myc* or *ras* proto-oncogenes (Thompson et al. 1989), disruption of p53, retinoblastoma (Rb) and *pten* tumor suppressor genes (Colombel et al. 1995; Thompson et al. 1995; Wang et al. 2000; Kim et al. 2002), disruption of Mxi1 gene (Schreiber-Agus et al. 1998), and disruption of Nkx3.1 homeobox gene (Bhatia-Gaur et al. 1999; Abdulkadir et al. 2002). However, only a few GM models that develop prostatic carcinoma have been described. These include models with coexpression of *ras* and *myc* proto-oncogenes in mouse prostate (Thompson et al. 1989), targeted overexpression of SV 40 T antigen in mouse and rat prostate (Greenberg et al. 1995; Perez-Stable et al. 2002), deregulated expression of insulin-like growth factor 1 (Digiovanni et al. 2000), and disruption of Rb-gene (Wang et al. 2000).

4
Analyzing the Female Phenotype

4.1
General Principles

As with the males, analyzing the fertility by setting up a mating colony is a powerful tool to analyze reproductive function. Also in the GM female mice, a disrupted reproductive tract function often results in subfertility or infertility, and
several tests are available for preliminary analysis of female reproductive tract
function (summarized in Table 1). The cyclic ovarian function (4- to 5-day-long
estrus cycle) is a feature to be taken into account in analyzing the female phenotype. During the different days of the cycle, there are significant changes in the
structure and function of the reproductive tract also in WT females.

4.2
Ovarian Function

Ovarian folliculogenesis is under similar control of the gonadotropins in mice
and humans, and circulating estradiol (E2) and progesterone levels are good indicators of ovarian function. Our analyses of LuRKO mice confirmed that no
ovulation in mice occurred without LH action, and no significant pubertal E2
production was found in these mice (Zhang et al. 2001). Basic ovarian phenotype analysis involves histological evaluation of the two central ovarian structures: the presence of ovarian follicles with different maturation stages (with the
presence of theca cells and granulosa cells), and the corpora lutea (CL). Dramatic histological changes in these ovarian structures are readily detectable (Fig. 4).
For example in LuRKO mice no corpora lutea are formed, as their folliculogenesis never reach the pre-ovulatory stage, and no ovulations occur without LH action (Zhang et al. 2001). Another example of a well-distinguishable phenotype is
the presence of large cystic follicles in LH/hCG overexpressing mice with highly
increased production of both T and E2 (Risma et al 1995; Rulli et al. 2002). However, the analysis of a possible imbalance in proportion of follicles at the different follicular stages is a demanding task. Durlinger et al. (1999) divided the follicles in different classes based on the mean follicular diameter. This was determined by measuring two diameters in the section in which the nucleolus of the
oocyte was present, and the growing follicles were divided into two classes, i.e.,
small and large follicles. However, also more detailed grading have been used
(Morita et al. 1999). Nonatretic and atretic follicles are also detectable in sections with standard histological staining. The criteria for atresia typically involve the presence of pyknotic nuclei in the granulosa cells and/or degeneration
of the nucleus of the oocyte (Durlinger et al. 1999).

The CL with typical morphological features are easily detectable ovarian
structures, and fresh CL can be distinguished from the older ones by their
smaller size of luteal cells. The lack of CL in LuRKO mice ovaries evidently indi-

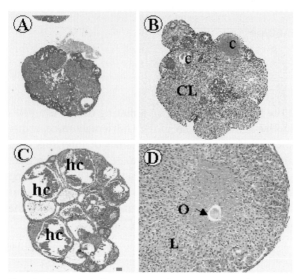

Fig. 4A–D Histological appearance of various ovarian phenotypes: **A** Normal wild type ovary, **B** Enlarged, highly luteinized ovary with large corpora lutea (*CL*) and hemorrhagic cysts (*c*). **C** Ovary present with large hemorrhagic cycts (*hc*). **D** Histology of a luteal structure (*L*) with an trapped oocyte (*O*), as an indicator of the ovulation failure in the mice

cates a failure of luteinization and ovulation in these mice. However, the formation of CL-like structures is not necessary an indicator of normal ovulation of the oocyte, while several GM mice exist with abnormal luteinization process. One of the indicators of an abnormal luteinization process is the presence oocyte trapped inside the luteal cell mass. Such a phenotype has been reported, e.g., in mice with disrupted function of progestin receptor (Lydon et al 1995) and the RIP140 (White et al 2000), a co-regulator of ERα, and recently we found an identical feature in TG mice constitutively expressing high levels of the hCGβ-subunit with elevated LH bioactivity (Rulli et al. 2002).

4.3
Onset of Puberty in Females, Estrous Cycle, and Mating Frequency

Fertility is dependent on regulation by a complex network of endocrine and paracrine factors, and targeted disturbance of their function frequently results in reduced reproductive performance in GM mice. The onset of puberty in female mice is determined by daily examination of vaginal opening, e.g., from day 21 onwards, and puberty is defined as the day of vaginal opening. It normally occurs at around the age of 26–30 days. However, the hormonal imbalance in GM mice can also cause precocious puberty: e.g., at 21–22 days of age, as found for the hCG overexpressing mice (Rulli et al. 2002). In contrast, in LuRKO mice the vaginal opening was delayed to 35–38 days (Zhang et al. 2001), as an indicator of a delayed pubertal development.

After puberty, the estrous cycle is regulated by the hormonal influences within the hypothalamic–pituitary–ovarian axis. The estrous cycle and its regularity are analyzed by daily vaginal smears for a continuous period of time. Dried vaginal smears can be examined microscopically, and the stage of the estrous cycle can be determined on the basis of the cell types present. Mating behavior in mice is regulated by the cyclic hormonal changes and mating normally occurs only at estrous, which is entered on average every 4–5 days. If fertilization is unsuccessful after mating, the coital stimuli alone trigger pseudopregnancy in healthy normal female mice, in which case new mating will resume only after about 12 days. Ovarian dysfunction in GM mice frequently results in disrupted estrus cycle, resulting in frequent mating without pseudopregnancy, or in the lack of mating. Because of the lack of ovulatory LH peak, LuRKO females never ovulate. Hence, they do not show cyclic periodicity in estrus cycle, and totally lack estrus type of pattern of vaginal smear, and do not mate (Zhang et al. 2001). Hence, the altered mating behavior of LuRKO mice is connected with ovarian dysfunction in the form of the lack of the luteal phase. As another example: after vaginal opening during the precocious puberty, a period of constant estrus-type pattern with cornified epithelial cells was present in hCG overexpressing mice, followed by a constant diestrus-type (luteal) pattern with persistent leucocyte infiltration (Rulli et al. 2002).

4.4
Analyzing Ovulation and Implantation

After ovulation, the oocytes can be recovered from the oviduct using standard embryo manipulation techniques (Hogan et al. 1986), and the number of oocytes can be calculated to determine successful ovulations and to analyze number of oocytes ovulated. The number of ovulated oocytes per mouse is strain-dependent, and hence, proper controls with identical genetic background are important. Ovulation can also be induced by gonadotropin stimulation consisting of one injection of PMSG (2–10 IU), followed by an injection of 2–5 IU of hCG, 46–48 h after the PMSG injection (Hogan et al. 1986). The procedure gives proper information about the gonadotropin responsiveness of the ovaries. In a severe case of luteal dysfunction, ovulation does not occur even with high doses of gonadotropins. As expected, this is the case in the LuRKO mice lacking the functional LH receptor.

The inability of a female mouse to carry out pregnancy may be caused by problems in implantation or in restoring the hormonal environment essential for pregnancy. The putative reasons for infertility can be addressed experimentally. For example, oocytes collected from the oviduct of a GM female mouse after normal, or gonadotropin-stimulated, ovulation could be transferred into pseudopregnant WT females using routine embryo transfer techniques used also in TG mouse production (Hogan et al. 1986). The ability of the GM oocytes to develop in WT females indicates a putative defect in the uterine implantation or in pregnancy of the GM females (Mikola et al. 2003). To further address whether the ovarian failure in GM mice is caused by defects in the ovary or systemic causes, ovary transfer experiments can be performed. If pregnancies occur after implanting WT ovaries into mutant females, the study demonstrates that the uterus, hypothalamus, and pituitary are able to support reproductive functions of the mutant ovary. Similarly, GM ovaries can be implanted into WT females to further analyze the role of local and endocrine factors as a cause of the infertility. The ability of the sperm to fertilize oocytes in vitro is also frequently analyzed.

5
Promoters Available for Expressing Transgenes in Reproductive Axis

Searching for tissue-specific promoters to drive transgenes to specific target organs of interest is of key importance for the development of specific disease models and models for drug development. The efficient use of transgenic technology in analyzing the reproductive function has been hindered by the limited amount of gene-regulatory regions efficiently targeting transgene expression into gonadal somatic cells. However, certain options are available, and more are likely to be developed in the near future. One of the most widely used promoters is that of the mouse mammary tumor virus (MMTV). In female mice, the promoter is especially useful for directing transgene expression to the mammary gland epithelial cells (Hennighausen 2000), but expression is frequently seen also in the ovary (Daphna-Iken et al 1998). In male mice, MMTV promoter directs TG expression to the urogenital region including testis, epididymis, seminal vesicles, and prostate epithelium (Kitsberg and Leder 1996; Korpelainen et al 1998).

For gonad-specific expression, a 6.0-kb and 2.1-kb fragments of the mouse inhibin-α subunit promoter has been successfully used to express genes in several cell types of the ovary (theca and granulosa cells and interstitial cells) and testis (Sertoli cells, Leydig cells; Hsu et al. 1995; Kananen et al. 1995). Hence, the inhibin-α promoter is relative broadly activated in different gonadal cell types of male and female mice. Furthermore, we have evaluated the possible use of the mouse LH receptor promoter to direct TG expression to testicular Leydig cells, and to ovarian granulosa luteal and theca cells. In these studies 7.0-kb, 2.1-kb, and 173-bp 5'-fragments were tested. In the testis the two shortest LH receptor promoter fragments directed weak TG expression in adult-type Leydig cells. However, the promoter was also activated during the germ cell development and is not considered optimal for targeted transgene expression in Leydig cells (Hämäläinen et al. 1999, 2000, 2002). Furthermore, the regulatory regions involved in ovary-specific expression were not identified. Hence, there is an ongoing active search for more efficient promoters to be used for expressing transgenes specifically in the somatic cells of gonads. The recent development in the use of large bacterial artificial chromosome (BAC) fragments in TG mice production should give new tools for identifying such promoters.

Interestingly, relatively large number of promoters have been shown to be active at certain stages of spermatocyte development (Venables and Cooke 2000), and there are several options for expressing a transgene in the male germ cells. Some of these include promoters for: (1) mouse acrosomal protein SP10, directing the transgene expression into round spermatids (Reddi et al. 1999); (2) protamine 1 (Prm-1), directing transgene expression into round and elongated spermatids (Fajardo et al. 1997); (3) phosphoglycerate kinase 2 promoter (Pgk-2), directing gene expression into spermatocytes and spermatids (Higgy et al. 1995). Recently, we found that a 3.8-kb $5'$-flanking region of mouse cysteine-rich secretory protein 1 (CRISP-1) gene is a new useful tool for expressing genes in the late meiotic and post-meiotic spermatogenic cells (Lahti et al. 2001). It should also be emphasized that a large number of endogenous and TG genes are expressed in the various developmental stages of spermatogenic cells without clear physiological function (endogenous genes). In addition, several TG promoters are expressed during the germ cell development for an unknown reason. Therefore, the reason for TG expression in spermatogenic cells should be inspected with caution.

Targeted transgene expression in the epididymis has been impossible until very recently when two different promoters were found to efficiently direct gene expression to this organ. These are the murine epididymal retinoic acid-binding protein (mE-RABP) promoter (Lareyre et al 1999), and mouse glutathione peroxidase 5 (GPX5) promoter (Lahti et al. 2001). However, the GPX5 and mE-RABP promoters seem to direct transgene expression differentially in the caput epididymidis. The 5-kb $5'$-fragment of the mE-RABP gene directs transgene expression into segments 2 to 5, while the 5-kb GPX5 promoter directs transgene expression especially into segment 4 of the caput epididymidis, but the transgene is also expressed at low level in other epididymal areas and in various other tissues (Sipilä et al. 2002).

In addition to the MMTV promoter mentioned above, at least two other promoters are useful for expressing transgenes in the prostate, namely a 5.7-bp $5'$-fragment of the prostatic steroid binding protein [C3(1)] gene (Maroulakou et al. 1994) and a modified probasin promoter (Zhang et al. 2000a) have been used successfully. Furthermore, in addition to the MMTV promoter, especially the whey acidic protein (WAP) promoter (Andres et al. 1987; Zhang et al. 2000b) has been used for targeted overexpression in mammary gland.

6
Manipulating Reproductive Hormone Concentrations by TG Technology

Generating TG mouse models with enhanced levels of polypeptide hormones consisting of one gene product is a straightforward approach. Basically, any tissue capable of the polypeptide processing, post-translational modification needed and secretion could be used for effective hormone production. For efficient over-production of a heterodimeric hormone or paracrine factor of interest usually needs a bi-TG model with two transgenes expressed in the same cell. However, if one of the monomers is expressed endogenously in excess, TG mice overexpressing only one subunit also lead to highly elevated hormone production. This was nicely demonstrated by a model overexpressing the bovine LH β-subunit under the mouse α-subunit promoter (Risma et al. 1995). In these TG mice, enhanced production of dimeric LH (consisting of a α/β-heterodimers) was obtained by overexpressing the β-subunit only. The endogenous α-subunit is produced in excess in the pituitary, and overexpressing the LH β-subunit by a transgene resulted in highly enhanced hormone secretion from the pituitary. Interestingly, there is a sex difference in the feedback regulation of the α-subunit promoter used for the β-subunit expression, resulting in the finding that gonadotropin concentrations were highly induced in females only. We recently produced TG mice expressing the hCG β-subunit under the human ubiquitin-C promoter, which is expressed in a broad range of tissues including the pituitary gland. In this model where the transgene expression was not affected by hormonal changes, even higher levels of circulating LH/hCG bioactivity was detected (Rulli et al. 2002). Hence, by using TG technology, any promoter leading to increased β-subunit expression in pituitary (FSH, LH, TSH) will distinctly increase the production of the corresponding hormone.

The human ubiquitin-C promoter is one of the options for constitutive expression in multiple tissues. The other option is to use CMV-enhanced chicken β-actin promoter. Of these two universal promoters, in our experience, the CMV-enhanced chicken β-actin promoter is far stronger than that of the ubiquitin-C. However, for highly elevated circulating hormone production, a weaker promoter is suitable as well. This was demonstrated by the TG mice overexpressing the hCG β-subunit under the ubiquitin-C promoter, which resulted into microgram per milliliter concentration of circulating β-subunit, being about 10,000-fold higher than the normal serum value (Rulli 2002). By the TG technology we can also enforce basically any tissue of interest to be the major endocrine organ responsible for the secretion of reproductive peptide hormones. For example, we recently generated a mouse model with enhanced expression of the hCG subunits in the liver by using a 700-bp-long PEPCK-promoter (S. Rulli et al., unpublished results). In these mice we could demonstrate a similar hCG β-subunit concentration to those produced by applying the ubiquitin-C promoter. In contrast to the straightforward approach for expressing at high-level peptide hormones or growth factors in TG mice, a direct manipulation of hormones consisting of small organic molecules such as steroids, for example, is a more complex issue. Any steroid hormone produced results from a steroid biosynthetic machinery involving several biosynthetic enzymes, and the biosynthesis is under a feed back regulation via gonadotropins. Overexpressing a certain enzyme in the pathway does not necessary lead into enhanced formation of the end product. However, certain manipulations of the steroidogenic pathway have also been successful, such as the AROM+ males present with enhanced estrogen-to-androgen ratio. In addition, hormonal manipulation of the gonadotropins often leads into over-stimulation of the steroid biosynthetic machinery, and to enhanced sex steroid production. This has been evidently shown in TG mice with high LH bioactivity (Risma et al. 1995; Rulli et al. 2002).

References

Abdulkadir, S.A., Magee, J.A., Peters, T.J., Kaleem, Z., Naughton, C.K., Humprey, P.A. and Milbrandt, J. (2002) Conditinal loss of Nkx3.1 in adult mice induces prostatic intra-epithelial neoplasia. Mol Cell Biol 22:1495–1503

Andres AC, Schonenberger CA, Groner B, Hennighausen L, LeMeur M, Gerlinger P (1987) Ha-ras oncogene expression directed by a milk protein gene promoter: tissue specificity, hormonal regulation, and tumor induction in transgenic mice. Proc Natl Acad Sci USA 84:1299–1303

Bhatia-Gaur R, Donjacour AA, Sciavolino PJ, Kim M, Desai N, Young P, Norton CR, Gridley T, Cardiff RD, Cunha GR, Abate-Shen C, Shen MM (1999) Roles for Nkx3.1 in prostate development and cancer. Genes Dev 13:966–77

Behringer RR, Finegold MJ, Cate RL (1994) Müllerian inhibiting substance function during mammalian sexual development. Cell 79:415–425

Birk OS, Casiano DE, Wassif CA, Cogliati T, Zhao L, Zhao Y, Grinberg A, Huang S, Kreidberg JA, Parker KL, Porter FD, Westphal H (2000) The LIM homeobox gene Lhx9 is essential for mouse gonad formation. Nature 403:909–913

Chua SS, Zhi-Qing M, Gong L, lin SH, DeMayo FJ, Tsai SY (2002) Ectopic expression of FGF-3 results in abnormal prostate and Wolffian duct development. Oncogene 21:1899–1908

Colombel M, Radvanyi F, Blanche M, Abbou C, Buttyan R, Donehower LA, Chopin D, Thiery JP (1995) Androgen suppressed apoptosis is modified in p53 deficient mice. Oncogene 10:1269–1274

Couse JF, Korach KS (1999) Estrogen receptor-null mice: what have we learned and where will they lead us? Endocr Rev 20:358–417

Daphna-Iken D, Shankar DB, Lawshe A, Ornitz DM, Shackleford GM, MacArthur CA (1998) MMTV-Fgf8 transgenic mice develop mammary and salivary gland neoplasia and ovarian stromal hyperplasia. Oncogene 17:2711–2717

DiGiovanni, J., Kiguchi, K., Frijhoff, A., Wilker, E., Bol, D.K., Beltrán, L., Moats, S., Ramirez, A., Jorcano, J. and Conti, C.(2000.): Deregulated expression of insulin-like growth factor 1 in prostate epithelium leads to neoplasia in transgenic mice. Proc natl Acad Sci USA, 97:3455–3460.

Durlinger AL, Kramer P, Karels B, de Jong FH, Uilenbroek JT, Grootegoed JA, Themmen AP (1999) Control of primordial follicle recruitment by anti-Mullerian hormone in the mouse ovary. Endocrinology 140:5789–96

Emmen JM, McLuskey A, Adham IM, Engel W, Verhoef-Post M, Themmen AP, Grootegoed JA, Brinkmann AO (2000) Involvement of insulin-like factor 3 (Insl3) in diethylstilbestrol-induced cryptorchidism. Endocrinology 141:846–849

Fajardo MA, Haugen HS, Clegg CH, Braun RE (1997) Separate elements in the 3 untranslated region of the mouse protamine 1 mRNA regulate translational repression and activation during murine spermatogenesis. Dev Biol 191:42–52

Gingrich JR, Barrios RJ, Kattan MW, Nahm HS, Finegold MJ, Greenberg NM (1997): Androgen-independent prostate cancer progression in the TRAMP model. Cancer Res 57:4687–4691.

Greenberg, N.M., DeMayo, F., Finegold, M.J., Medina, D., Tilley, W.D., Aspinall, J.O., Cunha, G.R., Donjacour, A.A., Matusik, R.J. and Rosen, J.M.(1995): Prostate cancer in a transgenic mouse. Proc Natl Acad Sci USA, 92:3439–3443.

Haavisto AM, Pettersson K, Bergendahl M, Perheentupa A, Roser JF, Huhtaniemi I (1993) A supersensitive immunofluorometric assay for rat luteinizing hormone. Endocrinology 132:1687–1691

He WW, Kumar MV, Tindall DJ (1991) A frame-shift mutation in the androgen receptor gene causes complete androgen insensitivity in the testicular-feminized mouse. Nucleic Acids Res 19:2373–2378

Hennighausen L (2000) Mouse models for breast cancer. Breast Cancer Res 2:2–7

Hess RA, Zhou Q, Nie R (2002) The role of estrogens in the endocrine and paracrine regulation of the efferent ductules, epididymis and vas deferens. In: Robaire B, Hinton BT (eds) The epididymis, from molecules to clinical practice, Kluwer Academic/ Plenum Publishers, New York Boston Dordrecht London Moscow, p 317–337

Higgy NA, Zackson SL, van der Hoorn FA (1995) Cell interactions in testis development: overexpression of c-mos in spermatocytes leads to increased germ cell proliferation. Dev Genet 16:190–200.

Hogan BL, Constantini F, Lacy E (1986) *Manipulating the Mouse Embryo*, Cold Spring Harbor Press, NY

Hughes IA (2001) Minireview: sex differentiation. Endocrinology 142:3281–3287

Huhtaniemi I, Nikula H, Rannikko S (1985) Treatment of prostatic cancer with a gonadotropin-releasing hormone agonist analog: acute and long term effects on endocrine functions of testis tissue. J Clin Endocrinol Metab 61:698–704

Hsu SY, Lai RJ, Nanuel D, Hsueh AJ (1995) Different 5'-flanking regions of the inhibin-alpha gene target transgenes to the gonad and adrenal in an age-dependent manner in transgenic mice. Endocrinology 136:5577–5586

Hämäläinen T, Poutanen M, Huhtaniemi I (1999) Age- and sex-specific promoter function of a two-kilobase 5'-flanking sequence of the murine luteinizing hormone receptor gene. Endocrinology 140:5322–5329.

Hämäläinen T, Poutanen M, Huhtaniemi I (2001) Promoter function of different lengths of the murine LH receptor gene 5'-flanking region in transfected gonadal cells and in transgenic mice. Endocrinology, 142:2427–2434

Hämäläinen T, Kero J, Poutanen M, Huhtaniemi I (2002) Transgenic mice harboring murine LH receptor/β-galactosidase fusion gene: Different structural and hormonal requirements of expression in testis, ovary and adrenal gland. Endocrinology 143:4096–4103

Jarred RA, McPherson SJ, Bianco JJ, Couse JF, Korach KS, Risbridger GP (2002) Prostate phenotypes in estrogen-modulated transgenic mice. TRENDS Endocrinol Metab 13:163–168

Kananen K, Markkula M, Rainio E, Su JG, Hsueh AJ, Huhtaniemi IT (1995) Gonadal tumorigenesis in transgenic mice bearing the mouse inhibin alpha-subunit promoter/ simian virus T-antigen fusion gene: characterization of ovarian tumors and establishment of gonadotropin-responsive granulosa cell lines. Mol Endocrinol 9:616–627

Kero J, Poutanen M, Zhang FP, Rahman N, McNicol AM, Nilson JH, Keri RA, Huhtaniemi IT (2000) Elevated luteinizing hormone induces expression of its receptor and promotes steroidogenesis in the adrenal cortex. J Clin Invest 105:633–41

Kero J, Savontaus E, Mikola M, Pesonen U, Koulu M, Keri RA, Nilson J, Poutanen M, Huhtaniemi I (2003)   Obesity in transgenic female mice with constitutively elevated luteinizing hormone secretion. Am J Physiol Endocrinol Metab (in press)

Mikola M, Kero J, Nilson JH, Keri RA, Poutanen M, Huhtaniemi I (2003) High levels of luteinizing hormone analog stimulate gonadal and adrenal tumorigenesis in mice transgenic for the mouse inhibin-alpha-subunit promoter/Simian virus 40 T-antigen fusion gene. Oncogene 22:3269–78

Kim MJ, Cardiff RD, Desai N, Banach-Petrosky WA, Parsons R, shen MM, Abate-Shen C (2002) Cooperativity of Nkx3.1 and Pten loss of function in a mouse model of prostate carcinogenesis. PNAS 99:2884–2889

Kitsberg DI, Leder P (1996) Keratinocyte growth factor induces mammary and prostatic hyperplasia and mammary adenocarcinoma in transgenic mice. Oncogene 13:2507–15

Koskimies P, Suvanto M, Nokkala E, Huhtaniemi IT, McLuskey A, Themmen APN, Poutanen M (2003) Female mice carrying a ubiquitin promoter-Insl3 transgene have descended ovaries and inguinal hernias but normal fertility. Mol Cell Endocrinol, in press

Korpelainen EI, Karkkainen MJ, Tenhunen A, Lakso M, Rauvala H, Vierula M, Parvinen M, Alitalo K (1998) Overexpression of VEGF in testis and epididymis causes infertility in transgenic mice: evidence for nonendothelial targets for VEGF. J Cell Biol 143:1705–12

Kreidberg, J., Sariola H, Loring JM, Maeda M, Pelletier J, Housman D, Jaenisch R (1993) WT-1 is required for early kidney development. *Cell* 74: 679–691

Lahti PP, Shariatmadari R, Penttinen JK, Drevet JR, Haendler B, Vierula M, Huhtaniemi IT, Poutanen M (2001) Evaluation of the 5'-flanking regions of murine glutathione peroxidase five (GPX5) and cysteine-rich secretory protein-1 (CRISP-1) genes for directing transgene expression in mouse epididymis. Biol Reprod 64:1115–1121

Lareyre J-J, Thomas TZ, Zheng W-L, Kasper S, Ong DE, Orgebin-Crist M-C, Matusik RJ (1999) A 5-kilobase pair promoter fragment of the murine epididymal retinoic acid-binding protein gene drives the tissue-specific, cell-specific, and androgen-regulated expression of a foreign gene in the epididymis of transgenic mice. J Biol Chem 274:8282–8290

Lei ZM, Mishra S, Zou W, Xu B, Foltz M, Li X, Rao CV (2001) Targeted disruption of luteinizing hormone/human chorionic gonadotropin receptor gene. Mol Endocrinol 15:184–200

Li X, Nokkala E, Yan W, Streng T, Saarinen N, Wärri A, Huhtaniemi I, Santti R, Mäkelä S, Poutanen M (2001) Altered structure and function of reproductive organs in transgenic male mice overexpressing human aromatase. Endocrinology 142:2435–2442

Lukyanenko YO, Chen JJ, Hutson JC (2001) Production of 25-hydroxycholesterol by testicular macrophages and its effects on Leydig cells. Biol Reprod 64:790–796

Luo X, Ikeda Y, Parker KL (1994) A cell-specific nuclear receptor is essential for adrenal and gonadal development and sexual differentiation. Cell 77:481–490

Lyon MF, Hawkes SG (1970) X-linked gene for testicular feminization in the mouse. Nature 227:1217–1219

Lydon JP, DeMayo FJ, Funk CR, Mani SK, Hughes AR, Montgomery CA Jr, Shyamala G, Conneely OM, O'Malley BW (1995) Mice lacking progesterone receptor exhibit pleiotropic reproductive abnormalities. Genes Dev 9:2266–2278

Mahendroo MS, Cala KM, Hess DL, Russell DW (2001) Unexpected virilization in male mice lacking steroid 5 alpha-reductase enzymes. Endocrinology 142:4652–4662

Maroulakou IG, Anver M, Garrett L, Green JE (1994) Prostate and mammary adenocarcinoma in transgenic mice carrying a rat C3(1) simian virus 40 large tumor antigen fusion gene. Proc Natl Acad Sci USA 91:11236–11240

McPherson SJ, Wang H, Jones ME, Pedersen J, Iismaa TP, Wreford N, Simpson ER, Risbridger GP (2001) Elevated androgens and prolactin in aromatase-deficient mice cause enlargement, but not malignancy, of the prostate gland. Endocinology 142:2458–2467

Morita Y, Perez GI, Maravei DV, Tilly KI, Tilly JL (1999) Targeted expression of Bcl-2 in mouse oocytes inhibits ovarian follicle atresia and prevents spontaneous and chemotherapy-induced oocyte apoptosis in vitro. Mol Endocrinol 13:841–850

Muller, W.J., Lee, F.S., Dickson, C., Peters, G., Pattengale, P. and Leder, P. (1990) The int-2 gene product acts as an epithelial growth factor in transgenic mice. EMBO J, 9:907–913.

Mulryan K, Gitterman DP, Lewis CJ, Vial C, Leckie BJ, Cobb AL, Brown JE, Conley EC, Buell G, Pritchard CA, Evans RJ (2000) Reduced vas deferens contraction and male infertility in mice lacking P2X$_1$ receptors. Nature 403:86–89

Nef S, Parada LF (1999) Cryptorchidism in mice mutant for Insl3. Nat Genet 22:295–299

Nef S, Parada LF (2000) Hormones in male sexual development. Genes Dev 2000 14:3075–86

Nef S, Shipman T, Parada LF (2000) A molecular basis for estrogen-induced cryptorchidism. Dev Biol 224:354–361

Ogawa S, Lubahn DB, Korach KS, Pfaff DW (1997) Behavioral effects of estrogen receptor gene disruption in male mice. Proc Natl Acad Sci USA 94:1476–1481

Olson GE, NagDas SK, Wifrey VP (2002) Structural differentiation of spermatozoa during post-testicular maturation. In: Robaire B, Hinton BT (eds) The epididymis, from molecules to clinical practice, Kluwer Academic/ Plenum Publishers, New York Boston Dordrecht London Moscow, p 371–387

Parr BA, McMahon AP (1998) Sexually dimorphic development of the mammalian reproductive tract requires Wnt-7a. Nature 379:707–710

Perez-Stable CM, Schwartz GG, Farinas A, Finegold M, Binderup L, Howard GA, Roos BA (2002) The G gamma/T-15 transgenic mouse model of androgen-independent prostate cancer: target cells of carcinogenesis and the effect of vitamin D analogue EB 1089. Cancer Epidemiol Biomarkers Prev 11:555–563

Plant TM, Marshall GR (2001) The functional significance of FSH in spermatogenesis and the control of its secretion in male primates. Endocr Rev 22:764–786

Prins GS, Birch L, Couse JF, Choi I, Katzenellenbogen B, Korach KS (2001) Estrogen imprinting of the developing prostate gland is mediated through stromal estrogen receptor alpha: studies with alphaERKO and betaERKO mice. Cancer Res 61:6089–6097

Reddi PP, Flickinger CJ, Herr JC (1999) Round spermatid-specific transcription of the mouse SP-10 gene is mediated by a 294-base pair proximal promoter. Biol Reprod 61:1256–1266

Risma KA, Clay CM, Nett TM, Wagner T, Yun J, Nilson JH (1995) Targeted overexpression of luteinizing hormone in transgenic mice leads to infertility, polycystic ovaries, and ovarian tumors. Proc Natl Acad Sci USA 92:1322–1326

Rulli SB, Kuorelahti A, Karaer Ö, Pelliniemi LJ, Poutanen M, Huhtaniemi I (2002) Reproductive disturbances, pituitary lactotrope adenomas and mammary gland tumors in transgenic female mice producing high levels of human chorionic gonadotropin. Endocrinology 143:4084–4095

Shawlot W, Behringer RR (1995) Requirement for Lim1 in head-organizer function. *Nature* 374: 425–430

Schreiber-Agus N, Meng Y, Hoang T, Hou Jr H, Chen K, Greenberg R, Cordon-Cardo C, Lee HW, De Pinho RA (1998) Role of Mxi1 in ageing organ systems and the regulation of normal and neoplastic growth. Nature 393:483–487

Sipilä P, Cooper T, Yeung C-H, Mustonen M, Penttinen J, Drevet J, Huhtaniemi I, Poutanen M (2002) Epididymal expression of Simian Virus 40 large T-antigen leads to angulated sperm flagella and infertility in transgenic mice. Mol Endocrinol 11:2603–2617

Song Z, Wu X, Powell WC, Cardiff RD, Cohen MB, Tin RT, Matusik RJ, Miller GJ, Roy-Burman P (2002) Fibroblast growth factor 8 isoform b overexpression in prostate epithelium: a new mouse model for prostatic intraepithelial neoplasia. Cancer Res 62:5096–5105

Sonnenberg-Rietmacher E, Walter B, Riethmacher D, Gödecke S, Birchmeier C (1996) The c-ros tyrosine kinase receptor controls regionalization and differentiation of epithelial cells in the epididymis. Genes Dev 10:1184–1193

Stanbrough M, Leav I, Kwan PWL, Bubley JB, Balk SP (2001) Prostatic intraepithelial neoplasia in mice expressing an androgen receptor transgene in prostate epithelium. Proc Natl Acad Sci USA 98:10823–10828

Teixeira J, Maheswaran S, Donahoe PK (2001) Mullerian inhibiting substance: an instructive developmental hormone with diagnostic and possible therapeutic applications. Endocr Rev 22:657–674

Thompson TC, Southgate J, Kitchener G, Land H (1989) Multistage carcinogenesis induced by ras and myc oncogenes in a reconstituted organ. Cell 56:917–930

Timms BG, Mohs Tj, Didio LJ (1994) Ductal budding and branching patterns in the developing prostate. J Urol 151:1427–1432

Tutrone, R.F. Jr., Ball, R.A., Ornitz, D.M., Leder, P. and Richie, J.P.(1993): Benign prostatic hyperplasia in a transgenic mouse: a new hormonally sensitive investigatory model. J Urol, 149:633–639

Vainio S, Heikkilä M, Kispert A, Chin N, McMahon AP (1999) Female development in mammals is regulated by Wnt-4 signalling. Nature 397:405–409

van Casteren JI, Schoonen WG, Kloosterboer HJ (2000) Development of time-resolved immunofluorometric assays for rat follicle-stimulating hormone and luteinizing hormone and application on sera of cycling rats. Biol Reprod 62:886–94

Wang Y, Hayward SW, Donjacour AA, Young P, Jacks T, Sage J, Dahiya R, Cardiff RD, Day ML, Cunha GR (2000) Sex hormone –induced carcinogenesis in Rb-deficient prostate tissue. Cancer Res 60:6008–6017

Weihua Z, Mäkelä S, Andersson LC, Salmi S, Saji S, Webster JI, Jensen EV, Nilsson S, Warner M, Gustafsson JÅ (2001) A role for estrogen receptor beta in the regulation of growth of the ventral prostate. Proc Natl Acad Sci USA 98:6330–6335

Venables JP, Cooke HJ (2000) Lessons from knockout and transgenic mice for infertility in men. J Endocrinol Invest 23:584–91

Wennbo H, Kindblom J, Isaksson OG, Tornell J (1997) Transgenic mice overexpressing the prolactin gene develop dramatic enlargement of the prostate gland. Endocrinology 138:4410–4415

White R, Leonardsson G, Rosewell I, Ann Jacobs M, Milligan S, Parker M (2000) The nuclear receptor co-repressor Nrip1 (RIP140) is essencial for female fertility. Nature Medicine 6:1368–1374

VomSaal FS, Timms BG, Montano MM, Palanza P, Thayer KA, Nagel SC, Dhar, MD, Ganjam VK, Parmigiani S, Welshons WV (1997) Prostate enlargement in mice due to fetal exposure to low doses of estradiol or diethylstilbestrol and opposite effects a high doses. Proc Natl Acad Sci USA 94:2056–2061

Yeung CH, Sonnenberg-Riethmacher E, Cooper TG (1998) Receptor tyrosine kinase c-ros knockout mice as a model for the study of epididymal regulation of sperm function. J Reprod Fert, Supplement 53:137–147

Yeung C-H, Sonnenberg-Riethmacher E, Cooper TG (1999) Infertile spermatozoa of c-ros tyrosine kinase receptor knockout mice show flagellar angulation and maturational defects in cell volume regulatory mechanisms. Biol Reprod 61:1062–1069

Yeung C-H, Wagenfeld A, Nieschlag E, Cooper TG (2000) The cause of infertility of male c-ros tyrosine kinase receptor knockout mice. Biol Reprod 63:612–618

Zhang J, Thomas TZ, Kasper S, Matusik RJ (2000a) A small composite probasin promoter confers high levels of prostate-specific gene expression through regulation by androgens and glucocorticoids in vitro and in vivo. Endocrinology 141:4698–710

Zhang M, Shi Y, Magit D, Furth PA, Sager R (2000b)Reduced mammary tumor progression in WAP-TAg/WAP-maspin bitransgenic mice. Oncogene 19:6053–8

Zhang F-P, Poutanen M, Wilbertz J, Huhtaniemi I, (2001) Normal prenatal but arrested postnatal sexual development of luteinizing hormone receptor knockout mice. Mol. Endocrinol 15:172–183

Zhao L, Bakke M, Krimkevich Y, Cushman LJ, Parlow AF, Camper SA, Parker KL (2001) Steroidogenic factor 1 (SF1) is essential for pituitary gonadotrope function. Development 128:147–54

Zimmermann S, Steding G, Emmen JM, Brinkmann AO, Nayernia K, Holstein AF, Engel W, Adham IM (1999) Targeted disruption of the Insl3 gene causes bilateral cryptorchidism. Mol Endocrinol 13:681–91

Zirkin BR (1998) Spermatogenesis: its regulation by testosterone and FSH. Semin Cell Dev Biol 9:379–91

Part 7
Toxicology

Understanding Molecular Mechanisms of Toxicity and Carcinogenicity Using Gene Knockout and Transgenic Mouse Models

G. Elizondo[1] · F. J. Gonzalez[2]

[1] Sección Externa de Toxicología, CINVESTAV-IPN, PO Box 14–740,
07000 México, D.F., México
[2] National Institutes of Health, Building 37, Room 3E-24, 9000 Rockville Pike,
Bethesda, MD 20892, USA
e-mail: fjgonz@helix.nih.gov

Abstract An exponential increase of new chemical agents came with the industrial revolution. Since then, thousands of new compounds have been released to the environment with an important negative impact on human health. Understanding the mechanisms by which xenobiotics induce toxicity is crucial to prevent potential health hazards. However, the complex mechanism of action of chemical toxins has made it extremely difficult to evaluate the precise toxic mechanism as well as the role of specific genes in either potentiating or ameliorating toxicity. Among the different strategies, the problem can be addressed with genetically engineered animal models where genes have been manipulated to study their roles in chemical toxicity. Xenobiotic-metabolizing enzymes and xenobiotic receptors are considered the interface between chemicals and the environment. In particular, the cytochromes P450 (P450) have an important role in metabolic activation and detoxification of xenobiotics through oxidative metabolism. P450s can activate inert compounds to electrophilic derivatives that are capable of damaging and transforming cells. Other enzymes such as the various transferases can inactivate reactive intermediates. Xenobiotic receptors including the aryl hydrocarbon receptor (AHR), peroxisome proliferator-activated receptor α (PPARα), pregnane X receptor (PXR), and constitutively androstane receptor (CAR), which bind to foreign chemicals and induce enzymes, including P450s, responsible for metabolizing xenobiotics. The study of the roles of P450s and receptors in toxicity and carcinogenicity has been complicated by the marked species differences in these enzymes, making the prediction of human toxicity based on rodent data difficult. During the past seven years, several lines of xenobiotic metabolism-null mice have been produced to address the role of P450s and xenobiotic receptors in whole animal carcinogenesis and toxicity. More recently, humanized mouse models have been developed to aid in human risk assessment to toxic chemicals. The use of transgenic models should lead to a much greater understanding of potential risks associated with exposure to xenobiotics.

Keywords Cytochrome P450s · Nuclear receptors · Peroxisome proliferator-activated receptor (PPAR) · Gene knockout mice · Humanized mice · Drug and carcinogen metabolism

1
Introduction

With the large and growing number of chemical compounds found in the environment, the study of molecular mechanisms of chemical toxicity is essential to develop reasonable human risk assessment guidelines. Cytochromes P450 (P450s) comprise a large superfamily of proteins that are of central importance in the activation and detoxification of a wide variety of foreign compounds, including many therapeutic drugs, chemical carcinogens, and environmental pollutants. In most cases, toxins and carcinogens are inert chemicals and require P450s for conversion to electrophilic derivatives capable of binding to cellular nucleophiles (DNA, RNA and protein) and causing damage. Other xenobiotic-metabolizing enzymes can conjugate and inactivate metabolites produced by P450s.

Many strategies have been used in an attempt to understand the role of P450s in toxicity and carcinogenicity. In vitro systems have established that metabolism is, in most cases, required to convert chemicals to electrophilic metabolites that are capable of binding to cellular nucleophiles (Miller 1998). Recombinant enzymes have proved to be of great value in determining enzyme specificity toward specific classes of chemical agents (Gonzalez and Korzekwa 1995). Animal models, particularly rats and mice, have been widely used to understand the relationship between metabolism of xenobiotics and their toxic and carcinogenic effects in vivo. However, there are marked species differences in the way animals activate or inactivate chemicals, and thus rodents are not always the most suitable models to understand the molecular mechanisms of chemical toxicity in humans (Gonzalez and Nebert 1990). Despite the large amount of data generated using in vitro systems and correlative studies in animal models, the role of xenobiotic metabolism in toxicity and carcinogenicity in intact animals has not been demonstrated using genetically defined models.

Transgenic and gene knockout mouse models have been developed in an attempt to understand the role of xenobiotic-metabolizing enzymes and xenobiotic receptors in modulating chemical toxicity and carcinogenicity in an intact mouse model. The present review summarizes the most important results derived from these models.

2
Knockout Mouse Models

2.1
The Xenobiotic Receptors

2.1.1
The Aryl Hydrocarbon Receptor

The aryl hydrocarbon receptor (AHR) is a member of the basic helix-loop-helix/PAS transcription factor superfamily that is ligand activated and induces gene expression through dimerization with the AHR nuclear translocator (ARNT) (Hankinson 1995; Safe 2001). AHR mediates the transcriptional activation of genes encoding xenobiotic-metabolizing enzymes such as P450s (CYP1A1, CYP1A2, and CYP1B1), nicotinamide adenine dinucleotide phosphate, reduced [NAD(P)H]:quinone oxidoreductase, and uridine diphosphate (UDP)-glucuronosyl-transferase 6. It also mediates most of the toxicological effects of the halogenated aromatic hydrocarbons such as polychlorinated dibenzo-p-dioxins, polychlorinated dibenzofurans, and polychlorinated biphenyls, all of which are widely present in the environment and are known to cause toxicity and birth defects in humans.

To examine the role of AHR in toxicity and cancer, the AHR-null mouse was developed. Inactivation of the AHR yielded a mouse line that was reproductively viable but suffered from a number of abnormalities (Fernandez-Salguero et al. 1995; Schmidt et al. 1996; Mimura et al. 1997). Induction of CYP1A1, CYP1A2, CYP1B1, and other xenobiotic-metabolizing enzymes by 2,3,7,8-tetra-chlorodibenzo-p-diozin (TCDD) is abolished in AHR-null mice, demonstrating that AHR is required for induction of these gene products in liver. The absence of AHR is also associated with decreases in the constitutive expression of CYP1A2 and Ugt^*06 mRNA in liver, indicating that AHR controls basal gene expression. The AHR-null mouse model was used to establish that the toxic effects of TCDD are mediated by the AHR (Fernandez-Salguero et al. 1995) and that TCDD-induced teratogenicity is due to the AHR (Mimura et al. 1997; Peters et al. 1999) as well as the carcinogenic effects of benzo[*a*]pyrene (Shimizu et al. 2000).

In addition to these results, new insights for the role of AHR in cellular homeostasis were discovered. AHR-null mice have pronounced liver fibrosis and a highly reduced liver-body weight ratio. This is due in part to an alteration in vascular structure in the developing AHR-null mouse where the embryonic vascular structure persist to adulthood (Lahvis et al. 2000). High levels of retinoic acid and retinyl esters are also found in AHR-null mouse liver, suggesting that the mechanism by which AHR controls transforming growth factor (TGF)-β levels may be through increasing retinoic acid-responsive genes such as transglutaminase II, which activates TGF-β (Andreola et al. 1997). This may contribute to the lower cell proliferation and elevated apoptosis rates observed in AHR-null mouse embryonic fibroblasts (Elizondo et al. 2000) leading to liver fibrosis and smaller liver size (Fernandez-Salguero et al. 1995). Furthermore, the immune system of the AHR-null mice displayed a lower population of splenic lymphocytes (Fernandez-Salguero et al. 1996) that also could be due to elevated rated of spontaneous apoptosis. These abnormalities suggest that AHR is involved in liver and immune system development.

Other AHR-null mouse lines have been generated (Schmidt et al. 1996; Mimura et al. 1997). All lines exhibit consistent similarities such as small livers, and some differences in phenotype such as neonatal lethality and immune cell dysfunction have been described; however, no explanation for these differences is immediately apparent. It has been proposed that different gene-targeting strategies can result in altered products with unexpected function or can alter the function of neighboring genes (Lahvis and Bradfield 1998). In addition, the phenotype may be acutely sensitive to environmental variables, such as pathogen and chemical exposure. Further, genetic background can have an influence on phenotype due to the type of embryonic stem cells and mouse lines used for propagation of the null alleles. Therefore, design of the targeting construct and, most importantly, genetic background can be viewed as critical steps in generating and characterizing genetically engineered animal models.

2.1.2
Peroxisome Proliferator-Activated Receptor α

The peroxisome proliferator-activated receptor (PPAR) family includes three receptors designated PPARα, PPAR$\beta(\delta)$, and PPARγ. This family of receptors appears to be involved in regulating metabolism, transport, and storage of fatty acids and cholesterol. PPARα activates target genes that encode enzymes involved in mitochondrial and peroxisomal fatty acid ω and ω-1 oxidation. PPARγ is required for the differentiation and function of adipocytes and is the cellular target for the thiazolidinedione anti type 2 diabetes drugs (Fajas et al. 2001;

Kliewer et al. 2001; Rosen and Spiegelman 2001). It is also involved in macro-phage function where it mediates fatty acid and cholesterol transport (Moore et al. 2001). The precise function of PPAR$\beta(\delta)$ has not been established, although it is ubiquitously expressed and appears to modulate differentiation of the epidermis during phorbol ester treatment (Peters et al. 2000). This is probably due to the presence of an activator protein (AP)-1 site upstream of the PPAR$\beta(\delta)$ promoter (Tan et al. 2001). In this regard PPAR$\beta(\delta)$ was found to modulate would healing (Michalik et al. 2001).

PPARα is responsible for mediating the effects of peroxisome proliferators (Gonzalez et al. 1998; Devchand et al. 1999). These compounds include hypolipidemic drugs (chlofibrate and fenofibrate), plasticizers (diethylheylplthalate), solvents (trichloroethylene), and endogenous hormones (dehydroepiandroster-one sulfate, leukotriene B4). In susceptible species of rodents, peroxisome proliferators, as the name implies, cause peroxisome proliferation, and when administered chronically in the diet, they induce marked hepatomegaly and the development of hepatocellular carcinomas. However, humans are resistant to the carcinogenic effects of fibrate drugs (Choudhury et al. 2000). This reflects the known species differences between humans and rodents. Despite years of study of peroxisome proliferators, the mechanism of species difference is not known. Introduction of human PPARα into PPARα-null mice restores target gene induction, indicating that the human receptor is functional (Yu et al. 2001). However, human liver PPARα levels are 1/10 of that found in susceptible mouse and rat species (Palmer et al. 1998). In order to determine the mechanism of action of peroxisome proliferators, PPARα-null mice were developed. PPARα-null animals are resistant to peroxisome proliferation and hepatocellular carcinomas, demonstrating that PPARα is required for the toxic and carcinogenic effects of these chemicals (Peters et al. 1997). This is due in part to a lack of peroxisome proliferator-induced cell proliferation (Peters et al. 1998). These mice should be of use in uncovering the mechanism of action of peroxisome proliferator and the dissection of the species differences in response to these chemicals.

2.1.3
Pregnane X Receptor

Pregnane X receptor (PXR) is a member of the nuclear receptor superfamily and mediates the action of pregnanolone 16α-carbonitrile (PCN), dexamethasone, and other lipophilic xenobiotics that induce transcriptional activation of the CYP3A family of P450s (Kliewer et al. 1998). Similar to the retinoic acid receptor, PXR requires the retinoid X receptor (RXR) as an obligate heterodimer-ization partner in order to activate target genes having PXR response elements. The human counterpart of the mouse receptor, designated steroid X receptor (SXR) (Blumberg et al. 1998), exhibits distinct and overlapping ligand specificity with mouse PXR (Jones et al. 2000). Mice lacking PXR are viable and exhibit no deleterious phenotypes but are unresponsive to induction by pregnenolone

16α-carbonitrile (PCN), dexamethasone, and probably all other PXR ligands (Xie et al. 2000; Staudinger et al. 2001). These observations suggest that PXR serves no role in mammalian development or physiological homeostasis and is only present to respond to dietary signals to elevate rates of xenobiotic metabolism. The null mouse models were used to establish that PXR is a sensor for bile acids; upon superphysiological levels of toxic bile acid lithocholate, PXR is activated resulting in induction of a P450 that metabolizes the bile acid (Staudinger et al. 2001; Xie et al. 2001).

2.1.4
Constitutive Androstane Receptor

Constitutive androstane receptor (CAR), originally characterized based on its ligand independent binding to retinoic acid response elements (Baes et al. 1994), was subsequently found to mediate the action of phenobarbital (Honkakoski et al. 1998). The mechanism of action of CAR in activating gene transcription is unique from other nuclear receptors (Sueyoshi and Negishi 2001). While it requires RXR for activity, inducers such as phenobarbital apparently do not directly bind the receptor and, unlike other RXR partners, CAR is located in the cytoplasm. Phenobarbital appears to stimulate nuclear translocation of CAR. Mice lacking CAR do not respond to this inducer and another more potent inducer 1,4-bis[2-(3,5-dichloropyridyloxy)]benzene (TCPOBOP) (Wei et al. 2000). They are resistant to phenobarbital-induced cocaine toxicity and do not exhibit typical hyperplastic responses to phenobarbital and the potent inducer TCPO-BOP. Otherwise, the CAR-null mice appear normal. It is interesting to note that the *cis*-acting elements in the CYP2B1 (direct repeat 4) and CYP3A1 (direct repeat 3) genes in rats are activated by both PXR and CAR (Smirlis et al. 2001). Thus, these nuclear receptors have distinct ligand-binding specificities but promiscuous DNA binding properties.

2.1.5
Farnesoid X Receptor

Farnesoid X receptor (FXR) was isolated as an RXR partner (Seol et al. 1995) and then designated the farnesoid X receptor because it is activated by farnesoids, precursors in the pathway of cholesterol synthesis (Forman et al. 1995). However, the concentrations required for induction by these chemicals are superphysiological. The natural high-affinity ligands for FXR are bile acids (Makishima et al. 1999; Parks et al. 1999; Wang et al. 1999). The FXR might be a suitable target for new generation low-density lipoprotein (LDL)-cholesterol lowering drugs, since it is the cellular target for the cholesterol-lowering effects of the natural product guggulsterone, a plant sterol from the guggul tree (*Commiphora mukul*) (Urizar et al. 2002). The FXR-null mouse was used to establish that FXR is a bile acid sensor in vivo that controls both bile acid and lipid homeostasis through regulation of genes that encode bile acid biosynthesis and transport in the liver and gut (Sinal et al. 2000). Interestingly, mice lacking FXR have a marked increase in expression of CYP3A P450s, suggesting the possibility that they are producing endogenous ligands for other nuclear receptors such as PXR and CAR (Schuetz et al. 2001).

3
Cytochromes P450

While there are a large number of P450s, it is not practical to attempt to disrupt most P450 genes. Many are present in subfamilies containing up to five members. P450s in the CYP2 family exhibit a high degree of species differences in catalytic activity and regulation. Only a limited number of P450s are conserved in catalytic activity between mice and humans. These were chosen for gene disruption experiments. To date, four lines of P450-null mice have been developed, CYP1A1 (Dalton et al. 2000), CYP1A2 (Pineau et al. 1995; Liang et al. 1996), CYP1B1 (Buters et al. 1999), and CYP2E1 (Lee et al. 1996). All lines are reproductively viable and physiologically normal, indicating that these P450s play no role in mammalian development and physiological homeostasis. This is surprising since the CYP1A P450s and CYP1B1 are all conserved in mammals and exhibit no polymorphisms in which the enzymes are not expressed or inactive.

3.1
CYP1A2

CYP1A2 is constitutively expressed in liver and is induced by ligands of the AHR. This P450 is involved in the metabolic activation of arylamines, heterocyclic amine carcinogens, and aflatoxin B1 (Guengerich and Shimada 1998). It is also able to produce catechol estrogens (Aoyama et al. 1990). To define more clearly the role of CYP1A2 in toxicity and carcinogenesis in an intact animal model, the CYP1A2-null mouse was developed. The CYP1A2-null mice exhibit altered metabolism of CYP1A2 substrates such as caffeine. Pharmacokinetic analysis revealed that caffeine had an eightfold longer plasma half-life in CYP1A2-null mice compared to wild-type; 87% of the elimination of caffeine is due to CYP1A2 (Buters et al. 1996). These data support the use of caffeine metabolism to estimate human CYP1A2 activity and the individual capacity to activate carcinogens (Kadlubar et al. 1992; Tang and Kalow 1996). CYP1A2 is also a major regulator of clozapine pharmacokinetics and pharmacodynamics (Aitchison et al. 2000). Clearance of clozapine is slower in mice lacking CYP1A2 when compared to wild-type, having exaggerated responses when administered the drug.

Mouse bioassays have been performed to assess the role of CYP1A2 in chemical carcinogenesis and toxicity using CYP1A2-null mice. The potent carcinogen 4-aminobiphenyl (4-ABP) is a constituent of tobacco smoke and in vitro studies have shown that CYP1A2 is responsible for the metabolic activation of 4-ABP (Eaton et al. 1995). However, in a neonatal carcinogen bioassay using 4-ABP, the incidence of adenomas and carcinomas is not different between CYP1A2-null and wild-type mice (Kimura et al. 1999). This study demonstrated that the CYP1A2 is not the only enzyme involved in activation of 4-ABP in mice. CYP1A2 is also the major enzyme required for PhIP N2-hydroxylation in mouse, the initial metabolic activation of PhIP that is thought to lead to tumor formation. However, there is no significant difference in cancer incidence when PhIP was applied in the neonatal mouse bioassay (Kimura et al. 2003). Thus, although the metabolic activation of PhIP is carried out primarily by CYP1A2, an unknown pathway unrelated to CYP1A2 appears to be responsible for PhIP carcinogenesis in mouse when examined in the neonatal bioassay. Similarly paradoxical results were obtained when phenacetin was tested. Phenacetin is an analgesic, commonly used between 1970 and 1980, that causes renal and urinary tract tumors in experimental animal models (Johansson 1981; Nakanishi et al. 1982). Although CYP1A2 has been implicated in phenacetin detoxification (Sesardic et al. 1990), no evidence was found supporting the hypothesis that phenacetin is more carcinogenic in CYP1A2-null mice (Peters et al. 1999). However, phenacetin-induced toxicity in liver, kidney, and spleen is exacerbated in the null mouse, indicating that metabolism of the drug by CYP1A2 reduces its toxicity.

Based on in vitro studies, CYP1A2 has been postulated to have a role in uroporphyrin accumulation (Sinclair et al. 1987; De Matteis et al. 1988), a disease usually associated with hepatic cirrhosis and a mild increase in body iron stores. As a model to study this disease, treatment with iron and 5-aminolaevulinic acid has been used to induce hepatic uroporphyrin accumulation in mice (Constantin et al. 1996). After prolonged treatment, CYP1A2-null mice do not develop uroporphyria, indicating that CYP1A2 is essential in the development of this disease (Sinclair et al. 2000; Smith et al. 2001).

3.2
CYP1B1

CYP1B1 is expressed constitutively in steroidogenic tissues like the adrenal, ovary, and testes. CYP1B1 is also expressed in steroid-responsive tissue such as the uterus, breast, and prostate and is inducible by adrenocorticotropin, cyclic adenosine monophosphate (cAMP), peptide hormones, and aryl hydrocarbon receptor ligands (Murray et al. 2001). CYP1B1 metabolically activates polycyclic aromatic hydrocarbon carcinogens, such as 7,12-dimethylbenzo[*a*]anthracene (DMBA) and benzo[*a*]pyrene. The pathway for DMBA metabolism by CYP1A1 and CYP1B1 is shown in Fig. 1. CYP1B1 carries out the critical epoxidation step at the DMBA-3,4 position. In addition to its metabolic activation of carcinogens, autosomal recessive mutations in CYP1B1 have been linked with the human congenital glaucoma (Stoilov et al. 1997).

The CYP1B1-null mice are fertile and produce normal-size litters (Buters et al. 1999). Histopathological analysis revealed no abnormalities, showing that CYP1B1 is not required for mammalian development and physiological homeo-

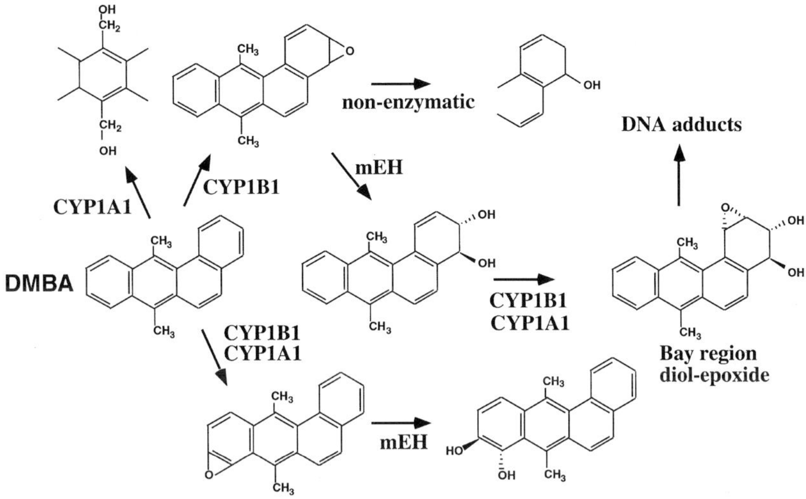

Fig. 1 Metabolic activation of DMBA. DMBA is metabolized by CYP1A1, CYP1B1, and mEH. CYP1B1 has a higher activity toward oxidation at the 3,4 position of DMBA than does CYP1A1. Both P450s have similar capacity to oxidize the 1,2 position of the DMBA-3,4 *trans* dihydrodiol

stasis, contrary to what was expected based on the conserved nature of this P450, its inducibility by hormones, and its role in development of glaucoma. CYP1B1 expression is absent in the lung, liver, kidney, uterus, and embryo fibroblast cells from CYP1B1-null mice. CYP1B1-null embryo fibroblasts are more resistant to DMBA toxicity than cells from wild-type mice, and CYP1B1-null mice are protected against DMBA-induced tumors, while wild-type mice develop malignant lymphomas, suggesting that CYP1B1 is an essential enzyme for metabolic activation of DMBA (Buters et al. 1999, 2002). DNA-binding studies using embryonic fibroblasts isolated from these animals provided further evidence that CYP1B1-catalyzed formation of fjord region DB[a,l]PDE-DNA adducts is the critical step in DB[a,l]P-mediated carcinogenesis in mice (Buters et al. 2002). Through the use of this mouse line, it was also demonstrated that bone marrow CYP1B1 is required for DMBA-induced pre-B cell apoptosis (Heidel et al. 1999) and a preleukemic effect (Heidel et al. 2000). Because human CYP1B1 activates many precarcinogens to mutagenic metabolites, it is thus possible that human bone marrow cytotoxicity is dependent on CYP1B1-mediated metabolism of polycyclic aromatic hydrocarbons.

An autosomal recessive mutation in CYP1B1 has been associated with development of primary congenital glaucoma in humans (Stoilov et al. 1997). Interestingly, examination of the CYP1B1-null mice revealed no evidence of glaucoma. However, these mice have drainage structure abnormalities matching those reported in human patients. When CYP1B1-null mice that are genetically identical except for their tyrosinase genotypes were analyzed, the protective role of tyrosinase activity against ocular defects caused by CYP1B1 deficiency was uncovered (Libby et al. 2003). These data indicate that lack of CYP1B1 is only one factor required for development of glaucoma and suggest that additional genes may contribute to the progression of the disease.

3.3
CYP2E1

CYP2E1 is highly conserved in mammals, and is constitutively expressed in various tissues with the liver having the highest level (Tanaka et al. 2000). It is the principal P450 responsible for the metabolism of many low-molecular weight compounds including alcohols, nitrosamines, and industrial solvents. In vitro data have indicated that many of these chemicals, some of them toxins and carcinogens, are metabolized by CYP2E1. To investigate the in vivo role of CYP2E1 in these toxic processes, a CYP2E1-null mouse line was produced (Lee et al. 1996). CYP2E1-null mice reproduce normally with no differences in litter size and growth rates as compared to wild-type animals, indicating that CYP2E1 is not required for mammalian development or physiological homeostasis. Initially the CYP2E1-null model was characterized by treating mice with acetaminophen (APAP). APAP is a widely used analgesic and antipyretic drug that in rare instances can lead to severe centrilobular hepatic necrosis in humans. The main P450s thought to be responsible for APAP bioactivation and hepatotoxicities include CYP2E1, CYP1A2, and CYP3A4. Using CYP1A2-null, CYP2E1-null, and CYP1A2/CYP2E1 double null- mice, it was established that CYP2E1 is the main P450 that mediates the hepatotoxicity of APAP at low doses, while CYP1A2 does at high doses (Zaher et al. 1998). All three null mice were resistant to APAP toxicity when compared to wild-type mouse with the order of sensitivity wild-type>CYP1A2-null>CYP2E1-null>CYP1A2/2E1-null mice (Fig. 2). These find-

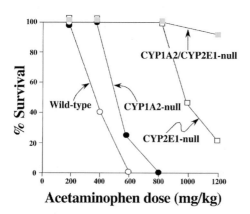

Fig. 2 Hepatotoxicity of acetaminophen. APAP was administered intraperitoneally at various doses and the survival of mice after 48 h was determined. Mice lacking CYP1A2 were partially resistant and mice lacking CYP2E1 were very resistant. Double-null mice not expressing CYP1A2 and CYP2E1 were almost totally resistant to the lethal affects of APAP

ings demonstrate the utility of the double-null mouse in assessing the overall role of P450 in xenobiotic-induced toxicity.

CYP2E1 also modulates benzene metabolism and toxicity. Benzene is an industrial chemical and environmental contaminant. In humans, benzene exposure has been associated with an increased incidence of aplastic anemia and acute myelogenous leukemia. It is generally agreed that benzene toxicity results from the biotransformation of the parent compound to a reactive species. Immunoinhibition studies of in vitro microsomal metabolism suggest that CYP2E1 is the major oxidative enzyme involved in benzene metabolism (Gut et al. 1996). The in vivo role of CYP2E1 on benzene metabolism and toxicity was investigated using the CYP2E1-null mouse. Benzene metabolism is significantly reduced in CYP2E1-null mice, demonstrating that CYP2E1 is responsible for benzene metabolism and the in vivo conversions to hydroquinone, muconic acid, and catechol (Valentine et al. 1996). In addition, the lack of benzene-induced cytotoxicity and genotoxicity in bone marrow, blood, and lymphoid tissues from CYP2E1-null mice indicates that benzene biotransformation by CYP2E1 is required for benzene-induced toxicity.

CYP2E1-null mice have also been useful to determine the role of this P450 in the biotransformation of several toxic compounds such as carbon tetrachloride (CCL_4). In animals, CCL_4 has been shown to produce liver damage and fatty degeneration (Recknagel et al. 1989). In humans, many cases of acute CCL_4 poisoning have been documented, mostly following occupational exposure to the solvent. The in vivo role of CYP2E1 in CCL_4 hepatotoxicity was investigated using the CYP2E1-null mouse. Mice lacking CYP2E1 are resistant to liver damage after exposure to CCL_4 (Wong et al. 1998). This indicates that CYP2E1 is the major factor involved in CCL_4-induced hepatotoxicity and that the CYP2E1-null mouse model will be useful to study the role of CYP2E1 in CCL_4-induced lipid peroxidation. CYP2E1, through the CYP2E1-null mouse, was also used to determine that CYP2E1 is involved in the bioactivation of several toxic compounds such as methacrylonitrile (Ghanayem et al. 1999), chloroform (Constan et al. 1999), and gasoline ethers (Hong et al. 1999).

Under fasting conditions or diabetes, acetone is produced and used in mammalian glucose metabolism. In vitro, acetone is metabolized by CYP2E1 to acetol and then to methylglyoxal, both intermediates in the gluconeogenesis pathway (Casazza et al. 1984). Consistent with the reports that acetone oxidation is catalyzed by CYP2E1 in vitro, a significant elevation of blood acetone was found in CYP2E1-null mice, suggesting an inability of these animals to catabolize the excess acetone produced during fasting (Bondoc et al. 1999). These results demonstrate that CYP2E1 plays an important role in the catabolism of acetone under fasting conditions where acetone metabolites and ketone bodies are used as source of energy, particularly in the brain.

4
Microsomal Epoxide Hydrolase

Microsomal epoxide hydrolase (mEH) catalyzes the reduction of reactive epoxides, most of which are formed by P450s (Fretland and Omiecinski 2000). In most cases, mEH inactivates epoxides that could cause cellular damage. However, it is required for the metabolic activation of polycyclic aromatic hydrocarbons to the bay region diol epoxides that are considered to be the ultimate reactive carcinogenic form of compounds such as benzo[a]pyrene and DMBA (Fig. 1). mEH catalyzes the hydrolysis of DMBA to the DMBA trans-3,4-diol. To study the function of mEH and its role in cancer and toxicity, mEH-null mice were produced. Mice lacking mEH reproduce normally and show no deleterious phenotype, thus establishing that this enzyme is not essential for mammalian development and physiological homeostasis (Miyata et al. 1999). This result is surprising, since mEH is widely expressed in mammals and no polymorphism resulting in lack of enzyme activity is known to exist, although there is a thermal stability polymorphism in mice (Lyman et al. 1980) and an allele with two amino acid substitution polymorphism in humans that produces an enzyme with only modest differences in catalytic activity compared to the wild-type allele (Omiecinski et al. 2000). Since mEH is required for the formation of diol epoxides of polycyclic aromatic hydrocarbons, a skin carcinogenesis bioassay was carried out. Mice lacking mEH show resistance to the experimental DMBA exposure (Miyata et al. 1999). In the initiation-promotion protocol using the 12-O-tetradecanoylphorbol-13-acetate (TPA) as a tumor promoter, mEH-null get papillomas but a lower frequency than wild-type mice. However, in the complete carcinogenesis assay, mEH-null mice are totally resistant to tumors. These data indicate that (1) the DMBA diol epoxide may be required for tumor promotion in the complete carcinogenesis assay and (2) other metabolites can function as initiators when TPA is used as a promoter. mEH had also been implicated in benzene myelotoxicity. mEH converts benzene oxide, produced by CYP2E1, to benzene dihydrodiol, which is then converted to a catechol by a dehydrogenase (Ross 2000). Male mice deficient in mEH exhibit resistance to benzene-induced toxicity (Bauer et al. 2003b).

5
NADPH: Quinone Oxidoreductase 1

NADPH: quinone oxidoreductase 1 (NQO1) is involved in the two-electron reduction of potentially toxic quinines, many of which are produced by P450s, to hydroquinones. Thus, this enzyme offers protection against cellular nucleophiles that can cause toxicity. Mice lacking NQO1 reproduce and appear normal, indicating that this enzyme while conserved in mammals is not required for development and physiological homeostasis (Radjendirane et al. 1998). NQO1-null mice exhibit increased susceptibility to menadione and benzo[a]pyrene-3,6-quinone toxicity as measured by lipid peroxidation, thus demonstrating an important role for NQO1 in toxicity derived from quinone metabolites (Joseph et al. 2000). Skin cancer bioassays were used to establish a role for NQO1 in the inactivation of polycyclic aromatic hydrocarbons. Mice lacking NQO1 were more susceptible to benzo[*a*]pyrene (Long et al. 2000) and DMBA (Long et al. 2001) induced papilloma formation. These data indicate that the quinones of these compounds may be efficient initiators of carcinogenesis. Alternatively, NQO1 may serve to alter the oxidative stress induced by polycyclic aromatic hydrocarbon carcinogen treatment. NQO1 deficiency in humans is associated with an increased risk of leukemia, specifically acute myelogenous leukemia, and benzene poisoning (Rothman et al. 1997). The benzene metabolites hydroquinone and catechol are converted by bone marrow myeloperoxidase to reactive quinones. However, 1,4- and 1,2-bezoquinones can each be readily converted to hydroquinone and catechol by NQO1; these metabolites are substrates for conjugating enzymes (Ross 2000). The role of NQO1 in benzene-induced myelotoxicity was confirmed by analysis of the NQO1-null mice which were found to be more susceptible to benzene-induced toxicity than wild-type mice. However, the specific patterns of toxicity differed between the male and female mice (Bauer et al. 2003a). It should be noted that the role of NQO1 in protection against cancer may be non-metabolic. NQO1 can bind to and stabilize p53 as demonstrated in cell-free systems (Anwar et al. 2003). Whether this occurs in vivo remains to be investigated.

6
Glutathione *S*-Transferase Pi

Glutathione *S*-transferase pi (GSTP1) and GSTP2 expression was abolished without serious consequence (Henderson et al. 1998). GSTP1 is the most actively expressed between two tandemly arranged genes. When the GSTP-null mice were subjected to DMBA skin cancer bioassay, they exhibited an increase in papilloma frequency, suggesting that GSTP1 is involved in hydrolysis of DMBA epoxides that lead to the ultimate carcinogenic form of DMBA.

Analysis of acetaminophen toxicity led to paradoxical results; GSTP-null mice were more susceptible to the drug than wild-type mice (Henderson et al. 2000). This result is surprising given the known role of the GST enzymes and its substrate (glutathione) in inactivating quinines that are the activated form of acetaminophen. Glutathione depletion was similar in both lines of mice treated with the drug, indicating that GSTP1 is not involved in acetaminophen conjugation. However, the rate of recovery of glutathione levels was greater in the null mice. A role for GST in acetaminophen toxicity was suggested in studies with the CAR-null mice (Zhang et al. 2002). CAR-null mice were resistant to acetaminophen toxicity, and this resistance was correlated with the lack of induction of GSTP1. Inhibition of CAR in wild-type mice also reduced acetaminophen-induced hepatotoxicity, suggesting a possible mechanism for therapeutic intervention of acute acetaminophen toxicity.

7
Humanized Mouse Models

P450 studies are essential to understand the mechanisms of toxicity. However, there are important species differences in the regulation, expression, and activities of P450s that may have an impact when using animal models to assess the potential risks of xenobiotics in humans. Transgenic mice can be produced that express human P450s (humanized mouse transgenic models). The main problem with this strategy is the presence of endogenous mouse P450s. However, introducing human P450 genes into P450-null mice can circumvent this disadvantage. Alternatively, the P450 expression could be generated using a construct containing the P450 cDNA under the control of a tissue-specific promoter. Such is the case of the CYP1A2 humanized mouse model (Ueno et al. 2000). The human CYP1A2 gene was introduced into mice under the control of the mouse elastase I promoter. This promoter was chosen to express CYP1A2 because is not expressed naturally in the pancreas, thus establishing a transgenic mouse model by the introduction of human CYP1A2 into a tissue-null background. Pancreatic microsomes from this transgenic model can be used to study the metabolism of chemicals by human CYP1A2, but more importantly to study human CYP1A2-mediated chemical toxicity and carcinogenesis in vivo.

Others used a similar strategy to produce a CYP3A7 transgenic mouse (Li et al. 1996). CYP3A7 is expressed specifically in human fetal liver and catalyzes the 16α-hydroxylation of dehydroepiandrosterone 3-sulfate, a precursor of estriol. It also activates mycotoxins as well as some mutagens produced by protein pyrolysis. Since CYP3A7 is the major form of P450 in human fetal liver, and to elucidate its toxicological significance, a human CYP3A7 transgenic mouse line was produced. This was accomplished by introducing a construct containing the CYP3A7 cDNA under the control of mouse metallothionein promoter. CYP3A7 protein was expressed in various organs including the liver, kidney, and testis. Through mating CYP3A7 transgenic mice with p53 knockout mice, the authors produced immortalized hepatocytes expressing CYP3A7 (Shimoji et al. 1995). This cell line, together with the CYP3A7 transgenic mouse, will be useful to study fetal toxicities of chemicals in humans.

The human CYP4B1 cDNA was expressed in mouse liver using the liver specific apoE gene promoter (Imaoka et al. 2001). These mice catalyzed lauric acid ω-hydroxylase activity and were able to activate 2-aminofluorene, showing that they may be a useful tool to study human CYP4B1 and its relation to chemical toxicity and carcinogenesis.

Human P450 genes can be also introduced into mice with their own regulatory elements. This has recently been accomplished using a λ phage clone containing the wild-type CYP2D6 gene. Wild-type mice do not significantly metabolize the prototypical CYP2D6 substrate debrisoquine, while humanized CYP2D6 mice readily metabolize this substrate as indicated by pharmacokinetic and urine metabolite analysis (Corchero et al. 2001) (Fig. 3). Additional breeding was done with the hepatocyte nuclear factor-α (HNF)-4α conditional liver-null mice

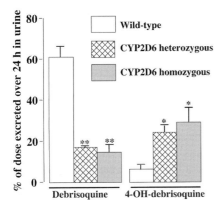

Fig. 3 Percentage of a single oral dose of DEB (2.5 mg/kg) excreted in urine over 24 h from wild-type, *CYP2D6* humanized heterozygous, and *CYP2D6* humanized homozygous mice. *Columns* represent the mean and standard error of mean (SEM) of debrisoquine and 4-OH- debrisoquine from 3–4 mice. *, Values of 4-OH-debrisoquine levels from *CYP2D6* humanized mice that are different ($p < 0.05$) from wild-type mice; **, values of debrisoquine levels from *CYP2D6* humanized mice that are significantly different ($p < 0.05$) from wild-type mice

(Hayhurst et al. 2001). HNF-4 liver-null/humanized CYP2D6 mice expressed lower levels of CYP2D6 than the control transgenics, thus establishing, in an intact animal model, that this transcription factor controls CYP2D6 gene expression. These mice should prove to be of great value in the study of the pharmacokinetics and pharmacodynamics of CYP2D6 substrates. For example, the humanized CYP2D6 was used to determine that CYP2D6 converts 5-methoxytryptamine, a metabolite and precursor of melatonin, to serotonin (Yu et al. 2003).

Humanized mice have also been produced for xenobiotic receptors. Since mouse PXR has different ligand specificity than its human counterpart, a PXR humanized mouse was produced from the PXR-null mouse (Xie et al. 2000). For example, mice do not respond to the CYP3A4 inducer rifampicin. Mice expressing human PXR in place of the mouse receptor respond to rifampicin and other ligands to human PXR.

8
Conclusions

The power of transgenic animals in understanding the mechanisms of chemical toxicity as well as identifying the enzymes involved in mediating toxic response have been illustrated. However, potential problems such as background activity, overlapping substrate specificities between gene families, species differences in gene regulation and toxicological response should be taken into consideration. Finding solutions to the above problems is important in order to avoid confounding the process of risk assessment. It is also critical not to ignore the complexity of mammalian organ systems in the interpretation of data collected from transgenic animals, because animals do not passively receive the experimenter's manipulation, and endogenous gene activities may be altered in response to the introduction of exogenous DNA sequences. Therefore, in addition to the technical advancement, a greater amount of basic information about the control of specific gene expression in animals is required to achieve the highest level of specificity in transgenic animals experiments.

Transgenic mouse models have proved to be a powerful tool in delineating and understanding the mechanism of chemical toxicity and carcinogenesis as well as identifying the role of P450s in these processes. The use of transgenic mice should lead to a much greater understanding of potential risks associated with exposure to xenobiotics and will provide new tools to facilitate preclinical drug development.

References

Aitchison KJ, Jann MW, Zhao JH, Sakai T, Zaher H, Wolff K, Collier DA, Kerwin RW, Gonzalez FJ (2000) Clozapine pharmacokinetics and pharmacodynamics studied with Cyp1A2-null mice. J Psychopharmacol 14:353–359

Andreola F, Fernandez-Salguero PM, Chiantore MV, Petkovich MP, Gonzalez FJ, De Luca LM (1997) Aryl hydrocarbon receptor knockout mice (AHR-/-) exhibit liver retinoid accumulation and reduced retinoic acid metabolism. Cancer Res 57:2835–2838

Anwar A, Dehn D, Siegel D, Kepa JK, Tang LJ, Pietenpol JA, Ross D (2003) Interaction of human NAD(P)H:quinone oxidoreductase 1 (NQO1) with the tumor suppressor protein p53 in cells and cell-free systems. J Biol Chem 278:10368–10373

Aoyama T, Korzekwa K, Matsunaga T, Nagata K, Gillette J, Gelboin HV, Gonzalez FJ (1990) cDNA-directed expression of rat P450s IIA1 and IIA2. Catalytic activities toward steroids and xenobiotics and comparison with the enzymes purified from liver. Drug Metab Dispos 18:378–382

Baes M, Gulick T, Choi HS, Martinoli MG, Simha D, Moore DD (1994) A new orphan member of the nuclear hormone receptor superfamily that interacts with a subset of retinoic acid response elements. Mol Cell Biol 14:1544–1551

Bauer AK, Faiola B, Abernethy DJ, Marchan R, Pluta LJ, Wong VA, Roberts K, Jaiswal AK, Gonzalez FJ, Butterworth BE, Borghoff S, Parkinson H, Everitt J, Recio L (2003a) Genetic susceptibility to benzene-induced toxicity: role of NADPH: quinone oxidoreductase-1. Cancer Res 63:929–935

Bauer AK, Faiola B, Abernethy DJ, Marchan R, Pluta LJ, Wong VA, Gonzalez FJ, Butterworth BE, Borghoff SJ, Everitt JI, Recio L (2003b) Male mice deficient in microsomal epoxide hydrolase are not susceptible to benzene-induced toxicity. Toxicol Sci 72:201–209

Blumberg B, Sabbagh W, Jr., Juguilon H, Bolado J, Jr., van Meter CM, Ong ES, Evans RM (1998) SXR, a novel steroid and xenobiotic-sensing nuclear receptor. Genes Dev 12:3195–3205

Bondoc FY, Bao Z, Hu WY, Gonzalez FJ, Wang Y, Yang CS, Hong JY (1999) Acetone catabolism by cytochrome P450 2E1: studies with CYP2E1-null mice. Biochem Pharmacol 58:461–463

Buters JT, Mahadevan B, Quintanilla-Martinez L, Gonzalez FJ, Greim H, Baird WM, Luch A (2002) Cytochrome P450 1B1 determines susceptibility to dibenzo[a,l]pyrene-induced tumor formation. Chem Res Toxicol 15:1127–1135

Buters JT, Sakai S, Richter T, Pineau T, Alexander DL, Savas U, Doehmer J, Ward JM, Jefcoate CR, Gonzalez FJ (1999) Cytochrome P450 CYP1B1 determines susceptibility to 7, 12-dimethylbenz[a]anthracene-induced lymphomas. Proc Natl Acad Sci U S A 96:1977–1982

Buters JT, Tang BK, Pineau T, Gelboin HV, Kimura S, Gonzalez FJ (1996) Role of CYP1A2 in caffeine pharmacokinetics and metabolism: studies using mice deficient in CYP1A2. Pharmacogenetics 6:291–296

Casazza JP, Felver ME, Veech RL (1984) The metabolism of acetone in rat. J Biol Chem 259:231–236

Choudhury AI, Chahal S, Bell AR, Tomlinson SR, Roberts RA, Salter AM, Bell DR (2000) Species differences in peroxisome proliferation; mechanisms and relevance. Mutat Res 448:201–212

Constan AA, Sprankle CS, Peters JM, Kedderis GL, Everitt JI, Wong BA, Gonzalez FL, Butterworth BE (1999) Metabolism of chloroform by cytochrome P450 2E1 is required for induction of toxicity in the liver, kidney, and nose of male mice. Toxicol Appl Pharmacol 160:120–126

Constantin D, Francis JE, Akhtar RA, Clothier B, Smith AG (1996) Uroporphyria induced by 5-aminolaevulinic acid alone in Ahrd SWR mice. Biochem Pharmacol 52:1407–1413

Corchero J, Granvil CP, Akiyama TE, Hayhurst GP, Pimprale S, Feigenbaum L, Idle JR, Gonzalez FJ (2001) The CYP2D6 humanized mouse: effect of the human CYP2D6 transgene and HNF4alpha on the disposition of debrisoquine in the mouse. Mol Pharmacol 60:1260–1267

Dalton TP, Dieter MZ, Matlib RS, Childs NL, Shertzer HG, Genter MB, Nebert DW (2000) Targeted knockout of Cyp1a1 gene does not alter hepatic constitutive expression of other genes in the mouse [Ah] battery. Biochem Biophys Res Commun 267:184–189

De Matteis F, Harvey C, Reed C, Hempenius R (1988) Increased oxidation of uroporphyrinogen by an inducible liver microsomal system. Possible relevance to drug-induced uroporphyria. Biochem J 250:161–169

Devchand PR, Ijpenberg A, Devesvergne B, Wahli W (1999) PPARs: nuclear receptors for fatty acids, eicosanoids, and xenobiotics. Adv Exp Med Biol 469:231–236

Eaton DL, Gallagher EP, Bammler TK, Kunze KL (1995) Role of cytochrome P4501A2 in chemical carcinogenesis: implications for human variability in expression and enzyme activity. Pharmacogenetics 5:259–274

Elizondo G, Fernandez-Salguero P, Sheikh MS, Kim GY, Fornace AJ, Lee KS, Gonzalez FJ (2000) Altered cell cycle control at the G(2)/M phases in aryl hydrocarbon receptor-null embryo fibroblast. Mol Pharmacol 57:1056–1063

Fajas L, Debril MB, Auwerx J (2001) Peroxisome proliferator-activated receptor-gamma: from adipogenesis to carcinogenesis. J Mol Endocrinol 27:1–9

Fernandez-Salguero P, Pineau T, Hilbert DM, McPhail T, Lee SS, Kimura S, Nebert DW, Rudikoff S, Ward JM, Gonzalez FJ (1995) Immune system impairment and hepatic fibrosis in mice lacking the dioxin-binding Ah receptor. Science 268:722–726

Fernandez-Salguero PM, Hilbert DM, Rudikoff S, Ward JM, Gonzalez FJ (1996) Aryl-hydrocarbon receptor-deficient mice are resistant to 2,3,7,8-tetrachlorodibenzo-p-dioxin-induced toxicity. Toxicol Appl Pharmacol 140:173–179

Forman BM, Goode E, Chen J, Oro AE, Bradley DJ, Perlmann T, Noonan DJ, Burka LT, McMorris T, Lamph WW, et al. (1995) Identification of a nuclear receptor that is activated by farnesol metabolites. Cell 81:687–693

Fretland AJ, Omiecinski CJ (2000) Epoxide hydrolases: biochemistry and molecular biology. Chem Biol Interact 129:41–59

Ghanayem BI, Sanders JM, Chanas B, Burka LT, Gonzalez FJ (1999) Role of cytochrome P-450 2E1 in methacrylonitrile metabolism and disposition. J Pharmacol Exp Ther 289:1054–1059

Gonzalez FJ, Korzekwa KR (1995) Cytochromes P450 expression systems. Annu Rev Pharmacol Toxicol 35:369–390

Gonzalez FJ, Nebert DW (1990) Evolution of the P450 gene superfamily: animal-plant 'warfare', molecular drive and human genetic differences in drug oxidation. Trends Genet 6:182–186

Gonzalez FJ, Peters JM, Cattley RC (1998) Mechanism of action of the nongenotoxic peroxisome proliferators: role of the peroxisome proliferator-activator receptor alpha. J Natl Cancer Inst 90:1702–1709

Guengerich FP, Shimada T (1998) Activation of procarcinogens by human cytochrome P450 enzymes. Mutat Res 400:201–213

Gut I, Nedelcheva V, Soucek P, Stopka P, Tichavska B (1996) Cytochromes P450 in benzene metabolism and involvement of their metabolites and reactive oxygen species in toxicity. Environ Health Perspect 104 Suppl 6:1211–1218

Hankinson O (1995) The aryl hydrocarbon receptor complex. Annu Rev Pharmacol Toxicol 35:307–340

Hayhurst GP, Lee YH, Lambert G, Ward JM, Gonzalez FJ (2001) Hepatocyte nuclear factor 4alpha (nuclear receptor 2A1) is essential for maintenance of hepatic gene expression and lipid homeostasis. Mol Cell Biol 21:1393–1403

Heidel SM, Holston K, Buters JT, Gonzalez FJ, Jefcoate CR, Czupyrynski CJ (1999) Bone marrow stromal cell cytochrome P4501B1 is required for pre-B cell apoptosis induced by 7,12-dimethylbenz[a]anthracene. Mol Pharmacol 56:1317–1323

Heidel SM, MacWilliams PS, Baird WM, Dashwood WM, Buters JT, Gonzalez FJ, Larsen MC, Czuprynski CJ, Jefcoate CR (2000) Cytochrome P4501B1 mediates induction of bone marrow cytotoxicity and preleukemia cells in mice treated with 7,12-dimethylbenz[a]anthracene. Cancer Res 60:3454–3460

Henderson CJ, Smith AG, Ure J, Brown K, Bacon EJ, Wolf CR (1998) Increased skin tumorigenesis in mice lacking pi class glutathione S-transferases. Proc Natl Acad Sci U S A 95:5275–5280

Henderson CJ, Wolf CR, Kitteringham N, Powell H, Otto D, Park BK (2000) Increased resistance to acetaminophen hepatotoxicity in mice lacking glutathione S-transferase Pi. Proc Natl Acad Sci U S A 97:12741–12745

Hong JY, Wang YY, Bondoc FY, Yang CS, Gonzalez FJ, Pan Z, Cokonis CD, Hu WY, Bao Z (1999) Metabolism of methyl tert-butyl ether and other gasoline ethers in mouse liver microsomes lacking cytochrome P450 2E1. Toxicol Lett 105:83–88

Honkakoski P, Zelko I, Sueyoshi T, Negishi M (1998) The nuclear orphan receptor CAR-retinoid X receptor heterodimer activates the phenobarbital-responsive enhancer module of the CYP2B gene. Mol Cell Biol 18:5652–5658

Imaoka S, Hayashi K, Hiroi T, Yabusaki Y, Kamataki T, Funae Y (2001) A transgenic mouse expressing human CYP4B1 in the liver. Biochem Biophys Res Commun 284:757–762

Johansson SL (1981) Carcinogenicity of analgesics: long-term treatment of Sprague-Dawley rats with phenacetin, phenazone, caffeine and paracetamol (acetamidophen). Int J Cancer 27:521–529

Jones SA, Moore LB, Shenk JL, Wisely GB, Hamilton GA, McKee DD, Tomkinson NC, LeCluyse EL, Lambert MH, Willson TM, Kliewer SA, Moore JT (2000) The pregnane X receptor: a promiscuous xenobiotic receptor that has diverged during evolution. Mol Endocrinol 14:27–39

Joseph P, Long DJ, Klein-Szanto AJ, Jaiswal AK (2000) Role of NAD(P)H:quinone oxidoreductase 1 (DT diaphorase) in protection against quinone toxicity. Biochem Pharmacol 60:207–214

Kadlubar FF, Butler MA, Kaderlik KR, Chou HC, Lang NP (1992) Polymorphisms for aromatic amine metabolism in humans: relevance for human carcinogenesis. Environ Health Perspect 98:69–74

Kimura S, Kawabe M, Ward JM, Morishima H, Kadlubar FF, Hammons GJ, Fernandez-Salguero P, Gonzalez FJ (1999) CYP1A2 is not the primary enzyme responsible for 4-aminobiphenyl-induced hepatocarcinogenesis in mice. Carcinogenesis 20:1825–1830

Kimura S, Kawabe M, Yu A, Morishima H, Fernandez-Salguero P, Hammons GJ, Ward JM, Kadlubar FF, Gonzalez FJ (2003) Carcinogenesis of the food mutagen PhIP in mice is independent of CYP1A2. Carcinogenesis 24:583–587

Kliewer SA, Moore JT, Wade L, Staudinger JL, Watson MA, Jones SA, McKee DD, Oliver BB, Willson TM, Zetterstrom RH, Perlmann T, Lehmann JM (1998) An orphan nuclear receptor activated by pregnanes defines a novel steroid signaling pathway. Cell 92:73–82

Kliewer SA, Xu HE, Lambert MH, Willson TM (2001) Peroxisome proliferator-activated receptors: from genes to physiology. Recent Prog Horm Res 56:239–263

Lahvis GP, Bradfield CA (1998) Ahr null alleles: distinctive or different? Biochem Pharmacol 56:781–787

Lahvis GP, Lindell SL, Thomas RS, McCuskey RS, Murphy C, Glover E, Bentz M, Southard J, Bradfield CA (2000) Portosystemic shunting and persistent fetal vascular structures in aryl hydrocarbon receptor-deficient mice. Proc Natl Acad Sci U S A 97:10442–10447

Lee SS, Buters JT, Pineau T, Fernandez-Salguero P, Gonzalez FJ (1996) Role of CYP2E1 in the hepatotoxicity of acetaminophen. J Biol Chem 271:12063–12067

Li Y, Yokoi T, Kitamura R, Sasaki M, Gunji M, Katsuki M, Kamataki T (1996) Establishment of transgenic mice carrying human fetus-specific CYP3A7. Arch Biochem Biophys 329:235–240

Liang HC, Li H, McKinnon RA, Duffy JJ, Potter SS, Puga A, Nebert DW (1996) Cyp1a2(-/-) null mutant mice develop normally but show deficient drug metabolism. Proc Natl Acad Sci U S A 93:1671–1676

Libby RT, Smith RS, Savinova OV, Zabaleta A, Martin JE, Gonzalez FJ, John SW (2003) Tyrosinase alleviates ocular defects caused by two glaucoma genes. Science 299:1578–1581

Long DJ, 2nd, Waikel RL, Wang XJ, Perlaky L, Roop DR, Jaiswal AK (2000) NAD(P)H:quinone oxidoreductase 1 deficiency increases susceptibility to benzo(a)pyrene-induced mouse skin carcinogenesis. Cancer Res 60:5913–5915

Long DJ, 2nd, Waikel RL, Wang XJ, Roop DR, Jaiswal AK (2001) NAD(P)H:quinone oxidoreductase 1 deficiency and increased susceptibility to 7,12-dimethylbenz[a]-anthracene-induced carcinogenesis in mouse skin. J Natl Cancer Inst 93:1166–1170

Lyman SD, Poland A, Taylor BA (1980) Genetic polymorphism of microsomal epoxide hydrolase activity in the mouse. J Biol Chem 255:8650–8654

Makishima M, Okamoto AY, Repa JJ, Tu H, Learned RM, Luk A, Hull MV, Lustig KD, Mangelsdorf DJ, Shan B (1999) Identification of a nuclear receptor for bile acids. Science 284:1362–1365

Michalik L, Desvergne B, Tan NS, Basu-Modak S, Escher P, Rieusset J, Peters JM, Kaya G, Gonzalez FJ, Zakany J, Metzger D, Chambon P, Duboule D, Wahli W (2001) Impaired skin wound healing in peroxisome proliferator-activated receptor (PPAR)alpha and PPARbeta mutant mice. J Cell Biol 154:799–814

Miller JA (1998) The metabolism of xenobiotics to reactive electrophiles in chemical carcinogenesis and mutagenesis: a collaboration with Elizabeth Cavert Miller and our associates. Drug Metab Rev 30:645–674

Mimura J, Yamashita K, Nakamura K, Morita M, Takagi TN, Nakao K, Ema M, Sogawa K, Yasuda M, Katsuki M, Fujii-Kuriyama Y (1997) Loss of teratogenic response to 2,3,7,8-tetrachlorodibenzo-p-dioxin (TCDD) in mice lacking the Ah (dioxin) receptor. Genes Cells 2:645–654

Miyata M, Kudo G, Lee YH, Yang TJ, Gelboin HV, Fernandez-Salguero P, Kimura S, Gonzalez FJ (1999) Targeted disruption of the microsomal epoxide hydrolase gene. Microsomal epoxide hydrolase is required for the carcinogenic activity of 7,12-dimethylbenz[a]anthracene. J Biol Chem 274:23963–23968

Moore KJ, Fitzgerald ML, Freeman MW (2001) Peroxisome proliferator-activated receptors in macrophage biology: friend or foe? Curr Opin Lipidol 12:519–527

Murray GI, Melvin WT, Greenlee WF, Burke MD (2001) Regulation, function, and tissue-specific expression of cytochrome P450 CYP1B1. Annu Rev Pharmacol Toxicol 41:297–316

Nakanishi K, Kurata Y, Oshima M, Fukushima S, Ito N (1982) Carcinogenicity of phenacetin: long-term feeding study in B6c3f1 mice. Int J Cancer 29:439–444

Omiecinski CJ, Hassett C, Hosagrahara V (2000) Epoxide hydrolase-polymorphism and role in toxicology. Toxicol Lett 112–113:365–370

Palmer CN, Hsu MH, Griffin KJ, Raucy JL, Johnson EF (1998) Peroxisome proliferator activated receptor-alpha expression in human liver. Mol Pharmacol 53:14–22

Parks DJ, Blanchard SG, Bledsoe RK, Chandra G, Consler TG, Kliewer SA, Stimmel JB, Willson TM, Zavacki AM, Moore DD, Lehmann JM (1999) Bile acids: natural ligands for an orphan nuclear receptor. Science 284:1365–1368

Peters JM, Aoyama T, Cattley RC, Nobumitsu U, Hashimoto T, Gonzalez FJ (1998) Role of peroxisome proliferator-activated receptor alpha in altered cell cycle regulation in mouse liver. Carcinogenesis 19:1989–1994

Peters JM, Cattley RC, Gonzalez FJ (1997) Role of PPAR alpha in the mechanism of action of the nongenotoxic carcinogen and peroxisome proliferator Wy-14,643. Carcinogenesis 18:2029–2033

Peters JM, Lee SS, Li W, Ward JM, Gavrilova O, Everett C, Reitman ML, Hudson LD, Gonzalez FJ (2000) Growth, adipose, brain, and skin alterations resulting from targeted disruption of the mouse peroxisome proliferator-activated receptor beta(delta). Mol Cell Biol 20:5119–5128

Peters JM, Morishima H, Ward JM, Coakley CJ, Kimura S, Gonzalez FJ (1999) Role of CYP1A2 in the toxicity of long-term phenacetin feeding in mice. Toxicol Sci 50:82–89

Peters JM, Narotsky MG, Elizondo G, Fernandez-Salguero PM, Gonzalez FJ, Abbott BD (1999) Amelioration of TCDD-induced teratogenesis in aryl hydrocarbon receptor (AhR)-null mice. Toxicol Sci 47:86–92

Pineau T, Fernandez-Salguero P, Lee SS, McPhail T, Ward JM, Gonzalez FJ (1995) Neonatal lethality associated with respiratory distress in mice lacking cytochrome P450 1A2. Proc Natl Acad Sci U S A 92:5134–5138

Radjendirane V, Joseph P, Lee YH, Kimura S, Klein-Szanto AJ, Gonzalez FJ, Jaiswal AK (1998) Disruption of the DT diaphorase (NQO1) gene in mice leads to increased menadione toxicity. J Biol Chem 273:7382–7389

Recknagel RO, Glende EA, Jr., Dolak JA, Waller RL (1989) Mechanisms of carbon tetrachloride toxicity. Pharmacol Ther 43:139–154

Rosen ED, Spiegelman BM (2001) Ppargamma : a nuclear regulator of metabolism, differentiation, and cell growth. J Biol Chem 276:37731–37734

Ross D (2000) The role of metabolism and specific metabolites in benzene-induced toxicity: evidence and issues. J Toxicol Environ Health 61:357–372

Rothman N, Smith MT, Hayes RB, Traver RD, Hoener B, Campleman S, Li GL, Dosemeci M, Linet M, Zhang L, Xi L, Wacholder S, Lu W, Meyer KB, Titenko-Holland N, Stewart JT, Yin S, Ross D (1997) Benzene poisoning, a risk factor for hematological malignancy, is associated with the NQO1 609C–>T mutation and rapid fractional excretion of chlorzoxazone. Cancer Res 57:2839–2842

Safe S (2001) Molecular biology of the Ah receptor and its role in carcinogenesis. Toxicol Lett 120:1–7

Schmidt JV, Su GH, Reddy JK, Simon MC, Bradfield CA (1996) Characterization of a murine Ahr null allele: involvement of the Ah receptor in hepatic growth and development. Proc Natl Acad Sci U S A 93:6731–6736

Schuetz EG, Strom S, Yasuda K, Lecureur V, Assem M, Brimer C, Lamba J, Kim RB, Ramachandran V, Komoroski BJ, Venkataramanan R, Cai H, Sinal CJ, Gonzalez FJ, Schuetz JD (2001) Disrupted Bile Acid Homeostasis Reveals an Unexpected Interaction among Nuclear Hormone Receptors, Transporters, and Cytochrome P450. J Biol Chem 276:39411–39418

Seol W, Choi HS, Moore DD (1995) Isolation of proteins that interact specifically with the retinoid X receptor: two novel orphan receptors. Mol Endocrinol 9:72–85

Sesardic D, Cole KJ, Edwards RJ, Davies DS, Thomas PE, Levin W, Boobis AR (1990) The inducibility and catalytic activity of cytochromes P450c (P450IA1) and P450d (P450IA2) in rat tissues. Biochem Pharmacol 39:499–506

Shimizu Y, Nakatsuru Y, Ichinose M, Takahashi Y, Kume H, Mimura J, Fujii-Kuriyama Y, Ishikawa T (2000) Benzo[a]pyrene carcinogenicity is lost in mice lacking the aryl hydrocarbon receptor. Proc Natl Acad Sci U S A 97:779–782

Shimoji M, Hattori K, Itoh S, Nakayama K, Katsuki M, Aizawa S, Yokoi T, Kamataki T (1995) Establishment of immortal hepatocytes from a CYP3A7-transgenic/p53-knockout mouse. Biochem Biophys Res Commun 217:1001–1005

Sinal CJ, Tohkin M, Miyata M, Ward JM, Lambert G, Gonzalez FJ (2000) Targeted disruption of the nuclear receptor FXR/BAR impairs bile acid and lipid homeostasis. Cell 102:731–744

Sinclair P, Lambrecht R, Sinclair J (1987) Evidence for cytochrome P450-mediated oxidation of uroporphyrinogen by cell-free liver extracts from chick embryos treated with 3-methylcholanthrene. Biochem Biophys Res Commun 146:1324–1329

Sinclair PR, Gorman N, Walton HS, Bement WJ, Dalton TP, Sinclair JF, Smith AG, Nebert DW (2000) CYP1A2 is essential in murine uroporphyria caused by hexachlorobenzene and iron. Toxicol Appl Pharmacol 162:60–67

Smirlis D, Muangmoonchai R, Edwards M, Phillips IR, Shephard EA (2001) Orphan receptor promiscuity in the induction of cytochromes p450 by xenobiotics. J Biol Chem 276:12822–12826

Smith AG, Clothier B, Carthew P, Childs NL, Sinclair PR, Nebert DW, Dalton TP (2001) Protection of the Cyp1a2(-/-) null mouse against uroporphyria and hepatic injury following exposure to 2,3,7,8-tetrachlorodibenzo-p-dioxin. Toxicol Appl Pharmacol 173:89–98

Staudinger JL, Goodwin B, Jones SA, Hawkins-Brown D, MacKenzie KI, LaTour A, Liu Y, Klaassen CD, Brown KK, Reinhard J, Willson TM, Koller BH, Kliewer SA (2001) The nuclear receptor PXR is a lithocholic acid sensor that protects against liver toxicity. Proc Natl Acad Sci U S A 98:3369–3374

Stoilov I, Akarsu AN, Sarfarazi M (1997) Identification of three different truncating mutations in cytochrome P4501B1 (CYP1B1) as the principal cause of primary congenital glaucoma (Buphthalmos) in families linked to the GLC3A locus on chromosome 2p21. Hum Mol Genet 6:641–647

Sueyoshi T, Negishi M (2001) Phenobarbital response elements of cytochrome P450 genes and nuclear receptors. Annu Rev Pharmacol Toxicol 41:123–143

Tan NS, Michalik L, Noy N, Yasmin R, Pacot C, Heim M, Fluhmann B, Desvergne B, Wahli W (2001) Critical roles of PPAR beta/delta in keratinocyte response to inflammation. Genes Dev 15:3263–3277

Tanaka E, Terada M, Misawa S (2000) Cytochrome P450 2E1: its clinical and toxicological role. J Clin Pharm Ther 25:165–175

Tang BK, Kalow W (1996) Assays for CYP1A2 by testing in vivo metabolism of caffeine in humans. Methods Enzymol 272:124–131

Ueno T, Tamura S, Frels WI, Shou M, Gonzalez FJ, Kimura S (2000) A transgenic mouse expressing human CYP1A2 in the pancreas. Biochem Pharmacol 60:857–863

Urizar NL, Liverman AB, Dodds DT, Silva FV, Ordentlich P, Yan Y, Heyman RA, Mangelsdorf DJ, Moore DD (2002) A natural product that lowers cholesterol targets the farnesoid X receptor. Science 296:1703–1706

Valentine JL, Lee SS, Seaton MJ, Asgharian B, Farris G, Corton JC, Gonzalez FJ, Medinsky MA (1996) Reduction of benzene metabolism and toxicity in mice that lack CYP2E1 expression. Toxicol Appl Pharmacol 141:205–213

Wang H, Chen J, Hollister K, Sowers LC, Forman BM (1999) Endogenous bile acids are ligands for the nuclear receptor FXR/BAR. Mol Cell 3:543–553

Wei P, Zhang J, Egan-Hafley M, Liang S, Moore DD (2000) The nuclear receptor CAR mediates specific xenobiotic induction of drug metabolism. Nature 407:920–923

Wong FW, Chan WY, Lee SS (1998) Resistance to carbon tetrachloride-induced hepatotoxicity in mice which lack CYP2E1 expression. Toxicol Appl Pharmacol 153:109–118

Xie W, Barwick JL, Downes M, Blumberg B, Simon CM, Nelson MC, Neuschwander-Tetri BA, Brunt EM, Guzelian PS, Evans RM (2000) Humanized xenobiotic response in mice expressing nuclear receptor SXR. Nature 406:435–439

Xie W, Radominska-Pandya A, Shi Y, Simon CM, Nelson MC, Ong ES, Waxman DJ, Evans RM (2001) An essential role for nuclear receptors SXR/PXR in detoxification of cholestatic bile acids. Proc Natl Acad Sci U S A 98:3375–3380

Yu S, Cao WQ, Kashireddy P, Meyer K, Jia Y, Hughes DE, Tan Y, Feng J, Yeldandi AV, Rao MS, Costa RH, Gonzalez FJ, Reddy JK (2001) Human peroxisome proliferator-activated receptor alpha (PPARalpha) supports the induction of peroxisome proliferation in PPARalpha-deficient mouse liver. J Biol Chem 276:42485–42491

Yu AM, Idle JR, Byrd LG, Krausz KW, Kupfer A, Gonzalez FJ (2003) Regeneration of serotonin from 5-methoxytryptamine by polymorphic human CYP2D6. Pharmacogenetics 13:173–181

Zaher H, Buters JT, Ward JM, Bruno MK, Lucas AM, Stern ST, Cohen SD, Gonzalez FJ (1998) Protection against acetaminophen toxicity in CYP1A2 and CYP2E1 double-null mice. Toxicol Appl Pharmacol 152:193–199

Zhang J, Huang W, Chua SS, Wei P, Moore DD (2002) Modulation of acetaminophen-induced hepatotoxicity by the xenobiotic receptor CAR. Science. 298:422–424

Subject Index

Printing: Saladruck Berlin
Binding: Stürtz AG, Würzburg